The Mount Sinai School of Medicine Complete Book of Nutrition

The Mount Sinai School of Medicine Complete Book of Nutrition

Victor Herbert, M.D., J.D.
and Genell J. Subak-Sharpe, M.S., Editors
Delia A. Hammock, M.S., R.D.
Associate Editor

■

St. Martin's Press / New York

Design by Amelia R. Mayone

Library of Congress Cataloging-in-Publication Data

The Mount Sinai School of Medicine complete book of nutrition / edited by Victor Herbert & Genell J. Subak-Sharpe.
  p.   cm.
  ISBN 0-312-05129-8
    1. Nutrition—Handbooks, manuals, etc. 2. Diet therapy—Handbooks, manuals, etc.
  I. Herbert, Victor. II. Subak-Sharpe, Genell J.
  III. Mount Sinai School of Medicine.
  RM217.2.M68   1990
  613.2—dc20   90-8624
                                          CIP

First Edition: November 1990

10 9 8 7 6 5 4 3 2 1

To William Bosworth Castle, first George Richards Minot Professor of Medicine at Harvard Medical School, one of the first "establishment" professors to recognize and teach the importance of nutrition science, mentor to Victor Herbert and a legion of other leaders in world medicine. Dr. Castle died in Boston at the age of 92, on August 9, 1990. His nutrition self-experimentation, along with that of his disciple, Dr. Victor Herbert, was recounted by Lawrence K. Altman in his 1987 book *Who Goes First: The Story of Self-Experimentation in Medicine* (Random House).

To Morley R. Kare, Ph.D., gentleman, scholar, fellow gourmet, close personal friend, international authority on taste and smell, and Founding Director of the Monell Chemical Senses Center in Philadelphia—whose untimely death on July 30, 1990, was mourned in a July 31 obituary in *The New York Times*.

And to those we love and cherish, in the bosom of our lives, that they may have at their fingertips what is true about nutrition as a science, to confirm their common sense.

Contents

Acknowledgments

Over the last three years, scores of people have devoted their efforts towards making this the most comprehensive and authoritative book on nutrition for the general public. A special thanks is due Mount Sinai's Dean, Dr. Nathan Kase; without his support, the project would never have gotten off the ground. Of course, the major credit goes to the more than sixty physicians, dietitians, researchers, and other health professionals at the Mount Sinai School of Medicine who are the book's major contributors. Without the knowledge, expertise, and unstinting cooperation of these busy professionals, this book would not have been possible.

More than a dozen writers and editors have also lent their talents to creating this book. They include Brenda Becker, Susan Berkman, Susan Carleton, Josh Eppinger, Ann Forer, Marjorie Joyce, Jane Margaretten-Ohring, Joy Nowlin, Julia Peace, George Ryan, Allen Scheiman, Rebecca Smith, Hope Subak-Sharpe, Norra Tannenhaus, Antonia van der Meer, Josleen Wilson, and Tom Zauber. Everton Lopez, Sarah Subak-Sharpe, and Peter Gannon have spent long hours typing, fact checking, and tracking down reference material. Ellen Felton of Mount Sinai's Medical Arts Studio created the illustrations.

We are particularly indebted to our editor at St. Martin's Press, Hope Dellon, and her assistant, Abigail Kamen. Both have provided invaluable help in whipping a massive manuscript into shape and keeping us on the right track. Amelie Littell has also been invaluable in keeping all the pieces together in her role as managing editor.

Finally, we want to thank our respective families, whose forbearance and support have seen us through three years of this book's "creative process."

Contributors

Donald Bergman, M.D.
Clinical Assistant Professor of Medicine
(Endocrinology)
Mount Sinai School of Medicine

Richard Berkowitz, M.D.
Professor and Chairman
Department of Obstetrics/Gynecology and
Reproductive Sciences
Mount Sinai School of Medicine

Susan Bershad, M.D.
Clinical Instructor of Dermatology
Mount Sinai School of Medicine

W. Virgil Brown, M.D.
President of Medlantic Research Foundation
Washington, D.C.
Lecturer in Medicine
Mount Sinai School of Medicine
President-Elect (1990)
American Heart Association

Ellen M. Buchbinder, M.D.
Clinical Instructor in Medicine
Mount Sinai School of Medicine

Neville Colman, M.D., Ph.D.
Medical Director for Clinical Laboratories
Mount Sinai Medical Center

Director, Blood Bank and Hematology
Laboratory
Bronx Veterans Affairs Medical Center

Mitchell Conn, M.D.
Instructor in Medicine
Mount Sinai School of Medicine

Kenneth Davis, M.D.
Professor and Chairman
Department of Psychiatry
Mount Sinai School of Medicine

David Gentili, M.D.
Attending Surgeon
Mount Sinai School of Medicine

Sheldon Glabman, M.D.
Clinical Associate Professor of Medicine
Mount Sinai School of Medicine

Ludwik Gross, M.D.
Veterans Administration Distinguished
Investigator
Chief of Cancer Research Unit
Bronx Veterans Affairs Medical Center
Emeritus Professor of Medicine
Mount Sinai Medical Center

Fran C. Grossman, R.D., M.S.
Supervisor of Clinical Nutrition
Director of Nutrition Education
Mount Sinai Medical Center

Delia A. Hammock, M.S., R.D.
Associate Director, Good Housekeeping
    Institute
Director, Nutrition, Diet and Fitness Center
Good Housekeeping Magazine

Leonard Handelsman, M.D.
Assistant Professor of Psychiatry
Mount Sinai School of Medicine
Director of Chemical Dependency Program
Mount Sinai Medical Center
Medical Director, Drug Dependency
    Treatment Program
Bronx Veterans Affairs Medical Center

Victor Herbert, M.D., F.A.C.P., J.D.
Professor of Medicine
Chairman, Committee to Strengthen Nutrition
Mount Sinai School of Medicine
Director, Nutrition Research Center
Mount Sinai Medical Center and Bronx
    Veterans Affairs Medical Center

Thomas John Iberti, M.D., F.A.C.P.
Associate Professor of Surgery, Medicine, and
    Anesthesiology
Director of Surgical Intensive Care Unit
Mount Sinai School of Medicine

Andrew Kaplan, D.M.D.
Assistant Clinical Professor of Dentistry
Coordinator, Department of Dentistry
Mount Sinai School of Medicine

Yair Karni, B.Sc.
Director of Nutrition
Wingate Institute for Physical Education
Natania, Israel

David P. Katz, Ph.D.
Research Assistant Professor of Pediatrics and
    Surgery
Codirector of Surgical Support Services
Mount Sinai School of Medicine

Leslie D. Kerr, M.D.
Assistant Professor of Medicine
Mount Sinai School of Medicine

Jerome L. Knittle, M.D.
Professor of Pediatrics and Director
Division of Nutrition and Metabolism
Mount Sinai School of Medicine

Rosalinda Lawson, R.D.
Executive Dietitian
Mount Sinai Medical Center

Neal LeLeiko, M.D., Ph.D.
Associate Professor of Pediatrics
Mount Sinai School of Medicine
Chief, Division of Pediatric Gastroenterology
Mount Sinai Medical Center

S. Robert Levine, M.D.
Clinical Instructor in Medicine and Cardiology
Mount Sinai School of Medicine
Medical Director, Heart-Health Promotion, Inc.

Charles S. Lieber, M.D.
Professor of Medicine and Pathology
Mount Sinai School of Medicine
Chief, Section of Liver Disease and Nutrition
Director, Alcohol Research and Treatment
    Center and G.I.-Liver Nutrition
Bronx Veterans Affairs Medical Center

David T. Lowenthal, M.D., Ph.D.
Formerly at Mount Sinai Medical Center, and
    now Professor of Medicine,
    Pharmacology and Exercise Science
University of Florida College of Medicine
Gainesville, Florida

Director, Geriatric Research, Education, and
    Clinical Center
VA Medical Center
Gainesville, Florida

Bernard Mehl, D.P.S.
Associate Professor
Mount Sinai School of Medicine
Mount Sinai Medical Center
Director, Department of Pharmacy

Peggy O'Sullivan, M.S., R.D.
Senior Dietitian
Mount Sinai School of Medicine

Elliot J. Rayfield, M.D.
Clinical Professor of Medicine
Mount Sinai School of Medicine

Denise Rollinson, M.S., R.D., C.N.S.D.
Pediatric Nutrition Support Nutritionist
Mount Sinai Medical Center

David B. Sachar, M.D.
Professor of Medicine
Director, Division of Gastroenterology
Mount Sinai School of Medicine

Carol Schreiber
Research Associate
Division of Medical Oncology
Mount Sinai School of Medicine

Artemis P. Simopoulos, M.D.
Vice President and Director
The Center for Genetics, Nutrition and Health
American Association for World Health
Washington, D.C.

Robbyn E. Sockolow, M.D.
Fellow, Pediatric Gastroenterology
Mount Sinai Medical Center

Elyse Sosin, R.D., M.A.
Supervisor of Clinical Nutrition
Mount Sinai Medical Center

Harry Spiera, M.D.
Clinical Professor of Medicine
Mount Sinai School of Medicine
Chief, Division of Rheumatology
Mount Sinai Medical Center

Barry Stimmel, M.D.
Dean for Academic Affairs
Mount Sinai School of Medicine

David V. Valauri, D.D.S.
Clinical Instructor in Dentistry
Coordinator, Department of Dentistry
Mount Sinai School of Medicine

Samuel Waxman, M.D.
Clinical Professor of Medicine
Division of Medical Oncology
Head, Cancer Chemotherapy Foundation
    Laboratory
Mount Sinai School of Medicine

Rosemary Wein, R.N.
Diabetes Coordinator
Department of Obstetrics and Gynecology
Mount Sinai School of Medicine

Stuart H. Young, M.D.
Associate Clinical Professor of Medicine and
    Pediatrics
Mount Sinai Medical Center

Ts'ai-fan Yu, M.D.
Research Professor of Medicine, Emeritus
Mount Sinai School of Medicine

How to Use This Book

The Mount Sinai School of Medicine Complete Book of Nutrition has been compiled by a team of distinguished physicians, dietitians, researchers, and other health professionals working under the guidance of Dr. Victor Herbert, one of the nation's most distinguished nutrition scientists. It is intended to give you authoritative and up-to-date nutrition information as well as practical guidelines to achieve a healthful—and pleasurable—diet.

The book is divided into six major sections. In Part I, you will learn the basics of a healthy diet, and how to separate food facts from myths and misinformation. Part II is devoted to specific categories of nutrients or dietary components—proteins, carbohydrates, fats, vitamins, minerals, fiber, sugar, salt, water, and other fluids. Food additives and preservatives also are covered in this section.

Part III deals with nutrition at different life stages, from before birth to old age. Part IV covers nutrition-related problems, including weight control, eating disorders, food/drug interactions, and the effects of alcohol, tobacco, caffeine, and other mood-altering substances. Special nutrition needs are also covered in Part IV. You'll find chapters on the nutrition problems faced by hospitalized patients, as well as chapters on the needs of athletes and vegetarianism.

Part V—the largest single section in this book—addresses the role of nutrition in various categories of disease. Cardiovascular diseases, cancer, diabetes, blood disorders, gastrointestinal diseases, liver diseases, and kidney diseases are but a few of the major problems covered in this section.

Part VI tells you how to put the preceding information into practical everyday use. Included are chapters on restaurant eating, food shopping, and food storage and preparation. Finally, the Nutrient Values table provides a handy reference for hundreds of foods.

Throughout, we have attempted to remove the mystique from nutrition. We have tried to avoid the jargon as well as myths and hype, and to concentrate on solid facts and practical advice. Every effort has been made to reflect accurately the most recent knowledge regarding nutrition and health. Still, you should not use this book to alter any treatment regimen without first consulting your doctor. In fact, we urge readers to show this book to their doctors. Should they want further professional guidance or information, they can call Mount Sinai's special referral service (800-637-4624 or MDSINAI), which will put them in touch with a health professional who can answer their questions.

Preface

More than ever, Americans are aware that good health is, to a large extent, determined by our habits and lifestyle. Cigarette smoking, for example, is the leading cause of preventable death in this country. Excessive alcohol consumption and illicit drug use also claim many thousands of lives each year. Still, good nutrition is the single most important factor in establishing and maintaining good health. As noted in the 1988 *Surgeon General's Report on Nutrition and Health:* "For the two out of three adult Americans who do not smoke and do not drink excessively, one personal choice seems to influence long-term health prospects more than any other: what we eat." The 1989 National Research Council report *Diet and Health* confirms this, as does the 1990 International Life Sciences Institute–Nutrition Foundation book *Present Knowledge in Nutrition.*

Although Americans claim to be aware of the vital role nutrition plays in good health, most are woefully ignorant about what actually constitutes a healthful diet. This was the conclusion drawn from a 1989 survey of 1,000 adults, conducted by dietitians from Brown University's General Clinical Research Center. Even the researchers were surprised at some of the results. For example, despite all the recent medical and media attention devoted to cholesterol, 68 percent of those polled did not know that it is found only in animal products. Large numbers of people failed to correctly identify food groups: 61 percent thought broccoli (a vegetable) was a legume; 41 percent classified catsup (a condiment) as a vegetable; and 60 percent thought that honey, corn syrup, and molasses (all simple sugars) were complex carbohydrates (starches) and good for you.

Most of those polled did know that being overweight increases the risk of heart attack and diabetes, but most lacked the basic nutritional knowledge on how to maintain desirable weight. Many thought that pasta and potatoes were more fattening than steaks (whose fat content makes them much higher in calories than starches). Many assumed that if meat looks lean, it is devoid of fat, but many overlooked even visible fat—39 percent did not know that the marbling in a steak is actually fat. A 1990 Gallup survey showed many cling to popular misconceptions about food to determine their dietary intakes, opting for quick fixes and the latest supplement fads.

This is only a small sampling of the mistaken notions revealed by this survey. Of course, it doesn't take surveys to determine that many Americans who think they are nutrition-wise are actually very misinformed. People who are ignorant about good nutrition are easy targets of misleading advertising claims, food faddists, and quackery. Billions of dollars are spent every year on unneeded vitamin, mineral, and other supplements. Billions more are spent on a mind-boggling assortment of diets, potions, and "nutritional" remedies—many bordering on the bizarre—all in the mistaken belief that they will improve health.

This book is devoted to providing you with the facts you need not only to make healthful food choices but also to protect you from common misconceptions. You will learn that what is magic about nutrition is not true, and what is true is not magic. You will learn what constitutes a good diet, and the role nutrition plays in health and disease. Armed with the facts on the following pages, you will be able to judge for yourself whether an advertising claim or scary headline is accurate. You will learn how to shop and cook wisely and how to ensure that the foods you buy give you the most nutrition for your dollar.

Unlike many nutrition books directed to the general public, this one is based on solid facts, not "pop" opinions or questionable theories. The more than 50 contributors to this book are health professionals at New York's Mount Sinai Medical Center. There is a long-standing charge that doctors learn about disease, but that few are taught the basics of nutrition. Fortunately, this has changed in the past decade as more and more medical schools have incorporated nutrition into their curriculums. In this respect, the Mount Sinai School of Medicine is one of the nation's leaders in teaching nutrition in every year of medical school as well as incorporating nutrition into the program of training in every specialty. Medical school graduates today are thoroughly versed in nutrition as a science. What some lack is adequate knowledge of dietetics, which is made up for by working closely with registered dietitians.

Although scientific accuracy is emphasized throughout, the practical how-tos also are stressed. You'll find recipes and menus, and tips on how to incorporate the scientific information into your everyday eating habits. Food plays many roles in addition to providing nourishment. Our goal is to give you sound nutritional information without detracting from the very real pleasures of eating.

—The Editors

Part I

The Basics of Healthy Eating

■

1

What Is a Healthy Diet?

Victor Herbert, M.D., J.D.

∎

INTRODUCTION

Despite all the good food–bad food hype promulgated by enthusiasts, the basics of a healthy diet can be summed up in three key words: *moderation, variety, and balance.* If you follow the principles inherent in these words, you will not need vitamin pills, "health" foods, or complicated dietary regimens. What's more, you'll be able fully to enjoy the pleasures of good eating without worrying about cholesterol, salt, excess weight, and all the other dietary bugaboos that have become catchwords in today's nutrition-conscious circles. All food is health food in moderation. Any food is junk food in excess.

I can almost hear you say, Healthy eating *can't* be that simple. First, be assured that good nutrition is neither complicated nor restrictive. Unless you have some rare metabolic disease or other specific nutrition-related health problem, you can enjoy virtually every food known to humankind—so long as you practice the first principle: moderation. By eating a wide variety of foods, you will get all the nutrients you need to maintain good health. Balance in nutrition means both a balance of vitamins, minerals, and other nu-

trients as well as calories consumed versus energy expended.

To make these principles even easier to follow, nutrition scientists have devised four basic food groups from which to select your variety of foods, and seven dietary guidelines to ensure moderation, variety, and balance. Over and over in this book, you will see how these principles and guidelines apply to the prevention and treatment of nutrition-related problems in a spectrum of human diseases, as the Surgeon General of the United States indicated in his 1988 report to the nation on diet and nutrition in health promotion and disease prevention and the National Research Council did in its 1989 report *Diet and Health.* Equally important, you will learn how to apply them to day-to-day life—everything from wise food shopping to how to avoid nutrition quackery—and to stop worrying and enjoy eating. This chapter outlines these all-important basics.

THE FOUR BASIC FOOD GROUPS

If you are over the age of 40 or so, you probably were taught the Basic Seven food groups;

if you're a bit older, you may even remember the Basic Eleven. In the early 1950s, nutrition educators realized that even seven food groups are difficult for the average person to remember and deal with in daily meal planning. So in 1957, the U.S. Department of Agriculture, spurred by an article in the *Journal of the American Dietetic Association* by Harvard's Dr. Fredrick Stare and his team, combined the groups into today's Basic Four: milk and milk products; "meats" (meat, fish, poultry, eggs, nuts, legumes); fruits and vegetables; and grains (breads, cereals, and pastas). A fifth and nonbasic group (i.e., optional) consists of sweets, fats, and alcohol. These are items that do not add much in the way of essential nutrients (except for a few strict vegetarians who may not get enough essential fatty acids in their diets), but they make foods tasty and eating more enjoyable, which are also important aspects of healthful eating.

For the average adult, we recommend from the Basic Four a minimum of 12 daily servings: two each from the milk and meat groups (the "animal foods" groups) and four each from the fruit and vegetable group and the grain group (the "plant foods" groups). (Table 1.1 lists the recommended servings for different age groups from the Basic Four.)

In moderate portions, these 12 servings add up to about 1,200 calories, and provide all of the vitamins, minerals, and other essentials for maintaining good health. Most normal-weight adults will need more than 1,200 calories a day, and they will actually lose weight if they consume only this amount. You can fill out your day's needs with an extra serving or two from the Basic Four, preferably the two plant groups, and then from the optional group, with foods that provide calories and eating enjoyment but generally not much in the way of vitamins and minerals.

Table 1.1. How to Use the Basic Four Food Groups

Food Group	Servings per Day	Serving Size
TWO HIGH-PROTEIN GROUPS (GENERALLY HIGH IN CALORIES AND FAT, AND LOW IN FIBER)		
Milk and milk products	2–3 for babies and children under 9 3 for children 9–12 4 for teenagers 2 for adults 3 for pregnant women 4 for lactating women	1 cup (8 oz. or equivalent in cheese and other milk products)
Meat, fish, poultry, and meat substitutes	2	2–3 oz. lean cooked beef, pork, lamb, poultry, or fish. (Count the following as 1 oz. of meat: 1 egg, ½ to ¾ cup cooked legumes, 2 T peanut butter or ¼ to ½ cup nuts or sunflower or sesame seeds).
TWO PLANT GROUPS (GENERALLY LOW IN CALORIES AND FAT, AND HIGH IN FIBER)		
Fruits and vegetables	Total of 4 including: 1 serving of citrus fruit or other source of vitamin C daily and 1 serving of dark green or deep yellow vegetable or fruit frequently for vitamin A	1 piece of fruit or ½ cup cooked or 1 cup juice
Bread, cereal, pasta, and other grain products	Total of 4, whole grain, enriched or restored	1 slice bread or 1 oz. cold cereal or ½ to ¾ cup pasta or cooked cereal

Source: *Food.* HG228, 1980 U.S. Dept. of Agriculture, Washington, D.C.

In selecting foods from within these groups, you should strive for variety rather than limiting your diet to the same foods over and over, even as you get the proper number of servings from each of the four groups. Variety within the Basic Four will ensure not only that you get the proper amounts of essential nutrients but also that you will add to your eating pleasure. For example, you could fulfill the Basic Four recommendations by consuming the following foods over the course of a day: two glasses of milk, a glass of orange juice, two roast chicken sandwiches, a baked potato, a green salad, and a serving of carrots. This eating program also fulfills the criteria of moderation. However, in addition to being boring if the same regimen were followed every day, it would not provide much variety within each of the Basic Four. And, unless you are on a weight-loss regimen or are very sedentary, it will not provide adequate energy. (See Table 1.2 for sample menus that meet all the criteria of moderation, variety, and balance.)

Thus, to plan an eating program that is consistent with good health, you need to pay attention to all of the basic principles, not just one or two. (Of course, a generous helping of common sense is also important.) Whenever I try to explain these basics, I'm constantly asked questions such as: Aren't you making this too simple? or How do I know for sure I'm getting the full RDA (Recommended Dietary Allowance) of every vitamin and mineral? To answer these questions, let's take a look at the individual food groups and their nutrients.

Milk and Milk Products

For generations, mothers have urged their children to drink milk, claiming that it's nature's most "perfect" food. For the first few months of life, breast milk is, indeed, the "perfect" food for babies. Beyond that, however, if "perfect" is defined as providing all the essential nutrients, milk does not fit the bill, since it falls short in iron and vitamin C. Still, milk is a major source of protein, calcium, riboflavin, and many other nutrients. In the United States, milk also is fortified with vitamin D, and vitamin A is added to skim milk to replace what is lost when fat is removed. Since milk and milk products are our best source of calcium, adults should have two servings from this group a day, and growing children, teenagers, and pregnant or nursing mothers should consume even more.

Many people have the mistaken notion that nonfat milk is not as nutritious as whole milk. Actually, except for the lesser amounts of fat, calories, and cholesterol in skim milk, there is little difference between the two. (See Chapter 10.) Both provide animal protein.

Some nutrition faddists also claim that pasteurized milk is not as healthy as raw milk, when, in fact, the opposite is true. Pasteurization is necessary to kill disease-causing bacteria and other microorganisms in milk; drinking raw milk or eating cheese and other milk products made from raw milk carries a very real danger of contracting life-threatening diseases. This fact was recently emphasized by several deaths on the West Coast from eating cheese made from unpasteurized milk. Federal restrictions on interstate movement of unpasteurized milk recently went into effect, but there is no federal control of milk that does *not* cross state lines.

Of course, not everyone likes to drink milk, and cheese, yogurt, ice cream, or ice milk may be acceptable alternatives (although some have more calories and fat than milk). (Table 1.3 lists equivalents of milk and milk products.) There are also large numbers of people, especially among blacks, Orientals, and the elderly, who are what is known as "lactose-intolerant"; that is, they lack the digestive enzyme lactase, which is needed to digest milk sugar, or lactose. They also can find suitable substitutes. Some may be able to tolerate two to six ounces of milk at a time, or they often can eat yogurt and aged cheeses without difficulty. There also are special lactose-free brands of milk, as well as a variety of soy milk products, such as tofu, which provide calcium, protein, and other nutrients without lactose. (See Chapter 30.)

Meats, Fish, Poultry, Eggs, Nuts, and Legumes (the "Meat Group")

This food group is our major source of protein. It includes all types of meat, fish, shellfish, poultry, eggs, dried peas and beans, lentils, peanuts and other nuts. The animal sources of protein are good sources of a number of vitamins, and our best sources of absorbable iron, as well as of many other minerals. They are also our only source of vitamin B_{12}, as the Surgeon General of the United States pointed out in 1988.

This food group is one in which moderation and variety are particularly important. In

Table 1.2.   Sample Menus Using Basic Four Food Groups

Day 1		Day 2	
BREAKFAST	½ grapefruit (fruits/vegetables #1; day's vitamin C requirement) 1 oz. cereal (grains #1) with 1 cup low-fat milk (milk group #1) Coffee or tea	BREAKFAST	½ small cantaloupe (fruits/vegetables #1; day's vitamin A requirement) ½ cup oatmeal (grains #1) 1 cup low-fat milk (milk group #1) Coffee or tea
MID-MORNING SNACK	English muffin (grains #2) with butter and jam (extras) Coffee or tea	MID-MORNING SNACK	Orange juice (fruits/vegetables #2; day's vitamin C requirement) Whole-wheat crackers (grains #2)
LUNCH	Split-pea soup (meats #1) Cheese (milk #2) sandwich on rye bread (2 slices, grains #3 & 4) Beverage	LUNCH	Pita bread filled with tuna salad (grains #3; meats #1) Apple (Fruits/vegetables #3) 1 cup skim or low-fat milk (milk group #2)
MID-AFTERNOON SNACK	Low-fat flavored yogurt (milk #3) Beverage	MID-AFTERNOON SNACK	Small corn muffin (grains #4) Coffee, tea, or other beverage
DINNER	Flounder fillet (meats #2) Baked potato (fruits/vegetables #2) Broccoli (fruits/vegetables #3, vitamin A requirement) Green salad (fruits/vegetables #4) Stewed pears (fruits/vegetables #5) with cookies (extras) 1 glass white wine (optional extra) Beverage	DINNER	Minestrone soup (fruits/vegetables #4) Pasta (grains #5) White clam sauce (meats #2) Spinach salad (fruits/vegetables #5) Strawberry ice milk (milk #3) Beverage

Note: These menus include the recommended number of servings from all four groups (with additional servings from the milk and fruits/vegetables group), along with optional extras. Depending upon weight and level of activity, these meals should provide adequate calories and can easily be adjusted according to individual needs.

the past, many people have interpreted two servings from this group as meaning two generous servings of beef, pork, or some other meat. This is not the case. You should fulfill your dietary requirement with a wide variety of foods within this group—and keep the portions much smaller than the traditional hunk of steak or roast beef. One day, for example, you might meet the requirement with a serving of meat and a peanut butter sandwich; the next, you might have fish at one meal and a legume dish at another.

In recent years, many Americans have made a conscious effort to replace excess portions of meat, especially beef and other red meats, with poultry and fish. There are several reasons for this dietary variety.

Consuming large amounts of fatty meat, such as marbled steaks, ribs, hot dogs, fried chicken, and other all-American favorites, contributes excess calories to the diet. Meat and other animal products also contain cholesterol, and thus are among the foods linked to an increased risk of heart disease, even though it is *blood* cholesterol, not *dietary* cholesterol, that is the risk factor. (This is a point of continuing confusion; see Chapter 6 for a more detailed discussion.) Animal protein is more expensive than legumes, an important consideration for large numbers of middle- to low-income people.

Fruits and Vegetables

The fruits and vegetables group, which includes juices, is our major source of vi-

---

Table 1.2.   Sample Menus . . . (cont.)

Day 3 (weekend with altered meal pattern)

BRUNCH	Orange slices (fruits/vegetables #1; day's vitamin C requirement)
	Blueberry pancakes (grains #1) with fresh-fruit topping (fruits/vegetables #2)
	Canadian bacon (meats #1)
	Coffee or tea
LATE LUNCH	Gazpacho (fruits/vegetables #3)
	Mexican rice and beans with corn chips (grains #2 and 3; fruits/vegetables #4)
	1 cup skim or low-fat milk (milk #1)
COCKTAIL HOUR	Raw vegetable tray (fruits/vegetables #5)
	Cottage cheese/horseradish dip (milk #2)
	Glass of wine (optional)
DINNER	Lobster bisque (extras)
	½ Cornish game hen (meats #2)
	Couscous (grains #4)
	Broccoli with lemon (fruits/vegetables #6, day's vitamin A requirement)
	Chocolate angel food cake (extras)
	Beverage
BEFORE BED	1 cup skim or low-fat milk (milk #3)
	Graham crackers (grains #5)

Table 1.3.   Nutritional Equivalents of Milk and Milk Products

To get the approximate equivalent of calcium and other nutrients found in an 8-ounce serving of milk, you can substitute the following milk products and substitutes. Note the differences in calories.

	Calories
Milk (whole)	150
Milk (skim)	85
Milk, 2%-fat	120
Milk, 1%-fat	100
Cocoa, hot chocolate (made with milk)	220
Milk shake, vanilla (1 cup)	252
Soybean milk (8 oz.)	87
Yogurt, plain (8 oz.)	145
Yogurt, fruit (8 oz.)	230
Firm cheese (1½ oz. cheddar, colby, etc.)	172
American (1¾ oz.)	183
Cottage cheese, 2% fat (2 cups)	400
Ice cream, 11% fat (1½ cups)	405
Ice milk, vanilla (1½ cups)	270

tamins A and C. Each day, you should consume a serving of citrus fruit or other source of vitamin C, and every other day, a serving of a dark green vegetable (for example, broccoli or spinach) or dark yellow or orange vegetable or fruit (for example, carrots or cantaloupe) in order to get adequate vitamin A. Foods in this group also provide substantial amounts of other essential vitamins and minerals, as well as dietary fiber. According to the USDA Food Consumption Survey (1984), the average American eats 120 percent of the RDA of vitamins A and C each day, so getting an adequate supply of A and C is hardly a problem in the United States.

A variety of fruits and vegetables make eating more interesting. As any good cook or gourmet knows, these foods help add color, texture, and taste to meals. And since the nutritional content varies among the many different fruits and vegetables, variety is all the more important. All are good fiber sources.

Grains: Bread, Cereals, and Pastas

Throughout recorded history, grain products have been dietary staples of agrarian societies. Foods in this group provide B vitamins, iron, starch (complex carbohydrates), and protein; they also are a major source of dietary fiber.

Traditionally, the type of grains consumed depended upon the geographic area. In the United States and other Western nations, wheat, corn, oats, and rye have been the major grains. In much of Asia, rice is the traditional staple. Thanks to modern agriculture and worldwide food imports, we can now enjoy a wide variety of grain products—everything from couscous and bulgur wheat to a huge array of pastas—from all parts of the world.

Until the last few years, many Americans shunned pasta, bread, and other grain products because of a misconception that they were "heavy" and fattening. Fortunately, this is changing, at least in the more nutritionally enlightened circles where pasta is in and he-man-sized steaks (which are fattening) are out, replaced by a few ounces of beef in a pasta or an Oriental stir-fry dish. Remember, however, that any food, including pasta and other grain dishes, can be made fattening by adding slabs of butter or other calorie-rich sauces.

The fiber fad of recent years also has prompted Americans to increase their intake of grain products, particularly things such as bran cereals. Unfortunately, Americans are quick to hop on almost any nutrition bandwagon, assuming that if a little is good, then more must be better. Too much bran—or any other form of fiber—can create nutritional imbalances and may be as detrimental as too little. (See Chapter 9.) Again, the secret is variety and moderation. Moderate servings of a variety of breads, cereals, pastas, and other such products will provide the desired balance of nutrients and fiber, without too much or too little of any one kind.

The Question of Supplements

Many people have the notion that vitamin and mineral supplements are needed for "insurance" unless they strictly adhere to the recommended number of servings from each food group day in and day out. This simply is not true. If your average intake over the course of a week or two equals the recommended number of servings, it really doesn't matter whether you have, for example, two or three instead of the recommended four servings from one of the groups on a particular day. The liver is a storehouse for the body's vitamins and minerals. This organ can quickly compensate for a temporary dietary shortfall by releasing its stored nutrients as needed, and then replenishing its stores when the opportunity arises.

Contrary to what the purveyors of nutritional supplements would like you to believe, the fact is, otherwise healthy people have to consume a rather bizarre diet in order to develop a serious nutritional deficiency. Vitamin C is a good example. Millions of Americans regularly consume large doses of this vitamin in the mistaken belief that their diets do not provide enough of it. The fact is, as physicians, we rarely encounter scurvy—or any nutrient-deficiency disease other than iron deficiency—except in chronic alcoholics or people with an underlying illness that interferes with their food intake or metabolism. And when we do, it usually makes for an interesting article in a scientific journal. A few years ago, I did come across such a case when I was called in to see a 42-year-old unemployed man who was suffering from easy bleeding in the gums and skin. It turned out he had scurvy. He did not have a refrigerator, and thus was unable to buy in bulk and store a variety of foods. His daily diet consisted of rice and canned sardines in tomato sauce. This is hardly a healthy, varied diet, but even so, he would not have developed scurvy if he had eaten the sardines right out of the can: The 12 milligrams of vitamin C in the tomato sauce would have been sufficient to stave off a deficiency. However, he prepared his sardines in a skillet of boiling water, thereby destroying the vitamin C. Even so, it took eight months of this diet, which was devoid of vitamin C, to deplete his body's stores to the point where he developed scurvy. This amply illustrates that unless you live on boiled sardines or an equally bizarre diet—or have an underlying disease—you are not likely to need supplements. (See Chapter 7 for a more detailed discussion.)

THE SEVEN DIETARY GUIDELINES

These guidelines, first issued in 1980 by the U.S. Department of Agriculture and the Department of Health and Human Services, are intended to further elaborate upon the principles of moderation, variety, and balance. The U.S. Surgeon General stressed them again in 1988 in his report to the nation on diet and nutrition in health promotion and disease prevention. In introducing the guidelines, these government agencies stress that there is no single ideal diet that can be recommended for everyone. To quote the guidelines (2nd edition, revised 1985):

> People differ—and their food needs differ depending on age, sex, body size, physical activity, and other conditions such as pregnancy and illness. In those chronic conditions where diet may be important—heart disease, high blood pressure, strokes, tooth decay, diabetes, osteoporosis, and some forms of cancer—the roles of specific dietary substances have not been defined fully. . . . [Even so,] the following guidelines tell how to choose and prepare foods for you and your family. This advice is the best we can give based on the nutrition information we have now. Slight wording revisions for guidelines 2 through 6 were suggested in 1990 by the Dietary Guidelines Advisory Committee as follows:

1. Eat a Variety of Foods

To date, nutrition scientists have identified some 40 different nutrients that are needed to maintain health. As stressed earlier in this chapter, and throughout the rest of this book, the best way of getting adequate amounts of these nutrients is to eat many different foods from each of the Basic Food groups. (There are some exceptions in which supplements are advised; for example, pregnant women may need more iron than they are likely to get in their diets. These exceptions are discussed in subsequent chapters.)

2. Maintain Healthy Weight

Excess weight is associated with an increased risk of high blood pressure, excessive blood cholesterol, heart attacks, adult diabetes, osteoarthritis, and a number of other health problems, including psychological ones. It is not known why some people become obese and others who consume a similar diet stay slim, but most experts agree that a combination of genetics, diet, and physical activity is probably to blame. We do know that in order to lose weight, you must burn up more calories than you consume, either by increasing physical activity, eating less, or (preferably) a combination of the two. We also know that fad or crash diets can result in serious medical problems and are of little or no value in the long run. (See Chapter 17 on Weight Control.)

3. Choose a Diet Low in Fat, Saturated Fat, and Cholesterol

High blood cholesterol is one of several factors related to an increased risk of heart attacks. A number of factors raise blood cholesterol, including genetics and a diet high in calories, saturated fats, and high-cholesterol foods. As noted in the guidelines, "There is controversy about what recommendations are appropriate for healthy Americans. But for the U.S. population as a whole, it is sensible to reduce daily consumption of fat. . . . Many foods that contain fat and cholesterol also provide high-quality protein and many essen-

tial vitamins and minerals. You can eat these foods in moderation as long as your overall fat and cholesterol intake is not excessive." (See chapters 6 and 26 for more details.)

4. Choose a Diet with Plenty of Vegetables, Fruits, and Grain Products

About 55 to 60 percent of total calories consumed should come from carbohydrates, with emphasis on starchy foods (complex carbohydrates) such as breads, pastas, cereals, potatoes, dried beans, peas, and other legumes. People concerned with weight control are well advised to substitute starchy foods for those with large amounts of fats (which, ounce for ounce, have about twice as many calories as carbohydrates) and sugars (which contribute calories but no other nutrients). Plant foods also add dietary fiber, which helps prevent constipation and certain other bowel disorders. The guidelines caution, however, that fiber intake should be increased by "eating more of these foods that contain fiber naturally, not by adding fiber to foods that do not contain it."

5. Use Sugars in Moderation

Most of our foods contain some type of sugar, either added in the form of sucrose (common table sugar) and other sweeteners (for example, corn syrup) or naturally occurring, such as fructose (the sugar in many fruits) or lactose (milk sugar). In fact, sugar (glucose) is the body's major form of fuel and we would not survive long without it. Sugar is not the dietary evil that many food faddists would have us believe, but like any other food, it should be consumed in moderation. Contrary to popular myth, sugar does not cause diabetes, heart disease, or other major illnesses. However, frequent snacking on high-sugar foods—candy, cakes, dried fruits, sugary soft drinks—increases the likelihood of tooth decay. (See chapters 8 and 37.)

A diet high in sweets also is linked to weight gain. Although sugar per se is no higher in calories than other carbohydrates, it is often teamed up with fats in such high-calorie foods as candies, ice cream, and pastries.

6. Use Salt and Sodium in Moderation

Many foods contain varying amounts of sodium; small amounts occur naturally in some foods, but the greatest amount is added in the form of table salt (which is made up of sodium and chloride). Sodium is also used as a preservative and is a major ingredient in MSG, baking soda, baking powder, and other common ingredients. A small amount of sodium is essential to maintain health, but the typical American diet provides much more than is actually needed.

A high-sodium diet is associated with high blood pressure. It is doubtful that sodium actually causes this disease, but excess sodium increases the risk of developing it among people with a genetic predisposition to high blood pressure. Since about one out of four American adults have elevated blood pressure (and it is impossible to predict who is susceptible), and of these, one in three has sodium-sensitive hypertension, it makes sense to encourage everyone to have his or her blood pressure checked and consider reducing sodium intake if the pressure is borderline. (See chapters 8 and 26.)

7. If You Drink Alcoholic Beverages, Do So in Moderation

For most people, small amounts of alcohol—a glass of wine with a meal, an occasional cocktail or glass of beer—is not harmful, but chronic overindulgence can have very harmful effects. For starters, alcoholic beverages are high in calories and low in nutrients and thus can contribute to weight problems. Chronic excessive consumption can damage the liver, brain, heart, and other vital organs. Driving after drinking is a major cause of traffic fatalities in this country. Heavy drinkers have many nutritional deficiencies. Women who consume large amounts of alcohol during pregnancy are more likely to have a baby with birth defects. Since it is not known how much alcohol poses a risk to an unborn child, pregnant women are advised to avoid alcoholic beverages. (See Chapter 21.)

A Lifelong Eating Program

Obviously, the dietary principles outlined above are not "quick fixes"; instead, they are guidelines for a commonsense, lifelong eating program. On the surface, they appear simple and straightforward. A careful analysis will show, however, that these guidelines address some of our most persistent and difficult nutrition-related problems. Granted, considerable progress has been made in recent years in reducing the consumption of saturated fat and sodium and increasing the intake of complex carbohydrates. Millions of Americans still can benefit from modification of their eating habits, however. For example, the guidelines urge people to maintain desirable weight, but excessive weight remains the most common nutrition-related health problem in the United States.

In the following chapters, we will elaborate upon these dietary principles and tell how they can be used to modify present eating habits. In keeping with the national guidelines and the U.S. Surgeon General's 1988 report, we will stress the *positive* aspects of good nutrition. It is noteworthy that the guidelines do not urge eating *less* of any food; instead, they stress *avoiding eating too much*. The distinction is an important one. If you are not consuming too much sodium, sugar, fat, or other foods, there's no need for you to eat less, and, indeed, advice to do so would be unsound. Equally important, you can eat anything you like so long as you do so in moderation and it is part of a varied and balanced diet.

How Does Your Diet Rate?

The following quiz is adapted from the FDA *Consumer* (October 1986) and is intended to help you determine whether your diet is well balanced.

Check the line that best describes your eating habits.

How Often Do You Eat:	Seldom/ Never	1 or 2 Times a Week	3 or 4 Times a Week	Almost Daily
1. Four or more servings of bread, cereals, rice, pasta, or other foods made from grains per day?	___	___	___	___
2. Foods made from whole grains?	___	___	___	___
3. Three different kinds of vegetables per day?	___	___	___	___
4. Cooked dry beans or peas?	___	___	___	___
5. A dark green vegetable, such as spinach or broccoli?	___	___	___	___
6. Two kinds of fruit or fruit juice per day?	___	___	___	___
7. Two servings (3 or 4 if a teenager, pregnant, or breastfeeding) of milk, cheese, or yogurt per day?	___	___	___	___
8. Two servings of lean meat, poultry, fish, or alternates, such as eggs, dry beans, or nuts per day?	___	___	___	___

How to Score: Compare your answers to the best answer, listed below:

1. *Almost daily.* Many people believe that eating breads and cereals will make you fat. That's not true for most of us. Extra calories come from the fat and/or sugar you *may* eat with them. Both whole-grain and enriched breads and cereals provide carbohydrates and essential nutrients.

2. *Almost daily.* Whole-grain breads and cereals contain vitamins, minerals, and the dietary fiber that is low in the diets of many Americans. Select whole-grain cereals and bakery products—those with a whole grain listed first on the ingredient label, or make your own and use whole-grain flour.

3. *Almost daily.* Vegetables vary in the amounts of vitamins and minerals they contain, so it's important to include several kinds every day.

4. *Three to four times a week.* Dry beans and peas fit into two food groups because of the nutrients they provide. They can be used as an occasional alternate to meat, poultry, and fish. They are also an excellent vegetable choice.

5. *Three to four times a week.* Spinach and other dark green leafy vegetables are excellent sources of some nutrients that are low in many diets.

6. *Almost daily.* Fruits are nature's sweets, high in vitamins and minerals. They taste good and are good for you.

7. *Almost daily.* Adults as well as children need the calcium and other nutrients found in milk and milk products.

8. *Almost daily.* Most Americans include some meat, poultry, or fish in their diets regularly. Dry beans and peas, peanuts (including peanut butter), nuts and seeds, and eggs can be used as alternates. Animal-product iron is much better absorbed than plant-product iron.

2

Our Changing Food Supply and Eating Habits

Victor Herbert, M.D., J.D.

■

INTRODUCTION

In this century, the United States has evolved from a mostly rural, agricultural society to an urban culture. At the turn of the century, most Americans grew what they ate and their diets were determined in large measure by economic status, geographic location, and the season. Even in the 1920s and 1930s, housewives would spend much of their summer preserving the produce from their gardens and orchards to see their families through the nongrowing months. The idea that someone in Minnesota or Vermont, for example, could regularly enjoy fresh tomatoes, lettuce, or oranges in the dead of winter would have seemed an impossible dream for all except the very wealthy.

All of this began to change between the Great Depression and the time of World War II, when millions of Americans left rural areas to take jobs in industrialized cities. Advances in agriculture, transportation, and food storage made it possible to ship fragile fresh produce from one part of the country to another.

Today, of course, very few of us produce the foods we eat; even so, never before has a society as a whole been blessed with a greater abundance or variety of food. Even in rural areas, supermarkets have now replaced the small general stores that once stocked mostly nonperishable staples. One has only to walk into a typical supermarket and view the shelves laden with, according to some estimates, up to 10,000 different food items, many produced in distant parts of the world, to realize just how privileged we are when it comes to abundance and variety of food.

In addition to greater abundance and availability of foods, many other aspects of our national eating patterns have changed in recent decades. Up until World War II, most Americans ate three meals a day, usually at home and with all or most family members present. Today, we eat more meals outside the home, and those eaten at home are likely to be made from processed or convenience foods. Recent government surveys of eating patterns show that 40 percent or more of meals are consumed away from home, and that very few families eat breakfast or lunch together. In fact, the average family may have dinner together only four or five times a week.

Even the traditional three-meals-a-day pattern is changing: Recent surveys have found that half of all young adults regularly skip breakfast and 25 percent go without

14

lunch. In contrast, snacking or "grazing" is increasing: The last National Food Consumption Survey found that at least 60 percent of Americans snack, with 20 percent of their calories and varying amounts of other nutrients coming from between-meal eating.

INCREASED AWARENESS OF NUTRITION

Although we frequently hear that changes in our foods and eating habits have resulted in a decline in sound nutrition, there is no solid evidence to support this. (In fact, overnutrition, not undernutrition, is our major diet-related problem, as the Surgeon General of the United States said in his 1988 report to the nation.) In general, Americans today are more nutrition-conscious than in the past, and this is reflected in what they buy at the supermarket. Sales of foods generally perceived of as being healthy—chicken without the skin, fish, lean cuts of beef, pasta, fruits, vegetables, whole-grain products, low-fat and skim milk, and low-fat and low-salt foods of all kinds— are increasing. In contrast, Americans as a whole are eating less whole milk, eggs, butter, and fatty red meats—foods whose high calories from fats are linked to overweight, high blood cholesterol, and heart disease.

Increasingly, Americans say they select foods on the basis of wholesomeness and nutritional value. A Lou Harris poll conducted in the mid-1980s for the Food Marketing Institute found that more than 90 percent of those questioned expressed concern about nutrition, with half saying that cholesterol content of food was a major worry, even though dietary saturated fat raises serum cholesterol more than does dietary cholesterol, and it is high *serum* cholesterol rather than high *diet* cholesterol that is the problem. A Department of

Agriculture survey of 1,353 households in 1980 found that 60 percent had made dietary changes in the preceding three years for "health" reasons.

Still, there are contradictions. Surveys have found that although Americans may claim to be more conscious of nutrition, they don't always follow through when it comes to eating a healthful diet. Sales of soft drinks have increased by more than 300 percent since 1950, and beer and wine consumption is also up. Food manufacturers have responded to Americans' concerns over weight, salt, and cholesterol by offering a vast array of low-calorie, low-salt, and low-cholesterol foods. Still, consumption of fast foods—which tend to be high in fat, salt, and calories—continues to rise. Sugar is generally perceived as bad for you, yet consumption of sweets—including high-fat pastries—is up. What is bad for you, of course, is empty calories in any form if you are overweight. Americans also say they consider cost in selecting foods, yet sales of the more expensive processed, convenience, and gourmet foods are at all-time highs.

Contradictions aside, there are a number of healthy trends in our food buying and eating habits. For example, today's food shoppers are more sophisticated and knowledgeable about nutrition and food values. They are more likely to seek out nutritious foods in a supermarket than pay the extra prices for so-called health foods that have no nutritional superiority. A look at recent surveys of American eating habits by the United States Department of Agriculture, as well as the National Food Consumption Survey, pinpoint specific trends. These include:

Increased consumption of fresh fruits and vegetables. In 1989, Americans spent $507 billion on food, and a large portion of this went for fresh fruits and vegetables. The USDA, in its 1990 bulletin, *Food Consumption, Prices, and*

Expenditures, 1967–88, reported that the total per capita consumption of nine major commercial fresh vegetables reached a record high, and was 27 percent above the 1967 level. In 1984—the last year in which the USDA compiled data on total per capita buying *and* consumption—Americans bought 209.2 pounds of vegetables and 142.9 pounds of fruit per person, and more than half were fresh foods. (Not all of this is actually consumed, since the figures reflect the amounts purchased, and do not allow for what is discarded or wasted.)

Since then, consumption of fresh fruits and vegetables have risen even more, as reflected in statistics for selected foods. For example, in 1984 the per capita *consumption* of 19 of the most common fresh vegetables (excluding potatoes and legumes) was 79 pounds per person; in 1988, this had risen to almost 90 pounds. Consumption of fresh fruits also increased, but not as dramatically, going from 88 pounds in 1984 to 94.4 pounds in 1988.

In reviewing the changing patterns, the Food and Drug Administration noted that "the biggest trend in fruits and vegetables is in the . . . greater variety of produce." In 1972, the typical supermarket carried an average of 65 different fresh produce items; by 1983, this had nearly tripled to 173 items, and, according to an FDA report, "some larger stores may carry as many as 250 items. Foods that were considered 'exotic' yesterday are becoming today's staples." Conversely, some of yesterday's standbys such as potatoes—both white and sweet—are declining in popularity. In 1910, for example, the per capita consumption of white and sweet potatoes stood at 221 pounds; by 1984, it was down to 90 pounds. Most of these are in the fat-added form of chips, French fries, and other frozen or processed foods.

Why the renewed interest in fruits and vegetables? According to the FDA report,

"Consumers who are most concerned about nutrition, who exercise the most, and who are on diets are most likely to eat fresh fruits and vegetables."

A decline in the consumption of eggs, butter, and whole milk, and a rise in the consumption of low-fat milk, yogurt, and other dairy products. Although pound for pound, dairy products still lead in food consumption, the total is down, and within this category products considered low in fat and cholesterol are gaining in popularity. In 1967, the average American used 276 pounds of milk and 287 eggs per year; by 1988, this had dropped to 236 pounds of milk and 234 eggs.

Since the 1960s, organizations such as the American Heart Association and the National Institutes of Health have urged Americans to reduce their fat and cholesterol intake, and it seems that these messages have been heeded. Concerns over fat, cholesterol, and weight are cited as reasons for cutting back on dairy products, especially whole milk, butter, cheese, and eggs. At the same time, sales of skim or low-fat milk and milk products and margarine (as a substitute for lard and butter) have increased. For example, sales of low-fat milk have risen by a whopping 1,681 percent since the 1960s—the largest rise among all the foods tracked by the Department of Agriculture. In contrast, the per capita consumption of whole milk has declined from 159 quarts in 1945 to 51 quarts per person in 1987. Total milk consumption is also down, due in large part to the increasing popularity of soft drinks.

Although cheese is much higher in fat than milk (50 percent or more compared to 3.5 percent fat in whole milk), cheese consumption has increased. In 1950, each American consumed an average of 7.7 pounds of cheese; this rose to 24.0 pounds in 1987. (These figures do not include cottage cheese.)

The increase is attributed to the use of cheese in fast foods, especially pizza, and the image of cheese as a healthy food.

Yogurt also has been a big gainer over the last 20 years. Per capita consumption in 1965 was just over 5 ounces, or less than a small container. Americans each now consume an average of more than 4 pounds per year, and the figure is rising steadily.

Reduced consumption of red meat and increases in fish and poultry consumption. Meat, especially beef, has always ranked high as a favorite all-American food. Department of Agriculture figures show that in 1971, Americans consumed a record high of 169 pounds of red meat per person, and most of it was beef. Since then, red meat consumption has steadily declined, reaching an average of 144 pounds per person in 1987. In contrast, fish and poultry intake has increased. In 1987, Americans consumed an average of 77.8 pounds of chicken and other poultry—a new record. Fish consumption also reached a new record—15.4 pounds per person—in 1987.

These changes reflect an increased perception of the possible adverse health effects of fat in beef, bacon, sausage, and other fatty meats. This is reflected as well in the growing popularity of the leaner cuts of beef in preference to fatty prime cuts and marbled steaks. Price is also a factor: Beef and other red meats tend to be more expensive than poultry.

Increased intake of pasta, cereals, and other grain products as well as dried peas, beans, and other legumes. Pasta became the new health food of the 1980s, and other grain products enjoyed increased popularity. Part of the reason is economic: Grain products tend to be less expensive than meats and other dietary staples. The increased popularity of ethnic foods has resulted in Americans' consuming more pasta and legumes. Pasta, once considered fattening, is now perceived as a healthy substitute for meat and other high-fat foods. And the fiber fad of the 1970s helped raise American consciousness as to the importance of fiber in a healthy diet, and was a factor in the increased consumption of cereals, whole-grain breads, and other grain products.

Increased intake of vegetable fats at the expense of animal fats. Americans still consume a large amount of fats (about 37 percent of total calories), but the sources of fats are changing. In the late 1970s, vegetable fats such as corn and other cooking and salad oils exceeded animal fats for the first time in the American diet, and the gap between the two is steadily widening. This is due to reduced consumption of butter, lard, whole milk, and fatty meats and increased intake of margarine, salad, and cooking oils. A Lou Harris poll found that Americans cited concerns over weight and cholesterol as the major reasons for switching, although economics is also a factor: Vegetable fats are less expensive than butter and animal fats. Of course, "contains no cholesterol" is advertising overkill for any plant product, since only animal products contain cholesterol. Additionally, the statement "contains no cholesterol" is a literal truth that contains a false message when applied to a tropical oil. Tropical oils—palm, palm kernel, and coconut—contain saturated fat, and saturated fat raises blood cholesterol more than does dietary cholesterol. (See Chapter 6.)

SNACKING

As noted earlier, at least 60 percent of all Americans consume some food or beverages between meals. As might be expected, snacking is more common among younger people. The latest National Food Consumption Survey found that up to 70 percent of all children and teenagers have at least one snack a day, and many consume a fifth or more of their food in snacks.

Many people associate snacking with poor nutrition. While it is true that things such as candy, cookies, pastries, soft drinks, and other high-calorie, low-nutrient foods are popular for snacking, analyses of snacking patterns show that snacks also contribute significant amounts of vitamins and minerals. For example, according to data collected in the National Food Consumption Survey, snackers get an average of 13 to 14 percent of their daily iron, vitamin A, thiamine, niacin, B_6, and B_{12} and 16 to 17 percent of their vitamin C and riboflavin from snacks. Children and teenagers get significant amounts of calcium from between-meal milk drinking.

The types of foods favored as snacks may surprise many. For example, half of all fresh fruits consumed in this country are used as snacks. For children, the most popular snacks are, in descending order, bakery products, milk, soft drinks, fruit, milk desserts (i.e., ice cream or yogurt), candy, and bread. For older children, the order is: bakery products, soft drinks, milk, milk desserts, candy, fruit, salty snacks, and bread.

Studies have failed to document a prevalence of health problems like obesity or increased dental decay among snackers, but data from the National Food Consumption Survey shows that people of all ages who do the most snacking (seven snacks or more over a three-day period) consume more calories, fat, sodium, and sugar than nonsnackers or those who have six or fewer snacks in a typical three-day period. The more frequent snackers also had higher intakes of iron, calcium, vitamin B_6, and magnesium.

Clearly, snacks have to be judged in the context of a person's total diet. Some people who snack constantly on high-calorie foods will gain excessive weight, while others may turn to low-calorie snacking to prevent excessive hunger and overeating. Snacks can be used to help improve the nutritional quality of a diet or, conversely, add little more than calories.

FAST FOODS AND OTHER AWAY-FROM-HOME EATING

Forty percent or more of the American food dollar is spent on eating away from home, with fast-food restaurants enjoying increasing popularity. Between 1970 and 1980, spending for fast foods increased more than 300 percent, to a total of more than $23 billion in 1980. McDonald's, the nation's largest fast-food chain, opens a new outlet about every 17 hours. A decade ago, 10 percent of Americans ate fast foods more than five times a week, and the figure is believed to be higher today. This trend is likely to continue for several reasons. More women work today than in the past and have less time to prepare meals. Fast-food restaurants are less expensive than regular restaurants, making them affordable for teenagers and families who otherwise may not be able to afford regular eating out. They are conveniently located, and they cater to popular tastes.

Fast-food restaurants have often received poor marks from a nutritional standpoint because of their heavy emphasis on fatty hamburgers, hot dogs, French fries, pastries, and other high-calorie, high-fat foods. However, their fat content and even their menus are changing in keeping with the increased nutritional awareness of the general public. Many have added salad bars; others have made serious attempts to reduce the fat and salt contents of their food. By selecting these foods, it is possible to put together nutritious reduced-fat, low-calorie meals in keeping with the basics of good nutrition. (For more specific guidance, see Chapter 39.)

ECONOMIC FACTORS

Is there widespread hunger in America? Media reports and advocates for the homeless and other economically disadvantaged groups maintain there is. The growing number of homeless Americans and people—especially children—who live below the poverty level would indicate that many of these have inadequate diets due to economic reasons. Inadequate up-to-date quantitative data makes it difficult to document and assess the breadth and depth of the problem of hunger in America.

Without doubt, there are substantial numbers of people who either do not get enough to eat or the quality of whose diets are limited by economic facts. Repeated surveys show that their numbers are relatively small, however, certainly when compared to the less affluent nations. Of course, it can fairly be argued that any American who is denied an adequate diet because of economics is one too many.

Food-Assistance Programs

In recent years, there has been considerable controversy over the adequacy of government food-assistance programs. In both cities and rural areas, the demand for emergency food relief increased by more than 20 percent between 1983 and 1984, and many observers contend that the problem has worsened since then. The latest food-consumption survey found only three percent who reported they often or sometimes did not have enough to eat. As would be expected, substandard diets exist mostly among people in extreme poverty—the homeless, migrant workers, children of the very poor, people living on Indian reservations, and the aged poor.

In 1988, an average of 18.7 million participants received food stamps. This was a decline of 400,000 from the previous year—a drop attributed mostly to stricter eligibility requirements rather than to a drop in the number of people needing food assistance.

Effect of Food Prices on Middle-Income People

Despite the rising numbers of people requiring food assistance, the fact remains that most people in this country have adequate or even overly abundant diets, and too many Americans eat too much. Department of Agriculture studies show that, for the most part, what nutritional deficiencies exist in this country (primarily inadequate iron and calcium levels for many women and adolescent females) are not related to income.

People in almost every income group, however, are more aware of food costs and make efforts to economize. The typical middle-income family now spends 11.7 percent or more of its disposable income on food. The National Food Consumption Survey found that about two-thirds of the respondents said they had changed their eating or shopping patterns because of economic reasons. Food-industry studies show that shoppers do not have as much brand-name loyalty as in the past; instead, they look for what they consider the best value. Most supermarkets now offer regular and premium house brands of frozen or canned goods that are less expensive than name brands.

Rising meat prices are cited for at least some of the shift to lower-cost poultry and vegetable protein. And the National Food

Consumption Survey shows that people in the lowest economic groups eat somewhat less meat and fats than those in the highest levels. Still, there is not much nutritional difference in the overall diets consumed by people in different income groups.

Outlook for the Future

Recent trends are expected to continue, at least for the next few years. The number of children born into poverty is expected to increase, and in coming decades, the elderly population also will reach record highs. Barring major droughts (and the drought of 1988 was a close call), or other natural disasters, American agriculture is expected to continue to produce a surplus of food. Thus, the major-

ity of Americans will probably continue to enjoy an affordable abundance of food, even though eating may continue to consume more of the average family budget.

Public awareness of the role of nutrition in health is also expected to grow. Too much of what the public gets is unreliable and biased. Too many in the food industry tend to use literal truths to convey false messages that their specific product, rather than the total daily diet, is protective against disease. On the other hand, "nutrition terrorists," whose livelihood depends on "industry bashing" and creating a "killer food of the month," present speculations as proven facts. Indeed, the creation of this book is, in large part, an answer to the public's demand for reliable and unbiased nutrition information.

3

Separating Food Facts and Myths

Victor Herbert, M.D., J.D.

■

INTRODUCTION

Each year, Americans spend more than $25 billion on health quackery, of which about half goes for health-food pills, powders, and potions. The list includes everything from megadoses of vitamins and minerals to nostrums such as bee pollen, ginseng root, dried algae, and a wide range of homeopathic products. These various potions are falsely promoted as preventives and cures for everything from the common cold, chronic fatigue, and sexual problems to cancer, heart disease, diabetes, and other chronic diseases. In reality, none is more effective than doing nothing, and some are unsafe, with effects ranging from dangerous to lethal. One must always be aware that nutrition is not magic, that claims for magic cures from nutrition are simply not true.

Unfortunately, many, if not most, people regard these various nutrition rip-offs as essentially harmless and perhaps even helpful, despite ample proof to the contrary. The dangers of fraud were highlighted in a recent four-year investigation into health fraud and quackery conducted by the House Subcommittee on Health and Long-Term Care, a group chaired by the late Representative

Claude Pepper of Florida. The findings were unsettling, with considerable evidence of widespread harm caused by nutrition and health fraud. As Representative Pepper stressed, "Quackery can no longer be considered quaint and comic." The American College of Physicians elaborated on this theme in a 1986 issue of its *Observer* newsletter: "The flimflammer of yesteryear, driving through dusty towns with his tonics, is a memory but not without counterpart; in some cases, he is the health food salesman, the vitamin pusher, the 'nutrition counselor' of today."

Obviously, knowledge is the best protection against becoming an unwitting victim of nutrition quackery. A major objective of this book is to give consumers solid information they can use to judge for themselves the validity of a health claim. Specific types of nutrition fraud—for example, those aimed at cancer or arthritis patients—are discussed in chapters devoted to particular diseases or conditions. This chapter concentrates on the common characteristics of nutrition fraud and provides general guidelines on how a consumer can tell whether a claim is legitimate or fraudulent. It also lists the kinds of questions readers should ask *before* taking a supplement, engaging a nutritionist, or undergoing any nutrition therapy. Anyone who tells you what they "believe" about nutrition is talking nutrition as cult, not as science. Those who talk about nutrition as a science say, "Here are the facts about efficacy and safety."

For a definition of a quack, we can turn to the words of the late Representative Claude Pepper who said a quack is "anyone who promotes medical schemes or remedies known to be false, or which are unproven, for a profit." The two basic elements of fraud are deception and profit. Thus, quackery is a form of health fraud.

COMMON CHARACTERISTICS

Many people still think of nutrition quackery in terms of yesterday's snake-oil salesmen and believe that it's easy to detect charlatans. Even the term *quack* brings to mind a vision of a shady character operating in alleys or back streets. No intelligent consumer would fall for the sales pitches of such characters, right?

While it's true that there's not much trade in snake oil these days, business is booming for other forms of nutrition fraud. The notion that it is easy to spot nutrition quackery and charlatans is false. Today's quacks hide behind a cloak of science and respectability. They have impressive-looking certificates and degrees hanging on their office walls; they use "scientific" terms, appear on television talk shows, and write best-selling books touting their theories or products. They sound and look convincing. Their message is one that millions of people want to believe. To all, they promise better health and a longer life. They promise hope to those who are incurably ill, relief to those in pain, and solace to people worried about pollution, stress, and other undesirable aspects of modern life.

How can you or any other layperson tell the real expert with a genuine service or product from a deceiver? One of my colleagues in the National Council Against Health Fraud, Dr. Stephen Barrett of Allentown, Pennsylvania, and I have compiled a list of 20 characteristics to look for.*

1. *The nutrition quack uses anecdotes and testimonials to support claims.* We tend to believe what others tell us about their personal experiences. Separating cause and effect from coincidence can be difficult, however, especially for a layperson. For example, many people honestly believe that a massive dose of vitamin C will cure a cold, and they relate their personal experiences as proof. "I started to get better after taking only five or six tablets," one claims, or "I get fewer colds now that I take vitamin C." What they overlook is the fact that many cold symptoms disappear quickly, with no treatment, and that taking vitamin C or any other remedy is coincidental rather than causal to the natural healing process. Also, we all get fewer colds with the passing years because each time we get a cold, we build up immunity to that one of the many cold viruses. Similarly, most chronic diseases, such as arthritis, have long symptom-free periods, so anything we happen to take when such a period is starting will get the credit—coincidence masquerades as cause and effect. Personal experience alone cannot determine whether a particular remedy is responsible for the remission of symptoms, because it never separates cause and effect from coincidence, suggestibility, or spontaneous improvement. Rather, such a remedy must be demonstrated to be effective in carefully controlled scientific studies involving a number of people.

The placebo effect also must be considered in determining whether an improve-

*Adapted from "Twenty-one Ways to Spot a Quack," by Victor Herbert, M.D., and Stephen Barrett, M.D., *Nutrition Forum*, vol. 3, no. 9, 1986.

ment is indeed due to a particular treatment. A placebo is a harmless, inert substance prescribed for psychological effect. Symptoms often are relieved by any product or therapy that a person is convinced will help, because suggestion is a potent force, which we call "subhypnotic suggestion." Chronic fatigue, tension headaches, and other minor aches and pains often respond to any nostrum that is enthusiastically recommended. Even responsible physicians will often prescribe a placebo—for example, a sugar pill or vitamin tablet—in these instances, and with good results. However, this personal experience cannot be used to justify promoting the placebo as a legitimate cure. In fact, only by comparing a placebo to a claimed cure (i.e., a "controlled study") can we learn whether the claimed cure is better than a placebo.

2. *The quack promises quick, dramatic, or miraculous cures.* The promises are usually couched in double-talk or are very vague so they can be denied or "explained" if a regulatory organization such as the FDA decides to investigate. The relationship between the product and the results is often implied rather than stated. For example, a promotion that asks, Would you like to lose weight while you sleep? is quite different from one that says, Take product X and you will lose weight while you sleep. The promises of cure almost invariably are not printed on the product labels or package inserts, because, under American laws protecting free speech, the only illegal place to lie about nutrition is on the product label. Writing on the label is commercial speech, and fraud in commercial speech is a crime.

3. *Claims are couched in pseudomedical terms or jargon.* Instead of actually promising to cure an ailment, a quack will resort to medical-sounding jargon instead of specific claims. Common examples include claims that product X will "detoxify" your body, "correct chemical imbalances," bring your body into "harmony with nature," or "strengthen your natural immune defenses." The use of such pseudomedical terminology may sound legitimate to a person unfamiliar with genuine terms. Of course, the quack never identifies the nature of the toxin, imbalance, disharmony, or weakness or measures its quantity before and after treatment to show you what has been corrected.

4. *The quack often uses credentials and degrees not recognized by responsible scientists or educators.* We have a well-established system of accreditations by agencies recognized by the U.S. Secretary of Education or the Council on Postsecondary Accreditation. Degrees or certificates from unaccredited diploma mills may look impressive, but they're not worth the paper on which they are printed. As proof of this, I have official-looking certificates hanging on my office wall. One proclaims that Charlie Herbert is a "Professional Member of the International Academy of Nutritional Consultants, a professional organization dedicated to maintaining ethical standards in nutritional consulting," complete with a logo stating "Health Is Wealth." The other is for Sassafras Herbert, and it is even more elegant and official-looking, proclaiming her a "Professional Member of the American Association of Nutrition and Dietary Consultants." It has a handsome seal and is signed and dated. Nowhere do these certificates note that Charlie is a cat and Sassafras is a poodle! Still, they meet the requirements of these particular organizations, one founded by Kurt Donsbach, a California chiropractor who doesn't even have a license to practice chiropractic in any state. To get such a certificate, the applicant needs only three things: a name that can be inscribed on the credential, an address for mailing purposes, and $50.

Be wary of anyone who uses unfamiliar degrees (e.g., D.M. for doctor of metaphysics or C.N. for certified nutritionist). Not even a Ph.D. guarantees that a person is qualified as a nutrition counselor or health practitioner. For example, the late self-proclaimed nutritionist Carlton Fredericks had a Ph.D. and was called Dr. Fredericks in his radio nutrition shows. However, his Ph.D. was not in a health science but in the field of radio communications. Many nutrition diploma mills currently operate, turning out "Ph.D.," "certified nutritionist," and other specious credentials. In only a few states is it by law a criminal offense to call oneself doctor or Ph.D. with a degree from a nonaccredited institution.

5. *Nutrition fraud is based on the false contention that most diseases and symptoms are due to a faulty diet and can be treated with "proper" nutrition. This allows the huckster, as a preventive step, to recommend vitamin and mineral supplements for virtually everyone.* As stressed in this book, aside from deficiency diseases such as scurvy and pellagra, there is little legitimate evidence that most diseases and symptoms have any significant relation to diet. As is emphasized elsewhere here, the development of most diseases depends upon a combination of factors. For example, diet may play an important role in heart disease, but research indicates that this is so only if you also have a genetic predisposition to develop the disease. Common complaints such as chronic fatigue, minor aches and pains, malaise, and insomnia are usually related to stress, not diet. If such symptoms persist, a doctor should be consulted to see whether a physical illness is causing the problem. In any event, contrary to the hucksters' claims, taking vitamin or mineral supplements will not give extra energy or relieve stress.

Today's nutrition quack is also quick to "diagnose" rare or nonexistent fad diseases that can be "cured" by dietary means. Common examples of fad diagnoses include mercury-amalgam toxicity, candidiasis (yeast) hypersensitivity, hyperactivity, joint pains and other ailments caused by food allergies. Very often, the diagnosis is based on tests such as hair analyses or cytotoxicity tests, which are worthless for diagnosing a need for supplements or existence of food allergy but are falsely represented as diagnostic for such purposes. Purveyors of these tests often claim they have scientific evidence to support their value, but when challenged to produce this evidence, they are unable to do so. Despite the fact that such tests and cures have been declared worthless by the FDA and a number of reputable medical and scientific organizations, and warnings to consumers have been published repeatedly in the *FDA Consumer* magazine, the National Council Against Health Fraud's *NCAHF Newsletter*, as well as in unbiased publications such as *Consumer Reports*, Americans continue to spend millions of dollars on them each year. Avoid anyone who sells such tests and treatments for these purposes.

6. *Natural vitamins are purported to be better than synthetic ones.* Every vitamin is made up of a specific chain of atoms strung together as a molecule. Vitamin molecules manufactured by nature in foods are identical to those made by humans in factories. It makes sense to get your vitamins from foods, but if you insist on taking supplements, it doesn't make sense to pay extra for the so-called natural vitamins that are extracted from foods instead of the less expensive ones made in factories. Your body is unable to tell the difference, and the so-called natural ones have the same chemical makeup as synthetic ones. In addition, the latter are more likely to be subjected to better dose and quality control than the "natural"

varieties that are often made by small companies with little regard for standard procedures.

7. *The quack recommends a variety of substances similar to those found in the body and these are claimed to have rejuvenative powers.* Sometimes misnamed as "cellular therapy," these treatments are based on the primitive notion that eating certain animal parts (usually raw) will in some way rejuvenate their counterparts in the body. For example, patients with heart diseases are urged to eat raw heart; concoctions made from animal brains are promoted to improve memory or treat symptoms of senility; raw bull testicles are purported to improve sexual and athletic performance, and so forth. The fact is, when eaten (either raw or cooked), these substances, as well as all other foods, are digested and metabolized in the stomach and intestine before being absorbed. Therefore, they cannot possibly revitalize a specific organ or body part, because what is absorbed is completely broken down and no longer bears any resemblance to the food that entered the mouth, and carries no message saying "take me to the heart"—or brain, or any other specific location.

8. *The quack claims that a greedy and closed medical establishment shuns his or her methods from fear of competition.* Purveyors of medical quackery often portray themselves as innovators who are ignored or held back by a greedy and jealous medical or scientific establishment. The notion is that the establishment wants to protect its territory from competition by the unorthodox, whose remedies are promoted as being superior but blocked for competitive or other reasons. The fact is that, over the past 30 years, not one quack, when challenged under oath, has been able to produce a valid scientific paper that has been rejected by the scientific community and yet objectively

demonstrates the validity of what they do. A recent example involves so-called immunoaugmentive therapy, which was purported to cure cancers by stimulating the patient's immune system with injections of various blood products. The treatments were banned in the United States but offered in a clinic in the Bahamas.

The developer claimed that he had scientific evidence that his therapy worked, but that the medical establishment refused to print it. When challenged in court to produce the evidence and papers submitted to scientific journals, he admitted that none had been submitted since 1974. In fact, there was no evidence that the therapy was of any benefit, and, indeed, analysis of the serum showed that some was tainted with the deadly AIDS virus.

The American Medical Association, physicians in general, and agencies such as the Food and Drug Administration are special targets of health-fraud practitioners who need to undermine the credible in order to lend validity to themselves. People, especially those with AIDS, cancer, and other diseases for which there is no cure, often want to believe these fraudulent claims. They are, after all, desperate and frustrated by the time it takes to develop and test a new treatment. The process that must be followed is lengthy, but for a good reason: Many of the new drugs that look promising in a test tube turn out to be lethal or worthless when administered to a human. Sometimes it takes years for adverse effects to show up. This is why the FDA insists upon lengthy testing and proof of both efficacy and safety.

A century ago, new ideas and therapies from innovative thinkers were difficult to evaluate and were sometimes rejected by the medical community, only to be upheld later. Today, however, the scientific community welcomes innovation, asking only that proponents demonstrate their methods as more effective than and as safe as doing nothing, or if not as safe, that the potential for benefit exceeds the potential for harm. For example, the minute a new vaccine or treatment for AIDS is developed and proved safe and effective, the public can rest assured that it will be released with the same dispatch with which the polio vaccine was approved more than three decades ago. It will make no difference whether the innovator is a famous member of the establishment or an unknown researcher working in a basement laboratory—provided the discovery can stand up to scientific scrutiny. The notion that physicians band together to block new approaches out of greed or fear of competition is a malicious lie. Frequently, quacks will attempt to bypass the scientific community's demand that efficacy and safety be demonstrated by going directly to political bodies to legalize their practices and to insurance companies to pay for them. Fortunately for the medical consumer, this is not the way medical science operates.

9. *Frauds declare that foods should be natural or organic and that health-food stores are preferable to supermarkets or regular produce shops.* Quacks falsely claim that the soil has been depleted of nutrients and food grown in it is lacking in vitamins and minerals, and that the use of chemical fertilizers produces foods that are nutritionally inferior to those that are organically grown (i.e., with manure or compost). These claims ignore the simple fact that if soil is lacking in nutrients, the plants simply will not grow. It makes no difference whether fertilizers are natural or chemical—plants will convert both to the same chemicals in order to grow. There is no basis to the claim that products in health-food stores are somehow better than in stores not labeled as such. In fact, a comparison of the two reveals that both sell many of the same products. The only dif-

ference is that you will probably pay a lot more in the health-food store and have a much more limited selection. In fairness, it must be stated that nothing is wrong with the foods in health-food stores. It is their pills, powders, and potions that are the real rip-off, as are the books and magazines that promote fake nutrition cures.

10. *Quacks oppose fluoridation of water as cancer-causing or dangerous to health. They often also oppose any other protection of the public health, such as vaccination.* Fluoride is needed to build decay-resistant teeth and strong bones, and the best way to obtain it is to add small amounts to the water supply. There is no evidence that this is in any way harmful to health, and there is ample proof that widespread fluoridation has markedly reduced tooth decay in this country. Lies such as those that claim public-health measures cause harm are quack's weapons against all government control in the health area. They hate government regulation because it is the only protection the public has against them. Of course, there are also those who hate government regulation in any form except in conformity with their own personal views. However, this does not alter the fact that regulation is the only protection the public has against quackery.

11. *Food processing or storage is claimed to destroy foods' nutritional quality.* This is a common argument among purveyors of lucrative natural or organic foods who oppose practices such as milk pasteurization and modern food processing and preservation. Processing does alter the nutritional composition of some foods, reducing the amounts of some nutrients and increasing others. The changes usually are minor and have no effect on health so long as a person consumes a varied diet. Pasteurization kills harmful bacteria; using unpasteurized milk and milk products

can be dangerous, and has been lethal to a number of children and other susceptible persons.

12. *Food additives and preservatives are depicted as akin to poisons that cause a variety of symptoms, including hyperactivity and murderous rages.* This claim is simply another scare tactic used by nutrition quacks to undermine public confidence in our foods. By raising fears about most products on supermarket shelves, the quack creates a larger market for expensive so-called health or natural products. The recent scare over Alar, a growth retardant sprayed on apples to make them crisp and improve color, is a case in point. For weeks, the media was caught up in the "great apple scare" of 1989, after a well-meaning but basically misinformed consumer group released a report claiming that several thousand children who ate apples or drank apple juice would develop cancer. When heated, one of the metabolites of Alar has been shown to increase cancer risk in laboratory animals. There is no evidence that fresh apples that have been sprayed with the substance are harmful. Nor is there a valid scientific basis for the claim that thousands of children, including those who consumed large amounts of apple juice, are in danger of getting cancer. These claims were based on flawed data that had been carefully reviewed by scientific bodies and rejected as invalid. However, scientists who cited these facts were put down as apologists for the food industry. It is unfortunately true that the public usually prefers to take the word of popular, attractive, and genuinely concerned but misinformed celebrities such as Meryl Streep over that of scientists.

Since then, apple growers have bowed to public demands and voluntarily agreed not to use Alar. The point of this discussion is not to defend the use of Alar—after all, its basic purpose is cosmetic and it has little effect on the safety of the food. Invariably, however, when Alar was cited in the media, it was mistakenly identified as a pesticide, and, by association, public fear of all pesticides was fueled. The U.S. government forbids the use of any pesticide or preservative that may constitute a health hazard. When evidence is presented that a pesticide or preservative is harmful, it is removed from the market. What the public fails to realize is that all fruits and vegetables are loaded with their own natural pesticides, many of which are cancer-causing agents more potent than the amounts of the chemical ones permitted by the government for use on foods. Does this mean that you should shun plant foods because of these natural cancer-causing substances? No; fortunately, plant foods also are loaded with natural anticancer agents, and the two balance each other out. (For a more extensive discussion, see Chapter 11.)

13. *Quacks assert that stress and certain conditions increase the need for vitamin or mineral supplements.* The claim that mental stress calls for supplements is a lie. The New York Attorney General recently forced a major seller to withdraw ads implying that this was the truth. Physical stress and certain diseases slightly increase the need for some nutrients, but rarely above the amounts found in the average American diet. A person who really is in danger of illness-related deficiency (for example, from cancer, kidney, or liver diseases) should be under medical care, probably in a hospital.

14. *Megadoses of certain vitamins and minerals are urged to prevent cancer.* There is not a single responsible study demonstrating that large doses of any vitamin or mineral have ever prevented cancer in a human. The American Cancer Society recommends that the diet include in its variety some foods rich in vitamins A and C, but it specifically does not advocate supplements, let alone megadoses.

Indeed, large doses of vitamin A can be dangerous and even lethal, and as little as 25,000 IU, which is five times the RDA, taken just before and early in pregnancy may cause fetal deformities. Excessive vitamin C can cause bladder irritation, kidney stones, and other problems. (See Chapter 22).

15. *Hair analysis and other expensive but worthless diagnostic tests are urged for everyone in order to detect vitamin and mineral "deficiencies."* Hair analysis has a limited ancillary value in detecting late mercury and other heavy-metal poisoning, but it is worthless in detecting a need for nutritional supplements. Still, some health-food stores, mail-order labs, and a variety of practitioners make

quick money by urging that everyone have a hair analysis. Typically, the testing lab sends back an important-looking computer printout listing "values" and recommending specific supplements, often sold by the testing lab or practitioner.

16. *Be wary of practitioners who sell vitamins and minerals.* Scientific nutritionists and reputable physicians are not in the vitamin-selling business. Unscientific practitioners often do—usually at several times their real cost. Their economic interest is often disguised by sending you to a particular vendor to "fill the vitamin prescription." They don't tell you the vendor gives them a kickback. A number of coaches get "honoraria" and various perks for

Dos and Don'ts for Choosing a Nutritionist

In this era of increased awareness of fitness, health, and nutrition, having your own nutrition counselor or adviser has become very popular.

Many people are unaware that only half the states have a legal definition, licensing procedure, or standards for nutritionists. Thus, anyone can go into business as a nutritionist. (As noted elsewhere in this chapter, both my dog and cat are credited with being "professional nutritionists," with fancy certificates to prove it.) Given today's widespread concern about health and diet, business for these "nutrition practitioners" is booming. Unfortunately, many so-called nutritionists don't know the difference between fact and fiction, recite as truth the lies they read, and dispense advice that can vary from questionable to dangerous.

Before engaging the services of a nutrition counselor, you should ask yourself:

1. Do I really need a nutrition adviser?
2. If so, what should I expect from this person?
3. Does this counselor have an economic interest in selling tests and products?

For the vast majority of people, this book alone will provide all the nutrition information that

they need. People with special diet-related problems may decide they want to know more or can benefit from individualized instruction or diet planning. Remember, however, that even the best-qualified responsible nutritionists cannot prescribe a diet that will cure heart disease, cancer, or any other disease. Dietary modification can cure only nutritional-deficiency diseases. Dietary modification can have some health-promotion and disease-prevention value in people at risk for heart disease, and, in the overweight, weight reduction can help those at risk for hypertension, diabetes, and, to a small extent, cancer.

Assuming your expectations are realistic, the next question is, Where do I find a qualified nutrition counselor?

There are a number of possibilities.

1. Physicians with a background in nutrition

The old notion that doctors don't know anything about nutrition is falling by the wayside as nearly all institutions follow the lead of places such as Mount Sinai and make solid nutrition education an integral part of their programs. Physicians who feel they themselves are inadequately schooled in nutrition can recommend a reliable counselor.

pushing supplements none of their athletes need; few "nutritionally oriented" coaches know what they are talking about. *Nutritionally oriented* is a code phrase used by supplement pushers to identify other people who push supplements.

17. *Sugar is condemned as a poison.* As noted in Chapter 8, when sugar is used in moderation as part of a normal, balanced diet, it is perfectly safe. In fact, even if you eat no sugar, the liver will make a certain amount from other foods because the brain and other vital organs need it for fuel. An excessive amount of sugar—or any other food—is unhealthy, but there is no evidence that sugar per se is a poison. The claim that sugar causes diabetes is a misstatement, according to the American Diabetes Association.

18. *Be wary of practitioners who use computerized questionnaires to diagnose nutritional deficiencies.* Nutritional deficiencies are diagnosed by appropriate medical tests and examination, not by computers. Any computer used for this purpose is likely to be programmed to recommend supplements for virtually everyone.

19. *Unscrupulous practitioners will advocate very restrictive fad diets for everything from weight loss to controlling serious diseases such as diabetes and high blood pressure.* Imbalanced or restrictive diets can result in se-

---

Dos and Don'ts for Choosing a Nutritionist *(cont.)*

2. Registered Dietitians (R.D.s)

Registered Dietitians have been schooled in the principles of sound nutrition. Some specialize in problems such as heart disease, diabetes, obesity, and the like. You can find a qualified dietitian by consulting the dietetics department at your local hospital or medical center. You can also obtain names of registered dietitians in your area by contacting the public-relations department of the American Dietetic Association: 312–280–5000.

3. Ph.D.s with nutrition expertise

The American Society for Clinical Nutrition (9650 Rockville Pike, Bethesda, MD 20014) is a reliable source of Ph.D.s (and M.D.s) with nutrition expertise. Its monthly journal, the *American Journal of Clinical Nutrition,* is the most widely respected clinical nutrition journal in the United States. I do not trust, nor do I believe you should trust, "me too" organizations such as the Nutritionist Association of America, which turn out to be associated with the promotion of questionable (but lucrative) "nutrition" practices.

The interlocking network of organizations promoting lucrative but questionable nutrition practices is described in *The Unhealthy Alliance* by Stephen Barrett, published in 1988 by the American Council on Science and Health, 1995 Broadway, New York, NY 10023. It describes the American Quack Association (yes, there really is such a group!), the National Health Federation (NHF), the Coalition for Alternatives in Nutrition and Health Care (CANAH), Project Cure, and other lucrative promotions of questionable nutrition practices. In 1989, the NHF sent out a fundraising letter warning that the FDA "has indicated they are going on a 'quack attack . . .' It is imperative that we continue to defend and maintain our right to be a quack. . . ."

The National Council Against Health Fraud (P.O. Box 1276, Loma Linda, CA 92354) publishes a bimonthly newsletter that gives individuals the facts they need to protect themselves from charlatans and hucksters.

The Food and Drug Administration also has a monthly publication, *FDA Consumer* (HFW–40, Food and Drug Administration, 5600 Fishers Lane, Rockville, MD 20857). It describes both fraudulent or questionable products and practices, as well as sound health measures.

rious health problems and should be avoided. There are legitimate dietary treatments for diabetes and high blood pressure, but they stress moderation and balance, and do not entail following fad diets. Be wary, too, of any practitioner that tries to sell you on a fast, painless way to lose weight. Such diets are seldom, if ever, effective in the long run, and some can cause serious or even life-threatening complications.

20. *Quacks try to portray doctors as money-hungry or incompetent butchers.* Quacks want you to trust them, not your doctor. Like all human beings, doctors can *and* do make mistakes. However, your chances of encountering actual medical misconduct are close to 100 percent when dealing with a quack and less than 1 percent with a responsible physician. Legally, true medical misconduct is defined as the use of worthless diagnostic tests, representing them to be of value, and the use of worthless and potentially harmful therapies while representing them to be effective and safe.

For further information, see the following books:

Nutrition Cultism: Facts and Fictions by Victor Herbert. Philadelphia: Stickley-Lippincott, 1981.

Vitamins and Health Foods: The Great American Hustle by Victor Herbert and Stephen Barrett. Paperback. Philadelphia: Stickley-Lippincott, 1985.

Health Schemes, Scams, and Frauds by Stephen Barrett and the Editors of Consumer Reports Books. New York: Consumer Reports Books, 1990. Distributed by St. Martin's Press.

A publicly accessible database of nutrition research information funded by the federal government. This database can be accessed by a computer modem through DIALOG (on-line service of DIALOG Information Services Inc.) as File 60, CRIS (Current Research Information System), subfile HNRIM (Human Nutrition Research Information Management).

Part II

What's in Your Food:
An Overview

■

4

Protein

Delia A. Hammock, M.S., R.D.

■

INTRODUCTION

Protein, the body's major building material, is among the most complex and important substances consumed in the daily diet. Protein is often called the quintessential nutrient because, like oxygen, it is essential to every individual cell's metabolic activities. It is second only to water in overall abundance in the body. The word *protein* comes from the Greek word *proteios*, meaning "of prime importance." The name is well chosen. The brain, muscles, blood, skin, hair, nails, and the connective tissues that hold the body together are all made mostly of protein. The antibodies of the immune system that fight off disease are constructed of protein, as are all the enzymes and many of the hormones that regulate the body's biochemical activities.

As scientists have learned more about the many roles proteins play in maintaining the body's diverse functions, various myths, food fads, misunderstandings, and, sometimes, dangerous quackery have also evolved. Many people believe, for example, that high-protein foods should predominate in a healthy diet, when, in fact, only 10 to 12 percent of daily calories should come from protein, assuming that total caloric needs are also met.

As a general rule, the diet consumed by Americans and most people in industrialized countries—high in meat, eggs, poultry, seafood, and other animal products—actually provides more protein than is needed. Because many high-protein foods are also high in fat and calories, this kind of diet can promote overweight. It can also impose extra work on the liver and kidneys, which must get rid of unused and potentially toxic parts of the protein molecule. Diets high in animal protein also entail unnecessarily consuming expensive food items to obtain nutritional benefits that could be supplied by much cheaper vegetable proteins or carbohydrate foods, such as legumes and pasta. (See Table 4.1.)

A person seeking to untangle the web of confusion and misinformation about protein's role in the diet must begin by understanding what protein is and how it functions in the body.

WHAT IS PROTEIN?

Proteins are organic substances like carbohydrates and fats in that they contain the same building material: a carbon backbone with oxygen and hydrogen attached. However, proteins have another essential addition—nitrogen—that makes them unique. Some proteins have other minerals such as sulfur, phosphorus, and iron as part of their structures, as well.

Each protein molecule is composed of subunits called amino acids. Twenty different amino acids are found in body proteins, of which 9 are essential in the diet; the other 11 can be made in the body. Several others are synthesized in the laboratory or in the body after the proteins are formed, by modifying their side chains. Each amino acid has two key structural features suggested by the

Table 4.1. Cost of 20 Grams of Protein from Specified Meats and Meat Alternates at December 1989 Prices

Food	Market Unit	Price per Market Unit*	Part of Market Unit to Give 20 Grams of Protein**	Cost of 20 Grams of Protein
Turkey, ready-to-cook	lb.	0.95	0.33	0.31
Eggs, large	doz.	1.14	0.28	0.32
Peanut butter	18 oz.	2.04	0.16	0.33
Tuna, canned	6.5 oz.	0.84	0.41	0.34
Bread, white, enriched***	lb.	0.69	0.50	0.34
Chicken, whole, ready-to-cook	lb.	0.88	0.42	0.37
Pork shoulder, smoked, bone in	lb.	1.17	0.32	0.37
Ground beef, regular	lb.	1.50	0.27	0.40
Milk, whole, fluid****	½ gal.	1.37	0.31	0.42
Ground chuck	lb.	1.88	0.25	0.47
Chicken breasts, bone in	lb.	2.01	0.27	0.54
Chuck roast of beef, bone in	lb.	2.01	0.29	0.58
Round roast of beef, bone out	lb.	2.78	0.23	0.64
Ham, canned	lb.	2.62	0.26	0.68
Round beefsteak, bone out	lb.	3.17	0.22	0.70
Frankfurters, all meat	lb.	2.11	0.39	0.82
Sirloin beefsteak, bone in	lb.	3.46	0.26	0.90
Bologna	lb.	2.40	0.38	0.91
Pork chops, center cut, bone in	lb.	2.85	0.32	0.91
Pork sausage, bulk	lb.	2.12	0.47	1.00
Bacon, sliced	lb.	1.96	0.52	1.02
Rib roast of beef, bone in	lb.	4.21	0.32	1.35
T-bone beefsteak, bone in	lb.	5.04	0.30	1.51

*U.S. average retail price of food items estimated using information provided by the Bureau of Labor Statistics, U.S. Department of Labor.
**About one-third of the daily amount recommended for a 20-year-old man. Assumes that all meat is eaten.
***Bread and other grain products, such as pasta and rice, are frequently used with a small amount of meat, poultry, fish, or cheese as main dishes in economy meals. In this way, the high-quality protein in meat and cheese enhances the lower quality of protein in cereal products.
****Although milk is not used to replace meat in meals, it is an economical source of good-quality protein. Nationwide prices for cheese were not available.

Source: U.S. Department of Agriculture, Human Nutrition Information Service, Hyattsville, Maryland 20782.

name—an amino group (-NH$_2$), which is the chemical fragment containing nitrogen, and an acid group (-COOH).

Unique chemical linkages called peptide bonds join amino acids together in long chainlike structures to form proteins. A useful analogy is a long freight train made up of different boxcars linked together in a common manner. As cars can be uncoupled and regrouped to comprise a different train or trains, so can different amino acids be joined to make a larger—or smaller—protein unit.

To understand the vast number of possible combinations of amino acids that form proteins, think of all of the English words that can be made from the 26 letters of the alphabet. With proteins, there are 20 "letters" or amino acids. However, there are no rules as there are in our language that require the alternation of vowels and consonants or restrict the length of a word. Thus, amino acids can be arranged in an almost infinite number of ways. Some of the 50,000 or more proteins the body requires are composed of hundreds of amino acids, while others contain only a few.

The nature, number, and sequence of amino acids in a protein ultimately determines the form, function, and character of that protein. The amino acid sequence for every individual's own body proteins is predetermined by the DNA (deoxyribonucleic acid), the genetic material that resides in the nucleus of each body cell. DNA provides a code, or "blueprint," that directs both the frequency with which amino acids appear and the pattern of their appearance. This genetic code is different for every species and for every individual within a species.

Adding even more complexity is the cross-linking of sulfur and hydrogen atoms that occurs between side chains of various amino acids. These linkages, which are not as strong as peptide bonds, cause some protein molecules to be tightly coiled in a ball-like shape, while others are stretched out, forming threadlike structures. Individual chains of amino acids can also fold and intertwine with each other, adding yet another level of complexity and diversity and ensuring that each protein is tailor-made for its specific body function.

THE ROLES OF PROTEIN

Protein supplies the amino acids the body needs to carry out its myriad activities, one of the most essential of which is tissue growth and maintenance. Adequate protein is essential for the development of the fetus, the production of human milk, the height and weight increases of children, the healing of a wound, and the constant growth of hair and nails. Less obvious, but equally important, is the need for amino acids to replace and maintain body tissues such as muscles, blood, skin, body organs, and connective tissue, which are constantly being degraded and rebuilt in a process called protein turnover. It has been estimated that the average 150-pound man breaks down and synthesizes about 400 grams of protein each day. This means that about four times as much protein is turned over daily within the body than is ordinarily available from a typical American diet. This is possible because most of the amino acids that are liberated during the course of protein breakdown are recycled to build new proteins. However, while the protein recycling system is relatively efficient, proteins are still lost from the body and must be replaced daily through the diet.

In addition to forming major body tissues, amino acids are needed in smaller amounts to make the enzymes and some of the hormones that regulate body processes.

For example, the hormone insulin is a protein that regulates the level of glucose in the blood. Enzymes are protein molecules that direct and accelerate the thousands of chemical reactions that are constantly taking place in the body. Enzymes are essential for breaking down protein, fats, and carbohydrates during digestion, as well as for rebuilding new substances from the raw materials obtained from the diet. Each enzyme is highly specific for a particular reaction, and without the appropriate enzyme, an enzyme-dependent reaction cannot take place.

Proteins are also a critical component of the disease-fighting immune system. Antibodies, the substances manufactured by the immune system to repel an invasion by an infectious organism or other foreign body, are proteins. The great specificity by which proteins can be manufactured using the 20 amino acids allows the body to produce an antibody specific to each foreign substance that enters the body. For example, the antibody for rubella virus will inactivate only that virus. However, when protein supplies are limited, antibody formation is depressed and the body becomes more vulnerable to disease and infection.

Other proteins have the specific task of transporting nutrients and other molecules. Some transport proteins carry nutrients such as sodium and potassium in and out of cells, while others ferry substances in the blood. For example, hemoglobin, an iron-bearing protein containing 300 amino acids, carries oxygen from the lungs to all body tissues, while the formation of protein-containing complexes called lipoproteins permits fats and other lipids to be carried in the aqueous blood.

Proteins also play an essential role in maintaining the body's water balance. Since protein molecules are too large to pass through the semipermeable membranes of blood vessels, they create osmotic pressure, which shifts water toward them, drawing fluid from the tissues back into the bloodstream. If protein levels in the blood plasma fall too low, as in protein deficiency, fluid accumulates in the tissues, causing the condition known as edema. (Other factors unrelated to protein status can also cause edema.) Proteins also act as buffers to regulate the acid-base balance (pH) of the body fluids.

Finally, protein can be used for energy, although carbohydrates and fats are more efficiently used for this purpose. But when the diet does not contain enough carbohydrate and fat to meet caloric needs, proteins are stripped of their nitrogen and burned for energy instead of being used for other vital functions that can be carried out only by protein. Similarly, if protein intake exceeds the body's requirements, the excess is also broken down and then converted to either glycogen or fat and stored for future energy needs. When used for energy, each gram of protein supplies four calories.

AMINO ACIDS—ESSENTIAL AND NONESSENTIAL

Amino acids, not protein per se, are necessary to build all proteins. Therefore, the ultimate value of a food protein is in its amino-acid composition.

The amino acids can be divided into two groups: essential amino acids and nonessential amino acids. The nine essential amino acids are so designated because it is essential that they be derived from the food we eat. The remaining 11 are also required for life, but they are called nonessential because, if they are not available from our diet, they can be manufactured inside our own body cells. (Under certain conditions, as in liver disease, or in the premature infant, the body may be unable to make adequate amounts of certain nonessential amino acids, in which case these nonessential amino acids become essential and must also be supplied by the diet, which is why the number of essential amino acids varies from 9 to 11.) (See Table 4.2 for a list of the essential and nonessential amino acids.)

HOW THE BODY HANDLES PROTEIN

Since every individual must make his/her own unique body proteins, the whole protein found in animal or plant tissues is not used in its intact state. First, the body must break it down and reassemble it. This disassembling of protein involves breaking the cross-links that have formed between the side chains of the various amino acids and then breaking the peptide bonds that hold one amino acid to another.

This first step may begin during cooking. Heat is one of several factors that alters the configuration of the amino-acid chains within the protein. This process, which is called denaturation, usually makes the peptide linkages between amino acids more susceptible to attack by the digestive enzymes, thus increasing the protein's digestibility. For example, an egg white is one of nature's best and most concentrated sources of protein. Although it can be eaten raw, cooking denatures the protein and makes it more digestible as well as more appetizing. However, overcooking of food sometimes creates enzyme-resistant linkages within the protein chains, interfering with digestion and absorption. Alcohol and acid can also cause denaturation, which is why marinating meat in wine or lime juice before cooking can have a tenderizing effect. Commercial meat tenderizers are even more effective denaturers, since they contain natural enzymes that can actually break the peptide bonds that hold the amino-acid chain together. If not used sparingly, however, these products may lead to overtenderization and a mushy texture.

Once protein-containing foods are eaten, digestion begins. The sight, sound, smell, and taste of food trigger the stomach to secrete acid and enzymes that begin denaturing the protein and uncoiling its molecules. The acid also helps trigger the release and activation of enzymes whose special function is to cleave specific peptide bonds, dividing the long amino-acid chains into smaller chains called polypeptides.

Protein digestion continues in the small intestine. Here alkaline juices from the pancreas neutralize the acidic stomach juices, and other specialized protein-splitting pancreatic and intestinal enzymes take over to break down the polypeptides to dipeptides and single amino acids, which are absorbed through the intestinal wall and into the blood for transport to the liver.

Protein absorption is very efficient, although some proteins are more digestible than others. In general, about 97 percent of the protein from animal foods is digested and absorbed, while proteins from legumes, cereals,

Table 4.2.   Amino Acids

Essential	Nonessential
Isoleucine	Glycine
Leucine	Glutamic acid
Lysine	Arginine*
Methionine	Aspartic acid
Phenylalanine	Proline
Threonine	Alanine
Tryptophan	Serine
Valine	Tyrosine
Histidine	Cysteine
	Asparagine
	Glutamine

*May become essential in some circumstances.

vegetables, and fruits are digested and absorbed with an efficiency of about 78 to 85 percent.

Some of the amino acids that enter the bloodstream are not from food. The digestive enzymes are also protein, so after they have done their work, they, too, are broken down into their component amino acids to be absorbed and reused as needed by the body. Similarly, protein-containing cells from the lining of the intestines are continually being sloughed off and replaced by new cells. Some of the protein contained in these worn-out cells is also broken down and absorbed, while some is excreted.

The fate of an amino acid after it is transported to the liver is highly dependent upon the body's needs at that moment. Some of the amino acids are used by the liver to manufacture its own proteins as well as many of the specialized proteins such as liver enzymes, lipoproteins, and the blood protein, albumin. Other amino acids enter the bloodstream, where they join amino acids that have been liberated during the constant breakdown and synthesis of body tissues. As these amino acids circulate throughout the body, each cell, directed by its own DNA blueprint, draws from the common pool of available amino acids to synthesize all the numerous proteins required for its functions.

An adequate supply of both essential and nonessential amino acids is vital for protein synthesis to take place. If one of the nonessential amino acids is needed but not available, the cell will simply make it, using parts from other amino acids, and continue assembling the protein. But if one of the essential amino acids is missing, the assembly of the protein is halted. The partially constructed protein is disassembled and the amino acids returned to the blood, where they again circulate through the body to be taken up by other cells in need of specific materials for their pro-

tein-building project. Any amino acids that are not used within a short time cannot be stored for future use. Instead, they are delivered back to the liver, where they are stripped of their nitrogen, which is then incorporated into urea and sent to the kidneys for excretion. The remaining protein skeleton will be converted to glucose and burned as energy or converted to fat or glycogen for storage.

Under other circumstances, protein synthesis cannot take place even when adequate amounts of the essential amino acids are present. Although protein synthesis is very important, the body's number-one priority is to obtain sufficient energy to carry on vital functions such as circulation, respiration and digestion. Therefore, in the absence of adequate dietary carbohydrate and fat calories, the body breaks down not only dietary protein, but also protein from the blood, liver, pancreas, muscles, and other tissues in order to maintain vital organs and functions. Such a situation can arise when a person follows a very low-calorie crash diet to lose weight. In a normal balanced diet, however, carbohydrates and fats are used to meet energy needs, and protein and its amino acids are spread for their unique purposes.

Protein Quality

Every food except for pure fat (oil) or pure sugar contains at least some protein, and every food protein differs in its makeup of amino acids. Thus it's not surprising that some foods provide a better selection of amino acids than others. Foods that contain all of the nine essential amino acids in about the same proportions needed to make body proteins are sometimes referred to as complete or high-quality proteins. All animal proteins, with the exception of gelatin, fall into this category. Vegetable proteins are often called incomplete or lower-quality proteins because—with the exception of soybean, which is almost equal to animal protein—they are deficient in one or more of the essentials. Fortunately, all plant foods are not low in the same amino acids. Thus, by combining plant foods that are low in different essential amino acids, strict vegetarians obtain adequate protein nutrition without eating animal protein. Two incomplete proteins that compensate for one another's shortfalls in this way are called complementary proteins. Virtually every ethnic cuisine features complementary protein dishes. Mexicans eat beans and tortillas; Indians eat dahl (split peas) and rice; Middle Easterners enjoy chick-peas with bulgur wheat; Orientals eat tofu with vegetables and rice; and Americans eat "Hopping John" (black-eyed peas and rice), baked beans with corn bread, and peanut butter sandwiches. (See Chapter 25 for more information about vegetarianism.)

A small amount of animal protein will also supply enough essential amino acids to make up for any deficiency in a plant food. Dishes such as macaroni and cheese, cereal and milk, stir-fried vegetables garnished with bits of meat, and cheese-topped bean casseroles all represent such combinations.

Since the body does not store amino acids as it does carbohydrates and fats, it was once thought that complementary proteins had to be eaten in the same meal to ensure that all essential amino acids would be available simultaneously for the synthesis of body proteins. However, newer research suggests that timing is not so important for adults, although it may be more important for growing children. The reason for this is that amino acids are added to the circulation (amino-acid pool) not only from the digestion of dietary proteins, but also by the constant turnover of body tissue and the breakdown of digestive enzymes. Thus, if any essential amino acid is in short supply in the diet, amino acids from these other sources will temporarily even out the imbalance. Eating a complementary protein or a source of high-quality protein later during the same day will replenish the amino-acid pool before any shortage can interfere with the body's synthesis of new proteins.

Scientists often use sophisticated tests and calculations to rate the quality of the protein in the foods we eat. For example, they may talk about a food protein's "biological value" (BV), its "protein efficiency ratio" (PER), or its "net protein utilization" (NPU). All of these ratings give slightly to greatly different values for the same foods and all of the tests have shortcomings. These measures of protein quality are useful to the industry for, say, comparing the nutritive value of different lots of a single food (for example, infant formula or animal feed) or in research situations where a uniform test diet is needed for humans or animals. These measurements, however, give little useful information about the protein quality of complex human diets. The amino-acid patterns of the various protein-containing foods in a mixed diet will always complement each other to some extent, making more protein available than would be in the single foods alone. How efficient the body is in its use of dietary protein also depends on an individual's intake of both calories and protein.

For practical purposes, diets can be planned simply by considering the protein source—animal (complete protein) or vegetable (incomplete protein). There is no reason for healthy people eating adequate calories from a variety of foods to be concerned with the protein-quality ratings of individual animal or vegetable proteins. People who consume diets containing solely vegetable proteins require somewhat more protein than those whose diets contain animal foods, but in the United States, almost everyone exceeds his or her protein needs.

ESTIMATING PROTEIN NEEDS

Because only protein contains nitrogen, research to determine the amount of protein an adult needs has traditionally been based on studies of the body's nitrogen balance. Nitrogen is lost continually through urine, stool, skin, hair, and nails. Dietary protein is necessary to replenish these losses. Adults consuming adequate calories and as much (or more) protein as they need are in a state of nitrogen equilibrium, or, simply put, the amount of nitrogen in is equal to the amount of nitrogen out. However, during times of growth or rapid protein synthesis, nitrogen balance becomes positive, meaning that more nitrogen is coming into the body than is going out of it. Growing children and teenagers, pregnant and breastfeeding women, and adults engaged in muscle building or recuperating from surgery, injury, or disease should be in positive nitrogen balance. When nitrogen excretion exceeds intake, a condition of negative nitrogen balance exists. This condition indicates that the body is breaking down its own proteins faster than they are being replaced. Negative nitrogen balance is not normal or desirable. It occurs during starvation, fasting or crash dieting, or whenever injury, illness, or immobilization cause excessive breakdown of tissues.

RECOMMENDED DIETARY ALLOWANCE

The exact amount of protein one needs depends on age, body size, composition of diet, state of health, and other factors. The RDA for protein for a healthy adult is 0.8 grams for each kilogram (2.2 pounds) ideal body weight. (Ideal body weight is used rather than actual body weight because body fat contains little protein.) This figure is based on nitrogen-balance studies, but it also includes two separate safety factors. First, the minimum intake required for nitrogen balance has been increased by 30 percent to account for individual variability and to cover increases caused by the stresses of daily living. Second, since protein varies in its digestibility and quality, the value has been further increased to ensure adequacy even when the quality of the protein is less than perfect.

Recommended Dietary Allowances have also been issued to cover the special needs of pregnant and lactating women. An additional 10 grams of protein per day is recommended for the pregnant woman, while lactating women require an additional 15 grams of pro-

Table 4.3. Recommended Dietary Allowances for Protein

To estimate protein requirements, multiply weight (or ideal weight if overweight) by RDA for age. Weight × RDA (by age) = grams of protein per day

	Age	Protein RDA (gm./lb.)
INFANTS	0–0.5	1.10
	0.5–1	0.72
CHILDREN	1–3	0.54
	4–6	0.5
	7–10	0.45
	11–14	0.45 (male)
		0.45 (female)
	15–18	0.40 (male)
		0.36 (female)
ADULTS	19 and over	0.36
PREGNANT		+10*
LACTATING		+15*

*If pregnant, calculate protein RDA at nonpregnant ideal weight and then add 10 grams. If breastfeeding, add 15 grams.

Reprinted from *Recommended Dietary Allowances*, 10th edition, 1989, with permission of the National Academy Press, Washington, D.C.

tein per day during the first six months of nursing, and an additional 12 grams thereafter. Infants, children, and teenagers also require more protein per pound of body weight than do healthy adults. (Recommended protein intakes for different ages are given in Table 4.3.)

The nitrogen-balance technique upon which the adult RDA is based has several limitations, and scientists are currently studying newer, more precise methods of measuring protein and amino-acid requirements. While this research will probably have little influence on the recommended intake of protein for healthy individuals, it may be very important in determining exact amino-acid requirements of specific groups such as infants and chronically or acutely ill patients.

OVERCONSUMPTION OF PROTEIN

In recent years, protein has acquired a false mystique as a super nutrient, a substance that can improve athletic performance, aid in weight-reduction programs, and enhance overall health. Many people have assumed that if a moderate amount of protein in the diet is good, more must be even better.

Federal government surveys of American eating habits in recent years have found that approximately 16 percent of the total caloric intake is from protein—the equivalent of about 63 grams per day for adult women and about 90 grams per day for adult men. Since the protein RDA is considerably lower, most Americans, including those at the bottom of the socioeconomic scale, receive more than enough protein. Indeed, protein deficiency is exceedingly rare in the United States. (For a list of protein sources for the American diet, see Table 4.4.)

High-protein diets have never proven to

be a serious hazard for healthy people, although processing excess protein can overburden a liver or kidneys that are damaged by disease. That's why individuals with kidney or liver disease are often put on protein-restricted diets. Likewise, very high protein formulas can also be detrimental to very young or premature infants whose kidney function is not fully developed. Some nephrologists have also speculated that eating a high-protein diet throughout life may be the reason for the slight decline in kidney function that usually occurs with age, but this connection is still under investigation.

Our typically high-protein, high-meat diets have also been implicated as a factor in the development of osteoporosis, but these claims may be the results of misinterpreting scientific research. Studies have shown that adding *purified* protein supplements and amino-acid mixtures that have had their phosphate removed do increase excretion of calcium by the kidney in both animals and humans. However, several long-term controlled human studies carried out by Herta Spencer, M.D., at the Hines VA Medical Center in Illinois have shown that high intakes of protein from natural protein sources such as meat, which have their phosphate intact, do not significantly increase calcium loss.

Overconsumption of protein is not totally benign. Two-thirds of the protein in the American diet today comes from animal

Table 4.4. Dietary Sources of Protein in the American Diet in 1985

Meat, poultry, fish, eggs	47%
Dairy products	21%
Cereal products	19%
Fruits and vegetables	6%
Legumes, soy products, nuts	5%
All others	1–2%

Source: *National Food Review*, Winter–Spring 1987, U.S. Dept. of Agriculture, Washington, D.C.

sources, and most meat-based proteins come packaged with fat, particularly saturated fat, which, in excess, can contribute to the development of atherosclerosis as well as obesity.

For example, red meat has a reputation as a high-protein food, but only about 25 percent of the calories in a choice T-bone steak come from protein; the remaining 75 percent come from fat. Even a carefully trimmed cut of lean beef such as flank steak may contain 50 percent of its calories as fat. Similarly, only about 31 percent of the calories in an egg are protein; the rest are fat. Fish, poultry with skin removed, and low-fat dairy products provide a higher percentage of protein per ounce than the usual meat and eggs. (See Table 4.5 for a list of protein and fat content of selected foods.)

As discussed earlier, the body does not store excess protein except in the sense that amino acids are present in all tissues. Extra protein just adds calories to the diet, so eating a high-protein diet is often just overeating. A high-protein diet is also likely to crowd out other foods such as fruits, vegetables, and grains, reducing the diet's variety and balance.

The myths surrounding protein have led many athletes to follow high-protein diets in the belief that more protein will foster development of muscles and heighten physical condition. However, while some athletes such as body builders, weight lifters, and endurance athletes may require somewhat more protein than the RDA, mainly because they are building muscle, their needs are easily met by the typical American diet. There is no reason for a

Table 4.5. Protein Guide

Food (cooked)	Portion	Calories*	Protein (gm.)	Fat (gm.)	Percent of Calories from Fat
Sirloin steak, lean	3 oz.	170	26	7	36
Ground beef, lean	3 oz.	230	21	16	62
Bologna	3 oz.	260	10	24	83
Frankfurter	3 oz.	207	6	17	73
Pork loin, lean	3 oz.	190	27	9	43
Ham, boneless	3 oz.	150	19	8	48
Spareribs	3 oz.	338	25	26	77
Lamb, leg, lean	3 oz.	160	23	7	39
Chicken, light, w/o skin	3 oz.	140	26	4	25
Chicken, dark, w/o skin	3 oz.	175	23	8	41
Tuna, white, in oil, drained	3 oz.	158	23	7	40
Tuna, white, in water	3 oz.	116	23	2	16
Flounder	3 oz.	89	20	1	10
Shrimp	3 oz.	84	18	1	11
Cottage cheese, creamed	½ cup	110	13	5	42
Cottage cheese, low-fat	½ cup	100	16	2	18
American cheese	1 oz.	105	6	7	60
Cheddar cheese	1 oz.	144	7	9	56
Whole milk	8 oz.	150	8	8	43
Skim milk	8 oz.	85	8	0.5	5
Yogurt, plain, whole milk	8 oz.	150	8	8	43
Yogurt, plain, low-fat	8 oz.	145	12	4	25
Egg, large	1	80	6	6	68
Pizza	1 slice	290	15	9	28
Hamburger w/bun	1	445	25	21	42

high-protein diet or protein supplements of any kind. Actually, a high-protein diet can work against an athlete by increasing the risk of dehydration, as extra water is required to rid the body of the by-products of protein metabolism. Furthermore, eating too much protein can make it difficult for the athlete to eat enough carbohydrate to ensure adequate stores of glycogen in the muscles and liver. (For more information about nutrition and athletics, see Chapter 24.)

AMINO-ACID SUPPLEMENTS

The regular consumption of amino-acid supplements is another potentially dangerous fad that is often promoted in health-food stores as well as in fitness and body-building magazines. There is no need for these products and claims for them are deceptive and misleading. Advertisements promote these pills and powders for everything from relieving insomnia to aiding weight loss. Many of these exaggerated claims are misrepresentations of the meaning of research during the last decade that suggested a possible role for amino acids in the treatment of certain disorders. Researchers have found that by adjusting the amounts of some amino-acid concentrations in certain animals, the activity of some important brain chemicals can be altered. There is little if any evidence suggesting that amino-acid supplements offer any benefit in treating nonnutritional disorders in humans.

Table 4.5. Protein Guide *(cont.)*

Food (cooked)	Portion	Calories*	Protein (gm.)	Fat (gm.)	Percent of Calories from Fat
Enchilada	1	235	20	16	61
Almonds	1 oz.	165	6	16	85
Peanuts	1 oz.	165	7	14	76
Walnuts	1 oz.	186	4	18	87
Sunflower seeds	1 T	160	6	14	78
Sesame seeds	1 oz.	161	5	14	78
Peanut butter	2 T	190	8	16	76
Kidney beans	½ cup	112	8	0.5	4
Chick-peas	½ cup	134	7	2	13
Lentils	½ cup	115	9	0.5	4
Split peas	½ cup	115	8	0.5	4
Soybeans	½ cup	149	14	8	48
Tofu	½ cup	95	10	6	57
Broccoli, chopped	½ cup	25	2	Trace	Trace
Corn	½ cup	90	3	1	10
Green peas	½ cup	65	4	Trace	Trace
Spinach	½ cup	30	3	Trace	Trace
Potato	½ cup	73	1	Trace	Trace
Oatmeal	1 cup	145	6	2	12
Spaghetti	1 cup	55	6	1	16
Rice, white	1 cup	220	4	Trace	Trace
Rice, brown	1 cup	230	5	1	4
Bread, avg.	1 slice	65	2	1	14
Pita bread	1 large	165	6	1	5

*Calorie counts may vary slightly from those listed elsewhere in this book because of variations in brands tested and similar factors.

Moreover, while amino acids are natural food substances, when used in research studies, they are administered in quantities far beyond those normally ingested in the diet. Thus, instead of acting as foods, they act as drugs, and as with any drug, misuse can be hazardous.

Studies on laboratory animals have shown that, under some conditions, consumption of excessive doses of amino acids can have serious side effects. For example, L-tryptophan, which was sold as a sleep aid until it was taken off the market in early 1990, has been shown to cause a number of serious problems in both humans and animals. As of April 1990, there had been more than one thousand cases of eosinophilia myalgia, a serious muscle disorder, reported among users of L-tryptophan. As of that time, about 20 deaths from eosinophilia had occurred, prompting the FDA to ban all nonprescription tryptophan supplements. There are also several rare genetic diseases that cause heavy concentrations of one or more amino acids to build up in the blood, resulting in problems ranging from mental retardation to death.

Taking single amino-acid supplements can cause imbalances that also may interfere with normal absorption of food-derived amino acids. Certain groups of amino acids compete for carriers to transport them across the intestinal wall for entry into the bloodstream. When an amino-acid supplement is ingested, it floods the transport carriers with that particular amino acid, which may result in other amino acids not being absorbed in the proper amounts.

Because of the potential toxicity of large doses of single amino acids, the Food and Drug Administration (FDA) removed these substances from the agency's list of those generally recognized as safe (GRAS) in 1974.

Amino-acid mixtures are sometimes used to meet the special needs of people who have liver or kidney disease, or for individuals born with genetic disorders of protein metabolism, but these special amino-acid supplements must be used under medical supervision and are not legally available to the public. There is no reason for a normal, healthy person to take amino-acid or protein supplements.

PROTEIN AND WEIGHT LOSS

Periodically, claims are made for the effectiveness of high-protein, low-carbohydrate diets for weight loss. Such diets, however, are no more effective than more balanced regimens, and they can be dangerous.

The main fuel of the brain and central nervous system is glucose, which is most easily obtained from carbohydrates, less easily from protein, and very poorly from fat. When the body's limited carbohydrate stores become depleted, as when a person is fasting or is on a very low carbohydrate diet, protein is degraded to supply needed glucose. This protein will come from the diet, if available, or from the body's lean tissues, such as body organs and muscles. Of course, if the body continued to break down its tissue protein to supply all the required glucose, death would result within three to four weeks. So, if carbohydrate remains unavailable for several days, the body attempts to conserve essential protein by producing an alternative fuel source from the partial burning of fatty acids. These ketones, as they are called, serve as a glucose substitute, fueling some, though not all, central nervous system cells. As the breakdown of fat continues, these ketones build up in the blood, causing an abnormal condition called ketosis.

Diets that cause ketosis—ketogenic diets—are often popular because they usually cause a dramatic weight loss in the first week or so of the diet. However, this initial weight loss is not fat, but water, caused by the kidney's attempts to rid the body of the excess ketones and of the by-products of the breakdown of protein. The ketones that pass out in the urine are falsely represented as constituting a large loss of calories. This weight is quickly regained when carbohydrates are added back to the diet. Longer adherence to such diets usually does cause a loss of body fat, since caloric intake is reduced, but the high-protein regime is no more effective for weight reduction than a better-balanced diet of equal caloric value.

Ketogenic diets make the blood more acid, upsetting the body's chemical balance and causing potentially serious and certainly unpleasant side effects such as headache, bad breath, dizziness, fatigue, and nausea. Furthermore, since high-protein, low-carbohydrate diets are usually synonymous with high-fat, high-cholesterol diets, they may increase the risk of heart disease in susceptible people. Ketosis can be particularly dangerous for diabetics and pregnant women.

Another fad was the use of very low calorie, protein-supplemented formulas for weight loss. These products, often called "protein-sparing modified fasts," caused side effects similar to a ketogenic diet, but because caloric intake was lower, medical consequences were even more severe, including death. These diets were under study by physicians who hoped to eliminate the risks associated with fasting by preventing loss of body protein during rapid weight loss. However, soon this approach to weight loss became the basis of a best-selling book, and the liquid protein supplement was marketed as a self-prescribed, over-the-counter cure for obesity. The consequences were grim. During the late 1970s, close to 100 cardiac deaths were reported as related to liquid protein diets. Autopsy revealed many of these people had eaten their heart muscle for calories.

Improved versions of protein-sparing modified fasts are used today. However, these very low-calorie diets are reasonably safe only when administered under careful medical supervision. There are still risks involved and such diets are, therefore, best reserved for patients who are more than 50 pounds above their desirable weight for height, sex, and age. No one should purchase and use on their own any diet containing fewer than 1,200 calories per day for a man or 1,000 calories per day for a woman.

5

Carbohydrates

Victor Herbert, M.D., J.D.

■

INTRODUCTION

Although many Americans shun carbohydrates as fattening or too pedestrian to be interesting, worldwide they are our most important source of energy. Even in this country, large numbers of people are taking new interest in carbohydrates, as witness the booming market in foods such as pasta and oats.

With the exception of lactose (which comes from milk), most dietary sugars are derived from plants. They are formed from carbon, hydrogen, and oxygen through a complex process in which plants with green leaves transform energy from the sun. The plant uses some of the carbohydrate for its own needs; the rest is stored in various parts—seeds, leaves, stalks, roots, tubers, and so forth.

CLASSIFYING STARCHES AND SUGARS

At first glance, carbohydrates seem to include a bewildering array of foods, from those with a healthy image (such as whole-grain cereals, pasta, and bread) to those sometimes dis-

missed as so-called junk food (such as potato chips and sweets). All carbohydrates serve one major function, however: providing a ready supply of energy to the body's tissues. Beyond this basic role, it can be misleading to describe individual high-carbohydrate foods as nutritionally better or worse than others. The merit of any one food depends not just on nutritional content and its preparation but also on the proportion of other types of nutrients in the diet, overall calorie needs and intake, and many other factors. No one carbohydrate food (table sugar, for instance) can be viewed as an enemy of good nutrition, nor can another one (say, wheat bran) be touted as a panacea for an otherwise faulty diet. Whether sugar or starch, a carbohydrate food—like any other—must be evaluated in the context of the total daily diet.

Carbohydrates provide direct energy for the human brain, central nervous system, and muscle cells in the form of glucose, or blood sugar. (It's been estimated that the central nervous system uses about 140 grams, or 9 tablespoons, of glucose a day). Energy is also supplied from carbohydrates indirectly, after they've been converted in the body to starch or fat. Carbohydrate chemical structure consists of molecular chains of carbon, hydrogen, and oxygen, whose varying configurations produce foods of plant origin as diverse as wheat, peaches, honey, and potatoes.

Simple carbohydrates are sugars, organic compounds whose bonds are easily broken down by digestion. They tend to taste sweet, to form crystals, and to dissolve in water. Sugars occur in nature (as in fruits, berries, some vegetables, maple sap, and honey) and in processed form (as in table sugar, brown sugar, and molasses). There are two main types of sugars:

1. *Monosaccharides* (*Mono*—meaning one). *These* are the most basic sugar molecules, having only a single sugar unit. They include *glucose*, the essential sugar unit that provides energy to human cells; *fructose*, or fruit sugar; and *galactose*, which occurs in milk products in combination with other simple sugars.

2. *Disaccharides* (*Di*—two). These are two monosaccharide units linked together. They include *maltose* (two glucose units), present in germinating grain and used in fermentation to produce malted beverages such as beer and whiskey; *sucrose*, or common table sugar (glucose plus fructose), processed from sugarcane or beets; and *lactose*, or milk sugar (glucose plus galactose). Lactose, present in dairy foods, is the only sugar found in significant quantities in animal products. Cow's milk is about 5 percent lactose by volume, and derives about 28 percent of its calories from this sugar. Much of the world's adult population, especially in the Middle East, Asia, and Africa, lacks lactase, the digestive enzyme necessary to absorb lactose (a condition called lactose intolerance), resulting in gastrointestinal difficulties when more than a few ounces of milk are consumed past infancy. (See chapters 10 and 33).

Complex carbohydrates are defined chemically as polysaccharides, molecular chains of many simple sugars that can be strung together by the hundreds or thousands. The varying structures of these chains endow complex carbohydrates with their great range of distinctive textures, flavors, structures, and colors. The two chief types of complex carbohydrate in the human diet are starch and fiber.

Starches. These are polysaccharides that humans can digest, at least after cooking. The starch in rice, grains, beans, and some other foods occurs in the form of granules encapsulated by an indigestible cellulose coating. (Unlike cows and other grazing animals, humans lack the enzyme needed to break down cellulose for energy.) Cooking softens the cellulose coating, breaking its chemical bonds and releasing the starch particles. In this soluble state, starch can be digested; that is, converted into its component glucose molecules for use by the body. (Cooked starch, when cooled, also tends to form a gel, which accounts for the thickening action of flour or cornstarch in a soup or gravy.)

There's another type of carbohydrate that falls midway between sugars and starches, called *dextrin*. Dextrin is the by-product of digestive enzymes that split starches into sugars, and it can also be produced from starch by using heat or chemicals. Baking bread, for example, produces dextrin, which gives a loaf its brown crust.

HOW CARBOHYDRATES ARE FORMED

Carbohydrates originate, either directly or indirectly, from plants via a transformation of solar energy into forms the plant can utilize or store. This process is called photosynthesis. In photosynthesis, the sun's energy is used by chlorophyll, the green coloring matter in leaves, to synthesize water (from soil) and carbon dioxide (from the air) into glucose. The plant uses this glucose for its immediate growth and repair needs; any extra is converted to starch and stored.

Different parts of plants store varying amounts of starch, depending on their purpose. Roots and tubers (such as potatoes, cassava, and yams) are a concentrated storehouse of starch and this sustains the plant through a long winter without leaves to renew its energy. Seeds, whether grains, peas, beans, or the pits or pips in fruit are another high-energy source, since they must nourish the seedling until it germinates and grows

leaves of its own. (These plant parts include fat and protein in addition to starch.)

The biochemistry of plants explains many phenomena that a greengrocer or cook takes for granted. Some starchy vegetables become less sweet after harvesting, as the carbohydrate initially stored as sugar converts gradually into starch. (This is why corn right off the stalk is sweetest, and why carrots grow tougher and more bitter as their freshness wanes.) Most fruits, though, tend to grow sweeter as they ripen or after harvesting, as their starch reserves convert to sugar (bananas, cherries, and plums, for example).

CARBOHYDRATES IN THE DIET

As noted earlier, carbohydrates are our most prevalent source of energy, making up about half of the calories consumed in the average American diet (see Table 5.1). In some parts of the world, the percentage is much higher. For example, in developing countries where rice, corn, and other grains, as well as yams, cassava root, and other locally grown produce are major dietary staples, more than 80 percent of calories consumed may come from carbohydrates. On the other end of the spectrum, less than 10 percent of the calories consumed by Eskimos, who have little access to

Figure 5.1. Process of Photosynthesis

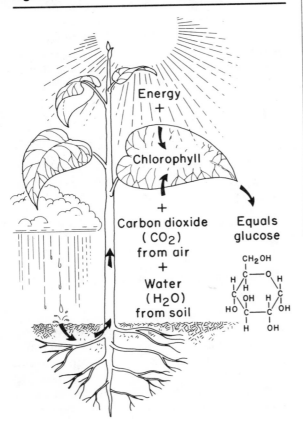

Energy
+
Chlorophyll
+
Carbon dioxide
(CO$_2$)
from air
+
Water
(H$_2$O)
from soil

Equals
glucose

Table 5.1. Where Americans Get Their Carbohydrates

Food	Percent
Sugar and sweeteners	40
Grain products	36
Fruits	7
Dairy products	6
Potatoes	5
Vegetables	4
Legumes and nuts	2

Source: *National Food Review*, 1987, vol. 36, U.S. Dept. of Agriculture, Washington, D.C.

plant foods, come from carbohydrates. (For a breakdown of the best food value for each dollar, see Table 5.2.)

In this century, there have been significant shifts in the types of carbohydrates consumed in the typical American diet. As we have gone from a mostly rural society to a more affluent, industrialized one, there has been a drop in consumption of complex carbohydrates and an increase in the intake of sugars, particularly corn syrup and other sweeteners (see Chapter 8), along with increased consumption of protein and fats.

Some epidemiologists have associated this shift in eating patterns with a rise in certain health problems such as obesity, heart disease, and some cancers and gastrointestinal disorders. The mere fact of these two simultaneous trends does not establish a cause-and-effect relationship; there is still no clear proof that changing patterns of carbohydrate consumption have triggered or worsened the spread of these diseases. Such epidemiological patterns have spurred further investigation, however; and various studies indicate that many cheap and humble carbohydrate foods, from beans to oatmeal, do indeed merit at least as prominent

a place in the diet as more expensive foods such as fatty meats and rich dairy products.

One reason for the decline in complex carbohydrates in our diet is the widespread, albeit false, notion that starchy foods such as potatoes, bread, and pasta are fattening. This misconception has been spurred by promoters of several fad diets who have urged millions of followers to forswear these foods in favor of meat and other high-protein foods.

In fact, starchy foods are no more fattening than protein: Ounce for ounce, both contain the same amount of calories. A person will gain weight whenever the calories consumed exceed those burned in daily activities, and it makes little difference whether the excess calories are from carbohydrates or protein. (There is some evidence that calories derived from fat are more easily stored as body fat than from the other two categories.)

Carbohydrates in general must be judged by the company they keep in their journey from the farm to the table. Anyone seeking to eat a well-balanced, varied, and wholesome diet can benefit from some understanding of the structure and function of carbohydrates, their different types, and the way the body uses them for energy. At the end of this chapter, we'll offer practical guidance for including adequate carbohydrates in meal plans and for making specific carbohydrate food choices.

Table 5.2. The Best Food Value per Dollar Spent

According to studies by the U.S. Department of Agriculture, families who spend their food dollars in the following manner get the best food value.

Food	Percent of Dollars
Meat, poultry, eggs, fish, dried beans and peas, peanut butter, nuts	35
Vegetables and fruits, fresh and processed	20
Other foods: fats, sugars, seasonings, dressings, beverages	20
Milk, cheese, yogurt, ice cream	13
Bread, cereal, pasta, rice, crackers, bakery goods	12

Source: U.S. Department of Agriculture.

HOW THE BODY USES CARBOHYDRATES

Carbohydrate foods are superbly designed to provide the human body with energy. That energy can be burned (or *oxidized*) in the form of glucose, or stored as glycogen for later use. Glucose is the only form of carbohydrate the body can use directly for energy; by the time a cell metabolizes glucose, its original source is indistinguishable. From this perspective, it makes little difference whether the glucose comes from a bowl of oatmeal or a piece of hard candy. Glucose is also the primary form of energy usable by the brain and nervous system, and is one of two types of fuel for the muscles (the other being fatty acids, a less-efficient source that is tapped only when glucose reserves are gone).

Burning carbohydrate for energy serves the body well in other, secondary ways. It spares protein for its prime role as a building block in cell growth and repair. If the body's supply of glucose runs low, stores of fat and protein must provide an alternate energy source. To metabolize fat efficiently, however, the body needs some carbohydrate to help. If it must burn fat without any carbohydrate present, the process releases toxic by-products called ketones, as discussed in the previous chapter. If ketones are allowed to build up, the result can be a dangerous biochemical imbalance called ketosis. Finally, many carbohydrate foods provide dietary fiber, which is not found in fat or protein.

It takes a little longer for the digestive system to break down the chemical bonds in a complex carbohydrate than in a simple one. This is partly why a sugary snack provides a quick lift in energy, and a bowl of cereal or a slice of bread gives a slower and more sustained one. This breakdown starts in the mouth with chewing and culminates in the small intestine. Various digestive enzymes split the molecular bonds in sugars and starches until only monosaccharides remain. Eventually, these sugar compounds are absorbed through the wall of the small intestine and then circulated into the bloodstream through the liver as blood glucose.

The body can put glucose to work in three ways:

1. It can burn the glucose immediately, splitting it into smaller fragments within individual cells and releasing carbon dioxide, water, and energy.

2. If the glucose isn't needed for energy right away, it's converted by the liver or the muscles into glycogen, which can be converted back to glucose later. Glycogen stored in muscles provides energy only to muscles; glycogen supplies from the liver can supply any part of the body. A burst of blood glucose is a part of our natural defense mechanism; when the hormone epinephrine, or adrenaline, is released as part of the body's "fight or flight" reaction, it triggers a flood of glucose from the liver as an emergency boost of energy.

The bloodstream holds only about an hour's supply of glucose, and the body can store only enough glycogen for half a day's needs. Thus, bodily carbohydrate reserves can be depleted in less than 24 hours without food. After all glycogen stores have been used, fat deposits are converted to fuel as an alternate energy source.

3. If the body has an excess of glucose, and all glycogen storage sites are full, the surplus glucose is converted to fat by the liver and stored in adipose-tissue deposits around the body. If needed, these fatty acids can be burned for fuel (although the fat cannot be converted back to glucose).

The body has a nearly unlimited ability to store excess calories from any food group as fatty tissue. The degree and pattern of fat buildup depend on a wide array of factors, including genetics and lifestyle, but are primarily related to whether a person consistently consumes more calories than are burned through activity.

The Blood-Sugar Connection

No food has a more direct influence on blood "sugar" (glucose) than carbohydrates, although various factors affecting that relationship are still being explored. The body's natural regulatory system automatically maintains close control over the level of blood glucose, because too high or low a level can quickly prove harmful or even fatal.

Blood glucose fluctuates dramatically after eating and must be stabilized by the action of two hormones: glucagon (a glucose-raising chemical) and insulin (a glucose-lowering one). In diabetes mellitus, the body releases inadequate insulin or is unable to use it effectively, resulting in elevated blood sugar. At this point, it is appropriate to note an important revision in how scientists believe carbohydrates affect the response of blood glucose, especially in people with diabetes.

It was long assumed that simple sugars provoked a rapid rise (and subsequent sharp fall) in blood glucose, while the more slowly digested complex carbohydrates caused a more gradual rise. In fact, complex carbohydrates appear to vary widely in the glycemic response they provoke; that is, the rise in blood sugar as compared to a baseline reaction to pure glucose. Some foods, such as rice, have a rather high glycemic index (with further variability among individuals), while other, sweeter-tasting foods, such as ice cream, have caused a relatively slow peak in blood sugar. (A low glycemic index alone doesn't qualify a food for frequent inclusion in a diabetic diet; other factors, such as caloric density, and fiber and fat content, come into play.)

Many variables seem to affect the glycemic index, including the form in which a food is eaten (e.g., flour in pasta versus flour in bread), duration and method of cooking (pasta *al dente* versus well-cooked pasta), timing of meals, and interactions with other foods. The role of the glycemic index in diabetic meal planning is under investigation, and our understanding of how carbohydrates fit into the picture will undoubtedly expand in years to come. (The dietary implications of diabetes are discussed in Chapter 28.)

DIETARY RECOMMENDATIONS

There is no RDA for carbohydrates, but nutrition scientists agree that a bit more than half of our calories probably should be derived from this class of nutrients. Research has demonstrated that it takes approximately 100 grams of carbohydrate a day to prevent ketosis in an adult, but most Western diets contain at least 200 grams, and usually about twice that.

It's also known that extremes of carbohydrate intake, at the high or low ends of the spectrum, can create problems. A diet very low in carbohydrates usually derives a proportionately greater share of its calories from fat; and a high-fat diet has been linked to obesity and an increased risk of heart attacks and some kinds of cancer. On the other hand, a diet extremely high in complex carbohydrates is likely to be high in bulk and low in caloric density. This may make it difficult to consume enough food to supply adequate high-quality protein or even adequate calories, especially for children or pregnant or nursing women. Excessive dietary fiber can also contribute to malabsorption of iron, zinc, and other minerals, as well as digestive disorders or discomforts. Finally, a diet that draws too high a proportion of calories from simple carbohydrates (sugar) is likely to fall short of dietary fiber, vitamins, and minerals, which are lacking in sugar. In addition, many sugar-loaded processed foods, such as candy bars, baked goods, and pastries, tend to be high in saturated fat as well.

What proportion, then, of the total calories in a normal diet should be allotted to carbohydrate, and what kinds of foods should be the source? The current recommendations are based not on a minimum carbohydrate intake but on a maximum fat intake, with carbohydrates taking the place of some of the fats. In other words, since excess fat has been targeted as a major problem in the American diet, we are being urged to replace some of those fat calories with carbohydrate calories.

According to a broad consensus of experts (including the American Heart Association and the National Cholesterol Education Committee), fat usually should supply not more than about 30 percent of total calories with not more than one-third of this from saturated fats. The need for protein, often overestimated by the American consumer, is usually no more than 10 percent of total calories; that leaves the remaining 55 to 60 percent to be drawn from carbohydrates, preferably mainly complex carbohydrates and the natural sugars in fruits and vegetables. Translating those percentages into actual meals will be discussed shortly.

Dietary Choices

If all carbohydrates are converted to glucose in the body, why choose mainly unrefined starches rather than refined sugars? There are several good reasons. Both contain what candy advertisers are fond of calling food energy—a raw supply of calories for fast glucose. Unrefined complex carbohydrates offer more, however: specifically, a wide assortment of vitamins and minerals necessary to good health. Many starchy foods also contain dietary fiber, unless they have been processed to remove it. Conversely, foods high in refined sugar also tend to be low in fiber and, often, high in added saturated fat. A product high in unrefined sugar is fruit, which is low in fat and provides varying degrees of vitamin C, other nutrients, and fiber.

Any fermentable carbohydrate food may contribute to tooth decay if teeth are not brushed soon after eating; enzymes in saliva break the starch down to sugar right in the mouth, given adequate time. However, the residue from sticky-sweet snacks (including "natural" ones such as raisins and honey-sweetened granola bars) may cling to tooth enamel with extra tenacity, giving the sugar time to be fermented to acid, which eats through the enamel. The tendency to snack intermittently for long periods on sweets such as hard candy further prolongs the cavity-producing cycle of bacterial growth that occurs in the mouth after eating. (See Chapter 37.)

Another advantage of starches over sugars, at least for the millions of Americans who are overweight or at risk for obesity, is their low caloric density (the number of calories per unit of weight). All carbohydrates contain four calories per gram. However, starchy foods tend to be relatively scant in calories per serving due to their bulk (thanks to the presence of indigestible cellulose), while relatively high in nutrients. Foods containing natural sugar, such as fruit, also contain a high water content that dilutes their caloric density, making them good choices to add sweetness to a weight-control diet. (Dried fruits, while low in fat, are dense in calories because the water has mostly evaporated from them.) In addition, starchy foods tend to be economical, versatile, easy to prepare, and available in great variety.

It's only recently that Americans have developed a renewed appreciation of complex carbohydrates as the mainstay of a good diet. As a nation, we eat fewer complex carbohydrates and more sugar, fat, and protein than we did several generations ago. In 1900, it's been estimated, carbohydrates (mostly complex ones) constituted some 56 percent of the calories in a typical American diet; in 1984, that percentage was closer to 45 percent, split about evenly between starches and sugars. (In those 84 years, sugar consumption per person roughly doubled when one balances the decline in refined sugar with the rise in corn-syrup sugar). Many social and technological changes have contributed to the shift: greater affluence, mass production of processed foods, changing tastes and perceptions, and ready availability of erstwhile luxuries such as beef, butter, and refined sugar and corn syrup.

A balanced diet has room for virtually every carbohydrate food one could desire, from whole-grain bread to sugar cookies. The relevant question centers on how often and in what amounts a certain food is consumed. There are no junk foods, only junk diets. Variety is a key goal in meal planning. A severely limited selection of foods increases the risk of nutritional deficiency; the more different foods eaten, from the carbohydrate and other food groups, the greater the range of nutrients consumed. Even a healthy food such as potatoes or corn cannot provide all the requisite vitamins and minerals, as proven by deficiency-prone populations who rely almost exclusively on one staple carbohydrate foodstuff. Even in affluent countries, where a glut of food choices is available, individuals may still put themselves at nutritional risk by circumscribing their diets due to lack of interest, money, or access (for example, an elderly person who subsists mainly on tea and toast).

According to the dietary goals advocated by Mount Sinai's experts and others, carbohydrates should take a prominent role at virtually every meal. For overindulgers, this means eating either more meatless meals or more meals in which meat is used in smaller portions than many Americans are accustomed to, often as a flavoring or side dish rather than a main course.

When carbohydrates dominate the menu, one pitfall is the time-honored American fondness for high-fat methods of preparation—which defeats the purpose and has burdened starchy foods with their fattening image. If a starchy main course means greasy fried rice, or pasta liberally doused with butter, eggs, and cream, one is calorically better off eating a grilled cut of lean meat. Low-fat carbohydrate cooking, contrary to some people's expecta-

tions, needn't be dry or dull. (The box on the next page suggests ways to modify favorite carbohydrate recipes to reduce their fat content and replace saturated fats with others.)

Increasing Carbohydrate Intake

It's easy to eat more complex carbohydrates; there are so many to choose from (see Table 5.3). A family's tastes, budget, and cooking habits will determine their choices. Try to develop a set of convenient, tasty meal plans centered on complex carbohydrates, to substitute for meat at least occasionally. Keep added fat to a minimum. (Chapter 6 offers advice on low-fat cooking and shopping.) These are the main carbohydrate food categories:

Grains and cereals. A nation's cuisine is characterized by its staple grain—rice in the Orient, corn in Mexico, wheat in much of Europe and America. Cereal grains, which also include barley, millet, oats, and rye, consist of up to 85 percent starch before cooking. That proportion is lower once water and other ingredients are added.

In general, whole-grain products are preferable to those made with refined flours. Whole grains include the outer cellulose layer, or *bran*, which contains fiber plus vitamins and minerals. If grain is milled to remove this layer (as in white flour and white rice), important nutrients are lost. Some lost nutrients may be replaced through the process of enrichment, although this doesn't replace the fiber. Recently, food manufacturers have begun offering a wider selection of whole-grain products, including everything from frozen waffles or English muffins to pasta and packaged dry cereals. Home cooks can mix half whole-wheat and half white flour in baking, or add wheat bran or oat bran to bake mixes and casseroles.

Bread and its many variations (including muffins, matzo, crackers, pizza dough, hamburger and hot-dog rolls) is one of our most popular sources of complex carbohydrates. Beyond bread, however, lies a vast selection of grains that can serve as the basis of a meal. They include:

- Rice, which can be simmered with broth as an Italian risotto; served with

Paring the Fat from Favorite Carbohydrate Dishes

Many high-carbohydrate foods and dishes have acquired a reputation of being rich, greasy, or calorie-laden, due mainly to the way they are prepared—with lots of added fat, especially saturated fat from butter, cream, and meats. With some recipe modification, though, these hearty family meals, favorite snacks, and desserts can often be served with less fat and fewer calories, with little, if any, loss in flavor or texture. In some cases, creative substitution of one food for another will provide a satisfying alternative. Herewith some examples:

Instead of:	Try:	Instead of:	Try:
Boston baked beans with pork fat and franks	Lean Canadian bacon to replace franks; eliminate pork fat or use half the amount the recipe calls for	Standard lasagna	Reduced-fat mozzarella and ricotta cheeses; substitute low-fat cottage cheese for half of the ricotta
Pancakes with butter and syrup	Pancakes topped with fresh or preserved fruit, low-fat yogurt, and chopped nuts	French fries	Cottage fries: cooked potatoes, sliced and browned in pan sprayed with nonstick oil
Macaroni salad with mayonnaise	A blend of half low-fat mayonnaise and half low-fat plain yogurt instead of regular mayonnaise	Potato chips	Plain, air-popped unbuttered popcorn with a sprinkling of chili pepper or other flavoring
Spaghetti and meatballs	Spaghetti with chunks of roasted eggplant and peppers	Strawberry thick shake	Fresh strawberries whipped in blender with skim milk, ice cubes, and low-fat yogurt (a small amount of honey or sugar can be added if desired)
Doughnuts	Whole-grain muffins (preferably homemade using polyunsaturated oil)		
Chocolate cake with icing	Angel food cake with sliced brandied fruits		
Filled cream cookies	Oatmeal cookies or fig bars	Croissants	Bagels, pita bread, English muffins
Fettucine Alfredo	Fettucine lightly dressed with clam sauce, made with olive oil		

Table 5.3. How to Increase Your Daily Intake of Complex Carbohydrates

This one-day menu, which adds up to about 1,800 calories, shows how easy it is to incorporate plenty of complex carbohydrates into your meals without making any drastic dietary changes. About 53 percent of the total calories come from carbohydrates, mostly complex, and the recommended 30 percent are contributed as fat. (The rest of the calories come from protein.) These foods also provide over 20 grams of fiber and fewer than 3 grams of sodium—the recommended limit for adults.

Food	Carbohydrate (gm.)*	Fat (gm.)*
BREAKFAST		
1 cup cornflakes	21.7	0.1
1 cup 2%-fat milk	11.7	4.7
½ banana	13.4	0.3
1 slice whole-wheat toast	11.4	1.1
1 t polyunsaturated margarine	NA	3.8
½ cup orange juice	12.9	0.3
LUNCH		
Roast beef sandwich		
1 T mayonnaise	0.4	11.0
2 oz. lean roast beef	NA	5.5
2 slices rye bread	24.0	1.8
lettuce leaf	NA	NA
¼ medium tomato	1.8	NA
1 cup black bean soup	19.8	1.5
½ cup grapes	7.9	0.2
MID-AFTERNOON SNACK		
1 apple	21.1	0.5
DINNER		
3½ oz. baked chicken breast, without skin	NA	4.1
4" corn on the cob	22.3	0.7
½ cup green beans	4.9	0.2
1 medium baked potato	25.2	0.1
2 t polyunsaturated margarine	NA	7.6
Tossed salad: 1 cup lettuce & ¼ cup each carrots, mushrooms, tomatoes, celery	7.2	NA
1 T salad dressing (French)	2.7	6.4
AFTER-DINNER SNACK		
2 oatmeal raisin cookies	17.8	5.2
1 cup 2%-fat milk	11.7	4.7

*To figure out the number of carbohydrate calories in a food, multiply the number of grams by 4. To compute the fat calories, multiply the number of grams by 9.

seafood as the Spanish dish paella; mixed with beans for a complete protein without meat; or topped with stir-fried vegetables, seafood, or meat. Rice cakes make a low-fat snack or sandwich base. Cooked rice can be *lightly* fried (preferably stir-fried in a wok, as the Chinese do) with added vegetables or protein, or added to a pudding made with low-fat milk.

- Kasha (buckwheat groats), a nutty-tasting grain used as a stuffing, side dish, or meat substitute.

- Couscous, a fluffy and quick-cooking grain dish used as the basis for spicy Mideastern stews.

- Polenta, an Italian cornmeal preparation not unlike American-style grits. Grits themselves should become as well known in the north as they are in the south.

- Pasta and noodles are another hearty option, available dry or fresh, colored and flavored with many vegetables and herbs, and in countless shapes and sizes. Pasta can be chilled and tossed with meats, vegetables, and seafood for a light and easy salad entrée.

Carbohydrates provide a rewarding alternative to the traditional American breakfast of eggs, bacon, and sausage. Since the news promotion of oat bran to help lower blood cholesterol, there has been a resurgence of interest in that old standby, hot oatmeal. Cold cereals, especially those with minimal added sugar, fat, and sodium, are a good choice, and also make excellent finger-food snacks for children and adults. (Granola, often processed with coconut oil, is an exception. Tropical oils largely deserve the bad reputation they have received.) Other breakfast options are pancakes or waffles made with whole-grain flour; homemade muffins with polyunsaturated vegetable oils, perhaps with added fruit or nuts; and quick breads. Of course, topping any of these foods with butter increases fat and calories; low-fat alternatives such as fruit purees and spreads are preferable.

Peas and legumes. The starchy members of the bean family have fallen out of favor with many busy cooks due to their long preparation time—first soaking, then cooking. However, since beans offer a tasty, low-cost meat alternative, high in protein, iron, and fiber, it's worth getting to know them better. The long cooking time can be avoided by using canned precooked beans. (Just wash off highly salted packing liquid before use.) Dry beans can be put down to soak in the morning, or quickly softened by parboiling before preparation. Their one undesirable side effect—an increase in intestinal gas caused by fermenting sugars in the lower digestive tract—can be controlled somewhat by changing the soaking water several times. This problem also tends to lessen by a gradual increase of beans in the diet.

Like pasta, cooked beans can be eaten hot or cold and combined with meats or vegetables. In addition to the familiar navy and kidney beans, try black and red pinto beans, split peas, chick-peas (garbanzos), lentils, lima beans, and black-eyed peas. Cooked beans can be seasoned, mashed, and used as a sandwich filling, dip, or spread.

Starchy vegetables. One reason for the decline in Americans' consumption of complex carbohydrates is that Americans eat fewer whole potatoes. The most popular incarnations of the potato—the potato chip and the French fry—are major vehicles for dietary fat. This is too bad, because potatoes can be a versatile, satisfying, and low-fat source of vitamins and minerals if served boiled, baked, or mashed, minus or minimizing fatty toppings such as

cheddar cheese or sour cream. (A plain baked potato has only 110 calories and 0.1 gram of fat; the same potato with 2 tablespoons of sour cream has 160 calories and 5 grams of fat!) Other choices in this group include sweet potatoes, yams, cassava, corn, and squash.

Fruits and vegetables. While not very high in starch, fruits and vegetables contain many vital nutrients such as vitamin C (especially high in citrus fruits) and beta carotene, a precursor of vitamin A found in dark yellow, orange, and leafy green produce such as winter squash, spinach, carrots, apricots, and kale. Most fruits have a sugar content of 10 to 25 percent, mostly from fructose. Since the edible peels of fruits and vegetables are high in fiber, they should be eaten unless they are tough or have been waxed. Fruits and vegetables are best eaten raw or quickly cooked by steaming, boiling, or stir-frying, to avoid losing the heat-sensitive vitamins. Most foods in this group contain virtually no fat, with the exception of avocados, nuts, coconuts, and olives.

Fruits are often suggested as a low-fat dessert, but their possibilities in this department go beyond the raw fruit eaten out of hand. Fruits such as pears and plums can be poached in a very light syrup; berries and other juicy fruits can be whipped with yogurt or pectin into frappés or spreads, or used to flavor water ices and low-fat sherbets; fruit juices can be frozen into Popsicles or cubes, or mixed with gelatin, to provide a treat for children. While many such preparations may have significant amounts of natural or added sugar, their big advantage over commercial baked goods and other desserts is their lack of saturated fat.

Dairy products. The lactose in milk is the only major carbohydrate from an animal source. Dairy carbohydrates supply a generous amount of calcium, needed by women (and men) to keep bone in shape and prevent osteoporosis, and needed by children to promote bone growth. Fortified milk is also a chief source of vitamin D. Since many dairy foods, such as hard cheeses and cream-based products, contain high levels of saturated fat, it's often preferable to choose skimmed or low-fat alternatives (replacing sour cream with low-fat or nonfat yogurt, for example, or switching gradually from regular milk to 2 percent or skim milk). Lactose-intolerant individuals can often tolerate milk in 4-to-6-ounce portions. As an alternative, they can buy milk pretreated with the enzyme lactase, which also can be added to milk products at home, or eaten with milk.

Sugars, natural and processed. Sugar is not a "poison," as some nutrition faddists erroneously claim, but any refined sugar by itself is a poor source of nutrition beyond the basic provision of calories for energy. For this reason, brown or "raw" sugar or honey offers no advantage over white table sugar except one of taste preference. (See Chapter 8 for a more detailed discussion.)

Keeping sugar intake in line isn't easy, considering the high levels of hidden sugars in soft drinks, condiments, and other processed foods. The consumer's best bet is to check labels, not just for sugar per se but for sugar in the form of dextrose, maltose, and high-fructose corn syrup. Appropriate sugar intake must be determined by an individual's calorie needs: Based on one's level of activity, age, and body size, is there room for nutrient-poor sugar calories once essential daily nutritional needs have been met? For athletes and others who burn calories at a high level, the answer is likely to be yes, in moderation; for people trying to reduce their weight, it's likely to be no.

Carbohydrates and Weight Control

The "carbohydrates are fattening" myth persists, perpetuated by many best-selling but unsound diet plans such as the Scarsdale diet, a low-carbohydrate, high-protein regimen. As explained earlier, such a diet can lead to nutritional deficiency and metabolic imbalance; furthermore, the diet is almost always doomed to failure since it leaves the person feeling weak, irritable, and hungry. Past eating habits return and so do lost pounds.

A high-carbohydrate diet has demonstrated in controlled studies that it is an effective means to weight control. In one study at Michigan State University, overweight students who ate 12 slices of bread a day for eight weeks, and were allowed to choose other foods freely, still lost weight at the end of the trial. The positive effect of complex carbohydrates goes beyond "filling you up"; it now appears that the body may actually less efficiently store carbohydrates as fat tissue than dietary fats, and the process of digesting carbohydrates itself burns more calories than the digestion of an equivalent amount of fats.

Studies at the University of Massachusetts indicated that the body uses up to 25 percent of excess carbohydrate to convert the carbohydrate to body fat—leaving only 75 percent of the extra carbohydrate calories for actual fat storage. By comparison, 97 percent of excess fat calories are stored as fat. In research by Elliot Danforth Jr., M.D., at the University of Vermont, men who overate both fats and carbohydrates gained weight more slowly than men who overate a high-fat diet alone. Studies such as these indicate fat is more fattening not only because it is converted to body fat more effectively but also because the "thermic effect" of carbohydrate food—the calories burned by the body after eating—is greater than it is for fats.

6

Fats and Cholesterol

W. Virgil Brown, M.D.

■

INTRODUCTION

Of all the components of the human diet, fats and cholesterol are among the most debated and misunderstood. We are constantly bombarded by advice and advertising claims, often conflicting, about both fats and cholesterol. With almost religious fervor, for example, middle-aged men are urged to consume fish-oil pills or follow some other regimen—often unproved—to lower their cholesterol and thereby reduce the risk of a heart attack. Similarly, women have been warned that consuming a high-fat diet not only can add unwanted pounds but also may increase their risk of breast cancer and other dreaded diseases—claims that also are unproved.

The fat-cholesterol controversy is complicated by the fact that we are dealing with an issue in which there is both a very strong basis for concern and a number of unresolved issues. There is general agreement that the typical American diet is too rich in fats and calories, as evidenced by recent recommendations from the American Heart Association, American Cancer Society, National Cancer Institute, National Academy of Sciences, and other highly respected and authoritative organizations.

Still, this issue is far from resolved. The media are filled with reports of new findings on the dangers or benefits of certain fats, many of which counter yesterday's claims. Food and nutritional-supplement manufacturers have hopped on the bandwagon by offering a mind-boggling assortment of products labeled cholesterol-free, low-fat, lite, low-calorie, and so on. It's little wonder that confusion abounds. What is often overlooked is the fact that certain issues are understood well enough to make recommendations, such as those regarding excessive intake of saturated fats and cholesterol. Other claims are based on incomplete or emerging data, and often need to be revised as more is learned. In this chapter, we will define the different types of fats, or lipids, to use their technical name, and review their roles in the human diet and health. We will also present up-to-date dietary guidelines, along with practical advice on lowering fat consumption. Although these guidelines are based on our best current understanding, it should be stressed that they may be revised in minor ways. In contrast, recommendations regarding consumption of saturated fats have not changed significantly in the last 25 years. The relationship between fats and cholesterol in heart disease, cancer, and other illnesses will be dealt with in the chapters on specific diseases.

ROLE OF FATS

With all the negative emphasis on fat and cholesterol consumption, we often overlook the fact that lipids, albeit in moderate amounts, are essential in maintaining health and, indeed, life itself. Specifically, fats are used to:

1. *Provide a ready source of energy.* Lipids supply a substantial portion of the energy used in basal metabolism, and stored body fat can be converted into energy in times of need.

2. *Supply the fatty acids necessary for many body chemical activities.* For example, linoleic acid, an essential fatty acid, is needed to ensure proper growth in children. It is used by the body to make sex hormones, prostaglandins (hormonelike substances that regulate a number of body processes), and cell membranes. It also prevents excessive skin dryness and flaking.

3. *Carry the four fat-soluble vitamins: A, D, E, and K.* An extreme low-fat diet can result in a deficiency of these vitamins, which, even if consumed in adequate amounts, cannot be properly absorbed by the body without some fat.

4. *Make eating more pleasurable. Fats lend foods flavor, aroma, and texture and satisfy feelings of hunger.* A fat-free diet would be extremely limited and boring, and probably even impossible, since most sources of protein and carbohydrate also contain at least some lipids. Fats are slow to digest, thus providing a feeling of satiety even after protein and carbohydrates have left the stomach. Lipids also stimulate the intestinal walls to release a substance called cholecystokinin, which appears to suppress the appetite and help prevent overeating.

Role of Stored Fat

When we talk about body fat, most people automatically think of obesity and all the problems associated with being overweight. Indeed, obesity is one of our most serious health problems (see Chapter 17). However, a moderate amount of body fat—about 18 to 24 percent of total weight for women and 15 to 18 percent for men—is normal and consistent with good health. In fact, the ability to store excess energy as fat has been an important factor in our evolution. In early times when food supplies were unpredictable, a reserve of body fat could spell the difference between starvation and survival. This may not be as important today as in prehistoric times, but even so, stored fat constitutes our major source of energy reserves. As noted in the previous chapter, glucose, or blood sugar, is the body's major fuel. A certain amount of glucose can be converted to glycogen and stored in the liver and muscle tissue. Since glycogen contains a substantial amount of water, however, it is rather bulky and not enough can be stored to carry a person through prolonged vigorous activity. Thus, a long-distance runner or other endurance athlete, for example, will need to call upon fat reserves for needed energy. Other specific functions of body fat include:

1. *Temperature regulation.* About half of the body's fat is deposited just beneath the skin (subcutaneous fat), which provides a layer of insulation to protect against changes in environmental temperature. Very thin people often are overly sensitive to the cold; in contrast, too thick a layer of subcutaneous fat can

lead to excessive discomfort during warm weather—as many overweight people know only too well.

2. *Protective cushion for organs.* The heart, kidneys, and other vital organs are surrounded by fat deposits, which help hold them in place and protect them from injury. This fat is about the last to be converted to energy in times of caloric need.

3. *Hormone production and regulation.* Hormones are the body's chemical messengers and are instrumental in virtually every body function. Most hormones are secreted by the endocrine glands (for example, the thyroid, adrenal glands, ovaries, testes, pituitary, among others). However, some hormones or hormonelike substances are produced in adipose tissue. For example, 7-dehydrocholesterol is a lipid found in the fat just beneath the skin surface. When the skin is exposed to the sun, the 7-dehydrocholesterol is converted to vitamin D_3, which has a number of hormonal functions, including a vital role in calcium metabolism.

Fatty tissue is also instrumental in regulating the production of female sex hormones. During puberty, girls begin to develop sexually and to menstruate after achieving a certain weight and percentage of body fat. Either too much or too little fat can interfere with normal menstruation, ovulation, and fertility. Thus, a woman who loses a large amount of weight often will cease menstruating; similarly, a very obese woman may have irregular periods and fertility problems. One of the adrenal hormones is converted to estrogen by the enzyme aromatase in the fatty tissue of both men and women, explaining why overweight older women may still have relatively high estrogen levels after menopause and why some obese men develop breast tissue. In contrast, teenage girls who are too thin often fail to fully develop secondary sex characteristics.

TRENDS IN FAT CONSUMPTION

Fats, after water and carbohydrates, are the most plentiful nutrient in the typical American diet. Almost all foods contain at least traces of fat, often in the form of invisible oils. The most abundant sources, however, are meats, poultry, dairy products, nuts, margarine and other spreads, shortening, salad and cooking oils, and fatty vegetables such as avocados, soybeans, and olives. Cholesterol, undoubtedly the most publicized of all the lipids, is found only in animal products, especially egg yolks, liver and other organ meats, and fat.

Exactly how much fat the average American consumes is open to debate, although most experts agree that the majority probably consumes too much. According to the United States Department of Agriculture, about 35 to 40 percent of calories in the average American diet come from fats. Stated another way, this adds up to an average of almost 100 grams, or one-fifth of a pound, of fat a day. Nutritionists point out that many people may not actually consume this much, since the Department of Agriculture figures are based on the amount of fat in foods purchased and do not take into consideration what may be trimmed away and discarded. Even so, nutrition surveys show that the average fat consumption is well above the 30 percent recommended by the American Heart Association.

Over the course of this century, Americans have gradually increased their consumption of fat. In 1910, for example, about a third of total calories came from fats. By 1960, the typical American diet derived 42 percent of its calories from fats. People consuming the traditional all-American diet—loaded with foods such as well-marbled red meats, bacon and eggs, ham, fried potatoes, well-buttered bread and vegetables, apple pie, ice cream, and whole milk—might well get 45 to 50 percent or more of their calories from fats.

This began to change in the 1960s as the American Heart Association and others concerned about the high toll of cardiovascular disease sounded the alarm linking diet and heart attacks. Since then, there has been a small but steady decline in consumption of animal fats, matched by increased carbohydrate intake. There also has been a marked change in the types of fats consumed. According to Department of Agriculture statistics, about 70 percent of fats consumed by Americans in 1960 came from animal sources—meats, poultry, fish, and dairy products. By 1982, this had dropped to 57 percent. To a great extent, the increased intake of vegetable fats is due to the use of margarine instead of butter, cooking oils instead of lard, and nondairy creamers instead of cream. Experts generally perceive this change as desirable but caution that balance and moderation are vital. Abruptly switching to an extreme low-fat diet may carry its own health hazards, as may a diet that provides only one type of fat. As you will see in the section on types of fats, some kinds of vegetable oils are no better for you than animal fats.

Of course, health perceptions are not the only factors in determining the makeup of fats in our diet; geographical, cultural, and economic considerations also are important. Japanese food, for example, tends to be low in fat, contributing less than 20 percent of calories. In contrast, a typical Italian diet may be 30 or 40 percent fat but since much of this is from olive oil, a monounsaturated fat, the diet is not considered as problematic as one high in animal (saturated) fats, which are associated with an increased risk of high blood cholesterol. Highly saturated oils, especially coconut and palm oils, are often used by American and other Western food processors because of their low cost. In addition, many Americans are willing to spend more for a well-marbled steak or a rich sauce. As a rule, the more developed a country, the higher its consumption of fats per person—and the greater its incidence of obesity, diabetes, heart disease, and other health problems linked to a high-calorie, high-fat diet.

DIETARY GUIDELINES

Although some fat is essential, only a very small amount is needed to meet basic nutritional needs. There is no RDA for fats, but as little as a tablespoon a day of (polyunsaturated) fat can provide all of the essential fatty acids the body needs. As noted earlier, most experts agree that you should consume more than this, and also, that you should eat a balance of different fats (see Kinds of Lipids, page 66). Even people who are trying to lose weight should get about 20 percent of their calories from fat. The 30 percent of calories recommended by the American Heart Association and other such organizations is probably a more realistic goal for most people. Even though a number of organizations and societies have settled on 30 percent of calories as a recommended goal, there are nutritionists who believe that 35 percent of calories is acceptable for people who are in good health, provided that the fat is low in saturates. The American Academy of Pediatrics recommends that 30 to 40 percent of calories in a normal child's diet should come from fat. Still others think that even 30 percent is too high for adults, and advocate 10 percent or less. Any benefits of these extremely low-fat diets, except in unusual circumstances, are unproved and highly controversial.

At Mount Sinai, we agree with the American Heart Association's 30 percent for adults and for children over two years of age. For younger children, higher fat diets may be needed to provide adequate calories. We also advocate—as do the American Heart Association, American Cancer Society, and others— that the major emphasis should be on reducing intake of saturated fats to less than 10 percent of total calories consumed. Polyunsaturates could be consumed in about the same amount as saturates, but more monounsaturates (up to 15 percent) are permissible. These recommendations may be altered in special circumstances, but given our present knowledge, they seem appropriate for the average person.

Dietary Versus Body Lipids

In talking about fats, it is important to distinguish between dietary lipids—what you consume in foods—as opposed to body fat or blood lipids—those that are stored in adipose tissue or that circulate in the blood. A person does not need to consume dietary fat in order to make body fat: Excess calories from protein or carbohydrates can be converted to fat by the body and stored. The minimum amount of body fat should be about 7 percent for males and about 12 percent for females. These are minimums, however; the ideal amount of body fat varies with the individual and may be twice as much as the minimum needed to maintain health.

Fat Storage and Conversion to Energy

All types of body cells can remove the triglycerides from circulating lipoproteins to use for energy or to store for future use. However, most cells can store only a limited amount of fat. Adipose, or fat, cells, are the exception—these cells simply enlarge to store more and more fat. In an obese person, the fat cells may be 50 or 100 times larger than a thin person's fat cells. In addition, an overweight person will have more of these fat cells than someone who is thin. At one time, it was thought that a person's total number of fat cells was established early in life; it is now known that the number can be increased in adulthood to accommodate extra weight gain. Once established, fat cells never disappear, but they will shrink if excess fat is removed for energy. Some researchers believe that these shrunken fat cells send out chemical hunger signals, which could explain why an overweight person tends to regain lost weight. (See Chapter 17.)

In recent years, a number of reports have appeared in the media describing the differences between white and brown fat, suggesting that people who can eat large amounts of food without gaining weight may somehow be blessed with a high amount of brown fat. Actually, this is an area of considerable controversy: Although some researchers think brown fat may be instrumental in weight control, this has not been proved. Most of what we know about brown fat has been gained from animal studies, and very little is known about it in humans. Infants appear to have a small amount of brown fat, mostly on the upper part of the body, but it has not been established that a significant amount is found in adults and that it plays any role in weight control.

Contrary to what one might suppose from the terminology, white and brown fat do not necessarily look different, although brown fat may have a reddish cast due to its increased blood supply. The major differences are in the cells' protein structures. There also are metabolic differences. Animal studies have demonstrated that brown fat is more active metabolically than white fat: To maintain body heat (thermogenesis), it burns calories at a faster rate than white fat, and also, it is quickly regenerated in a process that requires energy. Brown-fat metabolism is speeded up in response to cold; thus it is an important factor in temperature control, especially in hibernating animals. Animal studies also have found that brown fat becomes more active when the diet provides excessive calories; the fat's metabolism is speeded up and helps prevent weight gain. This has led some researchers to theorize that people who do not gain weight, even when they consume excessive calories, are lucky enough to have a high proportion of brown fat. They are assuming that what happens in animals also is a factor in human weight control, but so far, the theory is unproved.

The only way to reduce or eliminate stored body fat is to burn it for energy and this happens only when a person consumes fewer calories than are needed to meet physical and metabolic demands. Fat cells respond to deficit energy needs by breaking down stored triglycerides and releasing the resulting fatty acids into the blood. These free fatty acids travel in the circulation to other body tissues. Cells in need of energy break down these fatty acids and combine a lipid fragment with a glucose fragment to burn as energy. Without the glucose fragment, the fat will not break down completely, and the unused lipid products (ketones) will be excreted into the blood and urine. This can lead to a serious chemical imbalance known as ketosis. In short, some carbohydrate is needed in order to burn stored body fat. Thus, crash diets that exclude carbohydrates can be very dangerous because they promote the breakdown of lean body tissue to provide the glucose fragment needed for energy, as well as causing ketosis.

FATS AND CALORIES

Many people make the mistake of assuming that the recommendation that 30 percent of calories come from fat is the same as saying 30 percent of what you eat can be from fats. This is not true, because, gram for gram, fats contain more than twice as many calories as other major nutrients: A gram of fat has nine calories, compared to four for both protein and carbohydrates. Thus, fatty foods are a more concentrated source of calories than starches and other foods that may weigh more but pack fewer calories. For example, an ounce of roasted peanuts contains about 170 calories; for about the same number of calories, you could eat two medium-size apples, four large carrots, almost a cup of macaroni, or four ounces of lean chicken breast (without the skin). (See Table 6.1.) So even though excess calories from carbohydrates and protein can end up as body fat, a diet rich in fatty foods is more likely to result in weight gain than one made up mostly of starchy foods and a moderate amount of protein simply because of the larger number of concentrated calories of fat.

Recent studies also indicate that calories from fat may be more fully stored as body fat than calories from carbohydrates or protein. Studies by Dr. Jean-Pierre Flatt at the University of Massachusetts Medical School indicate that about a fourth of the calories in carbohydrates are burned up in the process of converting them to triglycerides for storage in the body's fat tissue. In contrast, only about 3 percent of dietary fat is burned in the process of converting it to body fat.

Another study—this one by Dr. Elliot Danforth, Jr., director of the University of Vermont Clinical Research Center—compared actual weight gain between two groups of evenly matched men. Both groups were fed diets that contained excess calories, but one group consumed a diet high in carbohydrates, with only a moderate amount of fat. The second group consumed fewer total calories, but with a higher proportion of fat than their counterparts. Men who ate the high-calorie, high-carbohydrate diet gained an average of 30 pounds in seven months. The second group also gained an average of 30 pounds, but it took them only three months to do so. As an explanation, Dr. Danforth postulates that the body is more efficient at storing calories from fat, and also, that the body burns

Table 6.1. Fat Content of Common Foods by Percent of Calories*

	Fat calories/ percent	Protein calories/ percent	Carbohydrates calories/ percent	Total calories
90 TO 100% FAT				
Italian dressing (1 T)	72/94	0/0	5/6	77
Lard (1 T)	126/100	0/0	0/0	126
Vegetable oil (Crisco)	122/100	0/0	0/0	122
Beef tallow (1 oz.)	252/100	0/0	0/0	252
Butter (1 T)	108/100	0/0	0/0	108
Margarine (1 T)	108/100	0/0	0/0	108
Mayonnaise (1 T)	99/98	1/1	1/1	101
Bacon/fried crisp (1 strip)	45/92	4/8	0/0	49
80 TO 89% FAT				
Pecans, shelled, no salt (12 halves)	99/89	8/7	4/4	111
Avocado, raw, peeled	144/82	8/5	24/13	176
Bologna (1 slice)	76/86	12/14	0/0	88
Coleslaw w/mayonnaise (3.5 oz.)	144/84	24/14	4/2	172
Cream cheese (1 oz.)	90/89	3/3	8/8	101
Frankfurter (beef)	121/83	20/14	4/3	145
Walnuts, black (2 T)	81/83	8/8	8/8	97
70 TO 79% FAT				
Chocolate, baking (1 oz.)	144/77	16/8	28/15	188
Peanut butter (1 T)	72/75	12/12.5	12/12.5	96
Spareribs, roasted (3 med. ribs)	90/74	32/26	0/0	122
Cheddar cheese (1 oz.)	81/72	28/25	3/3	112
Sardines in oil (8 med.)	225/73	84/27	0/0	309
50 TO 69% FAT				
Hamburger (1 patty)	137/61	87/39	0/0	224
Broiled tenderloin steak (1 oz.)	81/54	68/46	0/0	149
Corned beef (1 slice)	36/56	28/44	0/0	64
Egg, boiled (1 med.)	54/69	24/31	0/0	78
Tuna in oil (4 oz.)	189/66	96/34	0/0	285
Pound cake (1 piece)	81/58	56/40	4/2	141
Cream of chicken soup (1 serving)	81/69	28/24	8/7	117

calories at a higher rate when a person consumes a high-carbohydrate diet instead of a high-fat one. In more technical terms, this would indicate that a high-carbohydrate meal burns up more calories in thermogenesis than a high-fat meal.

Table 6.1. Fat Content of Common Foods by Percent of Calories* *(cont.)*

	Fat calories/ percent	Protein calories/ percent	Carbohydrates calories/ percent	Total calories
Roast chicken with skin intact (3½ oz.)	135/56	108/44	0/0	243
Pork chop (3½ oz.)	234/66	120/34	0/0	354
Potato chips (3½ oz.)	360/62	20/3	200/35	580
Canned salmon (⅖ cup)	90/53	80/47	0/0	170
Ricotta cheese (½ cup)	144/67	16/7	56/26	216
Ricotta cheese, part skim (½ cup)	90/53	24/14	56/33	170
Bass, striped, broiled (3½ oz.)	117/51	80/35	32/14	229
Pot roast (3½ oz.)	108/64	44/26	16/10	168
Lamb chop	54/53	48/47	0/0	102
30 TO 49% FAT				
Ice cream (1 cup)	126/47	124/46	20/7	270
Ham, boiled (1 slice)	21/32	45/68	0/0	66
Chocolate fudge (1" sq.)	45/33	4/3	88/64	137
Tuna in oil, 4 oz., drained	81/41	116/59	0/0	197
Whole milk (1 cup)	72/49	44/30	32/21	148
Creamed cottage cheese (1 oz.)	9/32	16/57	3/11	28
Regular yogurt (1 cup)	63/45	44/32	32/23	139
Lean ground beef (3½ oz.)	90/43	120/57	0/0	210
Cookies, assorted, commercial (1 avg.)	36/38	4/4	56/58	96
Corn muffin (1 avg.)	45/31	88/61	12/8	145
Chicken without skin (3½ oz.)	45/35	84/65	0/0	129
20 TO 29% FAT				
Beef liver (3½ oz.)	36/26	80/59	20/15	136
Wheat germ (1 T)	9/24	12/32	16/44	37
Crabmeat, steamed (3½ oz.)	18/20	2/2	72/78	92
10 TO 19% FAT				
Low-fat yogurt (1 cup)	27/19	68/48	48/33	143
10% OR LESS FAT				
Fruit ice (½ cup)	0/0	116/97	4/3	120

*Calorie contents may vary slightly from those listed elsewhere in this book.

KINDS OF LIPIDS

Lipid is the general name for a fat, oil, wax, sterol, ester, or similar substance that, for the most part, cannot be dissolved in water but that can be dissolved in an organic solvent such as cleaning fluid. There are a number of familiar examples to illustrate this. As every cook knows, water and fat simply do not mix. When cooking a stew, the liquid fat globules rise to the top but do not mix in with the water. Or if you drop margarine or some other fat on a tie, sponging with water will not remove the spot, but an organic cleaning fluid will take it out.

Lipids are built of the same three elements as carbohydrates—hydrogen, carbon, and oxygen—but the proportions are different. (The different kinds of lipids are listed in Table 6.2.) Energy is released when oxygen combines with carbon and hydrogen atoms in food. Fat contains very little oxygen, and therefore many oxygen atoms can combine with the carbon and hydrogen in fats. Carbohydrates already contain about half as much oxygen as they might ultimately utilize in the metabolic process, and they are less energy-rich than fats.

Fatty Acids

Fats found in the body or food are made up of a combination of one to three fatty acids and a molecule of glycerol, an alcohol. During the digestive process, the glycerol molecule can be broken off from the rest of the fat and used as a quick source of energy, similar to the way in which the body burns glucose.

Fatty acids may be looked upon as one of the major building blocks of fat. At least one fatty acid—linoleic acid—is essential, meaning it is not manufactured within the body and is therefore necessary to obtain in the diet. A linoleic-acid deficiency causes a drying and flaking of the skin, and occurs most commonly in infants bottle-fed on a formula lacking this essential fatty acid. A deficiency in linoleic acid occurs rarely in adults, and is seen mostly in hospitalized patients fed exclusively on intravenous fluids free of fats.

Table 6.2. Kinds of Lipids

Type of Lipid	Examples	Characteristics
SIMPLE LIPID		
Neutral fats	Triglycerides	Contains 3 fatty acids to 1 glycerol. Most abundant lipid in both dietary and body fat.
Waxes	Beeswax	Contains fatty acid esters with alcohol other than glycerol.
COMPOUND LIPIDS		
Phospholipids	Lecithin Cephalin Lipositol	Compounds of fatty acid, glycerol, a phosphoric acid, and a nitrogen base; generally water-soluble.
Glycolipids	Cerebroside Ganglioside	Fatty acid attached to a sugar plus a nitrogen-containing compound.
DERIVED LIPIDS		
Fatty acids	Palmitic acid Stearic acid Oleic acid Linoleic acid	Long chain of carbon atoms with a carboxy acid group at one end.
Steroids	Cholesterol Ergosterol Cortisol Bile acids Vitamin D Androgens, estrogen, and progesterone	Chemical structure is a series of rings. Many are referred to as steroid hormones.
Hydrocarbons	Terpenes (i.e., camphor and plant pigments such as beta carotene)	Compounds of hydrogen and carbon only.

(See list below for sources of linoleic acid.)

Fats made up of one or two fatty acids plus a glyceride are known as monoglycerides and diglycerides, respectively. During the digestive process, dietary fats may be broken down into mono- or diglycerides in the intestines. Although they do not occur naturally in most foods, these fatty acids often appear in the list of ingredients of baked goods or cake mixes. In this context, they are used as emulsifiers to give a smoother texture. Many people who are unfamiliar with the terms mistakenly think that mono- or diglycerides are harmful additives; actually, they are no more hazardous in a cake than those made naturally in the intestinal tract during digestion.

Fats formed from three fatty acids plus a glyceride molecule are known as triglycerides, which make up about 95 percent of dietary fat and 90 percent of body fat. Triglycerides also circulate in the blood. (See Cholesterol on page 74.)

Sources of Linoleic Acid

Safflower oil	Brazil nuts
Corn oil	Margarine
Cottonseed oil	Pumpkin and
Soybean oil	squash seeds
Sesame oil	Spanish peanuts
Black walnuts	Peanut butter
English walnuts	Almonds
Sunflower seeds	

Saturation of Fats

Increasingly, terms such as *saturated* or *polyunsaturated* are bandied about by food manufacturers to convey the message that saturation is the key in determining whether some fats or oils are more healthful than others. Often there is some justification for these claims, but consumers are uncertain as to what these labels really mean, and thus are easily misled.

Each fatty-acid molecule is a chain of carbon atoms, to which hydrogen atoms are bound. At the very end of this chain is a carbon atom attached to two oxygen atoms. This is an acid group called carboxy acid. The chains, which may be long, medium, or short, all have a backbone of carbon atoms. There are many types of triglycerides, due to the variety of fatty acids that may bind with glycerol. The structure of the fatty acid varies with chain length (usually 12 to 24 carbon atoms) and the degree to which the carbon atoms contain their full complement of hydrogen. If all the hydrogen atoms that can possibly bind are present, the fatty acid is referred to as saturated. When hydrogen atoms are missing from two adjacent carbon atoms, a stable second bond (double bond) is formed between these carbon atoms. Fatty acids containing one double bond are called monounsaturated and those with two or more double bonds are called polyunsaturated.

Of course, the average consumer does not need to know the chemical structure of fats. What is important is to remember that most fats contain varying amounts of saturated, monounsaturated, and polyunsaturated fatty acids, and the proportion of unsaturated to saturated fatty acids (after monounsaturates are eliminated) is expressed as the P/S ratio. This ratio is often cited in food promotion and labeling to guide consumers as to the nature of fats. In practical terms, a consumer usually can determine whether a fat is saturated or not by whether it is hard or soft at room temperature. With the exception of the tropical oils, palm and coconut, most saturated fats tend to be hard or solid at room temperature. In contrast, polyunsaturated fats are liquid both at room temperature and when refrigerated (unless extra hydrogen atoms have been added in a process called hydrogenation). Monounsaturated fats are liquid at room temperature, and semisolid or solid when refrigerated.

About half of the fat from beef and other hoofed animals is saturated; poultry fat is slightly less saturated, while two-thirds of fats in dairy products are saturated. In contrast, fish fats and oils are high in polyunsaturates. If they were not, the oil would harden when the fish was in its natural cold-water habitat and it would be unable to swim. (Table 6.3 lists fats according to saturation.)

For reasons that are not fully understood, most highly saturated fats interfere with the removal of cholesterol from the blood and are thus instrumental in raising blood-cholesterol levels. In contrast, polyunsaturated and monounsaturated fats lower blood cholesterol, hence the widespread recommendation that people concerned about cholesterol lower their intake of saturated fats and increase consumption of monounsaturates and polyunsaturates. While this is sufficient in most instances, there are exceptions that should be noted. Technically, the three types of saturated fats that are mostly to blame for raising blood cholesterol are lauric, myristic, and palmitic acids. Stearic acid, although saturated, does not raise blood cholesterol.

This may seem like just another confusing fine point, and one about which the average consumer does not need to bother. Are there really any practical applications of determining what type of fatty acid is in a particular food? In general, it is sufficient to simply look at the type or overall characteristic of a fat. If it is an animal fat that is hard at room temperature, it is likely to contain the cholesterol-raising fatty acids. The same is not true, however, of vegetable products, particularly margarine. In the past, we have recommended that soft margarines were preferable to those made from hardened or hydrogenated oils. We now know that many of the vegetable oils, such as corn oil, contain unsaturated fats that are converted to stearic acids when hydrogenated (see Hydrogenation on page 69). Consequently, they do not raise blood cholesterol. Thus, the key element in selecting a margarine is not whether it is soft or hard, but, instead, the source of the oil and its original fatty-acid content. Hence, a margarine made mostly from cottonseed oil, which is relatively high in palmitic acid, is not as good a choice as one made from corn, safflower, or soybean oil.

Table 6.3. Types of Fats According to Saturation

Type	Percent Poly-unsaturated	Percent Mono-unsaturated	Percent Saturated
MOSTLY POLYUNSATURATED			
Corn oil	62	25	13
Cottonseed oil	54	19	27
Safflower oil	78	13	9
Soybean oil	61	24	15
Sunflower oil	69	20	11
MOSTLY MONOUNSATURATED			
Canola oil	31	62	7
Margarine, hard	29	35–66	17–25
Margarine, soft	61	14–36	10–17
Margarine, tub	46	22–48	15–23
Olive oil	9	77	14
Peanut oil	34	48	18
Sesame seed oil	44	41	15
Vegetable shortening (e.g., Crisco)	33	44–55	22–33
MOSTLY SATURATED			
Beef fat	4	44	52
Butter	4	30	66
Coconut oil	2	6	92
Palm oil	10	39	51
Palm kernel	2	12	86

Source: U.S. Department of Agriculture.

Saturation and Calories

Many people mistakenly assume that a highly saturated fat contains more calories than one that is monounsaturated or polyunsaturated. This is not the case: All contain the same 9 calories per gram, or about 240 to 250 per ounce. There may be a difference, however, when fats are measured by volume rather than weight. A cup of oil, for example, usually weighs a bit more than a cup of solid fat, because the latter will contain some air. Also, water or air may be introduced in a food-manufacturing process. Thus, butter or margarine will not have as many calories as the same amount of oil or shortening, because up to 20 percent of either spread may be water. Reduced-calorie or imitation margarine has even more water, and thus fewer calories. Whipping butter or margarine results in a fluffy, air-filled product that will have fewer calories according to volume, but, ounce for ounce, the same as the regular spreads when measured by weight. (See Table 6.4.)

Hydrogenation

A normally soft or liquid polyunsaturated fatty acid can be transformed into a harder, more saturated fat via hydrogenation, also called saturation. There are several reasons for hydrogenating a polyunsaturated fat. For example, a polyunsaturated fat becomes rancid if oxygen atoms are allowed to occupy the empty links to carbon atoms. To prevent this from happening, and to thereby preserve the food, hydrogen gas is bubbled through the liquid oil. This hydrogenation process causes many more of the available links in the fat molecule's carbon chain to become occupied by hydrogen atoms, leaving fewer for oxygen atoms. (The addition of antioxidants, such as vitamins C or E, or additives such as BHT or BHA also prevent fats from turning rancid.) Food manufacturers also use hydrogenation to make a mostly polyunsaturated oil semi-solid or solid. A common example is margarine: By adding hydrogen to corn oil or other normally unsaturated oil, the product will be firm at room temperature. Similarly, vegetable oils are hydrogenated into shortening to give them the characteristics of lard.

Generally speaking, a person who wants to avoid saturated fats should cut down on all naturally occurring solid fats. For example, chicken fat is not as saturated as the harder fat in beef, and fish fats are even more liquid and less saturated. As noted in the preceding section, however, the hard versus soft test does not necessarily apply to artificially hardened vegetable fats, such as those in margarine.

In addition to making an unsaturated fat more saturated, hydrogenation often changes the shape of the fatty-acid molecule. Normally, the fatty acid has a folded, or *cis*, form. Hydrogenation can change this to an extended, or *trans*, form. The body does not create *trans* fatty acids, but there is little evidence of any harm from consuming *trans* fatty acids in quantities found in the American diet.

Table 6.4. Fat Calories by Weight and Volume

Type	Calories (tablespoon)	Calories (ounce)
Butter	108	203
Lard	117	255
Margarine (stick or soft)	108	203
Margarine (low-calorie or imitation)	55	102
Margarine or butter (whipped)	70	203
Vegetable oil	120	240
Vegetable shortening	111	250

Source: C. Adams, "Nutritive Value of American Foods in Common Units," *Agriculture Handbook No. 456*, 1975, U.S. Dept. of Agriculture, Washington, D.C.

A PRACTICAL APPROACH TO CUTTING DOWN ON FAT CONSUMPTION

Although Americans are repeatedly warned to eat less fat, as noted earlier, a reduction to 30 percent of calories (instead of the 35 to 40 percent in a typical diet) is sufficient for most people. Some extremists recommend a drop to 10 percent, to bring our diet more in line with the diet consumed in some nonindustralized societies where most of the calories come from complex carbohydrates. Such extreme fat restriction may be recommended for people with very rare diseases producing high blood-triglyceride levels, but for most Americans, this is neither necessary nor desirable. In fact, there is growing evidence to suggest that it is overconsumption of calories and not fats per se that is a contributing factor in many diseases. For example, several years ago, a number of cancer researchers suggested that a high-fat diet increased the risk of breast cancer, and women were urged to sharply reduce fat consumption. More recent evidence, however, suggests that fat consumption itself has little or no effect on the risk of breast cancer, but obesity and excessive caloric intake may be a predisposing factor. These questions need further study.

Moderation, variety, and common sense should prevail in determining how much and what kinds of fats should be included in an individual diet. For example, if an adult's ideal caloric intake is 2,200 calories a day, about 30 percent—or 660 calories—can come from fats. Since there are nine calories per gram, this adds up to a daily intake of about 73 grams of fat. (The boxed material on page 71 offers specific tips on cutting fat consumption, and Table 6.5 shows the calorie, fat, and cholesterol contents of common foods.)

In addition to watching total fat content, a person also should pay attention to the types of fats. A certain vigilance is required to achieve these goals, keeping in mind that fats contain twice the calories per weight as protein and carbohydrates, but it is not necessary to become an obsessive calorie counter. The first step must be to recognize foods that are high in saturated fats in particular, but also in poly- and monounsaturated fats.

It also should be remembered that fat and cholesterol content are not the same thing; foods low in fat may be high in cholesterol, or vice versa.

High-Fat Foods

All pure fats yield about 250 calories per ounce, or 9 calories per gram, regardless of type, or whether saturated or unsaturated. Determining calorie counts can be complicated.

Remember, not all fats are pure and not all counts are made by weight. When fats are measured by volume, instead of by weight, a liquid measure of oil provides slightly less than a weight measure of fat, which affects the calorie count.

Butter and Margarine

In a typical diet, butter or margarine is a major source of fats. Many people think that margarine has fewer calories than butter; in reality, however, they are about the same unless you use a reduced-calorie product. Butter and margarine are not pure fats; they are composed of 16 to 20 percent water. Addition of more water further lowers the calorie content—a common practice in low-calorie margarines. These products may be marketed as "lite," reduced-calorie, or imitation margarine. In any instance, the customer is actually buying additional water, not lower-calorie fats.

Similarly, butter or margarine can be whipped with air so that the volume contains fewer calories per tablespoon.

The use of margarine instead of butter re-duces the intake of saturated fat and cho-lesterol and is therefore desirable for anyone on a cholesterol-lowering diet. Margarines made from mostly corn, safflower, sunflower,

Tips on Low-Fat Cooking and Shopping

1. Choose lean cuts of meat and trim fat before cooking.

2. Roast, bake, broil, or simmer meat, poultry, and fish. Cook meat or poultry on a rack so that the fat will drain off.

3. Remove the skin from poultry before cook-ing. Avoid prebasted turkey, which is often injected with saturated coconut oil.

4. Chill meat or poultry broth, stews, and soups until the fat solidifies, rises to the top, and can be spooned off.

5. Sear meat quickly in a nonstick pan and then lower heat to cook to desired do-ness; if heated slowly, the meat will cook in its own fats. Vegetables absorb fat and therefore should never be browned with meat.

6. Nonstick cookware and nonstick vegetable cooking sprays reduce the need for oil and shortening.

7. Most salad dressings are high in fats and calories. Use fat-free or low-fat preparations or lemon juice; low-fat yogurt or cottage cheese whipped in a blender makes an ac-ceptable dressing.

8. A blender or food processor can be used to whip cold water with butter or margarine to produce a product lower in calories per tablespoon measure.

9. Allow butter or margarine to soften before use, so that it can be spread thinly.

10. Do not add oil to pasta water; butter or margarine to rice; butter or milk to mashed potatoes. The pasta does not need it. In-stead, flavor rice with parsley, onion, herbs, or spices; add low-fat yogurt or buttermilk to the potatoes.

11. Replace whole milk with low-fat or skim milk in all recipes. Evaporated skim milk can be whipped in a chilled mixing bowl and is a good substitute in dishes requiring cream.

12. Avoid nondairy creamers and nondairy top-pings, which are usually high in saturated fats (palm or coconut oils) and calories.

13. Reduce regular mayonnaise, which has 100 calories per tablespoon. Select low-fat brands or mix with an equal amount of low-fat yogurt to make a dressing for things such as potato salad. Use mustard in sand-wiches.

14. Sauté vegetables in chicken stock, bouillon, or wine instead of in butter, margarine, or oil.

15. Serve smaller portions of high-fat foods, while increasing portion sizes of pasta, veg-etables, fruit, and other low-fat items.

16. When shopping, look for the low-fat or re-duced calorie varieties of yogurt, cottage cheese, and processed foods.

17. Use low-fat plain yogurt, buttermilk, or low-fat cottage cheese instead of sour cream in dips or for baking. Adding a little corn-starch when cooking will prevent curdling.

18. In most recipes, the fat or oil can be reduced by a third without altering texture or taste.

(For other suggestions, see Tips on Lowering Cholesterol on page 85 and Chapter 17.)

rapeseed, or other highly unsaturated oils are preferred. As noted earlier, former recommendations that soft (tub) or liquid varieties were preferred over hard or stick margarines no longer hold, provided that the original oil is one that is converted to stearic acid (for example, corn, safflower, or soybean oils) instead of one of the cholesterol-raising fatty acids by the hardening process (for example, cottonseed oil).

Visible Versus Invisible Fats

Visible fats, which include the layers of fat in meat and poultry, butter, margarine, lard, salad oils, and cooking oils, are easily ap-

parent and can be readily measured. This is not true of the invisible or hidden fats that have not been separated from their source. These include marbled fat in meat and the fats of milk and dairy products such as cheese, nuts, eggs, and cereals. Invisible or hidden fats amount to up to 60 percent of the fats consumed and about 65 percent of the saturated fats. Red meat, poultry, and fish are the richest sources, accounting for about one-third of the invisible fats consumed.

The amounts and kinds of visible fat eaten by Americans have changed greatly since the turn of the century, with a decrease in animal fats and an increase in vegetable oils. Increased reliance on processed foods, especially things such as baked goods, and res-

Table 6.5. Cholesterol/Fat/Calorie Content of Common Foods

Food	Calories	Cholesterol (mg.)	Poly.	Fats (gm.) Mono.	Sat.
MEAT/FISH/POULTRY					
Beef (1 oz. lean chuck)	71	26	0.1	0.8	0.9
Beef (1 oz. fatty roast)	110	27	0.2	2.0	2.2
Beef liver (1 oz.)	46	83	0	0	0.1
Chicken (1 oz. dark)	58	26	0.6	1.0	0.6
Chicken (1 oz. white)	47	22	0.2	0.3	0.3
Fish (1 oz. lean—sole)	40	27	0.1	0.1	0
Fish (1 oz. fatty—trout)	58	25	1.1	1.1	0.9
Lamb (1 oz. lean)	53	17	0.2	0.2	0.1
Pork (1 oz. lean chop)	60	28	0.1	0.8	0.9
Tuna (1 oz. water pack)	45	11	0.1	0.1	0
Turkey (1 oz. white)	48	22	0.2	0.3	0.3
Veal (1 oz. cutlet)	51	28	0.1	0.8	2.2
DAIRY PRODUCTS					
Butter (1 T)	100	31	0.4	2.8	3.2
Cheese (1 oz. cheddar)	115	28	0.3	3.0	6.0
Cottage cheese 4% fat (½ cup)	110	16	0.1	1.0	1.6
Egg (1 large)	75	213	0.7	1.9	1.6
Ice cream 11% fat (1 cup)	270	56	0.3	9.6	16.8
Milk, whole (1 cup)	150	34	0.1	2.4	4.8
Milk, 2% fat (1 cup)	120	22	0.1	2.0	2.4
Milk, 1% fat (1 cup)	102	10	0.1	0.8	1.2
Milk, skim (1 cup)	85	4	0	0.1	0.3
Yogurt, plain, 1% fat (1 cup)	145	14	0.1	1.0	2.3

Note: A more extensive nutrient breakdown is in the Nutrient Values table at the back of this book. Exact values may vary somewhat, depending on the brand tested and similar factors.

taurant fast foods, which are often fried, are responsible for some of the increased intake of oil.

Animal Versus Plant Fats

Animal and plant fats are similar in that both are composed mainly of triglyceride mixtures. Plant fats do not contain cholesterol; they also lack certain vitamins and minerals associated with animal fats or provide them in less usable forms. (See Chapter 7.) In general, plant fats or vegetable oils are higher in polyunsaturated fatty acids than animal fats. There are exceptions: cocoa butter, coconut oil, and palm oils are among the most saturated of all fats; cod-liver oil and some fish contain high levels of unsaturated fats.

Fish and Shellfish

Fish and shellfish have more protein and fewer fats than many meats, and, ounce for ounce, usually have far fewer calories. The fat content of fish varies both by season and by species. (See Table 6.6.) In some fish, the fat content is four times higher in summer than in winter. As a general rule, the darker a fish's flesh, the higher the fat content. However, even fish with dark, oily flesh have lower levels of fat and fewer calories than many cuts of red meat or poultry with the skin intact.

Of course, the manner in which fish is prepared is a crucial factor in fat content. Fish prepared with butter, oil, margarine, sauces, or breaded or fried coatings, may contain four or five times as many calories as the fish broiled plain or with lemon juice, wine, or other low-fat ingredients. Canned fish packed in oil contains five times more fat and yields twice as many calories as the same fish packed in water.

Vegetable Oils

Virtually every supermarket offers a wide selection of oils, under many trade names and with often misleading labels and claims. Some are mixtures of animal and vegetable fats, some are mixtures of vegetable oils, and some are from a single source, such as safflower oil or olive oil. When the source is specified in the product's name—for example, corn oil—

Table 6.6. Fat Content of Fish

Fish	Fat (grams) in 3.5 oz., raw
Bass	3.7
Bluefish	4.2
Catfish	4.2
Cod	0.7
Eel	11.7
Flounder	1.2
Haddock	0.7
Halibut	Trace
Herring	9.0
Mackerel, Atlantic	13.9
Mackerel, Pacific	7.9
Monkfish	1.5
Mullet	3.8
Perch	0.9
Pompano	9.5
Salmon, Atlantic	6.3
Sea bass	2.6
Shad	13.8
Shark	4.5
Snapper	1.3
Surimi	0.9
Swordfish	4.0
Tilefish	2.3
Trout, rainbow	3.4
Tuna, bluefin	4.9
Shellfish	
Crab, king	0.6
Crab, blue	1.0
Lobster	0.9
Shrimp	1.7
Clams	1.0
Mussels	2.2
Oysters	2.5
Scallops	0.8

the product is likely to be pure. In contrast, a nonspecific name such as salad or cooking oil usually implies a mixture of oils, usually with soybean oil predominating, since it is inexpensive. Vegetable shortening is likely to be a mixture of partially hydrogenated cottonseed oil (i.e., partially saturated) and soybean oil.

Recently, canola oil has attracted considerable media attention. This is a hybrid variety of rapeseed oil, which has been in use in Europe for years but only recently introduced in the United States under the brand name New Puritan Oil. Canola oil, which contains the essential fatty acid linolenic acid and the omega-3 fatty acid linoleic acid, is very low in saturated fats and, like olive oil, high in monounsaturated fats. Thus, it is particularly useful as a fat source that can be used to cut intake of saturated fats.

The most desirable of these liquid vegetable oils are olive oil, corn oil, canola oil or rapeseed oil, soybean oil, safflower oil, and sunflower oil. While these are unsaturated and will not raise blood cholesterol, they should be eaten in limited quantities because they are high in calories.

Nonnutritive oils are mineral oils derived from petroleum and other hydrocarbons that are not digestible in the human gastrointestinal tract. Mineral oils are used mostly as laxatives, although they are sometimes used in place of regular oils by people who are trying to lose weight—a practice that should not be followed. These oils interfere with absorption of fat-soluble vitamins and can lead to deficiencies as well as other nutritional problems, not to mention the embarrassing problem of occasional bowel incontinence or leakage.

Artificial Fats

The idea of a substance that gives foods the flavor, texture, and the other benefits of fats without the calories obviously has tremendous appeal. One such artificial fat, Simplesse, is now being used in ice cream. It is made by heating and blending egg whites and milk protein to form tiny particles that, when eaten, are perceived as a fluid rather than individual particles. Their round, uniform shape creates a smoothness and richness that is associated with the "feel" of fats. Another artificial fat that is being tested for human use is sucrose polyester, often abbreviated to SPE, a substance that resembles a fat molecule except that a sucrose ester—a type of sugar—replaces the glycerol molecule. The *ester* refers to the nature of the bonding with fatty acids. Sucrose esters cannot be broken down and absorbed in the human digestive system. They have an added advantage of attracting lipophilic, or fat-loving, compounds such as cholesterol and excreting them from the body instead of entering the blood. Sucrose polyester can be used in cooking, and it is said to satisfy the craving for fats, while yielding no calories. As of this writing, sucrose polyester has not been approved for general use. Whether it will emerge as a safe means of reducing dietary fats is unknown.

CHOLESTEROL

In discussing fats and cholesterol, it is the latter that is of most concern to the general public. Americans are constantly being urged to watch their cholesterol by physicians and food advertisers alike, and most people know that excessive cholesterol is in some way related to heart disease. However, myths and misconceptions abound.

Technically speaking, cholesterol is a sterol, a compound in which the carbon, hydrogen, and oxygen atoms are arranged in rings; sterols, in turn, belong to the chemical family of steroids. Cholesterol is related to, but not synonymous with, fats. It is found only in animal products (see Table 6.7 for common sources of cholesterol), although, as stressed in the preceding section on fats in general, certain highly saturated vegetable fats, especially coconut and palm oils, raise blood-cholesterol levels in humans.

With so much negative publicity surrounding cholesterol, many people have the mistaken notion that it is all bad. In reality, cholesterol is essential to maintaining life. It is needed to build many body substances, including sex hormones and bile salts; it is an important structural part of nerve sheaths and cell membranes; in the skin, it is made into vitamin D with the assistance of sunlight. Still, we can get by without consuming any cholesterol; all that we need can be manufactured in the body. Most is made in the liver and in cells lining the small intestine, but every cell in the body has the capacity to make cholesterol to meet its own needs. As a rough guideline, about 15 percent of our blood cholesterol comes from our diet, and about 85 percent is made by the body.

One major source of confusion centers on the difference between dietary cholesterol—what you consume in foods—and blood or serum cholesterol—that which circulates in the blood. When a doctor says watch your cholesterol, he or she is referring to the level in your blood, not what is consumed in the diet. Although some experts think that a high intake of dietary cholesterol can contribute to high blood levels, the two are not closely related. Some people who consume very little dietary cholesterol can have high blood levels and, conversely, there are people who eat large amounts of cholesterol-rich foods and have low blood levels. Some believe that dietary cholesterol may not have as much of an impact on blood cholesterol as was assumed a few years ago, and that many other factors, including genetics, other dietary components, and physical activity, may be more important. However, it is premature to discount dietary cholesterol; consumption of cholesterol is statistically related to the development of heart disease in some fashion that is not explained by its effects on blood cholesterol.

High levels of blood cholesterol are causative in the development of atherosclerosis—the buildup of fatty deposits in the coronary arteries and other blood vessels. Atherosclerosis is the leading cause of heart attacks in the United States and other industrialized countries.

The fact that cholesterol is both manufactured in the body and supplied in the diet makes it difficult to determine the impact of each. Of the cholesterol in food, about 50 percent is absorbed by the body, with the amount varying from person to person from 20 to 90 percent. In recent years, the amount of cholesterol consumed in the average American diet has declined, but even so, we continue to consume about 300 to 600 milligrams of cholesterol per day, considerably more than the maximum of 300 milligrams a day recommended by the National Cholesterol Education Program. However, dietary cholesterol is not the major source of serum cholesterol; the body makes about 1,000 milligrams each day.

What is a "normal" blood cholesterol? New recommendations by the National Cholesterol Education Program provide practical guidelines. (See Chapter 26.) The Framingham Heart Study and other long-term population studies have consistently found

Table 6.7. Sources of Cholesterol in the American Diet

Eggs	36%
Meat, poultry, fish	38%
Dairy foods	15%
Lard and other animal-derived cooking fats	5%

that, among people below the age of 50, the risk of an early (before age 50 or 55) heart attack rises among people whose blood-cholesterol levels are above 200 to 220 milligrams per deciliter, and the higher the cholesterol, the greater the risk. Some experts now think that adults below the age of 50 should strive for blood-cholesterol levels in the 180-milligram-per-deciliter range, although there are others who think this is unrealistic. Be that as it may, people under the age of 50 whose total cholesterol is 180 or less have a low risk of a heart attack.

Cholesterol levels refer to the amount circulating in the blood serum, which is less than 10 percent of the total amount of cholesterol in the body. (The rest is in the cell membranes, nerve sheaths, and other body tissues.)

Although the total amount of circulating cholesterol is important, the type of molecule carrying the cholesterol is also an indicator of increased cardiovascular risk. As noted earlier, cholesterol and other lipids are not soluble in water. Since blood is mostly water, in order for a lipid to travel through the bloodstream, it must be attached to a lipid-carrying protein, or a lipoprotein. These lipoproteins come in different sizes and densities. The higher the proportion of protein, the greater the density of the lipoprotein. *Chylomicrons* are the least dense of the lipoproteins. They are formed in the intestines and are made up mostly of triglycerides, with only a very small amount of cholesterol.

The most abundant are the *low-density lipoproteins (LDL)*, which carry about 65 percent of the circulating cholesterol. LDLs are believed to carry cholesterol to the cells, and high levels of LDL cholesterol are associated with atherosclerosis. *High-density lipoproteins (HDL)*, the smallest and most dense of the lipid-carriers, are believed to pick up cholesterol from most of the body's tissues for transport to the liver. It may be returned to the plasma as a component of very low-density lipoproteins (see below) or, more importantly, excreted in the bile as cholesterol or as bile acids, its conversion product. HDL cholesterol—about 20 percent of the total circulating in the blood—is often referred to as the "good" cholesterol because it is actually thought to be protective against atherosclerosis.

Very low-density lipoproteins (VLDL) are triglyceride-rich particles made in the liver. They are converted to LDLs after depositing triglycerides in muscles for energy or in adipose tissue for storage. About 15 percent of the circulating cholesterol is carried on VLDLs.

In most individuals, receptors on the outer membranes of cells attract and hold the LDL, removing it from the bloodstream and taking it inside the cell to be broken down for the cell's chemical needs. When excess cholesterol accumulates inside these cells, they form fewer receptors to trap LDL particles, to match the lower needs. It is thought that in people who consume excess dietary fats and cholesterol over an extended period, the liver cells reduce the number of LDL receptors, allowing the blood LDL level to increase.

Monounsaturated fats, when substituted for saturated fats, lower LDL as much as polyunsaturated fats. The HDL cholesterol is not reduced significantly in some studies, as is the case with a high intake of polyunsaturated fats. Thus, it is not known whether this change in HDL is beneficial.

In recent years, there has been a good deal of media emphasis on "good" vs. "bad" cholesterol, which translates to HDL versus LDL cholesterol. These terms apply to the type of lipoprotein that circulates in the blood, and not dietary cholesterol, as many people mistakenly believe. In general, the higher the level of HDL cholesterol in the blood, the better, but this does not necessarily mean that a relatively high HDL level can completely eliminate the risk of elevated blood LDL cholesterol. HDL cholesterol, with its high percentage of protein, seems to be the transport mechanism for returning cholesterol to the liver to be broken down and either recycled or excreted from the body.

Even so, if the total cholesterol is above 275 milligrams per deciliter, the risk of a heart attack may be significantly increased, even if the HDL level is favorable. At lower levels, however, the proportion of HDL cholesterol may be of value in determining risk. In a 12-year study of 1,605 men, for example, the Framingham Study found that a low level of HDL cholesterol increases the risk of a heart attack, even if the total cholesterol is in the low-risk range. Unfortunately, a number of factors, including many of the strategies often suggested for reducing total cholesterol, also lowers levels of HDLs (see list on this page). Lowering LDL cholesterol should be the goal (see Chapter 26 for a more detailed discussion). The HDL level will help in choosing the goal for LDL reduction. Since current measurements of HDL levels are not as accurate as would be desirable, the focus should remain on getting LDL cholesterol below 130 in most adults.

Factors Influencing Cholesterol Levels

Most Americans have blood-cholesterol levels that are above what many experts consider ideal. For example, recent findings in the MRFIT (Multiple Risk Factor Intervention Trials) study show that about 80 percent of the 365,000 men studied over a six-year period had blood-cholesterol levels that may have increased their risk of a heart attack. Although there are still many unknowns regarding cholesterol metabolism, a number of factors that can alter blood levels have been identified.

These include:

Genetics

This is a very important factor, because the control signals for cholesterol absorption and synthesis are largely genetically controlled. Some people have inherited problems in lipoprotein metabolism. In one specific instance, this is called familial hypercholesterolemia, and people with this genetic disorder will have very high cholesterol levels—sometimes 400 to 600 milligrams per deciliter or more. This is usually due to inadequate numbers of LDL receptors. Unless identified and treated, many suffer severe heart attacks or sudden death at a very early age, sometimes even in childhood. Fortunately, familial hypercholesterolemia is relatively rare; far more common are the large numbers of people with moderate to high levels—say in the 240-to-350-milligram-per-deciliter range—whose bodies may contain a variety of minor genetic

Factors That Lower HDL (or "Good") Cholesterol

Obesity

Lack of exercise

Cigarette smoking

Drugs

Beta-blocking agents	Probucol
Thiazide diuretics	Neomycin
Anabolic steroids and androgens	Accutane (and other vitamin A
Progestational agents	derivatives)

Cholesterol-lowering regimens

High intake of polyunsaturated fats	Low-saturated-fat, high-polyunsaturated-fat diet
Low-fat, high-carbohydrate diet	

traits that add up to excessive LDL production or reduced LDL removal. Some of these people lower blood cholesterol through a low-fat, low-cholesterol diet, weight loss, and increased exercise, but with these conservative measures alone, many still may not be able to achieve the current minimum goal of less than 160 milligrams per deciliter for the LDL cholesterol level. In such cases, cholesterol-lowering drugs may be recommended as supplements to diet and lifestyle changes (see Chapter 26 for specific treatment strategies).

Weight

Excessive weight increases the likelihood of having high blood-cholesterol levels. Overweight people also tend to have low HDL levels, but the proportion of HDLs usually rises with weight loss. Recent studies have found that placement of the excess weight is also a factor in raising blood cholesterol. Weight centered in the abdominal area—the so-called potbelly that is so common among overweight men and postmenopausal women—seems to be more instrumental in raising blood cholesterol than the body fat that accumulates on the thighs or buttocks. The exact reason for this is unknown, but researchers speculate that the fatty acids released by abdominal fat are likely to flow directly into the portal vein, which flows to the liver, and thereby stimulate that organ to increase cholesterol output. Weight reduction often produces a substantial lowering of blood cholesterol.

Age and Gender

Cholesterol levels tend to rise somewhat with age: What is elevated for a child or young adult may be average for an older person. Men have lower HDL and higher LDL levels than women, especially before age 50. After 50, a woman's LDL cholesterol tends to rise more rapidly. This may explain why women have fewer heart attacks than men in middle life but tend to "catch up" after menopause. Postmenopausal estrogen supplements are believed to protect against rises in blood cholesterol and LDLs, but other factors, such as a possible increased risk of certain cancers, must be considered before prescribing hormone replacement. (See Levels in Childhood on page 79.)

Diet

Diet has long been associated with blood cholesterol. The Framingham Study and numerous other epidemiologic surveys have found that vegetarians or people who eat very little meat and other animal products tend to have low levels of blood cholesterol. For unknown reasons, highly saturated fats raise blood cholesterol probably more than any other dietary factor. Eating foods high in cholesterol—egg yolks, organ meats, and a diet high in animal products—also can raise blood cholesterol, but not as much as consuming large amounts of saturated fats. It is sometimes hard to separate the two because many animal products high in saturated fats also are high in cholesterol. Sometimes claims by food manufacturers tend to increase misunderstanding and confusion. "Contains no cholesterol" has become an almost standard label on a variety of foods: vegetable oils and shortening, margarines, peanut butter, cereals, baked goods, and numerous other nonanimal products that obviously contain no cholesterol. The implication that these foods are somehow healthier than those containing cholesterol or even comparable vegetable products that are not so labeled may be highly misleading, however, because it implies that the products will not raise blood-cholesterol levels. Remember, though, that highly saturated vegetable oils such as palm and coconut can raise blood-cholesterol levels even though they themselves contain no cholesterol. Thus, in reality, cookies, cereals, shortening, non-dairy creamers, and other foods made with coconut, palm, or other highly saturated oils may actually raise cholesterol more than similar products that contain less-saturated fats and cholesterol. However, when the product contains very little saturated fat, the implication is correct.

In contrast, unsaturated liquid vegetable oils lower blood cholesterol. Substituting these oils—for example, corn, safflower, sunflower, soybean, olive, or canola oils—for animal fats or saturated vegetable oils whenever possible is recommended as part of a cholesterol-lowering diet. Still, moderation and balance are important. The key word is *substitution* of saturated fats. Using larger amounts of polyunsaturated oils will not lower LDL cholesterol further. Interestingly, the HDL levels also tend to fall when saturated fats are removed from the diet. This is particularly evident when the replacement calories come from polyunsaturated fats or carbohydrates. Monounsaturated fats, such as olive or canola oils, and polyunsaturates have an equal effect on lowering LDL cholesterol, but the monounsaturates tend to lower HDL less than the polyunsaturates. The long-term effects of HDL reduction in this instance are not known. As a general guideline, if intake of saturated fat is reduced to less than 10 percent of calories, consumption of monounsaturates and polyunsaturates may be maintained at their current levels, which are about 15 and 7

Levels in Childhood

The American Academy of Pediatrics recommends cholesterol testing for children older than two years of age only if there is a family history (parent, grandparent, sibling, aunt or uncle) of high cholesterol or early heart attack. (Early is defined as 50 years or younger for men; 60 years or younger for women.) What levels might be predictive for later coronary heart disease have not been established, but the Academy recommends that children whose plasma cholesterol repeatedly tests in the 75th percentile (176 milligrams per deciliter) should undergo dietary modifications and counseling. Drug therapy for children with high cholesterol should be considered only for those children whose cholesterol levels are higher than 200 milligrams per deciliter (which would place them in the over-95th percentile), and whose levels have not been reduced by dietary changes.

Various health and government organizations have made recommendations regarding the amount and type of fat that children over two years of age should eat. Both the National Institutes of Health and the American Heart Association recommend that children over the age of two consume a fat intake equivalent to about 30 percent of their calories. Of this total amount, 10 percent or less should be from saturated fat; 10 percent from monounsaturated fat; and less than 10 percent from polyunsaturated fat. The American Heart Association recommends daily cholesterol intake should be 100 milligrams for every 1,000 calories, but not to exceed 300 milligrams per day. Similarly, the National Institutes of Health recommends between 250 and 300 milligrams or less of cholesterol daily. The American Heart Association set a goal for total serum-cholesterol values for children and young adults at an average of 140 milligrams per deciliter. This represents a 12.5 percent reduction from the current average levels of 160 milligrams per deciliter.

Because diet is only one factor in the risk of coronary heart disease, the Academy of Pediatrics advises that children also be counseled about lifestyle factors over which they have control—cigarette smoking, obesity, and exercise.

percent of calories, respectively. Increasing complex carbohydrates to 55 to 60 percent of total calories also is recommended.

Fish Oils, or Omega-3

Taking fish-oil supplements is the latest cholesterol-lowering fad. Like most fads, this one is based on the premise of "if a little is good, then a lot must be better." Of course, this does not necessarily follow, and, indeed, the opposite is more likely to be true. Although there is considerable evidence that substances in fish oils do indeed lower triglycerides—the most common form of lipids in the body—data so far do not indicate a specific reduction in LDL cholesterol, as compared to unsaturated vegetable oils.

Scientific interest in fish oils was sparked with the epidemiological observations that Greenland Eskimos, Japanese fishermen, and Indians of the Pacific Northwest—all groups that consume large amounts of fish—rarely develop coronary artery disease. Further studies found that Greenland Eskimos have low levels of LDL, especially when compared to population groups such as their neighboring Danes, who do not eat as much fish. Other studies also found that men who regularly consume fish, even only two or three servings a week or an average of an ounce a day, had significantly fewer heart attacks than men who ate none. (It should be noted that it is not known whether it is the oils or some other substance in saltwater fish that reduces heart-attack risk.)

Fish oils contain substances called omega-3 fatty acids. The two most common omega-3 fatty acids are EPA (eicosapentaenoic acid) and DHA (docosahexaenoic acid), and these are found in varying amounts in fish oils. A third omega-3, linolenic acid, does not occur in fish oils but is found in a number of vegetable oils. In fact, many fresh dark green vegetables, particularly uncultivated varieties, are rich in omega-3. (Linolenic acid is not to be confused with the essential fatty acid, linoleic acid.)

The omega-3 fatty acids are used by the body to synthesize prostaglandins, substances that mediate many chemical processes in the body. A marked increase of omega-3 fatty acids in the diet seems to increase the production of certain prostaglandins, which in turn increase specific chemical activities in the body. This interaction may explain some of the effects that have been tentatively attributed to a high intake of omega-3 fatty acids. For example, four areas have been identified in which omega-3 fatty acids change the body's metabolism:

1. They lower the rate at which the liver manufactures triglycerides.

2. They reduce the tendency for blood platelets to stick together, which can lead to formation of blood clots. This can be important in preventing heart attacks and thrombotic strokes, because blood clots often form in the coronary or carotid arteries, the vessels that nourish the heart and brain, respectively.

3. They may help repair the damage due to lack of oxygen to body tissue. This may be useful in people whose coronary arteries are severely narrowed by fatty deposits or other factors that can result in greatly reduced blood flow to a tissue.

4. They may lower blood pressure, a major risk factor for heart attacks and stroke.

In addition, omega-3 fatty acids are believed to assist in protecting the body when its tissues are attacked by its own immune system, as in rheumatoid arthritis. It should be stressed, however, that these claims are based on incomplete data, and none has been sufficiently established as yet for any general nutritional recommendations to be made. The benefits also must be weighed against potential adverse effects. For example, excessive omega-3 fatty acids may thin the blood too much, increasing the risk of bleeding problems. In fact, some observers believe that a possibly higher incidence of hemorrhagic strokes among Greenland Eskimos may be attributed to their high intake of fish oils. Some omega-3 supplements, particularly those extracted from liver, contain large amounts of vitamins A and D, which can be toxic when taken in large amounts.

It also should be noted that some fish oils are high in cholesterol as well, which may be a contraindication for people on low-cholesterol diets. Many experts consider plant sources of omega-3 fatty acids preferable to fish oils. Purslane, popular in salads in Mediterranean countries, is the richest known plant source of linolenic oil. Walnuts and walnut oil, wheat germ oil, rapeseed oil, soybeans, common beans, butternuts, and seaweed are other sources.

Purveyors of health foods and supplements have been quick to spot a huge potential market (estimated at $500 million a year), and there are now dozens of highly promoted fish-oil supplements on the market. There are instances in which these supplements may be taken under a doctor's supervision—in the same manner as any medication—but at present, we do not recommend them as self-medication for the general public. Not enough is known about possible long-term effects of taking large amounts of fish oil. It is known, however, that large amounts of omega-3 fatty acids (more than 4 grams a day) inhibit blood clotting. Aspirin and other drugs also reduce clotting, and it is not known whether fish-oil supplements along with these medications can lead to bleeding problems. It should be noted,

however, that the Pacific Northwest Indians and Greenland Eskimos, who suffer a tendency to hemorrhage, may consume 15 to 30 grams of omega-3s a day, which is far more than most supplements provide.

Also important is the fact that fish-oil supplements, although used as drugs, are marketed under regulations meant for foods. Thus they have not been subjected to the advance testing required of medications, and there is no uniformity as to dosage or contents. For example, cod-liver oil and certain other fish-oil supplements contain large amounts of vitamins A and D, and taking large dosages of them can result in a dangerous buildup of vitamin A in particular. Since the supplements are fats, they are high in calories—a factor that should be considered by anyone with a weight problem. Some products are promoted as being cholesterol-free, but others contain varying amounts of cholesterol. A recent report from Duke University Medical Center, for example, noted that cod-liver oil has 570 milligrams of cholesterol per 100 grams of oil, and that some of the fish-oil supplements contain as much as 600 milligrams of cholesterol per 100 grams.

As a prudent course, the American Heart Association recommends that fish be a regular part of the diet. Available evidence suggests that three servings a week is quite sufficient to obtain the benefits, whether or not they ultimately prove to be from omega-3s or some other substance in fish. (See Table 6.8 for omega-3 content of common fish and seafoods.) In addition, we go along with the Heart Association's recommendations that fish-oil supplements *not* be taken at this time unless under the careful supervision of a doctor.

Lecithin

Lecithin supplements are still another product that is widely promoted for lowering cholesterol, despite the fact that this has not been adequately demonstrated in scientific studies. In addition, what is sold as lecithin in health-food shops is almost always a commercial concoction that is only 3 percent pure.

Lecithin is a phospholipid—substances that are related to fats but have a phosphate group in place of one fatty acid and have either a nitrogen-containing or a carbohydratelike substance, which allows them to react with both water and fats. Phospholipids are important constituents of cell membranes and they also are important in the structure of the blood lipoproteins, and therefore, in the transport of the water-insoluble fats through the body's fluids. Lecithin helps to stabilize the cholesterol in bile and thus prevents gallstones from forming. It acts as a natural emulsifier in egg yolks and is widely used as a food additive to stabilize the fats in things such as margarine, salad dressing, baked goods, frozen desserts, and other foods. It is also used in soaps, paints, cosmetics, and other nonfood products.

Lecithin is consumed in a variety of foods, especially eggs, soybeans and other legumes, and commercial foods to which it has been added. In addition, the body makes all the lecithin it needs; thus it is not an essential nutrient. In short, there is no such thing as a lecithin deficiency.

For years, magical properties have been attributed to lecithin, mostly by purveyors of supplements and so-called natural or health foods. For example, lecithin supplements are promoted to prevent, treat, or cure high cholesterol, heart attacks, memory loss, arthritis, skin problems, gallstones, and nervous disorders, among other claims. Unfortunately, there is no scientific proof that lecithin supplements have any nutritional or health benefits. Take the claims that lecithin supplements lower cholesterol as an example. The theory is that dietary lecithin somehow breaks up lipids

and "washes" them out of the body. The cholesterol-lowering claims are bolstered by animal experiments showing that lecithin injected into rabbits reduced the effects of a high-cholesterol diet. Intravenous lecithin may alter plasma lipoproteins, causing them to be cleared by abnormal processes, which is not necessarily a good thing. Dietary lecithin does not have the same effects as that injected directly into the bloodstream, since the digestive process breaks it down into its component parts. Many claims of lecithin's benefits are based on one-time studies that have not been replicated. For example, one researcher also found that lecithin supplements raised HDLs in people with high blood lipids, but

Table 6.8. Omega-3 Fatty Acid and Calorie Contents of Fish and Seafood

FISH	Per 4-Ounce Serving	
	OMEGA-3 FATTY ACIDS (GRAMS)	CALORIES
Sardines (in fish oil)	5.83	278
Salmon (pink)	2.51	148
Tuna (albacore)	2.40	197
Mackerel (Atlantic)	2.17	201
Trout (lake)	1.60	185
Halibut (Atlantic)	1.49	131
Swordfish	1.03	139
Bass (striped sea)	0.80	107
Snapper (red)	0.69	126
Oysters	0.58	85
Mussels	0.49	91
Flounder	0.34	103
Clams (hard shell)	0.27	62
Shrimp	0.23	104
Perch (lake)	0.23	98
Haddock	0.23	95
Cod	0.23	86
Scallops (sea)	0.21	99
Scallops (bay)	0.15	91
Sole	0.11	101
Lobster	0.07	106

Adapted with permission from *Nutrition and Health*, vol. 9, no. 1, 1987, Columbia University College of Physicians and Surgeons, New York, NY.

other studies have not substantiated this. Since lecithin contains polyunsaturated fatty acids, many researchers feel that any cholesterol-lowering effect can be attributed to these substances rather than to any unique properties of lecithin itself.

A similar misinterpretation of research data applies to claims that lecithin can prevent memory loss. Lecithin contains a substance called choline, which is used in making acetylcholine, a neurotransmitter. As with lecithin, the body can make all of the choline it needs. But there are some neuromuscular disorders, such as tardive dyskinesia—a condition marked by uncontrolled tics and twitching—in which there is inadequate acetylcholine. Some studies have found that giving people with this disorder large amounts of lecithin (which releases choline) or choline itself may raise the levels of acetylcholine in the brain, and result in an improvement of symptoms. Other researchers have reported improvement in Alzheimer's disease after administering choline. Research into the possible beneficial effects of lecithin and choline are continuing, but to date, there is no evidence to support claims that taking lecithin supplements will prevent these disorders or improve memory loss. Furthermore, taking large amounts of either lecithin or choline produces a number of unpleasant side effects, most notably excessive sweating, appetite loss, intestinal distress, and drooling or excessive salivation. These side effects usually prevent people from taking potentially harmful amounts. Long-term high doses of lecithin can cause more serious effects, however, including mental depression and nervous-system disorders.

Dietary Fiber

There are many misconceptions about the possible role of fiber in lowering blood cholesterol. In the early years of the "fiber fad," people were urged to add large amounts of bran and other cellulose fibers to their diet on the premise that this would achieve a wide range of health benefits—everything from enhanced well-being to preventing constipation, diabetes, heart attacks, and a number of other serious diseases. Over the last decade, we have come to realize that many of these claims simply are not supported by scientific evidence. We now know that excessive dietary fiber can have harmful effects (see Chapter 9), and also, that different kinds of fiber have different effects. A number of studies have documented that the water-soluble fibers—pectin, guar and other gums, and the fiber found in legumes and oat bran—can lower blood cholesterol, mostly by lowering LDLs. It is important to remember that, while eating oat bran (or other soluble fibers) can lower cholesterol, you have to eat a lot of it, and it should be part of a low-fat diet. Eating more fruits and vegetables (particularly beans, peas, and other legumes) will incorporate additional sources of soluble fiber into a low-fat, low-cholesterol diet, and this may achieve a greater reduction of cholesterol than reducing fat and cholesterol intake alone. Studies have found less impressive effects among people with normal cholesterol levels. In contrast, wheat bran and other insoluble fibers have little or no effect on blood cholesterol, regardless of the level.

The water-soluble fibers are believed to lower cholesterol by increasing the excretion of cholesterol and bile acids and perhaps by also lowering the body's absorption of dietary cholesterol. Animal studies also suggest that the effect of the fibers on intestinal bacterial content may be a factor in reducing cholesterol, but the mechanism for this is unclear. A varied and balanced diet that includes foods high in all types of fiber makes good sense, but the same cannot be said for self-treating with high-fiber supplements or overloading the diet with one or two types of food, such as bran cereals.

Lifestyle Factors

As indicated earlier, diet and genetics are not the only factors that influence blood cholesterol; a number of lifestyle factors also play a role. These include:

Exercise. Vigorous exercise appears to increase HDL levels and lower LDLs, and some experts think this may explain why people who engage in regular strenuous exercise, either in their jobs or recreationally, have a lower risk of heart attacks. It also helps in weight control, which in turn helps keep blood pressure and cholesterol under control.

Stress. Studies have found that stress may contribute to elevated cholesterol, but how is unknown. Some researchers believe that the extra catecholamines, the adrenal hormones that are excreted in increased amounts during periods of stress, may signal the liver to increase cholesterol output. This appears to vary from person to person, so how an individual responds to stress may be more important than the nature of the stress itself.

Cigarette smoking. Tobacco use is linked with higher fibrinogen and other clotting factors in the blood, which may in part explain why smokers have an increased risk of heart attacks. Although smokers tend to have high levels of blood cholesterol, it is not known whether smoking actually increases cholesterol. Lower levels of HDLs are clearly associated with cigarette smoking and these appear to rise when smoking is stopped. Epidemiologic studies also indicate that people who smoke and have other cardiovascular risk factors, such as high blood cholesterol, have a greater risk of heart attacks than people who have only one risk factor. (See Chapter 26.)

Alcohol use. Moderate alcohol use, defined as an ounce to an ounce and a half a day, tends to raise HDL cholesterol. Although this effect has been widely reported in the media as beneficial, it is not known whether these alcohol-induced rises in HDLs do, indeed, help prevent heart disease. It has been demonstrated, however, that even moderate alcohol consumption can raise blood pressure and increase the risk of a stroke, so we would not recommend alcohol use as a possible means of increasing HDL cholesterol.

Miscellaneous factors. A number of other factors have been linked to elevated blood cholesterol or alteration of the LDL or HDL levels. For example, people with diabetes mellitus tend to have lower HDL levels, perhaps related to the obesity that is common among adult diabetics. A number of common medications, including certain diuretics used to treat high blood pressure, are known to either increase total cholesterol or, more commonly, to lower levels of the protective HDL cholesterol while raising LDL levels.

Lowering Cholesterol

There has been considerable debate over what constitutes an unhealthy cholesterol level and at what point a person should undertake a cholesterol-lowering regimen, but

Table 6.9.	National Cholesterol Education Program: Adult Treatment Panel Classification	
	Total Cholesterol (mg./dl.)	**LDL Cholesterol (mg./dl.)**
Desirable	<200	<130
Borderline high	200–239	130–159
High	≥240	≥160

Source: National Cholesterol Education Program, 1988.

much of this has been resolved by new guidelines by the National Cholesterol Education Program. (See Table 6.9.) This federally coordinated effort of government and private associations is recommending that adults strive for blood-cholesterol levels below 200 milligrams per deciliter of blood. Specifically, the program's guidelines recommend that if two blood tests confirm that a person's total cholesterol is above 200 but less than 240 milligrams per deciliter, he or she should go on a cholesterol-lowering diet. This would entail consuming a diet in which fat makes up no more than 30 percent of the calories consumed, mostly from vegetable oils, fish, and lean meats, and less than 300 milligrams of cholesterol per day.

A person whose blood cholesterol is more than 240 milligrams should be retested to determine the HDL and LDL levels and also the level of blood triglycerides. (The role of triglycerides in heart disease is not well understood, but very high levels are undesirable, especially if other lipids also are elevated. Depending upon the level of LDL cholesterol as well as results of the other tests, a strict diet, low in saturated fats and cholesterol, is prescribed. If adequate reduction in LDL cho-

Tips on Lowering High Cholesterol

1. Lose weight if you are above the desirable range. Although high cholesterol levels are not always associated with excess weight, overweight individuals typically have higher readings than normal-weight ones. Most of the suggestions for lowering cholesterol will also assist in doing this.

2. Use a low-fat, low-cholesterol cookbook for recipes or modify traditional ones to reduce saturated fat and cholesterol content. Reduce portion sizes of meat dishes, and always trim away visible fat. Cook meats so that fat can drain off, and discard or skim all fat from the drippings.

3. Use vegetables, pasta, and other low-fat, cholesterol-free foods to add quantity and variety to meals.

4. Markedly reduce consumption of cholesterol-rich foods, such as eggs and organ meats (liver, brains, and kidney). The American Heart Association recommends that a person consume no more than four egg yolks a week, including those used in baked goods.

5. Don't be misled by advertising claims of no cholesterol. Check the labels and avoid palm, palm kernel, coconut, lard, and other highly saturated fats and oils.

6. Exercise regularly. Frequent exercise helps in weight control and helps raise the HDL level in the blood.

7. Some types of dietary fiber can help lower cholesterol. These include the sticky or soluble fibers, such as pectin (found in apples and other fruits), guar (used in gum and as a thickener), and the fiber in oat or corn brans and dried beans and other legumes. Include foods containing these fibers in your regular diet.

8. Have meatless meals a few times each week, but avoid quiche and cheese, nut, and cream dishes that may be high in fat. (See Meatless Recipes on page 87, and in Chapter 6, the Tips on Low-Fat Cooking and Shopping on page 71 for additional suggestions for meatless meals.)

9. The butterfat found in milk and cheese contains more cholesterol-raising saturated fats than does the fat in red meat or poultry. Therefore, use skim or 1-percent-fat milk. Substitute margarine for butter, and use cheese sparingly unless it is made from skim milk. (Even part-skim-milk cheese tends to be high in fat.)

lesterol is not achieved in three to six months on this diet, cholesterol-lowering drugs may be added. Of course, any cholesterol-lowering program should include modifying any contributing lifestyle and miscellaneous other factors described in the previous section. (See Chapter 26 for more specific guidelines and a sample diet.)

In recent years, people with high blood cholesterol have been urged to cut down on egg yolks, butter, organ meats, and other rich sources of dietary cholesterol. The National Cholesterol Education Program's recommendation is that dietary cholesterol be limited to less than 300 milligrams a day for the average man. Some experts argue that these recommendations are unnecessarily stringent for healthy adults with blood-cholesterol levels of 200 to 220 milligrams or less, and others note that dietary cholesterol probably does not markedly affect blood cholesterol as much as saturated fat and excessive calories. Be that as it may, we agree with the National Cholesterol Education Program guidelines. Even though changing dietary cholesterol may not markedly alter blood cholesterol for everyone, consuming a prudent low-cholesterol, low-fat diet is consistent with the habits of population groups that enjoy a low incidence of cardiovascular disease. Perhaps most convincing is the evidence for large population studies that intake of dietary cholesterol correlates with the incidence of heart disease, independent of blood-cholesterol levels.

Cholesterol-Lowering Strategies

As noted earlier, confusion and conflicting advice abound regarding reducing consumption of dietary cholesterol. Many people assume, for example, that all red meats are high in cholesterol, and all poultry, fish, and other seafood low in cholesterol. In fact, lean red meat, poultry, and most fish vary little in cholesterol content. Lobster and shrimp contain more cholesterol than many red meats. Fish and shellfish, however, are low in saturated fats, as opposed to many red meats. Foods rich in saturated fats contribute to elevated blood-cholesterol levels even when their cholesterol content is low or nonexistent; therefore, following a low-fat diet will help reduce cholesterol more than restricting

Suggestions for Meatless Meals

Following are menus that feature meatless entrées.

Lunch or Dinner

Vegetarian chili
Rice
Tossed salad
Yogurt topped with fresh fruit
Beverage

Cold fruit soup
Ratatouille
Watercress and endive salad
Flan
Beverage

Green pea soup
Pasta bows with sun-dried tomatoes and herbs*
Fruit cup
Gingersnaps
Beverage

Zucchini soup
Mixed grain pilaf
Broccoli with lemon
Stewed pears
Beverage

Melon wedges
Pasta primavera*
Low-fat lemon sherbert or sorbet
Beverage

*Recipes included. For other suggestions and recipes, consult *The American Heart Association Cookbook,* fourth edition (New York: Random House, 1989), or any of a number of vegetarian cookbooks.

dietary cholesterol alone. (See Tips on Lowering High Cholesterol on page 85.)

Effectiveness of a cholesterol-lowering diet varies considerably from person to person. Generally, a person whose blood cholesterol is in the 200-to-300-milligram range can expect a 10 to 15 percent reduction by dietary measures alone. Not uncommonly, we will see a dramatic lowering of blood cholesterol by 30 percent after only a few weeks on a very strict diet low in saturated fat, calories, and cholesterol. The best-selling book *Eight-Week Cholesterol Cure* is based on this premise. (It should be noted that although this book claims to lower cholesterol by diet alone, it does recommend taking nicotinic acid, which is a drug when taken in doses large enough to lower cholesterol, and should be used only under a physician's supervision.) The important factor, however, is not how quickly blood cholesterol is reduced but, instead, how long the lower levels are maintained. The goal of any cholesterol-lowering regimen should be for the long term. Even though a crash diet will give dramatic short-term results, cholesterol levels will return to previous highs if former dietary habits are resumed. It may take six or eight months of gradually changing your eating habits to achieve lasting results, but these are more beneficial than a short-term yo-yo effect.

Meatless Recipes

Pasta Primavera

6–10 cauliflower florets
6–10 broccoli florets
1 zucchini, cut in rings
1 yellow or red pepper, sliced or diced
1 large white or red onion, cut in small wedges

16 oz. of high-protein pasta
15 black olives, sliced
3 cloves of crushed garlic
Juice of 1 lemon
2 T olive oil
8 T freshly grated Parmesan cheese
Pepper

1. Cook pasta until it is al dente. Drain.

2. While pasta is cooking, steam cauliflower, broccoli, and zucchini in boiling water until crisp or tender, depending upon preference. Drain and keep in pot with lid covered.

3. In a large bowl, toss vegetables and pasta and mix with diced pepper, onion, olives, and garlic. Add lemon juice, olive oil, Parmesan cheese and black pepper. Toss. Serve hot. Serves 4 to 6.

Pasta Bows with Sun-Dried Tomatoes and Herbs

16 oz. small pasta bows
10 to 12 fresh basil leaves, torn
1 T fresh parsley, chopped
Sun-dried tomatoes, drained and sliced
4 cloves garlic, crushed
¼ cup sesame seeds, lightly toasted (optional)

¼ cup sliced black olives
Black pepper
2 T olive oil
½ cup yogurt
¼ cup imitation mayonnaise
¼ cup grated Parmesan cheese

1. Cook the pasta bows in unsalted boiling water until firm, but not soft (*al dente*).

2. In a large bowl combine herbs, sun-dried tomatoes, garlic, sesame seeds, olives, and pepper. Heat oil, yogurt, and imitation mayonnaise over low heat. Do not boil. Pour sauce in a warmed bowl.

3. Drain pasta and pour sauce over. Toss. Add Parmesan cheese and fresh pepper. Serve hot or refrigerate to serve cold. Serves 4.

MODERATION IS THE KEY

Throughout this book, Mount Sinai experts stress the importance of moderation, variety, and balance in achieving a healthful diet. These guidelines certainly apply to saturated fat and cholesterol. Extreme regimens—especially in children—that severely restrict fat consumption or promote only one type of fat to the exclusion of all others can be as harmful as the excesses these diets purport to overcome. For the majority of people, modification of their present diets, as opposed to drastic change, is all that is needed to achieve the desired goals of reducing fat and cholesterol intake and thereby lowering blood cholesterol.

7

Vitamins and Minerals

Victor Herbert, M.D., J.D.

■

INTRODUCTION

For centuries, doctors have recognized that some diseases—for example, scurvy, beriberi, pellagra, and rickets—could be prevented by eating certain foods. It has been primarily in this century, however, that researchers have identified the specific food substances—vitamins and minerals—that are instrumental in preventing these deficiency diseases. As a result of this increased knowledge and the availability of a variety of foods rich in vitamins and minerals, deficiency diseases are now rare in the United States and other affluent industrialized nations. Despite this, millions of Americans believe that their foods do not supply adequate vitamins and minerals, and therefore they take nutritional supplements, often in potentially dangerous megadoses, and sometimes resulting in actual harm.

In this chapter, we attempt to put vitamins and minerals into their proper perspective. We describe the vitamins and minerals that are essential to human health, outline how much of each is needed, and list their best food sources. First, however, here are a few general principles about the role of vitamins and minerals in the body and for health.

1. Healthy adult men and healthy adult nonpregnant, nonlactating women who eat a varied diet get all the vitamins and minerals they need. Vitamin and mineral pills may be needed for some infants and for pregnant and lactating women. Supplements may also occasionally be useful for people with unusual lifestyles or modified diets, including certain weight-reduction regimens and strict vegetarian diets.

Proponents of vitamin supplements often argue that since many people don't eat a balanced and varied diet, they should take a daily vitamin pill "just to be on the safe side." The fact is, even a marginal diet will provide adequate vitamins and minerals; if you are an average, healthy American, you really have to follow an extremely limited or bizarre diet to develop vitamin deficiencies. As stressed in the 1989 National Academy of Sciences Report on Diet and Health, there is no evidence that supplements have *any value* for the average American. By the same token, there is no evidence that a daily supplement containing amounts specified in the Recommended Dietary Allowances (RDAs) does any harm, either. However, high doses can be harmful; supplements containing more than 150 percent of the RDA are strictly for disease treatment and should never be purchased unless a competent health professional has diagnosed a need for them.

2. Vitamins are organic (i.e., carbon-containing) molecules. They are necessary in tiny amounts to promote one or more specific and essential biochemical reactions. A lack of any one produces a unique deficiency disease that can be corrected only by supplying the missing vitamin.

3. Only very small amounts of vitamins and minerals are required to maintain health; this is why they are called micronutrients. More than adequate amounts of all the essential vitamins and minerals are easily obtained from a normal diet that includes a variety of foods selected from the Basic Four groups described in Chapter 1.

4. Aside from their specific metabolic functions, vitamins and minerals have no "super" medical properties. They do not improve appetite, confer immunity, relieve stress, boost energy, or cure colds—to cite but a few of the claims made by food faddists and purveyors of vitamin and mineral supplements.

5. When taken in megadose amounts, the vitamins and minerals that are in excess of those needed to saturate enzyme systems function as free-floating drugs (instead of as receptor-bound nutrients). Generally, vitamins function as coenzymes that attach to specific protein substances called apoenzymes in cells to become holoenzymes (enzymes, for short). Each cell has a limited maximum capacity to make apoenzymes, which are quickly saturated with vitamins, making it biochemically impossible for excess vitamins to function as vitamins. Thus, they act as drugs, and like all drugs, they have a potential for adverse side effects. In fact, chronic consumption of megadoses of some vitamins and minerals can be lethal. Thus, high-dose supplements should be taken only under a li-censed health professional's supervision for a specific medical purpose.

RECOMMENDED DIETARY ALLOWANCES

When determining how much of a particular vitamin or mineral is needed to maintain health, American nutritionists generally refer to the Recommended Dietary Allowances, or RDAs. These are standards established by the Food and Nutrition Board of the National Research Council, and consist of a table and a book of explanation of complex functions, such as absorbability, levels of inadequacy and of excess, and nutrient interactions. As defined by the board, RDAs "are the levels of intake of essential nutrients considered, in the judgment of the Committee on Dietary Allowances of the Food and Nutrition Board on the basis of available scientific knowledge, to be adequate to meet the nutritional needs of practically all healthy persons." (Table 7.1 lists the most recent RDAs.) RDAs are set by first determining the "floor" below which deficiency occurs, and then by determining the "ceiling" above which harm occurs. A number is selected that is sufficiently above the floor so that there is a substantial amount stored in the body as a reserve against possible weeks or months of inadequate intake, but not so high as to approach the ceiling.

The World Health Organization (WHO), through its expert committee, sets Recommended Dietary Intakes (RDIs), using the same experts used by the United States for its RDAs, and many more from other countries. The RDIs tend to be lower than the RDAs because WHO does not believe reserve stores need to be as high as are traditional in the United States.

The RDAs provide a guide for dietitians

and other nutrition professionals for planning and evaluating diets for specific population groups, such as hospital patients, pregnant women, schoolchildren, and so forth. They are not intended for specific individuals. In planning a family's eating program, the RDA table alone, without the book of explanation, is not of much help. Instead, a family's menu should be selected from a variety of foods from the Basic Four groups rather than by trying to calculate specific RDAs.

How, then, should the RDAs be used? Since the first RDAs were published in 1943 (they are reviewed and updated about every five years), they have been used to set standards and goals in food production and national nutritional programs. They also are used in food labeling, nutrition-education programs, and in the formulation and fortification of certain foods.

Many people have the mistaken notion that the RDAs are synonymous with dietary requirements, and that if you fail to get the full RDA of a particular nutrient every day, your diet is somehow deficient. This is not true; in reality, the RDAs actually allow far more than the average person needs to stay healthy. For example, the average person requires about 10 milligrams of vitamin C per day to prevent scurvy. The 1980 adult RDA of 60 milligrams is much higher than the basic requirement, and much higher than the RDI set by the WHO, but the Food and Nutrition Board has insisted on recommending amounts sufficient to produce quite substantial body stores for nonscientific reasons.

The Tenth Edition, published in 1989, reduced recommendations for some nutrients below those of the 1980 Ninth Edition. These lower levels for vitamins B_{12} and B_6, folate, iron, and zinc are more in accord with the international Recommended Dietary Intakes (RDIs) of the Food and Agriculture Organization/World Health Organization than were the 1980 RDAs. (The 1989 RDA text for B_{12}, folate, and iron is almost identical to recommendations I published as RDIs in 1987 in *American Journal of Clinical Nutrition.*)

U.S. RDAs

The FDA (Food and Drug Administration) created U.S. RDAs from the highest numbers in the 1968 RDAs. U.S. RDAs are used mainly for nutrition labeling on various food products. No one can be expected to remember the specific amounts of the 20 nutrients included in the U.S. RDAs, nor is it important that they should try. However, nutrition labels, which tell what percentage of U.S. RDAs will be satisfied by a particular product, can be used as general guidelines. For example, if a serving of a particular product provides 60 milligrams of vitamin C, or the full U.S. RDA, the label will list 100 percent for that nutrient. Thus, the consumer will know that more than enough vitamin C has been provided for that day's need, plus a substantial amount for storage. (Contrary to popular belief, the body does store some vitamin C—enough to last for several months.) (See Chapter 40.) On July 19, 1990, the FDA announced in the Federal Register that in 1992 it will replace the term "U.S. RDAs" with the term RDIs (Reference Daily Intakes), and that there will be 26 RDIs. The 20 U.S. RDAs are protein, 12 vitamins, and 7 minerals. The 26 RDIs will add vitamin K, manganese, molybdenum, selenium, fluoride, and chromium. The FDA will also establish a new category of reference values—DRVs (Daily Reference Values)—for food components that are associated with reduced rise of chronic diseases: fat, saturated fatty acids, unsaturated fatty acids, cholesterol, carbohydrate, fiber, sodium, and potassium.

PSEUDOVITAMINS

Pseudovitamins (false vitamins) include orotic acid ("vitamin B_{13}"), inositol, choline, methionine, paraaminobenzoic acid (PABA), carnitine ("vitamin B_4"), bioflavinoids ("vitamin P"), pangamate ("vitamin B_{15}"), laetrile ("vitamin B_{17}"), and gerovital ("vitamin H_3"). The use of the term *vitamin* to describe these substances has been described as health fraud, because it implies the substances have a specific role in maintaining health, but there is no scientific basis for these claims. Still, the substances are widely promoted and are sold in many health-food stores.

VITAMINS

Vitamins are organic substances, derived from animal or plant foods, that are essential to human health. There are 13 known for humans.

With the exception of vitamin D, which can be synthesized in the skin by exposure to sunlight for 1.0 to 30 minutes a day, biotin,

Table 7.1. Food and Nutrition Board, National Academy of Sciences—National Research Council Designed for the Maintenance of Good Nutrition of Practically All Healthy People in the

Category	Age (years) or condition	Weight[b] (kg)	Weight[b] (lb)	Height[b] (cm)	Height[b] (in)	Protein (g)	Fat-Soluble Vitamins Vitamin A (µg RE)[c]	Vitamin D (µg)[d]	Vitamin E (mg α-TE)[e]	Vitamin K (µg)	Vitamin C (mg)
Infants	0.0–0.5	6	13	60	24	13	375	7.5	3	5	30
	0.5–1.0	9	20	71	28	14	375	10	4	10	35
Children	1–3	13	29	90	35	16	400	10	6	15	40
	4–6	20	44	112	44	24	500	10	7	20	45
	7–10	28	62	132	52	28	700	10	7	30	45
Males	11–14	45	99	157	62	45	1,000	10	10	45	50
	15–18	66	145	176	69	59	1,000	10	10	65	60
	19–24	72	160	177	70	58	1,000	10	10	70	60
	25–50	79	174	176	70	63	1,000	5	10	80	60
	51+	77	170	173	68	63	1,000	5	10	80	60
Females	11–14	46	101	157	62	46	800	10	8	45	50
	15–18	55	120	163	64	44	800	10	8	55	60
	19–24	58	128	164	65	46	800	10	8	60	60
	25–50	63	138	163	64	50	800	5	8	65	60
	51+	65	143	160	63	50	800	5	8	65	60
Pregnant						60	800	10	10	65	70
Lactating	1st 6 months					65	1,300	10	12	65	95
	2nd 6 months					62	1,200	10	11	65	90

[a]The allowances, expressed as average daily intakes over time, are intended to provide for individual variations among most normal persons as they live in the United States under usual environmental stresses. Diets should be based on a variety of common foods in order to provide other nutrients for which human requirements have been less well defined. See text for detailed discussion of allowances and of nutrients not tabulated.

[b]Weights and heights of Reference Adults are actual medians for the U.S. population of the designated age, as reported by NHANES II. The median weights and heights of those under 19 years of age were taken from Hamill, et al. (1979) (see pages 16–17). The use of these figures does not imply that the height-to-weight ratios are ideal.

[c]Retinol equivalents. 1 retinol equivalent = 1 µg retinol or 6 µg β-carotene. See text for calculation of vitamin A activity of diets as retinol equivalents.

and pantothenate, which can be manufactured by bacteria that normally inhabit our intestines, all vitamins must be consumed in the diet. All 13 are essential for the normal growth, development, and maintenance of the human organism, and all can be harmful in excess.

Vitamins are generally divided into two categories determined by the way they are absorbed by the body. Vitamins A, D, E, and K are fat-soluble, which means they are absorbed with the help of fats or bile and are stored in fat. The eight B vitamins and vitamin C are water-soluble; fat is not needed to absorb them from the intestinal tract. Varying amounts are stored in the body to meet general daily needs, with a bit extra for periods when the individual's diet may be inadequate.

Contrary to popular belief, it is not necessary to consume water-soluble vitamins *every single day*; the body stores enough to provide reserves that last for a few weeks to months or even longer in some cases. It is important, however, that the *average* intake over a week or two provide the variety of foods that supply all the essential vitamins. The liver is the

Recommended Dietary Allowances,ª Revised 1989 United States

| Water-Soluble Vitamins | | | | | | Minerals | | | | | | |
Thiamine (mg)	Riboflavin (mg)	Niacin (mg ne)f	Vitamin B$_6$ (mg)	Folate (µg)*	Vitamin B$_{12}$ (µg)*	Calcium (mg)	Phosphorus (mg)	Magnesium (mg)	Iron (mg)*	Zinc (mg)	Iodine (µg)	Selenium (µg)
0.3	0.4	5	0.3	25	0.3	400	300	40	6	5	40	10
0.4	0.5	6	0.6	35	0.5	600	500	60	10	5	50	15
0.7	0.8	9	1.0	50	0.7	800	800	80	10	10	70	20
0.9	1.1	12	1.1	75	1.0	800	800	120	10	10	90	20
1.0	1.2	13	1.4	100	1.4	800	800	170	10	10	120	30
1.3	1.5	17	1.7	150	2.0	1,200	1,200	270	12	15	150	40
1.5	1.8	20	2.0	200	2.0	1,200	1,200	400	12	15	150	50
1.5	1.7	19	2.0	200	2.0	1,200	1,200	350	10	15	150	70
1.5	1.7	19	2.0	200	2.0	800	800	350	10	15	150	70
1.2	1.4	15	2.0	200	2.0	800	800	350	10	15	150	70
1.1	1.3	15	1.4	150	2.0	1,200	1,200	280	15	12	150	45
1.1	1.3	15	1.5	180	2.0	1,200	1,200	300	15	12	150	50
1.1	1.3	15	1.6	180	2.0	1,200	1,200	280	15	12	150	55
1.1	1.3	15	1.6	180	2.0	800	800	280	15	12	150	55
1.0	1.2	13	1.6	180	2.0	800	800	280	10	12	150	55
1.5	1.6	17	2.2	400	2.2	1,200	1,200	320	30	15	175	65
1.6	1.8	20	2.1	280	2.6	1,200	1,200	355	15	19	200	75
1.6	1.7	20	2.1	260	2.6	1,200	1,200	340	15	16	200	75

ᵈAs cholecalciferol. 10 µg cholecalciferol = 400 IU of vitamin D.

ᵉα-Tocopherol equivalents.

f1 NE (niacin equivalent) is equal to 1 mg. of niacin or 60 mg. of dietary tryptophan.

*The 1989 RDAs for folate, vitamin B$_{12}$, and iron are essentially copied from the RDIs (Recommended Dietary Intakes) of Herbert in the April 1987 *American Journal of Clinical Nutrition*. In July 1990, the FDA indicated that when it updates the U.S. RDAs (printed on cereal boxes, multivitamin pill labels, etc.) it will use RDIs (Reference Daily Intakes) rather than RDAs. An FAO/WHO (Food and Agriculture Organization/World Health Organization) panel established the latest (1988) RDIs (meaning Recommended Dietary Intakes) for vitamin A, folate, vitamin B$_{12}$, and iron. (Dr. Herbert was a member of that international panel.)

body's main nutrient storehouse. It absorbs and stores excess nutrients from the blood, and releases into the blood those nutrients that are not coming into the blood from the diet.

Pills Versus Food for Nutrition

Despite what millions of Americans believe, it is better to get your vitamins from food than from pills. Almost invariably, the high concentration in the intestine of a vitamin or mineral in pills interferes with the absorption of some other nutrients.

There also is a widespread misbelief that we need to take supplements to make up for what is lacking in food. This is not true, as is stressed in Chapter 2. For one thing, many foods already are enriched to compensate for the nutrients that may be lost in processing. Enriched and fortified cereals and breads are examples of processed foods that contain more of specific nutrients than their original unprocessed forms. This should not be misinterpeted as meaning the fortified versions are more healthful than the unfortified. The consumer should be aware when buying heavily fortified foods that this extra fortification is totally unnecessary and manufacturers may increase the price considerably for the additional vitamins and minerals.

Nutrition and Fertilizers

There also is no objective evidence to support claims put forth by proponents of nutritional supplements and "health foods" that foods grown with commercial fertilizers are any less nutritious than those grown with manure, compost, and other organic fertilizers. If a plant does not have adequate nutrition itself, it simply does not grow. Otherwise, the plant manufactures the molecules that comprise what it needs from the available soil nutrients. These molecules are identical in plants fed organic matter as opposed to commercial fertilizers. The composition of the soil itself can affect mineral content. For example, the lack of iodine in foods grown in the Alps and certain other areas is due to the lack of this mineral in the soil. However, deficiencies due to natural shortcomings in the local soil and growing process are rare because certain foods, such as iodized salt, are fortified and because we eat foods grown in many different places. As an example of this, it has been shown that people living in low-selenium areas in the United States are not lacking in this nutrient.

Individual Vitamins

Table 7.2 lists the various vitamins, their functions, sources, and signs of deficiency and overdose. Following is a brief overview of the 13 vitamins for humans.

Vitamin A. This vitamin, which has several active forms (i.e., retinol, retinoic acid, or retinyl esters) as well as precursors (most notably beta carotene), is fat soluble and available in liver, eggs, butter and fortified margarine, and a variety of yellow, orange, and dark green vegetables and fruits. It is needed to maintain normal vision, especially for seeing at night or in dim light. It also is required to build and maintain healthy skin and mucous membranes, and is essential for reproduction and for the formation of bones and teeth. In recent years, there have been studies suggesting that vitamin A may help prevent epithelial-cell (lining-cell) cancers, and promote other types of cancer, including prostate cancer. The American Cancer Society urges that smokers and others who are at high risk for developing cancer of the cells lining the breathing tubes include good sources of vitamin A in their diets. As a wiser course for smokers, however, they urge stopping smoking.

Vitamin A can withstand normal cooking temperatures as well as freezing and canning, so very little is lost in food preparation. When fresh foods such as spinach or carrots that normally are rich in vitamin A are allowed to wilt or dry out, however, the vitamin rapidly deteriorates. Rancidity also destroys vitamin A in butter and other fats.

Vitamin A deficiency is rare in the United States, but it is common in many Third World countries, where it is a major cause of childhood blindness. Since Vitamin A is stored in the body (particularly the liver) rather than excreted, excessive intake can cause serious liver damage and other toxicity problems, including birth defects when taken just before and in the first month or two of pregnancy. Toxicity from dietary sources is unlikely because it would be difficult to consume enough of foods high in the vitamin to cause a dangerous buildup. (Exceptions were some early polar explorers who ate large quantities of polar bear liver—a particularly rich source of the vitamin—and were believed to have died of vitamin A toxicity. Obviously, foods such as polar bear liver are not generally available, thus are not a problem.) However, consuming pills or solutions of vitamin A (including cod-liver oil and other fish oils) can be dangerous. No adult should ever eat daily more than 10,000 IU of vitamin A from all sources; no newly pregnant woman should ever eat more than a total of 8,000 IU daily from all sources; and no child should take any vitamin A supplement, except on the advice of a licensed health professional. (Many consumers are confused by the varying units of measurement for vitamin A. The preferred unit, which is used in the RDAs, is a retinol equivalent, or RE. Vitamin manufacturers continue to use the former measurement, which is an international unit, or IU. From animal sources, 1 RE is equal to 3⅓ IU; from plant sources (beta carotene), 1 RE equals 10 IU.) High doses of beta carotene or other vitamin A precursors have not been shown to cause short-term toxicity, although they may turn the skin yellow.

Care also must be taken when using drugs derived from vitamin A. For example, isotretinoin (Accutane), a prescription drug used to treat severe acne, is based on an active form of vitamin A. Although this drug can be highly effective against disfiguring acne, it also can cause serious birth defects when taken by women just before and during early pregnancy.

More recently, skin products formulated from retinols have been shown to reverse some wrinkling and sun-related skin damage in middle-aged women. FDA approval of Retin-A as an antiwrinkling drug resulted in a rush to dermatologists for prescriptions. It should be noted, however, that the drug does not erase deep lines, nor does it work for all women. Also, it can be so irritating to some skins that it cannot be used. It may prove to increase the frequency of sun damage, including skin cancer, since it thins the outer protective layer of skin.

Vitamin D. This fat-soluble vitamin is often referred to as the "sunshine" vitamin because ultraviolet light is instrumental in its formation. The plant form, D_2, is made when a substance in plants, ergosterol, is exposed to sunlight. The major form in human beings and other animals—vitamin D_3—is developed from a cholesterol derivative when the skin is exposed to sunlight. It has been estimated that 10 to 15 minutes of exposure to the midday sun two or three times a week will provide the daily need for vitamin D. Elderly persons need up to 30 minutes because they have less ability to synthesize the vitamin through the

Table 7.2. Vitamins and Minerals at a Glance*

Fat-Soluble Vitamins. These are vitamins that can be stored in the body and need not be consumed daily. It is difficult to overdose on vitamins from an ordinary diet, but consuming megadoses of most fat-soluble vitamins, especially A and D, can lead to dangerous buildups in the body.

Vitamin	What It Does	Signs of Deficiency	Signs of Overdose	Good Sources
Vitamin A	Keeps skin, hair and nails healthy. Helps maintain gums, glands, bones, teeth. Helps ward off infection. Promotes eye function, prevents night blindness. May help to prevent some cancers (i.e., lung cancer in smokers).	Night blindness. Reduced growth in children. Dry, rough skin. Lowered resistance to infection. Dry eyes.	Headaches. Blurred vision. Fatigue. Diarrhea. Irregular periods. Joint and bone pain. Dry, cracked skin. Rashes. Appetite loss. Hair loss. Itchiness. Possible birth defects if consumed in large amounts during pregnancy.	Low-fat or skim dairy products. Fortified cereals. Green and deep yellow or orange vegetables. Deep yellow or orange fruits. Organ meats.
Vitamin D	Helps build and maintain teeth and bones. Needed for body to absorb calcium.	Rickets (in children). Osteomalacia (bone softening in adults). Osteoporosis.	Calcium deposits, especially in heart, kidneys, blood vessels. Fragile bones. Hypertension. High cholesterol. Drowsiness. Diarrhea. Loss of appetite. Headache.	Egg yolks. Fish and cod-liver oil. Fortified milk and butter. Exposure to sun.
Vitamin E	Helps form red blood cells, muscles, and other tissues. Preserves fatty acids.	Unknown in humans.	Possible reduced sexual function.	Poultry and seafood. Seeds and nuts. Cooked greens. Wheat germ and fortified cereals. Eggs.
Vitamin K	Needed for normal blood clotting, bone metabolism.	Excessive bleeding. Liver damage.	Jaundice in infants.	Made by intestinal bacteria. Spinach and other green leafy vegetables. Oats, wheat bran, and other whole grains. Potatoes, cabbage. Organ meats.

Water-Soluble Vitamins. These vitamins are stored in smaller amounts than fat-soluble vitamins; therefore, they need to be consumed more often.

Vitamin	What It Does	Signs of Deficiency	Signs of Overdose	Good Sources
Thiamine (Vitamin B_1)	Enhances energy by promoting metabolism of carbohydrates. Promotes normal appetite, digestion, and proper nerve function.	Anxiety, hysteria, nausea, depression, muscle cramps, loss of appetite. Extreme cases: beriberi, marked by muscle wasting, heart failure,	Excess of one B vitamin may cause deficiency of others (excess B_1 can interfere with B_2 and B_6).	Pork. Fortified grains/cereals. Seafood.

Table 7.2. Vitamins and Minerals at a Glance* *(cont.)*

Vitamin	What It Does	Signs of Deficiency	Signs of Overdose	Good Sources
		paralysis. (Note: deficiency in U.S. occurs among alcoholics.)		
Riboflavin (Vitamin B₂)	Needed for metabolism of all foods. Instrumental in release of energy to cells. Maintains mucous membranes. Helps maintain vision.	Cracks and sores around mouth and nose. Visual problems. Sensitivity to light. Difficulty eating and swallowing.	Can interfere with B_1 and B_6.	Organ meats, beef, lamb, and dark meat of poultry. Low-fat dairy products. Fortified cereals, grains. Dark green leafy vegetables.
Niacin or Nicotinic Acid (Vitamin B₃)	Needed in many enzymes that convert food to energy. Promotes normal appetite and digestion. Promotes proper nerve function. In very large doses (which can lead to abnormal liver function, ulcers, elevated blood sugar and uric acid, and cardiac arrhythmias), lowers cholesterol.	Diarrhea, mouth sores. In extreme cases, pellagra, disease in which skin develops reddish rash, then turns dark and rough.	Hot flashes. Ulcers, liver disorders. High blood sugar and uric acid. Cardiac arrhythmias.	Poultry and seafood. Seeds/nuts. Peanuts, potatoes. Fortified whole grain breads and cereals.
Pantothenic acid ("Vitamin B₅")	Essential in converting food to molecular forms needed by body. Needed to manufacture adrenal hormones and chemicals that regulate nerve function.	Unknown in humans except when induced in experiments.	May increase need for thiamin. Megadoses may produce diarrhea and water retention.	Manufactured by intestinal bacteria. Also found in almost all plant and animal foods.
Pyridoxine (Vitamin B₆)	Essential to protein metabolism and absorption. Also important in carbohydrate metabolism. Helps form red blood cells. Promotes proper nerve function.	Depression, mental confusion. Inflammation of mucous membranes of mouth. Patches of itchy, scaling skin. Convulsions in infants.	Can lead to sensory nerve destruction (loss of feeling in fingers, legs, etc.).	Meats/fish/poultry. Grains and cereals. Spinach, sweet potatoes, white potatoes. Bananas, prunes, watermelon.
Cobalamin (Vitamin B₁₂)	Builds genetic material (nucleic acid) needed by all cells. Helps form	Blood and nerve damage. (Note: deficiency rare except	Only in infants with a rare genetic defect.	All animal products, including meats, poultry, eggs, and

Table 7.2. Vitamins and Minerals at a Glance* *(cont.)*

Vitamin	What It Does	Signs of Deficiency	Signs of Overdose	Good Sources
	red blood cells.	in strict vegetarians, the elderly, or people with malabsorption disorders.)		seafood. Low-fat dairy products.
Biotin	Needed for metabolism of glucose and formation of certain fatty acids. Essential for many bodily processes.	Rare except in infants. Scaling of skin. Muscle pain. Fatigue. Loss of appetite. Insomnia.	See B₁.	Made by intestinal bacteria. Meats, poultry, fish, and eggs. Nuts, seeds and legumes. Vegetables.
Folic acid (Folate or Folacin)	Needed to make genetic material (DNA and RNA). Needed in manufacture of red blood cells.	Impaired cell division marked by abnormal or oversized red blood cells. Anemia. Diarrhea. Bleeding gums. Weight loss, GI upsets. Irritability. (Note: Deficiency seen mostly in alcoholics, the pregnant, and the poor.)	Convulsions in epileptics (counteracts anticonvulsants). Megadoses damage zinc absorption.	Poultry and liver. Dark green leafy vegetables and legumes. Fortified whole-grain cereals and breads. Orange and grapefruit juice. One fresh uncooked fruit or vegetable or fruit juice a day keeps folate deficiency away.
Vitamin C (Ascorbic acid)	Helps bind cells together. Strengthens blood vessel walls. Keeps gums healthy. Helps resist infection. Promotes healing of cuts and wounds.	Bleeding gums, loose teeth. Easy bruising. Dry, rough skin. Loss of appetite. Slow healing. Extreme cases: development of scurvy.	Oxalate kidney stones, oxalate deposits in heart, other body tissues. Urinary-tract irritation. Diarrhea. Blood destruction.	Citrus fruits, citrus juices, strawberries, canteloupe, watermelon. Sweet potatoes, cabbage, cauliflower, broccoli, green or red pepper, plantains, snow peas.

Major Macrominerals. Macrominerals are those that the body needs in relatively large quantities but that are still measured in milligrams.

Mineral	What It Does	Signs of Deficiency	Signs of Overdose	Good Sources
Calcium	Helps build strong bones and teeth. Promotes proper muscle and nerve function. Helps blood to clot. Helps activate enzymes needed to convert food to energy.	Rickets in children; osteomalacia (soft bones) and osteoporosis in adults.	Calcium kidney stones and calcium deposits in body tissues. Mental confusion, lethargy. Muscle and abdominal pain. Hinders absorption of iron and other minerals.	Milk and milk products. Canned salmon (with bones). Oysters. Broccoli. Tofu.
Phosphorus	Works with calcium to build and maintain bones and teeth. Needed by certain enzymes to convert food to energy. Helps	Deficiency is rare; signs include weakness, bone pain.	Lowers blood calcium.	Dairy products and egg yolks. Meat, poultry, and fish. Legumes.

Table 7.2. Vitamins and Minerals at a Glance* *(cont.)*

Vitamin	What It Does	Signs of Deficiency	Signs of Overdose	Good Sources
	maintain body's chemical balance. Promotes proper nerve and muscle function.			
Magnesium	Activates enzymes needed to release energy in body. Promotes bone growth. Needed to make cells and genetic material.	Muscle weakness, twitching, cramps. Cardiac arrhythmias. (Note: Deficiency most common in alcoholics, people who take diuretics, or patients with kidney disease or severe diarrhea.)	Upset in calcium/magnesium balance, resulting in nervous-system disorders. Warning: Overdose can be fatal to people with kidney disease.	Green leafy vegetables. Beans and nuts. Fortified whole-grain cereals and breads. Oysters, scallops.

Trace Minerals. The following, although as essential to health as the macrominerals, are needed in very small amounts, hence are referred to as trace minerals.

Mineral	What It Does	Signs of Deficiency	Signs of Overdose	Good Sources
Iron	Essential to make hemoglobin, the red substance in blood that carries oxygen, and myoglobin, the substance that stores oxygen in muscles.	Weakness, fatigue, headache, shortness of breath, iron-deficiency anemia.	Toxic buildup in liver, pancreas and, in some instances, the heart. Diabetes, liver disease, arrhythmias. Damages zinc absorption.	Red meat and liver. Shellfish and fish. Legumes. Dried apricots. Fortified breads and cereals. Acidic foods cooked in cast-iron pots.
Zinc	Element in more than 100 enzymes that are essential to digestion and metabolism.	Slow wound healing. Loss of appetite. Retarded growth and delayed sexual development in children.	Nausea, vomiting, abdominal pain, gastric bleeding. Premature labor and stillbirth in pregnant women.	Beef, liver, and oysters. Yogurt. Fortified cereals and wheat germ.
Selenium	Interacts with vitamin E to prevent breakdown of fats and body chemicals.	Unknown in humans.	Nausea, abdominal pain, diarrhea, hair and nail damage, fatigue, irritability. Death.	Chicken, seafood. Whole-grain breads and cereals. Egg yolks. Mushrooms, onions, and garlic.
Copper	Component of several enzymes, including one needed to make body's pigment. Stimulates iron absorption. Needed to make red blood cells, connective tissue, and nerve fibers.	Rare in adults. Infants may develop a type of anemia marked by abnormal development of bones, nerve tissue, lungs, and hair coloring.	Liver disease, vomiting, diarrhea. (Note: Overdose may result from cooking in unlined copper pots.)	Lobster. Organ meats. Nuts. Dried peas, beans, prunes. Barley.
Iodine	Essential to normal thyroid-gland function.	Goiter. Cretinism in infants.	Disturbed thyroid function. Goiter.	Iodized salt. Seafood or vegetables grown in iodine-rich soil

Table 7.2. Vitamins and Minerals at a Glance* *(cont.)*

Vitamin	What It Does	Signs of Deficiency	Signs of Overdose	Good Sources
Fluoride	Promotes strong teeth and bones, especially in children. Improves body's uptake of calcium.	Tooth decay.	Mottling of tooth enamel.	Fluoridated water, food cooked in fluoridated water. Tea.
Manganese	Needed for normal tendon and bone structure. Component of some enzymes important in metabolism.	Unknown in humans.	Nerve damage.	Tea and coffee. Bran. Dried peas and beans. Nuts.
Molybdenum	Component of enzymes needed in metabolism. Helps regulate iron storage.	Unknown in humans.	Goutlike joint pain.	Dried peas and beans. Dark green leafy vegetables. Organ meats. Whole-grain breads and cereals.
Chromium	Works with insulin for proper glucose metabolism.	Diabeteslike symptoms.	Unknown for food (trivalent) chromium. Chromium salts toxic.	Whole-grain breads and cereals. Brewer's yeast. Peanuts.
Sulfur	Needed to help make hair and nails. Component of several amino acids.	Unknown.	Unknown for food sulfur. Sulfur salts toxic.	Wheat germ. Dried peas and beans. Beef. Peanuts. Clams.

Electrolytes. These are minerals essential to maintain proper body chemistry.

Mineral	What It Does	Signs of Deficiency	Signs of Overdose	Good Sources
Potassium	With sodium, helps to regulate body's fluid balance. Promotes transmission of nerve impulses and proper muscle contraction. Needed for proper metabolism.	Muscle weakness. Cardiac arrhythmias. Irritability. (Occurs most often among people taking diuretics or those with prolonged diarrhea.)	Nausea, diarrhea, cardiac arrhythmias that can progress to cardiac arrest.	Bananas, citrus fruits, and dried fruits. Deep yellow vegetables, potatoes, and legumes. Low-fat milk. Bran cereal.
Sodium	Helps maintain body fluid balance.	Rare in U.S.; loss of sodium via extreme perspiration may cause muscle cramps, headaches, weakness.	High blood pressure. Kidney disease. Heart failure.	Salt. Processed foods. Milk. Water in some areas.
Chloride	Helps maintain proper acid-base balance. Component of hydrochloric acid, found in gastric juices and important in digestion.	Upset in body's balance of acids and body fluids. (Note: Deficiency is very rare.)	Upset in acid-base balance.	Same as sodium.

*For a full range of toxicities and other harms from overdoses, see *Vitamins and Minerals: Help or Harm?* by Charles W. Marshall (New York: Consumer Reports Books, 1985).

skin. And people living in northern latitudes, such as New England, where the winter sun is too weak to produce vitamin D from November through March, may need extra portions of foods high in vitamin D (fortified milk or margarine, liver, or fatty fish) during winter months. A study has been proposed to have elderly people in a nursing home in winter get their exposure sitting around an ultraviolet lamp; whether this would do more good or more harm remains to be determined.

Vitamin D is essential for the body to absorb and metabolize calcium and phosphorus properly. Children who do not get enough vitamin D may develop rickets and other skeletal deformities as well as malformed teeth; adults may suffer from osteomalacia, or bone softening. Muscle twitching, cramps, and convulsions are other signs of deficiency.

In the United States, vitamin D deficiency is rare. Most people can make all the vitamin D they need simply by being out in the sun for an hour or so every week or two. Dietary sources may be needed by shut-ins, dark-skinned people living in cold or very cloudy climates, and others who are seldom exposed to the sun. In this country, milk is fortified with vitamin D; other good dietary sources include egg yolks, liver, tuna, and other cold-water fish.

Cod-liver oil is one of the richest dietary sources and has been recommended (although not widely used until this century) as a preventive against rickets since the Middle Ages. Vitamin D supplements are not needed except in special circumstances. For example, premature babies may need extra vitamin D to accommodate their growth rate and bone development. (Some pediatricians recommend vitamin D for normal full-term babies, but this usually is not needed.) The inability to absorb fat and certain liver and kidney disorders may interfere with vitamin D metabolism. In these instances, special vitamin D formulations may be recommended.

As with other fat-soluble vitamins, excessive intake of vitamin D can be toxic. Children are more susceptible to vitamin D overdoses than adults; certainly, parents should not give a youngster vitamin D supplements except under a doctor's supervision. Too much vitamin D can lead to kidney damage, calcification of the heart and other soft tissues, and other problems.

Vitamin E. A group of fat-soluble compounds called tocopherols are commonly lumped together under the term of vitamin E. Alpha-tocopherol is the most common and biologically active, thus this is the one most commonly associated with vitamin E. Nutrition scientists still do not fully understand the role of vitamin E. We do know that it acts as an antioxidant; that is, it protects certain tissues and substances from the effects of oxygen. For example, it prevents oxidation of vitamin A and polyunsaturated fatty acids (PUFA), thus helping maintain cell membranes, including those of red blood cells and their components. Although deficiency symptoms, including reproduction problems, have been produced in laboratory animals, these have not been demonstrated in humans.

In general, foods that contain polyunsaturated fatty acids contain all the vitamin E needed to use the PUFA. Consuming a diet that includes vegetable oils (especially safflower), whole grains, dark green leafy vegetables, nuts, and legumes provides adequate vitamin E. Dietary deficiency has never been seen in any American diet other than an artificial one deliberately created to exclude vitamin E for research purposes.

In recent years, there have been a number of claims that vitamin E can prevent cancer, slow down aging, prevent heart attacks, enhance sexual function, and relieve hot flashes and other symptoms of menopause. Despite the fact that none of these claims has been shown valid, large numbers of people take vitamin E supplements "just in case." It is not clear how harmful large doses of vitamin E are to humans, but a study of elderly Californians published a few years ago in the *Proceedings of the National Academy of Sciences* reported that those who took megadoses died twice as fast as those who took no supplements. (For more information see the book *Vitamins and Minerals: Help or Harm?* by Charles Marshall.)

Vitamin K. Also fat-soluble, vitamin K is used by the liver in the manufacture of prothrombin and other substances essential for proper blood clotting. It also appears to have a role in proper bone metabolism.

About half of our vitamin K is manufactured by bacteria in the intestinal tract; the remainder comes from the diet. Many foods contain vitamin K: Especially good sources include spinach and other green leafy vegetables, cabbage, potatoes, cereals, and liver. Because vitamin K is found in so many foods and is also made in the intestinal tract, deficiency is rare. Some newborn babies may be susceptible to vitamin K deficiency because they lack the intestinal bacteria needed to make it for the first few days of life. Most, however, are born with adequate reserves from their mothers. People on prolonged antibiotic therapy, which destroys the intestinal bacteria that make vitamin K, may develop deficiency symptoms of prolonged bleeding. People who do not properly absorb fats or who have underlying kidney disease, cancer, or other disorders that interfere with the production or absorption of vitamin K also may need extra vitamin K. Otherwise, supplements are not needed.

Vitamin C. Also called ascorbic acid, vitamin C is important in the production of collagen, the connective tissue that helps hold cells together. It helps maintain capillaries, cartilage,

bones and teeth; it also helps protect vitamins A and E and fatty acids from oxidation, as well as increase the body's absorption of inorganic iron.

Vitamin C is found in citrus fruit and many other fruits and vegetables. Of all the vitamins, C is one of the most fragile and is partly destroyed by chopping and overcooking, exposure to air, and by boiling or soaking foods in water. However, enough vitamin C survives cooking that if your only source of vitamin C were cooked potatoes, you still would get enough to prevent scurvy. Of course, fresh or lightly processed fruits and vegetables that have a minimum of handling or cutting are the highest sources of vitamin C.

Scurvy, the major manifestation of vitamin C deficiency, is now quite rare, except among dedicated alcoholics whose sole source of calories is alcohol. The symptoms—bleeding and swollen gums, easy bruising, poor healing, joint pain and disorders, muscle wasting, and so forth—are almost all due to the reduction in collagen production. Actually, very small amounts of vitamin C (5 to 7 mg., with an absolute maximum of 10 mg.) are needed to prevent scurvy symptoms. The average American gets about 120 percent of the RDA (i.e., about 72 mg.) of vitamin C per day in the diet.

Many millions of Americans take megadoses of vitamin C in the mistaken notion that it will prevent the common cold and other illnesses. Since 1970 when Dr. Linus Pauling first published his book claiming that large doses of vitamin C will prevent or cure colds, many studies have been conducted that have refuted this. There is no objective scientific study that supports the notion that a cold can be prevented or cured by taking this vitamin. However, large doses taken during a cold may ease the severity of the symptoms, because vitamin C has a mild antihistaminic effect.

Proponents of vitamin C megadoses often

argue that even if it has no medical effects, the pills aren't doing any harm and they may well produce a placebo effect. Megadoses of vitamin C are not harmless: They can produce unhealthy diarrhea, can cause nutritional imbalances, can deprive tissues of oxygen, and may produce a condition called metastatic oxalosis, with deposits of oxalate in the kidneys (kidney stones), the heart (producing abnormal rhythms), and so forth. Furthermore, if their only benefit is a placebo effect, then plain sugar pills would be just as beneficial and much less costly.

The vitamin B complex. The term *vitamin* (originally vitamine for vital amine) was coined in 1912 by the Polish chemist Casimir Funk to describe a substance in rice that prevented beriberi. Shortly thereafter, other researchers used the term *water-soluble B* to describe the substances that cured beriberi. Early nutrition researchers soon realized that there was a family of compounds, rather than a single substance, hence the term vitamin B complex.

In general, these individual B vitamins each come from food and attach to their own specific proteins made in cells to then become enzymes that carry out a variety of crucial metabolic functions. The eight B vitamins are thiamine (B_1); riboflavin (B_2); niacin (B_3, nicotinamide or nicotinic acid); B_6 (pyridoxine); B_{12} (cobalamin); folic acid (folate); pantothenic acid; and biotin.

Thiamine, or B_1, actually is the B vitamin that prevents beriberi, a condition caused by a deficiency of this and other vitamins and characterized by anemia, muscular atrophy, paralysis, and leg muscle spasms. It is important in converting carbohydrates into energy and fat. It also functions as a coenzyme to produce acetylcholine, needed for proper nervous-system functioning. Thiamine is found in greatest quantity in a variety of whole-grain or enriched cereals and breads, pork, liver, and soybeans. Moderate sources include all lean meats, poultry, eggs, milk, fish, and many fruits and vegetables. About 5 milligrams is the maximum quantity that can be absorbed from a given oral dose, so money spent on "stress tablets" containing more than 5 milligrams is wasted directly into the toilet.

Riboflavin, or B_2, is a key part of two coenzymes that are instrumental in oxidation-reduction reactions and energy production; it also helps maintain the skin, the mucous membranes, the cornea of the eye, and nerve sheaths. A deficiency can make the eyes overly sensitive to light; it also can produce skin and mucous-membrane disorders, especially around the mouth and nose. Good sources include whole-grain or enriched grain products, liver, milk, meat, eggs, and green leafy vegetables. Two to three times the RDA is so much more than the body can use that it pours out in the urine, giving it a bright yellow color. There is no wisdom in spending money to get yellow urine.

Niacin (nicotinic acid, nicotinamide, niacinamide), or B_3, is the B vitamin needed to prevent pellagra. This disease affects almost every cell in the body, especially those with a rapid rate of turnover, which include the skin, nerves, and gastrointestinal tract. In the past, it was a common cause of mental illness and death, especially among the very poor in the South. Its major symptoms are sometimes referred to as the three Ds, for diarrhea, dermatitis, and dementia, which ultimately led to a fourth D—death. The best sources of niacin are high-protein foods, such as meats, poultry, legumes, milk, eggs, and peanuts. Enriched grain products also contain niacin, but not as much as the high-protein sources.

Large doses of niacin are sometimes prescribed as a drug to lower blood cholesterol. Care must be taken in using high-dose niacin.

In addition to annoying side effects such as flushing and itching, headaches, cramps and nausea, gastrointestinal irritation, and wart-like spots on the skin, it can produce liver damage, disturbances of the heart rate and rhythm, and abnormal blood levels of sugar and uric acid.

Vitamin B_6 has three forms: pyridoxine, pyridoxal phosphate, and pyridoxamine. Rich sources include liver, herring, salmon, nuts, brown rice, wheat germ, yeast, and blackstrap molasses. Most vegetables, meats, fish, butter, and eggs contain moderate amounts of B_6. It is needed for proper protein, carbohydrate, and lipid metabolism and aids in the production of red blood cells. Symptoms that occur in B_6 deficiency include skin disorders similar to those of riboflavin and niacin deficiencies, irritability, mental confusion and nervousness, insomnia, poor coordination, and sometimes anemia. Epileptiform convulsions may occur, particularly in infants fed B_6-deficient formulas.

Certain drugs can interfere with B_6 absorption and utilization. Supplements may be recommended in these circumstances. Birth-control pills can reduce B_6 absorption moderately, but most people get enough B_6 from their diets that they need no supplements when taking such pills.

Premenstrual syndrome (PMS), a complex interrelation of normal premenstrual fluid retention and psychologic factors, with no specific relation to B_6, has been erroneously represented as being "cured" by B_6, when in fact the same 80 percent "cured" by B_6 are also "cured" by a placebo. Megadoses of B_6 produce nerve damage; large megadoses in a few months, small megadoses (50 mg. per day) in a few years.

Vitamin B_{12} is needed to make all blood cells, and a deficiency eventually produces severe anemia. B_{12} is necessary to make nerve sheaths, and, therefore, for proper nerve function. It is also needed for normal fatty acid and DNA synthesis. Since appreciable amounts of B_{12} can be stored in the liver, it may take years for a dietary deficiency to become apparent. B_{12} is produced by a limited number of bacteria, including some in the digestive tract of ruminant animals. All animal products (meat, fish, poultry, milk, milk products, eggs) are good sources, but nothing that grows out of the ground contains the vitamin.

People most at risk of developing a deficiency are strict vegetarians who eat no animal products and those who become unable to absorb B_{12} from food. This inability to absorb B_{12} from food or pills occurs with increasing frequency in each decade after 50, as we gradually decrease our ability to secrete stomach acid and enzymes. Everyone should have his or her vitamin B_{12} level measured at age 60 and each decade thereafter. If it is low, see a health professional to determine whether injections of B_{12} are necessary.

Caution: Vegetarians are often misled to believe that spirulina and tempeh are good sources of vitamin B_{12}, because their labeling claims significant B_{12} content. This is due to an unfortunate quirk in the labeling law, in which B_{12} content is determined by microbiological assay; that is, how well certain bacteria grow on the product. Our laboratory demonstrated by differential radioassay that most of the "B_{12}" in spirulina and tempeh is "false B_{12}." This is not B_{12} for humans, and some of it may even block B_{12} metabolism in humans. Additionally, 10 to 30 percent of the "B_{12}" in multivitamin and vitamin-mineral pills is "false B_{12}" created by the antioxidant action on "true B_{12}" of vitamins such as C, E, and thiamine, and minerals such as iron and copper. Whether "false B_{12}" is harmful to humans is under investigation. The scientific name for "false B_{12}" is "B_{12} analogue."

Folic acid (folate) interacts with vitamin B_{12} in normal synthesis of DNA and therefore in normal production of all cells, particularly blood cells. Deficiency produces anemia. Folate is required for practically all biochemical reactions involving one-carbon transfers. Folates are present in nearly all natural foods but are highly susceptible to destruction by prolonged cooking. Essentially, no one who each day eats one fresh uncooked fruit or vegetable or fruit juice is in danger of folate deficiency. However, folate deficiency is common in low-income people who may eat only well-cooked foods, and in alcoholics. Women are particularly vulnerable because of the drain by the fetus on maternal folate stores; it is particularly common in low-income pregnant women or low-income women with more than one child. Pregnancy is one of the few situations in which folate supplements are appropriate, in the form of 0.3 milligrams (300 mg.) commercial folic acid (pteroylglutamic acid) daily. Megadoses interfere with anticonvulsants, and can produce convulsions in epileptics taking anticonvulsant medications. Megadoses also interfere with zinc absorption, and, when taken by vegetarian pregnant women, can produce zinc-deficient babies.

Pantothenic acid is involved in the metabolism of lipids, carbohydrates, and some amino acids. It is synthesized by many microorganisms, including those in the small intestine; therefore, little is needed from food. Pure dietary pantothenate deficiency in humans has been shown to occur only on semisynthetic diets virtually free of the vitamin, which is widely distributed in foods and particularly abundant in animal products, legumes, and whole-grain cereals. Otherwise, pantothenate deficiency is only seen as part of the multiple-B-vitamin deficiency of severe generalized malnutrition or chronic alcoholism. Megadoses can produce diarrhea and should not be taken.

Biotin is provided in adequate amounts by our intestinal bacteria and is never needed in the diet by normal people unless they regularly consume a diet of raw egg whites, which prevent biotin absorption.

MINERALS

Minerals are inorganic (neither animal nor vegetable) elementary (atomic particle) substances that originate in soil and water and become incorporated in varying degrees in all plant and animal life. They form the ash when animal or plant materials are burned. Once considered contaminants of foods, certain minerals are now recognized as essential in the diet for a number of vital functions and body processes, and a few more may prove, in tiny quantities, also to be essential.

In the body, a number of minerals are found in larger amounts than vitamins. In a normal adult, they make up about 4 percent of total body weight—mostly in the bones—but only small amounts are essential in the diet. Minerals needed in the largest quantity, hundreds of milligrams a day—calcium, phosphorus, magnesium—are referred to as major or macro. Those that are required in much smaller amounts are called trace or micro minerals. These trace elements include iron, zinc, iodine, copper, manganese, fluoride, chromium, selenium, molybdenum, arsenic, boron, nickel, and silicon. Probably also essential in very tiny amounts are lithium and vanadium. Arsenic, an essential nutrient in the tiniest trace amounts but a deadly poison in larger amounts, is a perfect example of what's wrong with the cliché "If some is good, more is better."

Minerals are essential in almost every body process—everything from the transport of oxygen to every body cell to regulating the heartbeat and maintaining proper fluid and chemical balances. Some minerals combine with vitamins to produce enzyme activity; others are components of enzymes and hormones.

A varied diet that includes the recommended number of daily servings from the Basic Four food groups provides ample amounts of all essential minerals. RDAs have been established for seven minerals (calcium, phosphorus, magnesium, iron, zinc, iodine, and selenium, while estimated safe and adequate amounts have been established for five others—four metals, chromium, copper, manganese, and molybdenum, and one nonmetal, fluoride.

The body is very adept at regulating proper mineral balances within a rather narrow range. If you take in more iron than you need, for example, it will not be absorbed and will be excreted intact. If your iron stores are low, however, a greater percentage than normal will be absorbed from your food. However, some people have a genetic predisposition to retain excessive amounts of certain minerals. In such cases, eating too much can create problems. Perhaps the most well-known example is sodium. Some people, especially some blacks, have a genetic predisposition to sodium-sensitive high blood pressure. Thus, if they consume too much sodium (usually in the form of table salt), instead of excreting all that is not needed, the body will retain too much. To compensate for the extra sodium, the body must also retain extra water, and this increased fluid volume can promote high blood pressure.

Another example is a genetic predisposition to absorb too much iron, present to a small degree in about 10 percent of Americans and to a severe degree, producing iron over-

load disease, in about 1 of every 250 Americans.

Even so, the most common nutritional deficiency seen in this country is for iron. Some diets also may not provide adequate calcium, especially among people who do not drink milk or consume other milk products, particularly during the first 35 years of life. Other mineral deficiencies are rare in the United States, and very few people require mineral supplements except under special circumstances.

Individual Major Minerals

Calcium. Calcium is the most plentiful mineral in the human body. An average adult man has between 950 and 1,300 grams or between about 33 ounces and 45.5 ounces (over two pounds to nearly three pounds) of calcium; the average woman has between 770 grams and 920 grams or almost 27 ounces to over 32 ounces (over one and a half pounds to two pounds) of the mineral. About 99 percent of the body's calcium is in the bones and teeth. The rest is in soft tissues and body fluids and is essential for proper nerve and muscle function, blood clotting, and other body processes.

Many people think of bones as being inert tissue. In reality, bone tissue is metabolically active, with calcium and other substances constantly moving in and out, as each day the bone surface is resolving and re-depositing. When the blood level of calcium falls below a certain point (about 10 milligrams per milliliter of blood), the bones will release enough stored calcium to increase the blood levels. If the blood levels are above about 10 or 11 milligrams per milliliter, the bones tend to absorb the excess. Lesser amounts also will be absorbed from the intestinal tract, with the extra being excreted by the kidneys. All this is a complex process requiring a hormonal form of vitamin D as well as parathyroid hormone and calcitonin—two other hormones essential in maintaining a proper calcium balance.

Milk and milk products are our best sources of calcium, constituting 72 percent of the calcium in the average American diet. Canned sardines and salmon (with the bones) also are rich in calcium. Other sources include tofu processed with calcium, dried beans and peas, broccoli, and dark green leafy vegetables (except spinach).

Inadequate calcium absorption results in rickets (stunted bone growth) in children and osteoporosis (porous, fragile bones) or osteomalacia (soft bones) in adults. Osteoporosis affects about 25 percent of America's women after age 60, and about 7 percent of men.

In recent years, the popular media has carried numerous claims alleging widespread need for calcium supplementation by women, to protect them from osteoporosis. There also have been assertions that calcium may protect against heart attacks, colon cancer, and other disorders. While it is true that some women have low calcium stores, especially if they did not consume adequate milk and milk products during their growing years, calcium supplements alone later in life do not prevent the bone loss leading to osteoporosis. Many other factors—sex (men get less osteoporosis and get it later), estrogen levels, physical activity, cigarette smoking, alcohol intake, and other dietary components, such as phosphate, fluoride, boron, manganese, and magnesium—are involved in calcium metabolism. Race also is a factor. White women of Northern European extraction are at high risk, while blacks, who tend to have more bone mass than whites, have a relatively low risk of osteoporosis.

Taking a lot of calcium supplements is not the solution to osteoporosis. An increase in dietary calcium does not necessarily mean that it will be absorbed and, once absorbed, that it will be laid down in bone rather than lost in urine and feces. In general, a healthy adult absorbs about 30 to 40 percent of the calcium in an ordinary diet. If extra calcium is consumed, the total amount absorbed tends to remain about the same. Absorption increases in times of extra need, such as during growth, pregnancy, and breastfeeding. For reasons that are not fully understood, men absorb calcium more efficiently than women. Older women absorb less than younger women and use it less efficiently in laying down bone, presumably, in part, because of the lack of estrogen after menopause.

A number of dietary factors affect calcium absorption. Excessive phosphorus or the presence of oxalic acid (a substance in cocoa, spinach, chard, rhubarb) or phytic acid (a substance in soybeans and other legumes and bran) hinder calcium absorption, but an appropriate amount of phosphorus is needed to lay down bone. A high intake of dietary fiber also may reduce calcium absorption. Inactivity also disturbs calcium metabolism, as demonstrated by the fact that bedridden people are subject to rapid bone loss and increased formation of calcium kidney stones. Calcium supplements can interfere with iron absorption, and calcium-carbonate supplements are very poorly absorbed by the elderly, who have lost gastric acid. Adding vitamin D may increase the calcium absorption, but without estrogen, the vitamin D will not be converted into its active form. Adding the active form is dangerous and should be done only under medical supervision. Bone meal and dolomite have been found too often to contain toxic amounts of lead for them to be used as calcium supplements. Excessive calcium from supplements can cause loss of appetite, nausea, vomiting, weakness, dizziness, lethargy, kidney damage, and calcium deposits in many soft tissues, including the kidneys and eyes.

(See Chapter 34 for guidelines on calcium intake.)

Phosphorus. Phosphorus is the second most abundant mineral in the body, comprising about 1 percent of body weight. About 85 percent of phosphorus is in the bones and teeth, where, in combination with calcium and fluoride, it gives hardness to these tissues. The remaining 15 percent is distributed throughout the body's soft tissues, where it is instrumental in a wide variety of body functions. Many of these functions are carried out in combination with other substances. For example, phosphorus combines with fatty acids to form phospholipids, which are components of cell membranes that help regulate the movement of certain substances in and out of cells. The lipoproteins that carry fats through the bloodstream need phosphorus, as do the substances that provide the linkages in DNA and RNA—the materials that control heredity. Phosphorus is essential as high-energy phosphate bonds in the storage and release of energy, the activation of many enzymes and the B vitamins, and numerous other metabolic processes.

Most diets provide ample phosphorus. Good sources are milk, meats, whole-grain cereals and breads, and even soft drinks containing phosphates. Calcium and phosphorus are closely related; a rise or fall in one will be reflected by a similar change in the other. Typically, we consume more phosphorus than calcium; in addition, about 70 percent of phosphorus is absorbed, compared to 30 to 40 percent of calcium. A diet that provides much more phosphorus than calcium (for example, one high in meat and low in milk and other sources of calcium) may result in reduced absorption of calcium and poor laying down of bone. "Chelated calcium," consisting of calcium and amino acids, is well absorbed but tends to be excreted in the urine, because

there is no phosphorus with it to help it deposit in bone. Milk is a good source of both calcium and phosphorus.

Magnesium. Although all living cells require magnesium, the average human body contains only about an ounce of it. About 60 percent of the body's magnesium is in bones; the rest is in soft tissues or circulating in the blood. It is needed to build bones and also is essential in the transmission of nerve impulses, muscle function, the manufacture of protein and DNA, and the release of energy from glycogen stored in the muscles.

Dietary deficiency is rare because magnesium occurs so widely in foods and drinking water (except soft water). A diet that includes regular servings of green leafy vegetables, whole grains, meat, poultry, fish or eggs, and dried beans or peas will provide adequate magnesium. Nuts, seeds, and soybeans also are good sources. Even if the diet is a bit short of magnesium, symptoms of deficiency are unusual unless there is an underlying disease that damages magnesium absorption or metabolism. For example, alcoholism, prolonged diarrhea and/or vomiting, liver or kidney disease, and severe diabetes can promote magnesium deficiency. The use of diuretics or prolonged administration of intravenous fluids that do not contain magnesium also can lead to deficiency.

Symptoms of deficiency include nausea, apathy, loss of appetite, muscle tremor, convulsions, a prickling or burning sensation, insomnia, and irregular heartbeat. Because magnesium is one of the minerals whose levels fluctuate during the menstrual cycle, magnesium deficiency has been erroneously alleged to cause premenstrual syndrome. Megadoses of magnesium can be harmful to people with poor kidney function. Elderly people with a history of frequent use of magnesium-containing antacids and laxatives experienced drowsiness, lethargy, profuse sweating, slurred speech, unsteady gait, decreased tendon reflexes, and abnormal heart rhythms.

Potassium, sodium, and chloride. These minerals are electrolytes, substances that dissociate in water into their component ions, which conduct electrical currents. Sodium and potassium ions carry positive charges and chloride ions carry negative charges. The balance between tissue fluids inside and outside of cells is maintained by the potassium ions inside and the sodium ions outside.

Potassium is necessary for all living cells. Inside the cells, it is responsible for maintaining the proper fluid balance. As a component in the fluid surrounding cells, potassium is instrumental in conducting nerve impulses. It also is essential for proper muscle function, especially of the heart. Either too much or too little potassium can result in cardiac arrhythmias. While doing nutrition research on himself,* the author of this chapter developed an almost entirely flat ECG (electrocardiogram) from dietary deprivation of potassium, corrected by potassium added to the diet. Energy release and protein and carbohydrate metabolism also require potassium.

Dehydration and excessive loss of body fluids through vomiting, diarrhea, fasting, or long-term use of diuretics or laxatives can deplete the body's potassium reserves. Diabetes, kidney disease, and severe burns also can cause potassium loss. Symptoms of deficiency include muscle weakness and paralysis, nervous disorders, slowed heartbeat, and, if severe and uncorrected, death.

A diet that provides ample fruits and vegetables will provide adequate potassium. Especially rich sources include bananas, oranges, apricots, avocados, potatoes, bran, peanuts, and dried peas and beans. Lean

*The study is described in Lawrence K. Altman's 1987 book *Who Goes First: The Story of Self-Experimentation in Medicine.*

meats, coffee, tea, and cocoa also contain potassium.

Sodium and chloride form sodium chloride, commonly known as ordinary table salt. Deficiencies of these minerals are rare. Extreme fluid loss during starvation, prolonged vomiting, diarrhea, or profuse sweating can deplete body reserves of sodium. Symptoms include muscle weakness, inability to concentrate, dehydration, and acidosis.

Excessive loss of sodium usually means a loss of chloride, as well. Babies fed a formula deficient in chloride may suffer retarded growth and psychomotor defects, which can be reversed by adding chloride to the diet.

About 20 to 25 percent of Americans are subject to hypertension. About a third of these have "salt-sensitive" hypertension. These people should be on a low-salt diet to help control their disease. Everyone should have his or her blood pressure checked every year or two to find out whether or not to restrict salt intake.

Trace Minerals

As noted earlier, trace minerals are needed in very small amounts, but even so, they are essential to many vital processes.

Iron. This is the best known and most studied of the trace minerals; its deficiency is the most widespread in the United States. An adult male has about 4 grams of iron in his body, compared to about 2.5 grams for a woman. In both sexes, most of the iron—70 to 80 percent—is found in hemoglobin, the oxygen-carrying molecule in red blood cells. About 5 percent is in myoglobin, which serves as an oxygen reservoir in the heart and skeletal muscles. Much of the remaining iron is stored in the liver, spleen, and bone marrow.

An average of 10 percent of the iron in

the diet (from about 3 percent in plant products to about 15 percent in animal products) is absorbed. A number of factors influence how much iron from the diet will actually be absorbed into the body. Heme iron—the organic kind found in animal products, especially red meat, liver, and other organ meats—is more readily absorbed than the nonheme iron in vegetables. Vitamin C consumed in the same meal promotes nonheme iron absorption; the tannins in tea, phytates from grain products, and oxalic acid hinder iron absorption. As with calcium, iron absorption increases when the body's reserves are low. Thus, a pregnant woman or someone with iron-deficiency anemia will absorb two to three times as much iron as a person who has good iron reserves.

Iron-deficiency anemia is the most common nutritional deficiency in this country. About half of those who are deficient are sufficiently so that they have anemia. The most vulnerable are young women with heavy menstrual periods, pregnant women who need extra iron for the developing fetus, or people who lose blood, for example, through injuries, surgery, or a bleeding ulcer.

Although iron deficiency is our most common nutrient shortcoming, it is not as widespread as many people believe. Only about 3 percent of American women are iron deficient, as are some infants, children up to age four, and youths, briefly, at the onset of puberty. Large numbers of people, however, take iron supplements without establishing that they are needed. Contrary to popular commercials, that "tired blood" feeling is rarely due to iron deficiency; iron overload is one of the many other things that can cause it. Excess iron is usually excreted (and can cause constipation as a side effect). However, for those people who have a genetic tendency to accumulate iron, the excess is deposited in tissues and can cause serious liver and other organ problems. (See chapters 18 and 29.) Iron supplements should not be taken unless they are specifically prescribed by a responsible health professional to correct a deficiency diagnosed by measuring blood (not hair) iron, or to meet expanded needs, as during pregnancy. Hair is dead tissue.

Most people can get all the iron they need from their diets. Vegetarians or people who do not eat much meat can increase their dietary intake by cooking acidic foods such as tomato-based chili, soups, stews, and sauces in cast-iron cookware. The acid will leach out some of the iron from the cookware, and also will promote its absorption. (Practitioners of folk medicine have long known this. For centuries, pregnant women were advised to drink beer or wine from a keg in which a rusty nail had been placed. They may not have known that the nail increased the iron content, but they did observe that it produced healthier babies.) It should be stressed, however, that modern science does not recommend alcohol during pregnancy.

Iodine. Unlike many of the other essential minerals, iodine has only one known function; It is an essential part of the basic structure of thyroid hormones. Even though the body contains a very small amount—about 25 to 50 milligrams—and the amount needed is only 150 micrograms for adults, an iodine deficiency can result in goiter in adults. This may not produce symptoms of thyroid-hormone deficiency, but babies born to women with an iodine deficiency can develop cretinism—a form of severe mental retardation—and other abnormalities. Because iodine is added to salt and is also found in a variety of foods grown in other areas, iodine deficiency is rare in the United States, even though there are areas such as around the Great Lakes and in the Pacific Northwest where the soil (and, consequently, foods grown in it) contains very little iodine. Because of the use of iodophors in the decontamination of commercial milking apparatus, milk is often a source of substantial iodine. In some parts of the world, however, iodine deficiency is still common.

Fluoride (or fluorine). This is best known for its role in protecting teeth from decay. Small amounts are added to the drinking water in many areas of the United States. It also is an ingredient in many toothpastes and mouthwashes and can be applied directly to a child's teeth. The use of fluoride has resulted in an estimated 50 to 60 percent decline in childhood cavities.

Fluoride also plays a role in maintaining bones, and hardens them when incorporated in it. Some studies suggest it may be an aid in treating osteoporosis in the elderly; population studies also indicate that osteoporosis is less common among older people who live in areas with fluoridated water. Too much is harmful.

Zinc. Zinc is another trace mineral that is needed by all living organisms. It is an essential component of many different enzymes and is involved in a variety of metabolic processes. An interesting fact is that the daily dietary requirement is about the same as for iron, and, just as the greatest single iron loss in women is in menstrual-blood flow, the greatest single zinc loss in men is in semen.

Zinc deficiency was first observed in Egypt and Iran among adolescent boys with a particular type of dwarfism and a failure to develop sexually. These boys were found to have very low blood levels of zinc. Studies of their diet found they ate mostly unleavened whole-grain bread. Ordinarily, whole-grain products are good sources of zinc, but unleavened bread also has high amounts of phytate, which binds with the zinc and prevents the body from absorbing it. When zinc was added to the diets of these boys, their growth and sexual development increased.

Since then, many other symptoms have been noted in zinc deficiency. These include poor appetite, lethargy, poor wound healing and increased susceptibility to infection, hair loss, and abnormalities in taste and smell. People most likely to develop zinc deficiency in the United States are those with malabsorption syndromes, kidney or pancreatic diseases, sickle-cell anemia, and inflammatory bowel disease.

In recent years, zinc has received increased media attention. Zinc supplements have been added to the long list recommended by food faddists or self-styled nutritionists. They are marketed as remedies for acne, impotence, lack of energy, and a variety of other problems. Very few Americans have low living-tissue levels of zinc and there is no evidence that zinc will help any of these ailments in people who have adequate living-tissue levels of the mineral. (It is impossible to diagnose a need for zinc supplements from hair analysis.) Although zinc supplements are recommended for people with established living-tissue deficiency, there is no evidence that others will benefit from them. Very large doses of zinc can cause vomiting and diarrhea; long-term use of zinc supplements also may interfere with absorption of copper and iron.

The other trace minerals—*arsenic, chromium, cobalt, copper, manganese, molybdenum, nickel, selenium, silicon, tin,* and *vanadium*—have a variety of metabolic functions, some of which are not as well understood or studied as those described above. A diet that follows the rules of moderation and variety will automatically supply enough of all these trace minerals.

8

Sugar and Salt

Delia Hammock, M.S., R.D.

■

INTRODUCTION

Sugar and salt are by far our most popular food flavorings and additives. They are used in a wide variety of prepared foods and also are ingredients that can be found in virtually every kitchen and on every dining table. Americans are not unique in their liking for foods that are sweet or salty; large amounts of salt, sugar, and other sweeteners are consumed throughout the industrialized world.

Salt may be found in a greater variety of foods than sugar, but pound for pound, Americans consume more of the latter. There is considerable debate over the effects of high consumption of sugar and salt on general health. The Dietary Guidelines presented in the first chapter of this book urge that we avoid too much of both, but there is no clear agreement as to how much is too much. In this chapter, we will discuss the role of sugar and salt in our diet and what is known about how our liking for sweet and salty foods may affect health.

SUGAR

Sugar is a popular and versatile addition to many foods. It is inexpensive, plentiful, pal-atable, and easily digested. Almost pure, the white, crystalline substance that is in daily use in our kitchens and dining rooms provides sweetness without adding other flavors. It may be eaten raw or cooked and dissolves easily in water or other liquids. It enhances the flavor of jams, jellies, and marmalades and also prevents the growth of bacteria and mold in these products. In bakery products, sugar hastens yeast fermentation necessary for the product to rise, and contributes to the flavor and crust. Sugar adds texture, bulk, and body to many foods such as beverages, custards, and meringues.

There is little doubt that Americans have a sweet tooth. Except for salt, sugar is found in more foods than any other ingredient. Sweeteners are a common—and expected— ingredient in many of the foods we eat—soft drinks, cookies, and candy. However, they are also a hidden ingredient in many foods and even medications where we don't expect them—catsup, cereals, canned soups, salad dressings. Despite its virtues and prevalence in our diets, the consumption of sweeteners, especially sugar, has been linked to poor health, with critics alleging it leads to diabetes, behavioral disorders, tooth decay, and other maladies.

Sugars comprise a group of water-soluble

carbohydrates that, like other carbohydrates, are composed of carbon, hydrogen, and oxygen atoms. Sunlight, acting on the chlorophyll of green plants in the process called photosynthesis, converts these basic building blocks into molecules that have as their general formula 6 atoms of carbon, 12 of hydrogen, and 6 of oxygen ($C_6H_{12}O_6$). Every carbohydrate, whether it be starch, table sugar, or cellulose, is composed of this basic unit. Although these three elements are always present, the arrangement of atoms in the molecule varies, giving different carbohydrates different characteristics. The production of sugars in plants becomes the basis of the animal food chain.

Saccharides, the scientific term for sugars, are a group of carbohydrates, most of which are sweet-tasting. The simplest sugars—glucose, fructose, and galactose—are individual molecules known as monosaccharides. Disaccharides—sucrose, maltose, and lactose—are composed of two molecules of monosaccharide joined by chemical bonds. For example, sucrose is composed of one molecule of glucose plus one of fructose. (See list on page 114.)

Throughout the remainder of this chapter, the term *sugar* will be used to refer to any nutritive sweetener (one that adds calories) unless a specific saccharide is indicated.

THE BODY'S USE OF SUGARS

Regardless of the type or source, all digestible dietary carbohydrates are converted by the body to glucose, the primary fuel of cellular energy. Enzymes in saliva and the small intestine attack chemical bonds linking disaccharides or starches together in order to yield molecules of monosaccharides, primarily glucose. Consequently, simple sugars, the end products of digestion, are absorbed into the bloodstream from the cells of the small intestine. Glucose in the circulation elicits the release of the pancreatic hormone—insulin—which has an important function in controlling the metabolism of carbohydrates, protein, and fats. (For more information, see Chapter 28.) Glucose then enters the cells, where it can be used immediately for energy, converted by the cells of the liver or muscles to glycogen for storage, or metabolized into triglycerides, a form of fat. Unlike many substances, excess glucose is not excreted from the body; glucose not needed for energy production or body stores of glycogen is converted into body fat. Whenever external sources of food are not available and blood glucose falls below the optimal level, body reserves of glycogen are converted to glucose for energy. After stores of glycogen have been exhausted, fat stores may also be used as fuel energy.

THE HISTORY OF SUGAR

Studies of human infants and other animals species have shown that the taste for sugar and other sweeteners is innate and unrelated to the nutritive value of the sweetening agent. Because it is clearly pleasurable to eat them, people throughout history have eagerly and actively sought out sweet foods and beverages.

Although carbohydrates from plants and naturally occurring sugars from sources such as honey and dates have contributed to the diet of man since prehistoric times, the inclusion of refined sugars is more recent. Sugar was probably first produced in Southeast Asia from the juice of sugarcane, a giant grass. The first written records mentioning sugar can be traced to the time of Alexander the Great, who encountered it in India in 325 B.C.

Europeans first used sugar, like spices, for medicinal purposes during medieval times and later demanded greater quantities for dietary consumption. Sugar cultivation and refinement played a major role in the colonization of the Americas, particularly by the Spanish, English, Portuguese, and Dutch. In the 1700s, a brisk traffic (and slave trade) revolved around the increasing demands by the European market for sugar produced in the West Indies. Rum, produced from the residues of the sugar-making process, became a popular by-product. During the time of Napoleon, a European sugar industry based on the discovery of beet sugar reduced the dependence of Europe on maritime commerce and colonies that were by then largely controlled by the British.

SUGAR AND HEALTH

Theories concerning the relationship between sugar ingestion and disease abound. The association between sugary foods and dental caries (tooth decay), long suspected, has been proven. Sugars and other carbohydrates are converted by normal bacteria in the mouth to an acid that attacks tooth enamel. When such substances remain in contact with the teeth for a long period of time, an increase in dental caries results. Studies on infants showed that the practice of giving children bottles of juice, milk, and other fluids containing sugars (milk is high in lactose, or milk sugar, and juices contain fructose) at nap or bedtime correlated with tooth decay, whereas the consumption of sugar during normal mealtimes was not found to have a marked cariogenic effect.

A committee established by the Food and Drug Administration concluded that several factors contribute to dental caries: a caries-producing bacteria, a "susceptible target," and an environment that promotes the growth of bacteria. Good dental hygiene, reduction of snacks between meals, and fluoride—in water, toothpaste, mouthwashes, supplements, and applied to the teeth directly, which increases the decay-resistance of tooth

Monosaccharides and Disaccharides

The following is a list of the different sugars according to their chemical grouping.

MONOSACCHARIDES

Glucose: Also called dextrose, this is the substance measured in blood and urine laboratory tests. It is one of the sugars found in fruits, honey, and vegetables, but it is not very sweet.
Fructose: Sometimes called fruit sugar, this contains the same chemical formula as glucose, but its different arrangement of atoms stimulate the taste buds differently. It is perceived as being very sweet.
Galactose: Seldom found alone in nature, this sugar is one of the molecules that makes up disaccharide lactose.

DISACCHARIDES

Sucrose: Common table sugar, this disaccharide is composed of molecules of glucose and fructose bonded chemically. Its principal food sources are sugarcane and sugar beets, but sucrose is also found in honey, many fruits, and some vegetables.
Lactose: This is the principal carbohydrate in milk and dairy products. When broken down by the digestive enzyme lactase, molecules of glucose and galactose are produced.
Maltose: Also called malt sugar, this disaccharide, composed of two molecules of glucose, is present briefly during seed germination in plants.

enamel—have proven to be effective in reducing the problem. (See Chapter 37.)

Despite much research, the link between sugar and dental caries is the only detriment to health that has been substantiated by scientific evidence.

Effects on Behavior

In recent years, a number of claims have been put forth stating that a high intake of sugar can result in a variety of behavioral problems, ranging from hyperactivity and learning problems to criminal acts. Explanations of how sugar produces these behaviors vary. Some claim that it produces changes in the production of certain brain neurotransmitters that are associated with activity, resulting in the restlessness and other characteristics of hyperactivity. Others have proposed that a diet high in sugars stimulates excess insulin production, which then lowers blood sugar (hypoglycemia) and increases production of adrenaline, a hormone associated with hyperactivity. Despite the widespread publicity accorded these claims, numerous studies have failed to link hyperactivity in children and sugar consumption. The association between criminal behavior and ingestion of refined sugars, the so-called Twinkie defense, has also not been substantiated. In 1986, a task force commissioned by the Food and Drug Administration to investigate the health aspects of sugars concluded; ". . . there is no substantial evidence that the consumption of sugars is responsible for behavioral changes in children or in adults with the exception of relatively rare hypoglycemias due to abnormal metabolism."

If there is no valid evidence that sugar affects behavior, why do so many people insist that is does? There is no simple answer. For one thing, the behavioral symptoms attributed to sugar are vague and hard to pinpoint. If a complete medical examination and tests fail to find a cause for the symptoms, there's a tendency to seek an explanation in environmental factors, with diet (and more specifically, sugar) being only one of many. (Interestingly, the warm southern winds that sweep through parts of Europe in the summer often are blamed for the very same effects as sugar, and in some countries, these winds are accepted as a defense for murder!)

Historically, the notion that sugar has an effect on behavior goes back to before the turn of the century. Doctors of that era often advised their patients that eating refined sugar could trigger bad tempers and bring out "animalistic instincts." In a few years, however, the notion died out, only to be revived in the middle of this century by the actress Gloria Swanson's best-selling book *Sugar Blues* (written with her husband, Bill Dufty), in which she attributed her many emotional and medical problems to refined sugar, but said that raw cane sugar was fine. Robert Rodale, Adele Davis, and others picked up on the theme, and their large popular following can be credited with many of the misconceptions about sugar that persist to this day. It should be stressed that none of these writers conducted objective, scientifically controlled studies to demonstrate behavioral effects of sugar. Instead, they relied upon anecdotal accounts and personal impressions and opinions— highly subjective criteria that have no value as scientific proof.

In the early 1980s, Dr. Judith Rapoport and her colleagues at the National Institute of Mental Health set out to demonstrate whether or not sugar had any effect on behavior. They placed advertisements in Washington, D.C., papers seeking out parents who felt their children's hyperactivity or other behavior problems were due to sugar. As a result, 36 children were enlisted for a double-blind controlled study. In this type of study, neither the researcher nor the volunteer knows who is getting a placebo and who the real thing. The children were divided into groups; some were given high doses of sugar disguised with lemon, others were given drinks containing lemon but no sugar, and a third group was given a placebo. The groups were rotated, so eventually each child would have all three types of drinks.

Each child was put in a room where his or her behavior could be observed after each administration of the drinks. After receiving the sugar drinks, there was no increase in hyperactivity or other changes in behavior among any of the children. Indeed, the only noticeable difference was that some of the children receiving the sugar drinks were more drowsy afterward than the others—obviously, the opposite effect to that which the sugar was supposed to have.

Even though these results have been published in the scientific literature and noted in the popular media, many people remain unconvinced. However, until their beliefs can be confirmed by controlled studies, these beliefs have no more validity than the notion that a warm wind can bring on murderous rages.

Diabetes

Diabetes mellitus is a disorder of metabolism in which a deficiency of the hormone insulin or insulin receptors results in excess glucose in the bloodstream and in the urine. The disease is classified according to whether the patient requires insulin injections for control (commonly referred to as Type I or juvenile diabetes because it often appears in childhood) or can be managed by diet and oral drugs (Type II or adult-onset diabetes). Two factors—obesity and heredity—are thought to be key elements in determining whether an adult will develop diabetes. Although all insulin-dependent diabetics must adjust their intake of carbohydrates, especially sweets, to control blood sugar (or increase the insulin dosages to compensate for the added carbohydrates), there is no evidence to support the popular misconception that eating too much sugar *causes* this disease. (For more information see Chapter 28.)

Hypoglycemia

Ninety-five percent of healthy adults have normal blood-sugar (glucose) levels ranging between 70 and 120 milligrams per deciliter. Hypoglycemia, defined as blood-sugar levels below 40 milligrams per deciliter, is an uncommon occurrence that may be associated with several different disorders, only a few of which are related to diet. As the blood-glucose level decreases, the brain, which requires glucose for fuel, is affected, resulting in confusion, weakness, dizziness, tremors, irregular heartbeat, and nervousness.

The theory is that ingestion of a large amount of sugar can cause a sudden rise in blood-glucose levels, stimulating the secretion of excessive amounts of insulin. According to this theory, reactive (a reaction to food) hypoglycemia then occurs as the extra insulin rapidly lowers the blood glucose to hypoglycemic levels. In addition, adrenaline flow is stimulated by insulin, causing nervousness and hyperactivity.

To test this theory, numerous studies of glucose levels in individuals before and after consuming meals high in sugars and other carbohydrates were conducted. Hypoglycemic levels of blood glucose *accompanied by the other hallmarks* of this disorder were only rarely detected. Furthermore, studies show that table sugar causes no more of a rise in blood sugar than other carbohydrates, such as bread and rice. (See Chapter 28.) Thus, it is highly doubtful that normal, healthy persons are affected in this way by sugar consumption.

Obesity

Contrary to what many believe, eating foods high in sugar does not cause obesity, nor does the craving for sweet foods cause individuals to overeat, resulting in obesity.

When metabolized, carbohydrates, including sugar, produce four calories per gram, the same number as protein. In contrast, fats produce nine calories per gram. While sugar itself is no more fattening than protein or complex carbohydrates, it is often combined with fats to produce sweet, high-fat (and consequently, high-calorie) foods. Pastries, cookies, chocolate, candy, ice cream, and whipped cream are but a few examples. Remember, too, that when more calories are ingested than are needed for muscular, metabolic, and digestive activities, the excess calories are stored as fat. Thus, overeating foods of any type leads to the production and storage of body fat. Interestingly, several studies have shown that, on the average, obese individuals actually consume less sugar than thin people. (See Chapter 17.)

Cardiovascular Disease

Diseases of the heart and blood vessels, the leading cause of death in the United States, are associated with a number of risk factors, including some (e.g., high blood cholesterol) that are linked to diet. In the past, there have been claims that sugar may increase the risk of a heart attack, but research has failed to document this. Indeed, most researchers agree that studies fail to show any relationship between sugar intake and the risk of heart disease.

Effects on Healing

Folk medicine has long recognized that sugar, when applied to wounds, can halt infection and promote healing. Researchers in the United States have confirmed this effect. For the same reasons that sugar is effective in preventing bacterial growth in foods, sugar solutions applied directly to the infection site can promote healing, often with minimal scarring. (It should be noted, however, that sugar solutions should not be considered a medical alternative to prescribed antibiotics.)

SUGAR IN THE DIET

Despite what many people believe, sugar is not the villain that robs us of our health: Most claims identifying it as a harmful substance have been refuted by scientific evidence. Still, as stressed in Chapter 1, a diet high in sugars is not recommended, especially if sweets substitute for other, more nutritious foods. Sugar contains calories, and thus is a source of energy, but it is devoid of vitamins and minerals—essential components of a healthy diet. A pound of sugar contains about 2,000 calories—enough energy to see the average person through the day. However, sugar supplies little or none of the other important nutrients that we need each day. For this reason, sugar is said to provide only "empty calories," placing the nutrient burden on the remaining foods. Thus, a person whose diet consists mostly of candies and other sweets, soft drinks (or alcoholic beverages), cakes, cookies, and other sweets can quickly consume all the calories needed, but nothing else in the way of needed nutrition. Clearly, sweets should not replace dietary sources of carbohydrates such as grains, fruits, and vegetables, which help supply the daily requirements of protein, vitamins, and minerals.

How much sugar is acceptable? The Dietary Guidelines from the United States Department of Agriculture do not specify a recommended daily allowance for sugar. However, the U.S. Dietary Goals, written by a government-appointed committee in 1977, recommended that added sugar (and/or corn syrup and other sweeteners) should supply no more than 10 percent of daily calories. A 1986 study by the FDA based on a national food-consumption survey concluded that Americans receive an average of about 21 percent of their total calories from sugars, of which naturally occurring sugars, such as those in fruit, milk, and vegetables, contribute 10 percent, and added sugars 11 percent. It is important to note that average figures fail to distinguish individual differences in consumption; while some people consume very little sugar, heavy users derive about 20 percent or more of their total calories from added sugars.

Studies show that overall consumption of sugars and other sweeteners in the United States has increased approximately 14 percent between 1965 and 1985. (The consumption of noncaloric sweeteners tripled in the same period.) During these years, the types of sugars consumed and the pattern of usage have changed dramatically. As a result of increased consumer dependence on prepared foods, it is the food industry, not the individual, that to a large extent currently controls the sugars in the diet.

Prior to the 1970s, manufacturers relied almost entirely on cane and beet sugars for their products. An examination of food labels today reveals many varieties of sweeteners. One of these products, high-fructose corn syrup, now accounts for a substantial portion of the market, especially in the soft-drink industry, where it predominates. As its name implies, high-fructose corn syrup is derived from the starch in corn, which is treated with enzymes to form sugars, predominantly fructose and glucose. This sweetener, which costs 10 to 40 percent less than sucrose, accounts for more than half of the U.S. market for nutritive sweeteners. (See Table 8.1.)

What's in a Label?

The presence of added sugars is not always apparent by reading food labels. There are many different sweeteners—both caloric

Table 8.1.   Changes in Sugar Consumption

Refined Sugar (Sucrose) per Capita Consumption	
1909	73.7 lbs.
1930	109.6 lbs.
1951	94.0 lbs.
1960	97.6 lbs.
1970	101.7 lbs.
1980	83.7 lbs.
1985	63.4 lbs.
1987	62.4 lbs.
Corn Sweetener per Capita Consumption	
1960	11.6 lbs.
1970	19.3 lbs.
1980	40.2 lbs.
1984	57.8 lbs.
1985	65.0 lbs.
1987	68.8 lbs.
Noncaloric Sweetener (Tabulated according to sweetness equivalency to refined sugar. Sweetness is much greater than refined sugar; therefore, actual poundage consumed is much lower.)	
1955	2.0 lbs.
1960	2.2 lbs.
1965	5.7 lbs.
1970	5.8 lbs.
1975	6.2 lbs.
1980	7.7 lbs.
1981	8.2 lbs.
1982	9.4 lbs.
1983	13.0 lbs.
1984	15.8 lbs.
1985	17.0 lbs.
1987	19.0 lbs.

Note: All figures are based on USDA disappearance data. These statistics are an overestimate of actual consumption because they do not reflect food lost to spoilage or waste.

and noncaloric—that are added to foods. The box below lists some of the more common ones.

The terms *sugar-free* or *sugarless* on a food label means that the product contains neither sucrose nor any other calorie-containing sweetener. It may, however, contain one of the sugar alcohols, sorbitol, xylitol, or mannitol, which, though technically not sweeteners, contain the same number of calories as sugar.

REDUCING SUGAR IN THE DIET

Even though sugar may not be the evil that some would have us believe, many people may benefit from reducing its consumption. As noted earlier, the calories from sugar are nutritionally empty, so anyone who has a weight problem can benefit from cutting down on sweets, especially those that are also high in fats. Noncaloric artificial sweeteners can, in some applications, substitute for caloric sweeteners, but there are also other ways of cutting sugar calories. Food producers, responding to consumer demand, are marketing canned and frozen unsweetened fruits and fruit juices as well as low-sugar jams, jellies, and preserves.

Tasty sauces, breading mixtures, soups, and salad dressings can be prepared at home without added sugar. Fresh fruits and fruit purees can substitute for sugary desserts. Seltzer and club soda, plain or sweetened with fruit juices, are good low-calorie alternatives to sugar-laden, high-calorie soft drinks.

"Natural" sugars are superior to white sugar only when the natural sugar comes as a component of a nutrient-rich food. For example, fruit contains natural sugar, but this sugar comes packaged with vitamins, minerals, and fiber. Also, since fruit is 80 to 90 percent water, fruit provides an excellent nutritional return on your caloric investment. However, if the sugar from fruit is concentrated and this

Identifying Added Sugars

The following are sugars commonly encountered on product labels:

Corn syrups: Derived from cornstarch that has been enzymatically treated to yield sucrose, fructose, and glucose in varying amounts.

Dextrose: Another name for glucose, commercially produced from cornstarch that has been treated with heat and acids or enzymes.

Fructose: Naturally occurring fruit sugar.

Glucose: See dextrose. Also refers to blood sugar, the body's main fuel.

Honey: A distinctive-tasting sweetener, produced by bees from the nectar of flowers and consisting predominantly of fructose and glucose.

Lactose: Principal sugar found in milk, also used in pharmaceutical products.

Maltose: Disaccharide found in germinating seed.

Mannitol, Sorbitol, Xylitol: Sugar alcohol, derived from fruits or produced from dextrose, found in many foods accepted in diabetic diets.

Maple Sugar and Syrup: Products of the sap of the maple tree that turn sweet after boiling.

Molasses: Concentrates that remain after sucrose is extracted from sugarcane. Blackstrap molasses is the product that remains after the extraction process has been performed three times, leaving a strong-tasting syrup that is lower in sucrose content but higher in other nutrients.

Sucrose: Refined from beets or sugarcane. Comes in granulated and powdered forms. Includes raw sugar, turbinado sugar, brown sugar, and invert sugar.

fruit sugar or fruit syrup is used to sweeten such other foods as cookies and muffins, the benefits are lost. Contrary to popular belief, when fruit sugar is concentrated, the nutrients in the fruit are not concentrated in the fruit sugar. Thus, cookies sweetened with fruit-juice concentrate, for example, have no health benefits over cookies sweetened with table sugar.

Club soda with a splash of fruit juice is recommended over a sweetened carbonated beverage simply because the club soda and fruit-juice mixture supplies fewer calories ounce for ounce and the fruit juice supplies small amounts of nutrients, as well.

For some strange reason, people tend to think that foods that are white (white sugar, white bread, white flour, white rice) are bad, while foods that are brown (whole-wheat flour and bread, brown rice, honey, molasses, brown sugar, raw sugar, etc.) are good. This is nonsense. Aside from the fair amounts of some minerals in blackstrap molasses, none contributes significant amounts of any vitamins and minerals.

The FDA does not allow raw sugar to be sold in the United States because of the impurities it contains. The product Sugar in the Raw is not raw sugar.

Brown sugar is simple white sugar crystals coated with molasses.

Honey is another of those "natural" foods surrounded by more myth and mystique than reality. Actually, it differs very little from sucrose. While table sugar is pure sucrose, honey is a mixture of sugars (fructose, glucose, sucrose, etc.) formed from nectar by an enzyme—honey invertase—present in the bodies of bees. Honey varies in composition and flavor, depending on the source of the nectar (clove, orange blossom, etc.). It does contain trace amounts of some minerals, but the amounts are insignificant. A tablespoon of table sugar contains 46 calories; a tablespoon of honey contains 64.

ALTERNATIVE SWEETENERS

Worldwide, there is an enormous demand for substances other than sucrose that impart a sweet taste to foods. Concern about weight control has caused many to seek low-calorie alternatives to sucrose. Sugar's association with tooth decay has prompted a need for sweet substances that cannot be metabolized by the caries-producing bacteria of the mouth. In the United States alone, there are more than 6 million people with diabetes who must avoid concentrated sweets as part of their dietary regimen. There are also large numbers of people who turn to sugar substitutes in the belief (albeit mistaken) that these products will reduce the risk of heart attack, diabetes, and other diseases.

Sugar substitutes (which contain no sucrose) can be divided into two categories: nutritive sweeteners, which supply calories; and nonnutritive or artificial sweeteners, which do not add appreciable calories to the diet.

Nutritive Sweeteners

Nutritive sweeteners include corn syrup, fructose, invert sugar, maltodextrin, maltose, sorbitol, and xylitol. These products are primarily used in commercially produced food products.

Fructose

Fructose, or fruit sugar, a monosaccharide that along with glucose makes up sucrose, has the same number of calories as other carbohydrates. Since it occurs naturally in fruit, it is often touted as a natural replacement for ordinary table sugar. However, the powdered fructose available in stores is produced from sucrose or cornstarch—not from fruit.

Fructose's use as an aid to weight loss has also been greatly overstated. The argument posits that because fructose is sweeter than sucrose, less would be needed—and therefore fewer calories would be used—to achieve the same sweetening effect with fewer calories. However, the intensity of fructose's sweetness depends on how it is used in foods and beverages. For example, one study showed that while fructose was sweeter than sugar when used in lemonade, it was not perceived as sweeter in cookies, cakes, or pudding.

Fructose is sometimes recommended for use by certain diabetics because it is absorbed more slowly than glucose or sucrose, thereby producing a slower rise in blood sugar. Even so, fructose should not be used indiscriminately by those with severe insulin deficiency. Although its initial uptake does not require insulin, this hormone is required for metabolism of fructose.

Sugar Alcohols

Sugar alcohols, substances derived from monosaccharides, include xylitol, sorbitol, mannitol, and lycasin. These sweeteners also have the same number of calories as sugar, but because they are not metabolized by cavity-producing bacteria, they are noncariogenic. Some of them are less sweet than sugar and most have a laxative effect when used in substantial amounts. Sorbitol, the most commonly used sugar alcohol, is often the sweetener used in "sugar-free" candies. Sweets containing sorbitol are generally no lower in calories than their sugar-laden counterparts.

Nonnutritive (Artificial) Sweeteners

The major nonnutritive sweeteners—cyclamate, saccharin, aspartame—are many times sweeter than sugar and therefore add sweetness with only negligible calories. However, all have been the subject of intense public and scientific debate. Presently only aspartame has official FDA approval, although the use of saccharin is allowed under special congressional action pending further studies, and cyclamate is being reevaluated after having been removed from the approved list in 1969. Despite the controversy surrounding artificial sweeteners, the case against these products is considered by many to be unimpressive. All have been investigated thoroughly with regard to cancer-causing potential and a wide variety of other possible toxic effects. Numerous studies by private and governmental agencies have failed to link these sweeteners with adverse health effects in normal individuals.

Saccharin

Saccharin, discovered in 1879, has the distinction of being the first artificial sweetener. It is probably also the most widely distributed and is now available in approximately 80 countries. Despite the fact that millions of people have consumed this product and its safety has been scrutinized since the early 1900s, controversy still surrounds its use. Concern over experimental data showing a relationship between bladder tumors and consumption of massive amounts of saccharin by rats prompted the FDA to announce in 1977 plans to ban it. At that time, saccharin was the only artificial sweetener available in the United States, and public outcry was immediate and widespread. In response, Congress passed a moratorium on the FDA action, which has since been extended several times. The debate continues, but most experts feel that if there is a risk of cancer in people who consume saccharine-containing products, the risk is very small. In 1985, the American

Medical Association reiterated its support for the sweetener but recommended continual monitoring and evaluation of consumption, especially in young children and pregnant women, since data concerning the effect of saccharin on these groups is very limited.

Even though it is 300 times as sweet as sugar, saccharin provides no calories: It is a petroleum derivative that passes through the body and is not absorbed. Since it does not affect blood sugar, it is popular with diabetics and is widely used in dietetic foods, soft drinks, and nonnutritive table sweeteners. Although generally heat stable, saccharin does not provide the bulk and texture characteristic of sugar. Another drawback—its bitter aftertaste—is somewhat overcome by its use in conjunction with other sweeteners.

Aspartame

Aspartame, marketed under the brand names of Equal and NutraSweet, was discovered in 1965 but was not approved for use until 1981, following years of investigation. Composed of two naturally occurring amino acids—aspartic acid and phenylalanine—aspartame is 200 times as sweet as sugar, has a pleasant taste that enhances flavors, and does not promote tooth decay. Although aspartame cannot be used for cooking because it breaks down when heated, it is widely used in carbonated soft drinks, cereal, gelatin desserts, and instant coffee, tea, and cocoa mixes. Aspartame also is frequently used in conjunction with saccharin because it masks the aftertaste of that product.

Despite FDA approval, extensive testing, and acceptance by numerous health organizations here and abroad, questions still regularly arise about the safety of aspartame. A number of people have filed complaints about a wide range of symptoms that they have attributed to the consumption of this sweetener. The Centers for Disease Control (CDC) determined that a wide range of reported symptoms followed no specific pattern, were generally mild, and also common among people who do *not* use aspartame. The agency concluded that the data "do not provide evidence for the existence of serious, widespread, adverse health consequences," although they acknowledged the possibility that some people may be unusually sensitive to the sweetener. Therefore, people who experience symptoms that seem related to aspartame may be advised to avoid its use.

There also has been concern over the use of aspartame by people who suffer from seizures. Some scientists are concerned that large amounts of aspartame consumed with carbohydrates may affect certain brain neurotransmitters, causing subtle behavioral changes and possibly increasing the risk of seizure in epileptics. However, the Food and Drug Administration has concluded that the available data do not support this hypothesis. Furthermore, the Epilepsy Institute has found no increase in seizure activity among its patients, many of whom use aspartame regularly. Similarly, there have been claims that aspartame may cause brain changes and retardation, but there are no data with regard to humans to support these claims.

The FDA continues to review consumer complaints, and focused clinical studies are also being conducted in an attempt to identify any possible sensitivity to aspartame. The FDA has set an Acceptable Daily Intake of aspartame at 50 milligrams per kilogram (slightly over 22.7 milligrams per pound) of body weight. Under these guidelines, an 150-pound adult could consume about 20 cans of aspartame-sweetened soda and a 50-pound child could drink about 7 cans. Since the average person is unlikely to consume anywhere near this much, the amount would seem to have a large built-in safety factor.

There is one population group for whom aspartame does pose a hazard, namely those with the inherited metabolic disorder known as phenylketonuria (PKU). These individuals lack the enzyme necessary to metabolize the amino acid phenylalanine, one of the components of aspartame, and toxic levels can build up in their blood and tissues. Products containing aspartame contain a warning label to alert people with PKU to avoid them.

Acesulfame K

The calorie-free sweetener Acesulfame K was approved by the FDA in the summer of 1988 for use in the United States. Sold under the name Sunette, it is 200 times sweeter than sugar. It is available in packet form or tablets, and as an ingredient in chewing gums, gelatin, pudding mixes, dry beverage mixes, instant coffee, instant tea, and in nondairy creamers. It also can be added to food before cooking or baking.

New Low-Calorie Sweeteners

A number of new low-calorie sweeteners are undergoing safety testing aimed at achieving FDA approval for general marketing. These include L-Sugars, alitame, and sucralose. Several have been approved in other countries. Most of these substances are many times sweeter than sucrose, and do not cause dental cavities. These new substances have the added advantage of not breaking down when heated, allowing their use in cooking.

Other countries whose regulations differ from those in the United States have approved the use of several high-intensity natural sweeteners extracted from the leaves, fruits, or berries of certain South American or African plants. Included in this group are sweeteners such as stevioside, a substance 300 times as sweet as sucrose; miraculin, a protein extracted from a West African fruit that alters the taste of anything sour, making it taste intensely sweet; and thaumatin, also a protein sweetener, which has been approved for use in England and Japan.

SALT

Historical Perspective

Salt is essential for all animal life. Scientists theorize that life began in the primordial seas, which were less salty than today's oceans. When the first primitive animals climbed ashore, they took with them within their cells this dilute seawater environment. To this day, the salt content of the human body is about the same as that of these ancient seas.

History attests to man's dependence on salt through the ages. Settlements grew up around salt deposits and ancient caravans carried salt many miles across African deserts. In ancient Greece, laborers and soldiers took part of their wages in salt, and wars have been fought over salt taxes. During medieval times, herds were slaughtered in autumn and the meat preserved by salting or smoking, the only methods known to preserve food. More recently, in India, salt was the focus of one of Ghandi's most effective attacks on British rule, when he and his followers successfully protested a government monopoly on salt production.

Salt may be extracted from seawater or mined in the abundant deposits in the earth left by ancient seas. Modern methods of processing and refining make salt both inexpensive and widely available.

RELATIONSHIP BETWEEN SALT AND SODIUM

Salt is a mineral composed of sodium and chloride. By weight, 39 percent of salt is sodium and 61 percent chloride. While chloride is also of importance in the body, it is sodium that has received the most attention because of its link with high blood pressure.

The amount of sodium contained in a substance is usually expressed in grams, milligrams, or, in the case of prescription drugs, milliequivalents. (For a list of sodium conversions, see Table 8.2.)

Sodium occurs naturally in many foods. In addition, it is used in baking, as a preservative in foods such as sausages, pickles, and bacon, and as a flavor enhancer added during cooking or at the table. Drinking water and over-the-counter drugs may also contain significant amounts of sodium.

FUNCTION OF SODIUM IN THE BODY

Body fluids, composed primarily of water and salts, provide the medium in which most biochemical reactions take place. Although each of the fluids is continually being lost and replaced, their composition remains remarkably constant. The concentration of sodium is an important factor in controlling the movement of fluid in and out of cells.

When dissolved in water, salt separates into electrically charged particles of sodium and chloride called ions. Sodium ions are the major cations, or positively charged ions, of the body fluid found outside the cells. Sodium ions in the extracellular fluid must balance the number of potassium ions inside the cell in order to regulate the flow of fluids. When the level of either sodium ions or potassium ions

gets out of balance, water shifts by osmosis to the area of highest concentration of ions and proper cell function may be impaired.

In addition to its pivotal role in controlling fluid flow, sodium plays an important role in other body processes:

- Control of blood volume.

- Maintenance of body acid-base balance through chemical reactions that counteract acids formed during metabolism.

- Transmission of electrical nerve impulses.

- Muscle contractions, including heart muscle.

- Contraction of blood vessels in response to nervous stimulation or certain hormones.

- Absorption of glucose and transport of other nutrients across membranes, especially the intestine.

Table 8.2.   Calculating the Amount of Sodium

1 gram of salt = 0.39 gm. or 390 mg. of sodium (weight of salt × .39 = weight of sodium).

1 gram of sodium is contained in 2.5 gm. or 2,500 mg. of salt (weight of sodium × 2.5 = weight of salt).

1 milligram of sodium = 1/23 milliequivalents (mEq) sodium (weight of sodium ÷ atomic weight [23] of sodium = mEq sodium).

1 milliequivalent of sodium = 23 mg. sodium or 58.5 mg. salt (mEq sodium × 23 = mg. of sodium).

1 teaspoon salt = 2.1 gm. sodium.

REGULATION OF SODIUM LEVELS

Regulation of sodium in the body involves both the control of sodium retention and the control of sodium loss. Dietary sodium is absorbed primarily in the small intestine and from there passes into the bloodstream and throughout the body. Bone appears to be a storage site for approximately 40 percent of the body's sodium, with 50 percent circulating in the blood and 10 percent contained in cells. In healthy persons, only a small portion of the total amount of sodium consumed is needed and the excess is excreted primarily through the kidneys, although some sodium is also lost through perspiration. Thus, sodium loss is ordinarily balanced by daily intake and only the composition of the urine is affected by the amount of salt consumed.

In certain conditions, this equilibrium between salt and water may become unbalanced. For example, low concentrations of sodium in the blood, or hyponatremia, can occur as the result of prolonged vomiting, diarrhea, excessive sweating, or certain types of kidney disease. Both water and sodium must be replenished to maintain the balance between intracellular and extracellular fluids.

Hypernatremia, increased blood sodium, is seen when there is excessive water loss from the body, thus making the sodium more concentrated, or when excess sodium is retained. The high sodium level causes the body to conserve water in an effort to decrease the concentration. This explains why patients with kidney disease who cannot remove excess sodium have swelling (edema) of the face, legs, and feet. Hypernatremia does not occur in normal individuals who consume excess salt, because many body regulatory processes, including the thirst mechanism, maintain internal balance.

RECOMMENDED INTAKE OF SODIUM

Throughout the world, the consumption of sodium varies greatly, in part because of the variation in the cuisines of different cultures. Orientals, who use a great deal of soy sauce and monosodium glutamate, have very high levels of sodium intake. Some primitive groups living in nonindustrialized societies consume much less. The average American consumes from 2,300 to 6,900 milligrams of sodium daily, the amount in about one to three teaspoons of salt. Sources of sodium in the diet include naturally occurring sodium in food and water (25 to 40 percent), sodium added during processing of food (40 to 50 percent), and salt added during cooking or at the table (25 to 40 percent).

For healthy individuals, sodium requirements vary depending upon climate and humidity, physical activity, and the amount of potassium in the diet. People lose an estimated 115 milligrams per day in urine, feces, and sweat.

The daily dietary sodium requirement for humans has not been established; however, experts unanimously agree that the average American diet far exceeds the need for sodium. While only a relatively small percentage of people are sodium-sensitive, the total number runs in the millions. Since there is no test for sodium-sensitivity, the Food and Nutrition Board of the National Academy of Sciences considers 500 milligrams of sodium a safe minimum intake for adults, and 2.4 grams of sodium chloride (about one teaspoon of salt) a safe maximum for people not susceptible to hypertension.

Table 8.3. Common Foods High in Sodium

Food	Portion	Milligrams of Sodium
MEATS		
Bacon, cooked	3 slices	303
Canadian-style bacon	2 slices (1½ oz.)	711
Corned beef, cooked	3 oz.	964
Bologna	1 oz. slice	289
Ham, cured, roasted	3 oz.	908
Ham, chopped	1 oz.	387
Frankfurter, cooked	1 average	504
Pork sausage, cooked	1 oz. patty	349
Salami, cooked	1 oz.	302
Beef, dried, chipped	1 oz.	984
Pepperoni	5 slices (1 oz.)	560
FISH AND SHELLFISH		
Anchovies, canned	5 (20 gm.)	734
Caviar, black & red	1 T	240
Cod, dried and salted	1 oz.	1968
Lox	1 oz.	570
Salmon, pink, canned	3 oz.	471
Tuna, oil or water-packed	3 oz. (drained)	317
Herring, pickled	3 oz.	850
Sardines, packed in oil, drained	3 oz.	425
SOUPS		
(Canned, condensed, prepared with equal amount of water)		
Bean with bacon	1 cup	951
Beef broth	1 cup	782
Beef noodle	1 cup	952
Chicken noodle	1 cup	1106
Minestrone	1 cup	911
Mushroom	1 cup	1032
Tomato	1 cup	871
Vegetable beef	1 cup	956
VEGETABLES		
Asparagus, canned	6 spears	278
Beans, green, canned	½ cup	170
Corn, canned, kernels	½ cup	285
Corn, canned, cream style	½ cup	365
Mixed vegetables, canned	½ cup	122
Mushrooms, canned	½ cup	332
Peas, canned	½ cup	186
Potatoes au gratin (with cheese)	½ cup	530
Potatoes, mashed, with milk and margarine	½ cup	310
Spinach, canned	½ cup	342
Sauerkraut	½ cup	780
Tomato, canned	½ cup	196
Tomato juice	½ cup	440
Vegetable juice cocktail	½ cup	442

Table 8.3. Common Foods High in Sodium (*cont.*)

Food	Portion	Milligrams of Sodium
BREADS		
Rye, light	1 slice	175
White	1 slice	129
Whole-wheat	1 slice	180
Pita	1 6½ in. diam.	339
English muffin	1 whole	378
Bread stuffing	½ cup	568
CEREALS		
All-Bran, Kellogg's	1 oz. (⅓ cup)	320
Cheerios	1 oz. (1¼ cup)	307
Corn Flakes, Kellogg's	1 oz. (1¼ cup)	351
Product 19	1 oz. (¾ cup)	325
Rice Krispies	1 oz. (1 cup)	340
Total	1 oz. (1 cup)	352
Wheaties	1 oz. (1 cup)	354
DAIRY PRODUCTS		
American cheese	1 oz.	406
American cheese spread	1 T	218
Blue cheese	1 oz.	396
Cottage cheese, low-fat	½ cup	459
Cottage cheese, creamed	½ cup	425
Feta	1 oz.	316
Swiss, processed	1 oz.	388
Butter	1 T	116
Margarine	1 T	132
Milk, whole or low-fat	1 cup	121
Buttermilk	1 cup	257
Milk, condensed	⅓ cup	130
Milk, evaporated, canned	½ cup	140
Yogurt, plain, low-fat	1 cup	159
CONDIMENTS		
A.1. sauce	1 t	75
Catsup	1 T	156
Mayonnaise	1 T	80
Mustard, yellow	1 T	189
Soy sauce	1 T	1029
Tartar sauce	1 T	182
Teriyaki sauce	1 T	690
Worcestershire sauce	1 t	60
Relish, sweet	1 T	107
Olives, green, canned	4 medium	312
COOKING AIDS		
Baking powder	1 t	339
Baking soda	1 t	821
Bouillon cube, beef	1 cube	864

SALT AND PREGNANCY

Pregnant women were, until recently, advised to reduce their intake to reduce edema. It is now believed that pregnant women have an *increased* need for sodium because of their increased blood volume and tissues. However, the need for extra sodium is relatively small and is easily supplied by the usual diet consumed by nonpregnant women. (For more information, see Chapter 12.)

SALT NEEDS OF INFANTS AND OLDER PERSONS

Infants, young children, and older persons are less able to tolerate either excesses or deficiencies of water and electrolytes than people of other ages. Dehydration due to excess fluid loss in perspiration, diarrhea, or among older people who are taking diuretics (drugs that cause the kidneys to remove more salt and water from the body) can result in sodium and potassium depletion and even death. Another serious problem, particularly for the elderly, is increased fluid retention caused by an excess of salt. The decreased capacity of the heart to tolerate an increase in blood volume can result in congestive heart failure.

Table 8.3. Common Foods High in Sodium *(cont.)*

Food	Portion	Milligrams of Sodium
Bouillon cube, chicken	1 cube	1152
Garlic salt	1 t	1850
Meat tenderizer	1 t	1750
Salt	1 t	2132
Monosodium glutamate (MSG)	1 t	492
SNACKS		
Almonds, oil-roasted, salted	1 oz.	220
Mixed nuts, oil-roasted, salted	1 oz.	185
Peanuts, dry-roasted, salted	1 oz.	122
Peanut butter	1 T	75
Pickles, dill	1 pickle	928
Pretzels	1 oz.	476
Potato chips	1 oz.	133
Corn chips	1 oz.	233
DESSERTS		
Chocolate pudding, instant	½ cup	440
Vanilla pudding, instant	½ cup	375
DIGESTIVE AIDS		
Alka-Seltzer	1 tablet	567
Bromo Seltzer	1 tablet	761

SALT AND HIGH BLOOD PRESSURE

The relationship between sodium and hypertension, or high blood pressure, has been an area of intense investigation and controversy in recent years. Currently, the nature of the link between sodium intake and hypertension has not been clearly defined and the long-term effects of excess salt ingestion are not known with certainty. Studies show that 30 to 50 percent of those who have hypertension may be particularly sensitive to sodium. (Recent studies indicate that chloride also may be a factor.) In this susceptible population, sodium restriction may help reduce high blood pressure, and in some cases may eliminate the need for antihypertensive drug therapy or reduce the amount of drugs needed to control blood pressure. (See Chapter 26.)

SOURCES OF SODIUM

The largest single source of sodium in the diet is common table salt, about one-third of which is added by the consumer. In addition to the following, any product that lists on its label sodium, soda, or salt as part of its name contains sodium. (See Table 8.3 for a listing of common foods that are high in sodium and list below for food additives containing sodium.)

Fresh foods. Naturally occurring sodium is found in fresh foods from animal sources and,

Food Additives That Contain Sodium

Baking powder (baking soda plus an acid)—used as a leavening agent for muffins, cakes, and quick breads

Baking soda (sodium bicarbonate or bicarbonate of soda)—used as a leavening agent in breads and cakes; sometimes added as a color preservative to green vegetables

Brine—used to flavor corned beef, pickles, sauerkraut, and as a preservative

Disodium phosphate—used in processed cheese, meat, and some fast-cooking cereals to help retain fluids

Hydrolyzed vegetable protein—used as a filler in dried soups and other processed foods

Monosodium glutamate (MSG)—used as a flavor enhancer and tenderizer in cooking and preserving foods

Sodium alginate—used to give smooth texture to ice cream, chocolate milk, and other products

Sodium benzoate—a preservative used in many condiments, such as relishes and salad dressings

Sodium ascorbate—used as a preservative

Sodium caseinate—used in cake mixes and baked goods

Sodium citrate—used as a flavoring and preservative

Sodium cyclamate and sodium saccharin—used in some low-calorie drinks and desserts

Sodium hydroxide—used to soften and loosen skins of ripe olives, hominy, and other fruits and vegetables

Sodium nitrate and sodium nitrite—used in cured meats, sausages, ham, bacon, dried fish, etc. as preservatives

Sodium propionate—used to inhibit molds in cheeses, breads, cakes, and other baked goods

Sodium sulfite—used as a preservative in dried fruits and as a color preservative in fruits and wines

Soy sauce and soy isolates—used as flavorings, especially in Oriental dishes

Whey solids—used as a filler; the sodium is usually added during processing

to a lesser extent, nonanimal sources. The amount of sodium in these foods is, however, significantly less than that found in the same foods after they have been processed, cured, canned, or, in some cases, frozen.

Processed or preserved foods. Large amounts of sodium are often used in processing and preserving food. Products containing sodium are used to prevent the growth of bacteria and mold, as artificial sweeteners, to enhance the flavor of foods, as meat tenderizers, and as buffers and emulsifiers. Pickles and sauerkraut are cured in brine, peas are sorted by size in salt solutions, and skins are removed from tomatoes by sodium hydroxide.

Baked goods. Breads and cakes frequently contain baking soda or baking powder, leavening agents that contain sodium.

Drinking water. Sodium is found in varying amounts in public and bottled water. Soft water, although advantageous for laundry and bathing, contains more sodium than hard water, which usually contains high levels of calcium carbonate. Softeners added to water supplies exchange calcium ions for sodium ions, thus converting a water supply that is low in sodium to one that is high in sodium. Although the Environmental Protection Agency (EPA) does not regulate the maximum level of sodium in water, it indicates as op-

Table 8.4. Sodium-Free Herbs, Spices, and Flavorings That Can Be Used Instead of Salt

Herb, Spice, or Flavoring	For Use in:	Herb, Spice, or Flavoring	For Use in:
Allspice	Baked goods, some vegetables and fruits, seafood dishes	Nutmeg	Baked goods, meats, fruits, vegetables, quiches
Almond extract	Baked goods	Onion powder	Vegetables, meats, soups
Basil	Meat, fish, pasta, tomato and Italian dishes, vegetables, stews, soups	Oregano	Vegetables, pasta, Italian dishes, pizza, spaghetti sauces and other tomato dishes
Bay leaves	Stews, gravies and soups, fish, poultry		
Caraway seeds	Rye breads, cabbage and sauerkraut	Paprika	Eggs, creamed dishes and sauces, Hungarian dishes
Chives	Eggs, dips, soups, as garnish		
Cinnamon	Baked goods, spicy beverages, sweet potatoes	Parsley	Vegetables, salads, soups, pasta, as garnish
Cloves	Baked goods, baked beans, sauces	Pepper	Meats, eggs, vegetables, soups, stews
Curry powder	Meat, poultry and seafood dishes, sauces, creamed vegetable dishes	Peppermint extract	Baked goods, candies
		Poppy seeds	Baked goods, salads, noodles
Dill	Lamb, egg and cheese dishes, potato salads, cucumbers, tomatoes	Rosemary	Lamb, pork, vegetables
		Sage	Poultry, stuffings
Garlic	Vegetables, soups, garlic bread, eggs	Savory	Eggs, cheese, stuffings
Ginger	Baked goods, sweet and sour Oriental dishes, pickles	Sesame seeds	Breads, salads, casseroles
		Tarragon	Dressings, eggs, seafood, some vegetables
Lemon extract	Baked goods		
Mace	Baked goods, creamed dishes, cheese dishes	Thyme	Meats, poultry, fish
		Tumeric	Pickles, curries, chutneys
Maple extract	Maple syrup, baked goods	Vanilla extract	Baked goods
Marjoram	Meat and vegetable dishes, fish, soufflés, potatoes, tomatoes	Vinegar	Dressings
		Walnut extract	Baked goods, ice cream
Mustard powder	Salad dressings, deviled foods, pickles, sauces		

timal "sodium levels of 20 milligrams or less" per quart. Studies by the U.S. Public Health Department and others have indicated that 42 percent of the nation's water supplies provide sodium in excess of the optimal level.

Medications. Sodium is consumed in a wide variety of over-the-counter drugs and several prescription medicines. These products, ranging from analgesics to antacids, from sleep aids to antibiotics, often carry warnings to the consumer who is on a salt-restricted diet. Salt contents may be appreciable, ranging from 49 milligrams for a single aspirin tablet to 1,000 milligrams per dose for a commonly used antacid or laxative. Salt-conscious consumers are advised to consult their physicians or pharmacists when in doubt about the sodium content of any product that does not have its contents clearly stated on the label.

REDUCING SODIUM INTAKE

Although harmful effects of sodium have not clearly been established, reducing salt intake to moderate levels may prove beneficial, and, in any event, is not likely to be harmful. For a substantial number of the 60 million Americans who have high blood pressure, sodium reduction, along with exercise, weight loss, and the use of antihypertensive drugs, can be an important component in bringing blood pressure under control, thereby reducing the likelihood of heart disease, kidney disease, and stroke. People who are taking certain medications or who have conditions associated with fluid retention, such as congestive heart failure, cirrhosis with complications, or kidney failure, may have to restrict sodium intake.

The easiest and most effective way to reduce sodium intake is simply to cut down use of salt during cooking and at the table. Dietitians recommend gradually reducing the amount of salt added to foods during cooking and adding instead other seasonings. Fresh or dried herbs, spices, and extracts such as those listed in Table 8.4 add flavor and variety to the taste of many foods. Avoiding heavily processed convenience foods in favor of fresh fruits, vegetables, and meats is also beneficial. Recent FDA regulations regarding sodium labeling of food products can assist consumers in making informed choices about their diet. Beginning in July 1986, the FDA required sodium content of food on the nutrition label. Furthermore, the FDA has specified standards for label claims such as "low sodium," "very low sodium," and "sodium free." (See Table 8.5.)

Although a palatable diet can be planned without the use of special low-salt foods, a wide variety of products is now available in supermarkets. It is important to note that while the products add variety to the diet and convenience to food preparation, they are usually not sodium-free, so the amount of sodium they contain must be calculated in the diet.

Salt substitutes are also available. These products generally fall into one of three categories: those that are a mixture of sodium

Table 8.5. Interpreting Food Labels

The Food and Drug Administration has established the following criteria for labeling regarding sodium content.

When the Label Says:	It Means:
Sodium-free	Fewer than 5 milligrams per serving
Very low sodium	35 milligrams or fewer per serving
Low sodium	140 milligrams or fewer per serving
Reduced sodium	Processed to reduce the usual level of sodium by 75 percent
Unsalted	Processed without the normally added salt
Lite	Processed with less than the usual amount of salt

chloride and potassium chloride; those composed of potassium chloride only; and those that contain neither sodium nor potassium but instead are mixtures of spices and herbs. Many people find the flavor of potassium chloride bitter and more objectionable than no salt at all. Furthermore, increased potassium intake is not recommended for those with kidney disorders. People taking diuretics that conserve potassium or who are on potassium supplements also should not take potassium-containing salt substitutes unless specifically recommended by their doctors. For normal healthy individuals, these products used in moderation are not harmful.

9

Dietary Fiber

Victor Herbert, M.D., J.D.

■

INTRODUCTION

In recent years, there has been a renewed interest among both nutrition researchers and the general public in the dietary importance of fiber—the parts of plant foods that are not absorbed from the human digestive tract. Fiber's value in normal digestive function has been recognized for centuries, but today, almost mystical powers are attributed to it. While there is no doubt that fiber is an important component of the human diet, it is not the magic cure-all some promoters of high-fiber foods and diets would have us believe. In this chapter, we will present what is known about the role of dietary fiber in human health, as well as dispel some of the more popular fiber myths. The bottom line is that we should get not fewer than 15 nor more than 35 grams of fiber, and it should come from moderate amounts of a variety of fruits, vegetables, and grains (breads, cereals, and pastas) and not from pills.

WHAT IS DIETARY FIBER?

With one exception (lignin, a polymer that is found in plant-cell walls), the various fibers are complex carbohydrates. However, the human digestive tract lacks the enzymes to break down these carbohydrates into a form that can be absorbed and used for energy. (Table 9.1 lists the different kinds of dietary fiber, common sources, and important functions.)

Generally, fibers are classified as either soluble or insoluble and fermentable or nonfermentable. The soluble fibers are those that are sticky and mesh with water to form gels. They include pectin, guar, mucilages, and the fiber in oat bran, barley, dried beans, and other legumes. In recent years, the soluble fibers have gained increased attention because of their ability to lower blood cholesterol.

The insoluble fibers are those that pass through the digestive tract pretty much unchanged except for being broken up by chewing. They absorb large amounts of water—up to 15 times their weight—thus creating a soft, bulky stool. Cellulose is the most common soluble fiber; sources include wheat bran, whole-grain products, and the skins of fruits and vegetables. Insoluble fibers have little or no effect on blood cholesterol; instead, their major role seems to be to help move the stool through the colon and thus prevent constipation. There also has been speculation that insoluble fiber can help protect against colon cancer and other digestive disorders. (See the following discussion on specific diseases.)

Fermentable fiber is broken down (fermented) by bacteria in the lower small bowel and upper large bowel into volatile, short-chain fatty acids, which supply energy after being absorbed. Generally, the more soluble the fiber, the more fermentable it is.

Recent interest in the role of dietary fiber—defined as the sum of the unabsorbable crude fiber (mainly cellulose and lignin) remaining in the colon after digestion, plus the available (fermentable) fiber—can be traced to the 1970s and the work of Denis B. Burkitt and Hugh Trowell, British physicians who studied patterns of disease in Uganda, Africa. They noted that a host of diet-related diseases common in Western industrialized societies—colon cancer, appendicitis, gallbladder disease, diverticulosis, hemorrhoids, coronary disease, and diabetes—were rare among rural Africans. They concluded that diet, or more specifically, the intake of dietary fiber, was a major reason for the differences.

The traditional diet of rural Africa is high in grains, vegetables, and fruits and thus provides a large amount of fiber. In contrast, the typical diet of most industrialized countries is high in animal products, sugar, and processed foods that have little or no fiber. Their conclusion ignored the fact that not only was the fiber intake a different pattern from that in the Western world but almost everything else in the diet, water, air, and lifestyle was different; in short, there were many other possible explanations (i.e., "confounding variables").

Almost overnight, the great "fiber fad," which continues today, was born. From the prevention branch of the National Cancer Institute on down, enthusiasts urged that Americans eat more unprocessed bran as well as increase their intake of whole-grain products, fruits, vegetables, and other high-fiber foods. There also has been a flood of books and articles directed at both the general public and health professionals extolling the benefits of fiber, which often was interpreted as bran and bran products. More recently, the pendulum has begun to swing back, and a more moderate approach is being urged. For example, in the April 1990 issue of the *Journal of the National Cancer Institute*, the prevention branch of the institute conceded that the data on dietary fiber and colon cancer do not permit discrimination between effects due to fiber and non-fiber effects due to vegetables (and various substances vegetables do and don't contain).

What is important to remember is that there are many different varieties of fiber and all are good in moderation. Eat as wide a variety of fruits, vegetables, and grains as you can afford, adding up to a total of 15-35 grams of fiber per day.

Table 9.1. Functions and Sources of Different Kinds of Dietary Fibers

Type of Fiber	Sources	Functions
Cellulose	Bran, whole grains, nuts, white part of orange rind, etc.	Adds bulk to stool to reduce constipation, diverticulosis, hemorrhoids
Hemicellulose	Vegetables, fruits, nuts, whole grains	Same as cellulose
Pectin	Legumes, apples, pears and other fruits, some vegetables, nuts	May help lower blood cholesterol; normalize blood sugar; added to foods as a thickening agent
Lignin	Woody parts of bran, fruit skins, nuts, whole grains	Same as for pectin
Guar, carrageenan, etc.	Algae and seaweeds	Same as for pectin
Mucilages	Plant seeds and plant secretions	Same as for pectin

EFFECTS OF FIBER

Bowel Function

Certain fibers—especially cellulose and hemicellulose—act as tiny sponges, absorbing many times their weight in water. As a result, the feces become waterlogged, soft, and bulky. This bulky stool stimulates peristalsis—the rhythmic contractions of the bowel—and thus it passes more easily and rapidly through the digestive tract. This helps prevent constipation and related problems due to increased pressure in the gut, such as diverticulosis and hemorrhoids. Drs. Burkitt and Trowell accurately noted that the stools of rural Africans were more frequent and much larger and softer than the small, hard stools typical of many Britons and other Westerners.

Many of today's popular laxatives are fiber-based and people who suffer from chronic constipation are urged to consume a high-fiber diet. Moderation is important, however, especially for older, relatively inactive people whose bowel function may be sluggish. Consuming large amounts of bran and other high-fiber supplements actually can produce intestinal obstruction. In extreme cases, surgery may be required to relieve it. A case in point, reported in the *Archives of Surgery* in January 1988, is that of a 50-year-old man who ate two large bowls of bran cereal with milk and several hours later began experiencing cramping abdominal pain. X rays taken 18 hours later showed a typical bowel obstruction, and the thick, pasty bolus of bran required surgical removal. A commonsense approach of eating a variety of breads, cereals, pastas, fruits, and vegetables, each in moderation, is far preferable to taking bran supplements or high-fiber laxatives. There is nothing wrong with a portion of bran cereal as part of moderation and variety, but pouring bran on fruits and vegetables in addition is excessive. Drinking plenty of water and increasing physical activity also are important components of healthy bowel function. (See Chapter 30 for a more detailed discussion.)

Diverticular Disease

Diverticular disease is caused by the formation of small out-pouches or pockets in weakened segments of the intestinal wall. Excessive pressure within the colon worsens the condition by further weakening the pockets and forcing waste material into them. There is a danger that the pockets will rupture, spilling bowel contents into the pelvic cavity. This can lead to serious infection. More often, however, the pouches become inflamed without actually rupturing—a condition called diverticulitis—resulting in pain, fever, and increasingly impaired bowel function.

At one time, people with diverticular disease were put on a low-fiber diet on the assumption that a large, bulky stool would make matters worse. Today it is recognized that consuming a varied high-fiber diet is a better approach. The larger, bulkier stool produced by a high-fiber diet does not require as much intestinal muscle contraction pressure to push it through the bowel, thereby reducing the chances of fecal matter filling the diverticular pockets. The softer stool also passes more easily without excessive "straining at stool," which promotes hemorrhoids (dilated blood vessels).

Although diet is unlikely to "cure" diverticulosis and hemorrhoids, a high-fiber regimen can halt this progression and ease symptoms. Caution is needed, however. It should be stressed that too much fiber can be irritating to the colon and worsen diverticulosis. A doctor should be consulted before attempting any dietary change in the presence of diverticular disease. (See Chapter 30.)

Irritable Bowel Syndrome

Irritable bowel syndrome is characterized by spasmodic contractions of the bowel muscles, resulting in abdominal pain, gassiness, and alternating diarrhea and constipation. For many, stress is linked with irritable bowel syndrome; for others, the attacks may occur with no identifiable provocation. As with diverticular disease, a high-fiber diet is often recommended in treating irritable bowel syndrome. In fact, a large number of patients need only dietary treatment.

Colon Cancer

The role of a high-fiber diet in protecting against colon cancer is not as well established as many people believe. Drs. Burkitt and Trowell put forth their "fiber hypothesis"—namely, that a diet high in fiber protects against colon cancer, while a diet low in fiber promotes it—in the 1970s when they started writing about the epidemiology of certain diseases in Africa compared to Great Britain and other industrialized countries. They theorized that colon cancer may be caused by prolonged contact with certain carcinogens in the stool. Since the stool produced by a diet high in fiber moves more quickly through the digestive tract than one that is low in fiber, this hypothesis seems logical. In addition, the increased water in the bulkier high-fiber stool may help dilute cancer-causing chemicals. Researchers also have noted modest differences in the bacterial population of the intestinal tract of people who consume a high-fiber diet versus those who do not.

While all of this is logical, the fact remains that it has not been demonstrated that a high-fiber diet does, indeed, reduce the risk of colon cancer. The epidemiological studies comparing disease patterns in rural Africa and those of industrialized countries do not take into account the many other differences, or variables, that may affect the incidence of colon cancer. The first epidemiologic study that did account for most of the variables (called a "community-based case control study") was published in 1986 in the *Journal of the National Cancer Institute;* it showed that the Australian women who ate the most cereal also had the *most* colon cancer. (Women get colon cancer more often than men; men have a greater chance of getting rectal cancer than women.) As of this writing, two other studies have produced similar results. After reviewing the diet, nutrition, and cancer evidence to date, a panel of the National Academy of Sciences concluded that there is "no conclusive evidence . . . that dietary fiber . . . exerts a protective influence against colorectal cancer in humans." A 1987 study of fiber by the Life Science Research Office of the Federation of American Societies for Experimental Biology drew the same conclusion.

It may well be, however, that other substances in grains, vegetables, legumes, and other high-fiber foods do have a protective effect. In fact, the 1989 National Academy of Sciences Report on Diet and Health concluded that any cancer-protective effects of high-fiber food very likely do not come from dietary fiber but from other substances in these foods. Or it may be that a high-fiber diet may influence other factors—such as total caloric intake—and, in turn, these may reduce the risk of colon cancer. However, we do not have any evidence to state unequivocally that simply eating more fiber will cut the risk of colon cancer. (See Chapter 27.)

Heart Disease

Whether certain types of fiber can reduce the frequency of heart attacks, or more specifically, the development of coronary atherosclerosis, is another subject of intensive research and debate. There is sound evidence that some of the soluble fibers—pectin, oat bran, guar, and others—*can* have a cholesterol-lowering effect. Since high blood cholesterol is closely associated with the narrowing of coronary (and other) arteries from fatty plaque—the major cause of heart attacks—dietary means of lowering cholesterol can play a role in reducing the risk of heart attacks. The questions are: How much of a role? After all, half the heart attacks occur in people who do not have high serum cholesterol. Isn't it wiser first to measure serum cholesterol and see whether it's above 200? And to see if LDL (low-density lipoprotein) cholesterol is above 130? (In October 1987, the National Institutes of Health decided the answer to these last two questions was yes, although there is no harm in adopting a prudent diet, such as that recommended by the American Heart Association, even if there is no evidence of coronary disease.)

Again, there is considerable public confusion over the value of fiber in preventing heart disease. When a doctor urges a heart patient to eat substantial amounts of fiber to help lower cholesterol, it has to be soluble fiber; wheat bran and other insoluble fibers have little or no effect on blood cholesterol. Instead, it is the soluble fibers (the ones that become sticky when wet) that may be important in this regard. Several controlled studies have shown that adding oat bran or pectin, for example, to the diet will produce a modest lowering of blood cholesterol. The addition should be gradual, however; abruptly adding large amounts of oat bran (or any other fiber) can upset gastrointestinal function, resulting in bloating, diarrhea, abdominal pain, flatulence, and other symptoms. But just eating more fiber alone will not lower cholesterol unless you simultaneously reduce the fat content of your diet. For more details, see chapters 6 and 26, as well as How Much Fiber? on page 141.

Diabetes

The role of fiber in the control of blood-sugar levels is still another area of ongoing research. Studies have found, for example, that diabetic patients who ate moderate amounts of oatmeal as part of a high-carbohydrate, high-fiber diet had better control of blood sugar and did not require as much insulin as patients on a regular diet without the oat products. When these findings were first announced, some diabetes specialists began urging their patients to consume a high-fiber diet. Subsequent research has shown that not all dietary fiber has the same antidiabetes effect. In fact, wheat bran and other insoluble fibers have little or no effect on blood sugar. Again, it is the soluble fibers—oat bran, pectin, guar, etc.—that seem to improve diabetes control. It is not fully known how these soluble fibers help stabilize blood-sugar levels, but a number of studies have shown that, as part of a high carbohydrate, high-fiber diet, they benefit patients with both Type I and Type II diabetes. In addition, soluble fibers help lower cholesterol, in part by increasing the amount of bile acids that is excreted in the stool, thereby requiring the liver to remove more cholesterol from the blood in order to make more bile acids and salts. The fact that diabetics have an increased incidence of atherosclerosis and heart attacks is another reason to advocate a diet that includes good sources of these fibers. (See Chapter 28.)

Weight Control

The value of high-fiber foods in appetite and weight control has long been recognized. Indeed, many of today's so-called diet aids are simply concoctions of various kinds of fiber. In theory, at least, dietary fiber can help control weight in several ways. Since the human digestive tract does not break the crude-fiber portion of it down into forms that can be used for energy, that portion does not contain calories. However, fiber adds bulk to the diet and gives a feeling of fullness, and thus can help prevent overeating at a single sitting. Over the long haul, however, most people will simply increase their food intake at other times to maintain their weight. A familiar example involves Chinese or other mostly vegetable meals: You may feel full for an hour or so after eating, but the satiety is short-lived because the carbohydrates are absorbed and therefore metabolized relatively quickly compared to proteins and fats. Therefore, a meal

that includes modest amounts of these nutrients in addition to the high-fiber vegetables, fruits, and grains will have a more lasting effect on appetite and weight control than one that is only high-fiber carbohydrates.

High-fiber foods (especially cereal bran) seem to interfere moderately with the digestion and absorption of certain foods, and, as a result, may moderately reduce their total caloric value. Two possible mechanisms are believed to be responsible for this effect. When food moves through the digestive tract more rapidly, the body may not have time to absorb all of the contained nutrients before they

Table 9.2. Fiber Content of Selected Foods

Type of Food	Serving Size	Total Fiber (gm.)	Calories
CEREALS			
Bran (100%) cereal	⅓ cup	8.5	71
Oats, whole	¾ cup cooked	1.6*	108
Shredded wheat	⅔ cup	2.6	102
Wheat flakes	1 cup	2.0	99
Wheat germ	¼ cup	3.4	108
BREADS, ETC.			
Bran muffins	1 small	2.5	104
French bread	1 slice	0.7	102
Pumpernickel bread	1 slice	1.0	66
Whole-wheat bread	1 slice	1.4	61
Rye wafers	3	2.3	63
PASTA/RICE			
Brown rice	½ cup cooked	1.0	97
Macaroni	1 cup	1.6	144
Spaghetti (reg.)	1 cup	1.1	155
Spaghetti (whole-wheat)	1 cup	3.9	155
White rice	½ cup	0.2	82
FRUITS*			
Apple (with skin)	1 medium	3.5*	80
Apricots (fresh)	3 medium	1.8	50
Apricots (dried)	5 halves	1.4	240
Banana	1 medium	2.4	90
Blueberries	½ cup	2.6	40
Cherries	10	1.2	56
Grapefruit	½ large	3.1	60
Grapes	20	0.6	36
Orange	1 medium	0.8	45
Peaches	1 medium	1.9	40
Pear	½ medium	1.6	35

reach the colon. In addition, fiber may partially block the action of certain digestive enzymes, resulting in less efficient uptake of food. Studies have found, for example, that the stools produced from a high-fiber diet contain more fat than those of low-fiber meals. Again, caution is needed; too much fiber also hinders absorption of essential minerals and can lead to deficiencies, particularly of iron, zinc, and calcium, which are bound to the unabsorbed fiber that is excreted in the stool. This is one reason that vegetarians have more iron and zinc deficiencies than omnivorous people.

When attempting to lose weight, it is better to modify the diet to include a variety of high-fiber (and therefore low-calorie) foods than to rely on fiber diet pills and other supplements. As emphasized in Chapter 17, strict low-calorie regimens and crash diets are more likely to create rather than overcome weight problems. What one needs instead is the initiation of sensible, lifelong eating habits that will balance food intake and energy expenditure. This can be accomplished by increasing the intake of a variety of fruits and vegetables, legumes, and grains, including whole-grain products and other starchy foods—all good

Table 9.2. Fiber Content of Selected Foods *(cont.)*

Type of Food	Serving Size	Total Fiber (gm.)	Calories
Pineapple	½ cup	1.1	40
Prunes	3 medium	3.0	240
Strawberries	½ cup	1.5	22
LEGUMES (COOKED)*			
Dried peas	½ cup	4.7	115
Kidney beans	½ cup	7.3	110
Lentils	½ cup	3.7	95
Lima beans	½ cup	4.5	65
Navy beans	½ cup	6.0	110
VEGETABLES (COOKED)			
Asparagus	½ cup	1.0	15
Beans, green	½ cup	1.6	15
Broccoli	½ cup	2.2	20
Brussels sprouts	½ cup	2.3	30
Parsnips	½ cup	2.7	50
Peas	½ cup	3.6*	55
Potatoes (with skin)	1 medium	2.5	105
Spinach	½ cup	2.1	20
Squash, summer	½ cup	1.4	15
Zucchini	½ cup	1.8	10
VEGETABLES (RAW)			
Celery	1 stalk	1.1	15
Lettuce	1 cup sliced	0.9	10
Mushroom	½ cup	0.9	10
Pepper, green	½ cup	0.5	10
Spinach	1 cup	1.2	10
Sprouts, bean	½ cup	1.5	15

*High in soluble fiber.

Adapted from table 5 in "A Critical Review of Food Fiber Analysis and Data," by Elaine Lanza and Ritva R. Butrum. Reprinted by *Journal of The American Dietetic Association*, Vol. 86:732, 1986.

sources of different kinds of fiber—and going easy on alcohol, fatty foods, and other high-calorie items. Remember, carbohydrates and proteins are four calories a gram, alcohol is seven, and fat is nine. Unfortunately, many people still think that bread, pasta, potatoes, dried peas and beans, and other starchy foods are fattening. Although any calorie-containing food eaten in excess is fattening, the fact is, a diet high in starchy foods is more likely to accomplish good weight control than one emphasizing high-protein, high-fat foods (fatty meats, whole milk, cheese, etc.), fats, sweets, and other calorie-dense foods. (See Chapter 17 for more details on using fiber to control weight.)

Sample Menus for Adequate Fiber Intake

Day 1	Grams Fiber
BREAKFAST	
½ grapefruit	3.1
⅔ cup shredded wheat	2.6
Skim milk	
MID-MORNING SNACK	
Seltzer, fruit-flavored	
3 rye wafers or whole-wheat crackers	2.3
LUNCH	
Tuna sandwich on 2 slices pumpernickel bread	2.0
Spinach salad	2.3
AFTERNOON SNACK	
1 banana	2.4
Skim milk	
DINNER	
Fish poached with onions	
Brown rice, ½ cup	1.0
Cooked peas, ½ cup	3.6
Green salad	3.0
Gingerbread	
	Total: 22.3

Day 2	Grams Fiber
BREAKFAST	
Cooked oatmeal, ½ cup	0.9
Skim or low-fat milk	
Cantaloupe, ¾ cup of cubes	0.8
MID-MORNING SNACK	
Pears, 1 fresh	3.2
LUNCH	
Chunky vegetable soup, 1 cup	1.2
Carrot/raisin salad, ½ cup	1.7

	Grams Fiber
AFTERNOON SNACK	
Bran muffin	2.5
Skim milk	
DINNER	
Wheat bulgur, ½ cup	0.9
Roast chicken	
Yellow squash, ½ cup	1.8
Tossed salad	3.0
Baked apple	3.2
	Total: 19.2

Day 3	Grams Fiber
BREAKFAST	
Orange juice, 6 oz.	0.3
Grape-Nuts cereal, 1 oz.	3.5
Low-fat milk	
Strawberries, ½ cup	1.5
LUNCH	
Lentil soup, 1 cup	3.4
Rye crackers	2.3
Apple	3.5
AFTERNOON SNACK	
Fig bar	0.7
Skim milk	
DINNER	
Spaghetti, 1 cup	1.1
Vegetarian sauce with tomatoes, peppers, mushrooms and zucchini, ½ cup	1.6
Coleslaw, ½ cup	1.3
Peach with lemon sorbet	1.9
	Total: 21.1

HOW MUCH FIBER?

Since the typical American diet now provides about 12 grams of fiber a day, it is safe to say that the average American could benefit from increasing fiber intake. Unfortunately, many people have been misled to believe that a recommendation to take more fiber is synonymous with taking fiber supplements or sprinkling bran on your broccoli, neither of which is a wise idea. Health-food sellers and other food faddists capitalize on the fiber fad by pushing all sorts of fiber products—including such things as high-fiber bread made with sawdust or flour made from the white of orange peels. Avoid them.

Fiber should come from a variety of foods and intake should be spread throughout the day to avoid a sudden overload of the digestive system. Table 9.2 lists the fiber content of common foods. In general, however, it's not necessary meticulously to count up grams of fiber consumed. See Sample Menus on page 138. A diet that provides a variety of foods from the four food groups and includes fresh or lightly processed fruits and vegetables, whole-grain products, legumes, and starches will supply ample fiber and a balance of soluble and insoluble types, as well as other needed nutrients. Remember that both plant groups in the Basic Four (the fruit-vegetable and the grain groups) are the fiber groups, and you need a minimum of four portions daily from each of these two groups.

If your present diet is low in fiber, a gradual approach to increasing it is recommended. If, for instance, your diet now provides 10 grams or less of fiber and you suddenly increase this to 30 or 35, you may well experience unpleasant bloating, gassiness, and other symptoms. Also, some high-fiber foods—beans and other legumes are notorious examples—are more likely to produce gassiness than others. If a particular food creates symptoms, cut back on the portion or substitute some other choice that contains a similar fiber. People who can't tolerate beans may have no problems with oatmeal, apples, pears, or other sources of similar fiber.

10

Water and Other Fluids

Delia A. Hammock, M.S., R.D.

■

INTRODUCTION

Water is the most indispensable of all the six groups of nutrients necessary for survival. People can go without food for two months and live, and vitamin deficiencies take weeks or months to cause symptoms. Without water, however, death occurs within days.

Water is by far the most abundant substance in the body, as well as the most plentiful component in human diets. This colorless, calorie-free compound of two parts hydrogen and one part oxygen (H_2O) accounts for one-half to three-fourths of the body's weight, depending on age, sex, and body composition. The body of a newborn infant is 75 to 80 percent water, but a gradual process of water loss continues throughout life until, in old age, water accounts for only about 50 percent of body weight.

All tissues contain water in varying proportions. Water makes up about three-fourths of muscle tissue, but only about one-fourth of body fat. Thus, lean individuals and most men, with their greater muscle mass, have a higher percentage of body water than do obese individuals. Even bone, which seems to be dry, is more than one-fifth water.

FUNCTIONS

The reason that we can survive only a short time without water becomes evident when we consider that the body uses water for virtually all its functions: digestion, absorption, transporting nutrients, building tissue, and maintaining temperature. Every cell in the body depends on water to carry out its essential activities. Water in blood plasma (the liquid portion of the blood), as well as water inside the cells themselves and in the spaces between the cells, serves as a solvent to transport nutrients to each cell and to remove waste products to the lungs, kidney, gastrointestinal tract, and skin for elimination.

Water also acts as the climate-control system for the body, maintaining body temperature by releasing heat through perspiration, which then evaporates. In hot weather or during exercise vigorous enough to raise the internal temperature, heat sensors in the skin and in the brain's hypothalamus stimulate the sweat glands to release perspiration, reducing the body's core temperature. Even when there is no noticeable sweat, the body still regulates temperature through insensible, or undetected, perspiration. Expired air in the breath also contains some moisture and contributes to insensible water loss.

Watery synovial fluid also bathes joints, helping them to move smoothly. Other watery secretions lubricate the digestive tract, and cushion the delicate internal organs such as the lungs, spinal cord, and brain. Amniotic fluid surrounds and protects the fetus during pregnancy. Moreover, water acts as the medium for thousands of life-supporting chemical reactions that constantly occur throughout the human body.

BODY REGULATION OF WATER

The average adult consumes and excretes about two and a half to three quarts of water a day. Water balance is carefully regulated by the kidneys and the thirst center of the brain's hypothalamus so that the amount lost each day through perspiration, expiration of water vapor from the lungs, and elimination of water in urine and feces equals the amount taken in.

A decline in the body's water content is reflected in a decline in blood volume, which causes a slight rise in the concentration of sodium in the blood. These changes are quickly sensed by the brain's thirst receptors, triggering the sensation of thirst. Additionally, as blood volume decreases, there is a decrease in the secretion of saliva as well, producing a dry feeling in the mouth resulting in more fluid intake. Meanwhile, the hypothalamus signals the pituitary gland to release antidiuretic (antiurination) hormone (ADH), which causes the tubules of the kidney to reabsorb more water into the bloodstream, resulting in a less dilute urine. No matter how little water is consumed, however, healthy kidneys will excrete at least 10 to 17 ounces of water each day to rid the body of toxic waste products.

If more water is taken in than the body needs, blood volume increases and its relative sodium concentration falls. The hypothalamus quickly senses these changes and sends out signals that suppress the release of antidiuretic hormone, causing the kidneys to excrete the extra fluid.

ABNORMALITIES IN WATER BALANCE

Under normal circumstances, this constant interplay of regulatory forces maintains careful control over the body's water balance. Such fine tuning is essential, since a loss of just 5 percent of the body's water may cause symptoms of heat exhaustion such as a weak, rapid pulse, headache, dizziness, and general weakness. A 10-percent loss is extremely dangerous and can lead to heatstroke and death if not treated immediately.

However, the control mechanisms can be thrown off kilter, especially when large amounts of fluid are lost, as in severe vomiting, diarrhea, blood loss, high fever, or profuse sweating.

Dehydrating conditions can be especially dangerous for infants, not only because babies cannot communicate that they are thirsty but also because they have a large body surface area in proportion to their fluid volume, causing them to become seriously dehydrated in a short period of time. The elderly also can become dangerously dehydrated quickly, since they typically have a lower percentage of body water.

Athletes are also particularly prone to dehydration, because their thirst mechanism cannot always keep pace with the excessive water losses that sometimes occur in strenuous sporting events. (For more information regarding the fluid needs of athletes, see Chapter 24.)

Disorders such as kidney disease and various endocrine disorders that interfere with the body's ability to regulate sodium levels may also result in water imbalances. Excretion of too much sodium, which, by osmosis, pulls water along, is often associated with dehydration, while excessive sodium retention can lead to swelling (edema) or high blood pressure or both.

Although unusual, it is also possible to drink enough water in a short period of time to develop water intoxication. Such excessive water drinking is usually the result of a psychiatric disorder known as psychogenic polydypsia (poly means many; dypsia means thirst), but a few cases of water overload have been reported in people following fad diets that called for excessive amounts of water as part of a weight-loss plan. In such cases, the kidneys cannot keep pace with the volume of fluid being ingested. As a result, the cells take up the extra water, diluting the concentration of sodium and other electrolytes—elements that help balance the acidity-alkalinity of fluids within the body's cells. This prevents the cells from functioning properly. Water intoxication can lead to convulsions, coma, and death.

HOW MUCH WATER?

The requirement for water varies greatly from one person to another and there is no RDA. Climate, exercise, and individual differences in perspiration affect fluid needs. Normally, thirst is the best indicator of water need, but this mechanism is not perfect. People often consume only enough liquid to quench a dry or parched throat but not enough to cover all their losses. Thus the recommendation that we should drink six to eight 8-ounce glasses of liquid, or the equivalent, a day—thirsty or not—is a good one.

Fortunately, drinking beverages is not the only way to satisfy the body's fluid needs. Few of us drink enough to replace the daily losses of two and a half to three quarts or more. The remainder comes from chemical reactions within the body that release water and from solid foods. Most fruits and vegetables contain 80 to 95 percent water; like human muscle, meats are about 45 to 65 percent water, and even bread weighs in at about 30 to 37 percent water. (See Table 10.1.)

BEVERAGES

Water

Ninety percent of the drinking water in the United States comes from the country's 60,000 public water systems. About half of the water from municipal supplies comes from lakes, streams, rivers, and other forms of surface water; the other half comes from groundwater—reserves of water hidden beneath the earth in large areas of water-bearing rock, sand, or gravel that are called aquifers.

Regardless of its source, water is always two parts hydrogen and one part oxygen, but only distilled or demineralized water is really pure. Tap water also contains varying amounts of essential minerals such as calcium, sodium, magnesium, manganese, sulfur, potassium, iron, chromium, iodine, selenium, zinc, fluorine, copper, chloride, and traces of lithium, as well as varying amounts of bacteria and contaminants such as arsenic and lead. The exact composition depends on where the water came from and how it was processed.

The minerals found naturally in water come from the soil and rocks through which the water passes. Different kinds and amounts of minerals give water from different sources a taste unique to that source. Since the type of soil and rock varies from city to city and state to state, the taste of tap water—and its nutritional value—varies accordingly. Several years ago, a *Consumer Reports* taste panel found New York City municipal tap water tastier than most bottled waters, including the most famous.

Water Hardness and Softness

The mineral content of water gives it other properties, as well. Water that is naturally hard is given that designation because it has relatively high levels of calcium and magnesium, which leave a residue that can build up in home appliances, reducing their ability to transfer heat, and sometimes clogging pipes and parts. It's these mineral deposits that stay behind after the water has evaporated that also cause clothes to gray in the wash and water spots or film to appear on clean dishes.

Soft water is distinguished by higher levels of sodium. Many people prefer soft water because it leaves less residue and doesn't interfere with the lathering action of soap. As a result, some municipalities soften their water by removing calcium and magnesium and adding sodium.

While this process may lead to cleaner clothes, it has some drawbacks from a nutritional standpoint. While calcium, magnesium, and sodium are all essential nutrients, the average diet is often relatively low in calcium but quite high in sodium. The amount of sodium added to water supplies, although not large, may be undesirable for those on low-sodium diets.

Soft water also tends to dissolve toxic metals such as lead and cadmium that are in

the water pipes much more readily than hard water does. (See Lead and Drinking Water on page 146 for more information regarding this.)

Some investigators suggest there may be certain disease-protective effects to hard water. Many studies in the United States, Canada, and in other parts of the world indicate the death rates from cardiovascular disease for populations using soft water are up to 15 percent higher than for those using hard water, but other studies have failed to find this association. There are also many different speculations and theories about which specific factors may be involved in any association between water and health.

Water Pollution

Along with differences in mineral concentration, water as it comes from ground or surface supplies also contains varying levels of contaminants. Some of these such as sand, silt, gravel, and organic compounds from de-

Table 10.1.	Percent of Water in Common Foods
Celery	95
Mushrooms	92
Watermelon	92
Broccoli	91
Whole milk	88
Apples	84
Grapes	81
Eggs (hard-boiled)	75
Potato (baked)	71
Chicken breast (roasted)	65
Tuna (canned)	62
Ground beef (broiled)	55
Frankfurter	54
Cheddar cheese	37
English muffin	29
Pound cake	24
Graham cracker	5
Mixed nuts	2

caying vegetation affect mainly the clarity, taste, and odor of water, while others such as human organic waste carry disease-causing microorganisms that can result in epidemics of waterborne illness. While modern methods of water purification—particularly chlorination—have eliminated such infectious diseases as cholera, typhoid fever, and dysentery, problems still exist. Between 1971 and 1985, 445 outbreaks of waterborne illness affecting over 100,000 Americans were reported, but because many more cases often go unreported, the Environmental Protection Agency estimates the number of Americans affected

Lead and Drinking Water

In 1986, the Environmental Protection Agency reported that an estimated 40 million Americans may be drinking water containing an unacceptable level of lead. Excessive exposure to lead can cause serious damage to the brain, kidneys, nervous system, and red blood cells. Young children, infants, and fetuses are particularly vulnerable to lead poisoning.

Currently, the EPA sets a limit of up to 50 parts per billion for lead in drinking water, and, generally, local water-treatment plants have no problems meeting this standard; water leaving the treatment plant is usually relatively lead-free. However, lead levels can increase significantly after the water leaves the treatment plant, due to corrosion of lead-containing pipes or solder. Amendments passed in 1986 to the Safe Drinking Water Act require that only lead-free pipes and solder be used in new pipe construction and plumbing repairs in public water supplies and in residences connected to public water supplies. In June of 1988, the EPA also lowered the limits for lead in the drinking water to 20 parts per billion or fewer.

The major source of contamination of household water is the lead solder that, until recently, was used in joints of copper plumbing. Lead can also come from old lead pipes, which were frequently used for interior plumbing and in municipal water systems built before 1930. Whether or not lead is leached from pipes and joints depends on the corrosiveness of the water flowing through the pipes. The more acidic or "soft" the water is, the greater its ability to pull lead from the pipes. The local water-supply authority can provide information about the corrosiveness of the water.

The best way for homeowners or apartment dwellers to determine the lead content of drinking water is to have the water tested. This is particularly important if the plumbing was installed before 1930. Plumbing installed within the last five years—if lead solder was used—is also more likely to cause contamination, since leaching from lead solders diminishes after five years. Contact the local water utility or the local health department for information and assistance regarding water testing. Individuals should check their water pipes, looking for a dull gray color of the joints or pipes themselves. Silver indicates plumbing made of other metals. When in doubt, try scratching the metal with a key; lead is soft enough to be easily scratched.

The following steps can also be taken in the home to protect against excessive lead in the drinking water.

- In the morning or after any prolonged period of nonuse, let the cold water run until it becomes as cold as it will get. This should be done for each faucet in the household used for drinking or cooking. In this way, the water that has been standing in the pipes and accumulating lead will be flushed out. (This water can be used for bathing purposes.)

- Avoid using hot water from the tap for cooking or for mixing hot drinks or baby formula, as hot water tends to dissolve more lead from pipes than cold water.

- Avoid water softeners, or use them only on the hot-water line. Harder water leaches far less lead than does softened water.

was probably between 300,000 and 500,000.

In recent years, public-health professionals have become increasingly concerned about a whole new group of man-made compounds that can contaminate groundwater and surface water when used or discarded improperly. Detergents, pesticides, fertilizers, industrial by-products, nuclear wastes, and a wide variety of chemicals often seep into our water supply through storm runoff, industrial dumping, leaking underground storage tanks, and landfills.

While some of these contaminants pose no immediate health threat for short periods of exposure, others are harmful even in small amounts, if long-term exposure occurs. These compounds can be extremely difficult to remove once they have contaminated a water supply.

Ironically, certain disinfectants used to purify water can also create potentially hazardous by-products. Chlorine, for example, can react with natural and man-made chemicals in water to produce chemicals known as trihalomethanes (THMs). There is strong evidence that certain trihalomethanes, such as chloroform, can cause cancer and/or can cause genetic mutations that promote cancer.

To deal with the problem of water contamination, Congress passed the Safe Drinking Water Act of 1974, which requires the EPA to set minimum national standards for drinking-water quality. To meet these standards, many water supplies are disinfected and filtered to prevent bacterial contamination and remove impurities.

The Safe Drinking Water Act currently requires the EPA to set maximum contaminant levels (MCLs) for 26 potentially harmful substances that must be monitored in public water systems. These include certain radioactive compounds, trihalomethanes, pesticides, herbicides, and inorganic chemicals, as well as bacteria. Responsibility for monitoring the levels of contaminants in water falls to the water utilities, who, in turn, must periodically report the quality of the water supply to the state or, occasionally, federal government. If the water fails to meet the EPA's levels and poses a serious health risk, the municipality must also notify consumers of the problem and provide instructions on any necessary precautions.

In 1986, Congress passed several amendments to existing legislation that make the measures designed to protect our drinking water even more rigorous. Under these amendments, the EPA is in the process of issuing MCLs for a total of 83 contaminants. In addition, the EPA must identify candidates for future regulation and regulate 25 of these every three years. These amendments also require the EPA to set criteria for disinfection and filtration, as well as make it easier for the agency to enforce the standards.

Ensuring safe and adequate supplies of drinking water for all Americans has become an increasingly complex issue. Small municipal systems, in particular, have technical and economic difficulties in complying with EPA regulations. Fortunately, however, most reports of tainted tap water are fairly isolated and easily correctable. In general, the supplies of drinking water in America are among the world's safest. (See Ensuring a Safe Water Supply on page 148.)

Bottled Water

The increase in the consumption of bottled water has been dramatic. Until 1977, bottled water was barely a ripple on the surface of the U.S. beverage industry. Since then, it has become a wave. According to Beverage Marketing Corporation, a New York-based market research and consulting firm, Americans drank some 1,223 million gallons of domestic nonsparkling water; 183 million gallons of club soda and seltzer; 116 million gallons of domestic sparkling mineral water; and 37 million gallons of imported bottled water in 1987—more than double the total consumption in 1981. Wholesale sales of bottled water now exceed $2 billion annually.

Traditionally, the bottled-water business has catered to people who are concerned about the purity of tap water or who don't like its odor or taste, and today, bottled drinking water—bought in bulk for drinking and cooking—still makes up the largest share of the market.

Drinking bottled waters, especially foreign imports, has also become a fashionable alternative to alcoholic beverages, coffee, and soda. Although manufacturers cannot, by law, make health claims about their products, packaging and advertising cite the purity and

mineral content, with the implication that their water is more healthful than tap water.

Bottled water comes from a variety of sources: springs, spas, wells, geysers, or simply public water supplies. No government rule obligates companies to disclose the location of their water's source, though many brands do. After the Consumer's Union, an independent consumer group, rated New York City tap water tastier than most bottled water, entrepreneurs began bottling and selling New York City tap water to visitors.

All bottled water, except for purified or distilled water, naturally contain minerals, although the amounts differ from brand to brand. Some bottling companies either add or subtract minerals to source water during processing in order to achieve a desired flavor.

Ensuring a Safe Water Supply

If the water streaming from the tap becomes unusually brown, cloudy, or otherwise murky-looking, or if it develops a strange odor or unpleasant taste, immediately contact the local water utility or the local health department for information and assistance. In some instances, these authorities will test the water, or they can recommend a qualified laboratory.

Many toxic hazards are colorless, tasteless, and odorless. Laboratory analysis is the only way to be certain that drinking water meets safety standards. Since all municipal water supplies must, by law, be tested on a regular basis, first ask the local water superintendent for the latest test report.

Individuals whose water comes from a private well, or those concerned about contamination by chemicals that are not included in routine testing, may want to have their water analyzed by a commercial laboratory, listed in the Yellow Pages under Laboratories, Testing. Check with the state or local department of the environment or health to be sure that the company has been approved by the state for testing drinking water.

Water-Treatment Systems

Several types of home water-treatment systems are also available, but it's important to realize that no one type may treat all water problems. For example, activated carbon filters can improve the taste and odor of water as well as remove many chemicals, but they won't remove bacteria or toxic metals such as lead. In fact, unless the carbon-filter cartridges are changed regularly, they can provide a breeding ground for bacteria. All home water-treatment devices should be thoroughly researched for use and performance before purchase.

Further information is available from *Consumer Reports,* January 1990, "Fit to Drink," and the EPA's Safe Drinking Water Hotline: 1-800-426-4791 and 1-202-382-5533 (Washington, D.C., residents). The hotline provides information on the agency's drinking-water programs, including standards for contamination, survey results, and well-water regulations.

Although mineral water has enjoyed a long-standing reputation for its therapeutic effects or restorative powers, the small amounts of minerals in bottled water are seldom either helpful or harmful. One exception may be sodium, which is sometimes present in amounts high enough to be a problem for those on salt-free diets.

The safety and purity of bottled waters are regulated by the Food and Drug Administration. FDA standards for most bottled waters are in line with the Environmental Protection Agency's standards for drinking water. However, EPA regulations do not apply to products labeled *mineral water* because it is assumed—sometimes incorrectly—that they are not a long-term, regular source of water. Likewise, sparkling waters, including club soda and seltzers, are exempt from the bottled-water standards because, for regulation purposes, they are considered soft drinks, not water, and therefore come under different FDA regulations. (See Types of Bottled Water below.)

Because of these regulatory loopholes, some bottled water may contain levels of contaminants that are higher than those allowed for tap or bulk water. In January 1987, *Consumer Reports* reported that levels of arsenic exceeded the federal standards for tap and bulk waters in 3 of 28 brands of sparkling waters; they recommended that these three not be used as a sole source of water.

At the present time, there is no evidence that bottled water is safer or nutritionally superior to tap water.

Fluoridation of Water

Fluoride—an essential trace mineral—is present in at least trace amounts in all natural water supplies, although the concentration varies widely. Fluoride concentrations of about one part per million (ppm) are associ-

Types of Bottled Water

Drinking water is most often used as an alternative to tap water and is sold in bulk. It can be obtained from any approved source—a spring, a well, a river, or even a tap. It has been disinfected and filtered and may have been demineralized and then remineralized to achieve a specific composition and flavor.

Spring water comes from a natural spring. If a product is advertised as natural spring water, the mineral content has not been altered. Spring water may be naturally carbonated, have carbonation added, or it may be still—without gas bubbles.

Sparkling water is carbonated, or made bubbly by dissolved carbon dioxide gas. If a water is labeled natural sparkling, the carbon dioxide occurs naturally in the source water. Otherwise, the carbon dioxide gas is added by the manufacturer.

Seltzer is typically tap water that has been filtered and artificially carbonated. No minerals or mineral salts are added.

Club soda is the same as seltzer except that it is flavored with mineral salts such as bicarbonates, citrates, and phosphates of sodium.

Mineral water is defined by the International Bottled Water Association as natural water that contains at least 500 milligrams of minerals per liter. Natural mineral waters contain only naturally occurring minerals; in others, the manufacturer may add or remove minerals.

Purified water has had its minerals removed. Some water is purified by distillation. In this process, the water is first evaporated into steam and then recondensed. Only purified water that has undergone distillation can be labeled distilled water.

ated with a lower incidence of tooth decay. Since the mid-1940s, fluoride has been added to many public drinking water supplies that lack a desirable level of natural fluoride. This process of fluoridation has gained an impressive record as a safe and cost-effective measure to reduce the incidence of dental caries. Nevertheless, fluoridation continues to be a process that incites local community fervor and fears based on misinformation—often deliberately planted by people who sell expensive water purifiers or profit thereby.

Like many essential nutrients—sodium, potassium, iron, vitamins, and even water itself—fluoride can be toxic in excessive quantities. However, more than four decades of research have found no ill effects or symptoms resulting from drinking water containing natural or added fluoride at the desirable level of one ppm. Daily intakes of 20 to 80 milligrams or more for years are necessary to produce serious toxicity symptoms. The amount consumed from fluoridated water is typically about 1 to 2 milligrams a day, with another 0.2 to 0.6 milligrams coming from food.

In a few areas of the country, primarily Texas and South Carolina, naturally high concentrations of fluoride have been known to cause fluorosis, a discoloring of the tooth enamel that occurs prior to tooth eruption. The U.S. Surgeon General has determined fluorosis to be a cosmetic rather than a health problem, however.

Although the benefits and safety of fluoridation have been resoundingly demonstrated in more than 30 countries, 40 percent of the public water systems in the United States still contain suboptimal amounts of fluoride largely because of scare tactics used by the opponents of fluoridation. The continuing campaigning of these antifluoridation groups gives the illusion of scientific controversy over the safety of the process, but actually there is no controversy. The practice is safe, econom-

ical, and beneficial. The Consumers Union has called the survival of this fake controversy "one of the major triumphs of quackery over science in our generation." Leading antifluoridationists lost in court when they claimed the Consumers Union defamed them by indicating their "fluoridation causes cancer" statistics had no basis in reality.

Soft Drinks

The first carbonated beverage was produced in 1772 by a renowned British scientist, Joseph Priestley. However, carbonated water wasn't sold commercially in America until some 34 years later. Flavored soda water became popular in the early 1800s, and by 1860, 123 commercial plants were producing flavored carbonated drinks.

In 1886, a druggist named John Styth Pemberton created a carbonated beverage to be used as a remedy for headaches and hangovers by adding an extract from the African kola nut to an extract from coca. After Pemberton's death, Atlanta druggist Asa Candler became sole owner of the first carbonated cola beverage and formed the Coca-Cola Company in 1892.

Today the amount of soft drinks consumed per year continues to grow at a dizzying pace, having increased more than 300 percent since 1950. In 1971, sodas surpassed coffee as America's most popular beverage, and by 1987, per capita consumption totaled more than 16 ounces a day, amounting to 46.4 gallons per year.

Weight consciousness has also had a major impact on the carbonated beverage market. In 1987, diet sodas represented 23.5 percent of total soft drink consumption in America, up from 7 percent in 1970.

Multimillion-dollar advertising outlays fostering an alleged link between carbonated beverages and a youthful, active lifestyle may be responsible for the fact that those between 12 and 34 years consume more soft drinks than any other group. Those from 6 to 11 rank second in soft-drink consumption. A 1986 survey found that 25 percent of the one- to three-year-olds studied drank carbonated beverages, averaging 7 ounces a day.

This soaring popularity is of particular concern to nutrition professionals. Soft drinks are the number-one source of added sugar in the American diet and have surpassed tea as the second most important source of caffeine.

Actually, only cola and "Pepper" soft drinks are flavored with kola-nut extracts, a neutral source of caffeine. Some manufacturers also add caffeine extract to typically caffeine-free beverages, however. Food and Drug Administration regulations permit caffeine to be added at levels up to 6 milligrams per ounce, although caffeine-containing soft drinks generally fall between 2.5 and 4.9 mg., usually less than in either coffee or tea. Young children, however, consume more caffeine from soft drinks per body weight than adults and may be more sensitive to caffeine's stimulant effects, especially if they are unaccustomed to it.

There is also a growing selection of caffeine-free soft drinks on the market.

Ingredients

Regular soft drinks are 86 to 92 percent carbonated water and 7 to 13 percent sugar—often in the form of high fructose corn syrup. Each 12-ounce can contains the equivalent of 9 to 12 teaspoons of sugar, or 144 to 192 calories. Diet soft drinks are about 99 percent carbonated water and contain saccharin, aspartame (NutraSweet), or a blend of the two. Other soft-drink ingredients usually include natural and artificial flavors, and edible acids for tartness. Optional ingredients include caffeine, preservatives, caramel or artificial colors, and gums and thickeners to regulate consistency.

With an eye toward the health-conscious consumer, soft-drink manufacturers have introduced carbonated beverages with added fruit juice. While a few of these new varieties contain as much as 75 percent natural fruit juice, most are only about 10 percent juice—an amount that adds next to nothing to their nutritive value. The juice component of these beverages is often an inexpensive blend of fruit concentrates rather than a particular fruit juice. Some juice-added drinks contain added vitamins as well, but none is nutritionally equal to a glass of pure fruit juice.

In moderation, carbonated beverages can be an acceptable part of the diet, provided nutrient needs are met from other foods and that calories from soft drinks are taken into account. As the intake of soft drinks increase, however, so does the possibility that they will take the place of more nutritious beverages in the diet.

Coffee

Americans consume more coffee than any other national population, drinking almost a fifth of the world's 6.5 million ton production. In 1987, average daily consumption was about one and three-quarters cups per person—down 44 percent from the 1962 peak of slightly over three cups per person. The percentage of the population drinking coffee has also fallen—from almost 75 percent in 1962 to 52 percent in 1987.

Coffee is composed of at least 393 chemicals. Its principal ones are caffeine, tannins, caramelized sugar, carbon dioxide, and various aromatic constituents. A six-ounce cup of coffee contains trace amounts of several vitamins and minerals, as well as about four calories.

Coffee has been the major dietary source

of caffeine in the American diet since 1773. Presently it provides 75 percent of all the caffeine consumed in the United States. The amount of caffeine per serving varies with the variety of coffee bean used, the coffee grind, the method and length of brewing, and whether the coffee is regular or instant. (See Table 10.2 for the caffeine content of beverages.)

Recent concern has focused on the effects of moderate coffee consumption on health. It has been speculated that caffeine may cause cancer, coronary heart disease, high blood cholesterol, ulcers, and birth defects, but no hard evidence to support these speculations has appeared so far. Caffeine is a stimulant and a diuretic, and too much of it can be harmful because of these pharmacologic qualities. (See Caffeine and Related Substances on page 153.)

Decaffeinated Coffee

Health concerns about caffeine have spurred a considerable increase in the consumption of decaffeinated coffee. In 1962, only 4 percent of the population drank decaffeinated coffee; by 1987, 17.5 percent were choosing decaffeinated at least part of the time. Coffee is decaffeinated by exposing green coffee beans to steam and solvent in a rotating drum. The caffeine is absorbed by the solvent and then steam is used to wash out the caffeine-bearing solvent, leaving only trace amounts. Most American manufacturers use methylene chloride, ethyl acetate, water, or natural coffee oils as extracting fluids.

The use of methylene chloride, in particular, has been questioned because rats given extremely large dosages (equivalent to a person's drinking 12 to 24 million cups of de-

Table 10.2. Caffeine Content of Popular Beverages

Item	Caffeine Content (mg.)	Item	Caffeine Content (mg.)
Coffee (5 oz.)		Soft drinks (12 oz.) *(cont.)*	
Drip method	60–180	Mello Yello	52
Percolated	40–170	RC Cola	48
Instant	30–120	Diet RC Cola	48
Decaffeinated	1–5	Tab	46
		Coca-Cola (Cherry or Classic)	46
Tea (5 oz.)		Diet Coke (also Diet Cherry Coca-Cola)	46
1-min. brew	9–33	Shasta Cola	44
3-min. brew	20–46	Shasta Cherry Cola	44
5-min. brew	20–50	Shasta Diet Cola	44
Instant (5 oz.)	12–28	Sunkist Orange	40
Iced tea (12 oz.)	22–36	Dr. Pepper, regular and sugar-free	39.6
Hot cocoa (6 oz.)	2–20	Pepsi-Cola	38.4
		Diet Pepsi	36
Chocolate milk (8 oz.)	2–7	Pepsi Light	36
Soft drinks (12 oz.)		Canada Dry Jamaica Cola	30
Jolt	72	Canada Dry Diet Cola	2
Shasta Diet Cherry Cola	56		
Mountain Dew	54		
Shasta Citrus Mist	53		

Note: There are at least 200 flavors, varieties, and types of soft drinks, manufactured by the leading bottlers, that contain no caffeine.

Sources: Food and Drug Administration, Institute of Food Technologists, National Coffee Association, Consumers Union, and the individual soft-drink manufacturers.

caffeinated coffee virtually every day throughout a lifetime) developed cancer.

Current FDA regulations permit the decaffeination of coffee with methylene chloride as long as the residue does not exceed 10 parts per million. FDA calculations show that at the maximum residue level, the cancer risk over a lifetime of drinking decaffeinated coffee is between one in 100 million and one in 250 million. However, since the level of methylene chloride in most decaf coffee sold in the United States is considerably below the permitted maximum, the cancer risk is considered almost negligible. The methylene chloride method has been largely replaced by a water method in many decaffeinated coffees.

Tea

Tea, with its ancient and rich cultural heritage, is the most popular beverage in the world. In the United States, however, it ranks behind coffee, soft drinks, milk, and fruit juice.

Although tea leaves have a higher con-

Caffeine and Related Substances

Caffeine and the related substances theophylline and theobromine belong to a group of drugs called methylxanthines—or xanthines for short—that occur naturally in more than 60 species of plants, including coffee and cocoa beans, kola nuts, and tea leaves. These three chemicals have similar actions on the body, although they differ in the intensity of their actions.

Caffeine is absorbed rapidly, appears in all tissues and organs within about 5 minutes of ingestion, and reaches its peak in the blood within about 30 minutes. Caffeine is a relatively mild central nervous system stimulant; 85 to 250 milligrams of caffeine (the equivalent of one to three cups of coffee) suppress fatigue and improve alertness. Higher doses of caffeine, however, may produce nervousness, restlessness, and insomnia. Some individuals are sensitive to even small amounts of caffeine. (See Chapter 22 for more information.)

Theophylline (found in tea) is also a central nervous system stimulant, and theobromine (the main xanthine in chocolate) does not have any significant effect on the central nervous system.

The xanthines also affect the cardiovascular system, although the actions of these chemicals are complex and sometimes antagonistic. In general, caffeine and theophylline stimulate the heart muscle and dilate coronary arteries, increasing blood flow to the heart. In excess (sometimes only modest excess), however, these substances can also trigger irregularities in the heartbeat in some people, especially those with preexisting heart conditions.

In contrast to their dilating effect on other blood vessels, the xanthines constrict the blood vessels of the brain, reducing cerebral blood flow. For this reason, caffeine may relieve some types of headaches associated with dilation of cerebral arteries and is often a component of both prescription and nonprescription analgesics used to treat headaches. Conversely, individuals who do not regularly drink coffee may find that heavy caffeine consumption may cause a headache, while abstention from coffee by heavy coffee drinkers may trigger a caffeine-withdrawal headache.

The xanthines also relax various smooth muscles, particularly those of the air passages, or bronchi. Theophylline is most effective in opening up bronchial airways and is, therefore, often prescribed in the treatment of asthma. A therapeutic dose of theophylline, however, is much greater than the one milligram that is contained in a cup of tea. Caffeine is also an effective bronchodilator, and it has been reported that as little as three cups of coffee can increase the potency of asthma medication containing theophylline.

All the xanthines act on the kidney to increase urination, which limits their usefulness in fulfilling the body's fluid needs.

centration of caffeine than coffee by weight, more coffee than tea is required to make a cup. Tea also contains small amounts of the caffeine-related substances theophylline and theobromine. All three substances are chemically known as xanthines. (See Caffeine and Related Substances on page 153.)

Another component of tea—tannins—can irritate the digestive tract and cause constipation. Tannins also bind with iron, cutting iron absorption by as much as 87 percent. Tea-drinking vegetarians are especially susceptible to iron deficiency. Both caffeine and tannins can be reduced by limiting steeping time. Also, the addition of milk to tea binds the tannins, making them less available for binding to iron. Tea also comes in decaffeinated form, which contains less of the stimulant.

Herbal Teas

The focus on natural, caffeine-free alternatives to coffee and tea has resulted in the recent popularity of herbal teas. Herbal teas are not tea in the true sense of the word—that is, made from leaves of the tea bush—but drinks brewed from the flowers, leaves, seeds, bark, or roots of any plant or combination of plants.

Herbal teas were once available only in health-food stores, but supermarkets now stock a wide variety. Popular blends include the familiar ingredients cinnamon, ginger, mint, lemon, orange, and apple. Unfortunately, many exotic varieties found in health-food stores contain ingredients that can cause side effects that are much more serious than those of caffeine. Some of the most potent natural poisons—hemlock, curare, mandrake, belladonna—are also found among the herbs.

While many of the spices and herbs found in herbal teas are approved by the FDA

for use as seasonings, they have not been tested for safety as teas. For example, a pinch of nutmeg added to a cup of eggnog has no harmful effects, but when brewed into tea, it can cause rapid pulse, dizziness, disturbed vision, and hallucinations.

Herb teas made from some herbs such as lobelia, wormwood, root of pokeweed, foxglove, or mistletoe are toxic. Sassafras, comfrey, and coltsfoot contain cancer-causing substances. Some herbs such as senna, aloe, buckthorn bark, and dock roots can cause severe diarrhea if too much is consumed. Even the common chamomile and yarrow teas can cause serious allergic reactions in individuals sensitive to pollen from ragweed, asters, and chrysanthemums. (For more information, see Tips for Enjoying Herbal Teas Safely on page 155.)

Additional information can be found in: *The "New" Honest Herbal*, Varro E. Tyler, Ph.D., 2nd edition (Philadelphia: George F. Stickley Co., 1987); and in the appendix of *Vitamins and Health Foods: The Great American Hustle*, V. Herbert and S. Barrett, paperback (Philadelphia: George F. Stickley Co., 1985).

Cocoa

Cocoa contains only small amounts of caffeine, but much larger amounts of a related chemical, theobromine, which is similar to caffeine in its structure and biological effects. Cocoa and chocolate products contribute very little to per capita caffeine consumption in the United States.

Instant dry mixes contain varying amounts of cocoa, but sugar tends to be the primary ingredient in all but the low-calorie varieties. In contrast to the traditional cup of homemade cocoa—milk, sugar, cocoa and water—instant mixes may contain more than 20 ingredients, including several different sweeteners, sodium, saturated fat, thickening agents, artificial flavors, and other additives.

Mixes generally fall into two categories: those meant to be mixed with milk—either hot or cold—or water mixes that contain non-fat dry milk and need only to be mixed with hot water. Most of the nutrients in the milk-supplied mixes are from the added milk, although the mixes themselves provide substantial amounts of protein, calcium, and riboflavin, as well as a variety of other vitamins and minerals. The water mixes usually provide only half or less the protein and calcium supplied by cocoa made with milk, although some are fortified with calcium or other vitamins and minerals.

Milk

The popularity of other beverages, particularly soft drinks, has had a major impact on the consumption of milk, which dropped steadily from 1945 to 1983.

Currently, however, milk consumption is again on the rise, due at least in part to the heightened calcium consciousness of Americans. Within that rise, however, whole-milk sales have dropped markedly, reflecting a concern over fat, while low-fat milk has skyrocketed—jumping from less than half a pint per person in 1955 to more than 52 quarts per person in 1987.

Milk is one of our most nutritious foods. An eight-ounce serving of whole milk (3.3

Tips for Enjoying Herbal Teas Safely

Most popular varieties of herbal teas, when taken in moderation, are not harmful. To be on the safe side, follow these tips.

- Buy only tea bags manufactured by well-known companies. Avoid loose teas commonly sold in health-food stores. Often they are not clearly identified, and many of them are contaminated by other substances that may have harmful effects.

- Read the ingredient list. The names of teas often do not give any indication as to what they contain.

- Use a new variety of tea sparingly, taking only a small amount of a weak mixture. If there are no adverse effects, have more the next time.

- Don't substitute herbal teas for conventional medicines. The concentration of therapeutic (and toxic) ingredients in herbal teas varies depending on the plant the tea comes from, how the herb is stored, and the strength of the tea, making herbal treatment haphazard and possibly dangerous.

- People taking prescription drugs should check with a physician or pharmacist before drinking herbal teas. The druglike actions of some herbal compounds can counter or exaggerate the effects of the prescribed drug.

- Never gather leaves, roots, berries, seeds, or flowers to make tea, even if following a guidebook. Many plants have toxic look-alikes and mix-ups can be deadly.

- Since the long-term effects of drinking any herbal tea are unknown, don't drink more than two to three cups a day on a regular basis.

- Pregnant women should be particularly cautious when drinking any herbal tea, since effects of these generally untested substances on the fetus are unknown. The same warning holds for giving herbal teas to children.

percent fat) contains nearly one-fifth of the RDA for protein and calcium, as well as riboflavin, vitamin B_{12}, and phosphorus. Fat, at slightly more than eight grams, contributes nearly half of the 150 calories. Most milk is also fortified with vitamin D.

Low-fat and skim milk fortified with vitamins A and D have essentially the same nutrients as whole milk but with less fat, meaning fewer calories.

In contrast, powdered and liquid non-dairy creamers are generally high in calories and fat and contain few if any vitamins or minerals. Their use should be limited to a spoonful in an occasional cup of coffee, rather than as a constant substitute. Nonfat dry milk is an acceptable low-calorie alternative, as is skim or low-fat milk.

In an effort to compete with soft drinks, a dairy-association trade group has developed carbonated milk, in flavors such as peach, coconut, mint, strawberry, cola, and root beer. Made by bubbling carbon dioxide through skim milk and then adding flavorings and sweeteners, the product is designed to appeal to a younger, upscale market as a tasty drink combining milk's calcium, vitamins, and minerals with carbonation's light, fizzy taste.

Many adults cannot drink milk freely because of a deficiency of lactase—the intestinal enzyme necessary to break down the lactose in milk. This common condition, known as lactose intolerance, generally occurs after five years of age and is typified by gas, cramps, bloating, and diarrhea when milk is consumed. Many lactose-intolerant people can consume certain dairy products as well as small amounts (three to six ounces) of milk without incurring symptoms. (For more information about lactose intolerance, see Chapter 33.)

Raw Milk

Contrary to health-food claims, when consumed in its raw, unpasteurized state, milk is far from being a healthful food. On the contrary, unpasteurized milk is often contaminated with bacteria that can transmit disease to humans. Objective studies have shown no health benefits from the consumption of raw rather than pasteurized milk, nor are there any significant nutritional differences between raw milk and its pasteurized counterpart. Yet, due to heavy promotion, the sale of raw milk has persisted and even increased in recent years. The Food and Drug Administration has declared raw-milk consumption to constitute an unnecessary health risk and has banned interstate shipments of raw milk intended for consumer use.

Fruit Juices

Consumption of fruit juice has more than doubled since 1950, jumping from 2.1 to 5.4 gallons per person in 1986. This trend in fruit-juice consumption reflects the increased concerns about a healthy diet, but unfortunately misconceptions about the nutritional value of fruit juices abound.

Not all fruit juices are rich in vitamins and minerals, nor are they necessarily low in calories. The nutritive value of the juice depends on the fruit from which it is made. Although there is a myth that the juice is more nutritious than the whole fruit, this is not so. Usually, some of the nutrients and most of the fiber are left behind in the pulp.

Nevertheless, citrus juices are rich sources of vitamin C as well as lesser sources of several other nutrients such as potassium and folic acid. One cup of prune juice provides about three milligrams of iron (almost 17 percent of the RDA). Other popular juices such as apple, cranberry, or pineapple provide few vitamins unless they are fortified.

It does not matter whether juices are fresh-squeezed, because the differences among fresh-squeezed juice, juice reconstituted from frozen concentrate, and canned juice are insignificant if the juices have been stored properly. (For example, the frozen concentrate must remain frozen *hard* until it is reconstituted, or nutrients will be lost.) All juices quickly lose vitamins if they are not stored properly after squeezing, reconstituting, or opening.

Fruit juices are also a rich source of natural sugar (fruit sugar). Lemon juice has the lowest percentage at 6 percent; prune juice, at 19.5 percent, is the highest. Eight ounces of the most popular—orange juice—contains the equivalent of almost five teaspoons of sugar. In fact, fruit juices and soft drinks contain roughly the same amount of total sugar—and total calories; soft drinks, however, lack the vitamins and minerals of natural juices.

The popularity of fruit juices has given rise to a host of drinks with *fruit* in the title, but these contain little or no actual juice. These fruit drinks, ades, punches, nectars, breakfast drinks, and cocktails are generally mixtures of water, sugar, fruit juice (10 to 50 percent), coloring agents, artificial flavorings, citric acid, and preservatives, with vitamin C added. Some of them may contain no fruit juice at all. In addition to providing fewer nutrients, these beverages are often more expensive than the pure juices. (For the calorie content of different beverages, see Table 10.3.)

Alcoholic Beverages

Alcohol consumption has leveled off in recent years after increasing more than 60

Table 10.3. Beverage Calorie Counter*

Club soda or seltzer	0	Orange juice	109
Diet soda	2	Fruit punch drink	112
Tea (unsweetened, 6 oz.)	2	Apple juice	116
Coffee (black, unsweetened, 6 oz.)	4	Bloody Mary (5 oz.)	116
Tomato juice	42	Cocoa, instant (6 oz.)	120
Vegetable-juice cocktail	52	Orange-flavored carbonated beverage	120
Flavored coffees (instant, sweetened with		2%-fat milk	121
sugar, 6 oz.)	56	Tom Collins (7.5 oz.)	121
White table wine (4 oz.)	80	Whiskey sour (3 oz.)	123
Ginger ale	80	Pineapple juice	134
Tonic water	80	Cranberry juice cocktail	144
Red table wine (4 oz.)	84	Beer (12 oz.)	146
Skim milk	86	Whole milk	150
Iced tea (sweetened with sugar)	90	Grape juice	155
Grapefruit juice	97	Martini (2.5 oz.)	156
Carrot juice	98	Chocolate milk, low-fat	169
Lemon-lime carbonated beverages	99	Gin and tonic (7.5 oz.)	171
Kool-Aid (sweetened with sugar)	100	Screwdriver (7 oz.)	174
Lemonade (sweetened with sugar)	100	Prune juice	181
Light beer (12 oz.)	100	Piña colada (4.5 oz.)	262
Cola carbonated beverages	101	Shake (fast-food, 10 oz.)	331
1%-fat milk	102		

*All values are for 8 oz. unless otherwise indicated.

percent from 1962 to 1981. In 1987, total alcoholic-beverage consumption averaged 40.1 gallons per adult, down from the 1981 peak of 44.6 gallons per adult.

From a nutritional point of view, all alcoholic beverages may be classified as foods because they provide energy in the form of calories. Pure alcohol—which by volume makes up 4.5 percent of beer, 11.5 percent of table wine, and 40 to 50 percent of distilled spirits, including gin, whiskey, and vodka—contains seven calories per gram as compared to the four calories per gram contributed by any additional carbohydrates. Some wines contain iron and potassium as well as a number of other vitamins and minerals, and beer has substantial amounts of niacin, chromium, phosphorus, and vitamin B_6. However, in the amounts normally consumed, the contribution of beer and wine to daily vitamin and mineral requirements is very small. The vitamin or mineral content of distilled liquors is negligible unless fruit-juice mixers are used.

Heavy drinkers who often fail to eat regular meals consume alcohol calories empty of essential nutrients ("empty calories") rather than essential vitamins and minerals. Large amounts of alcohol also interfere with the absorption and metabolism of many nutrients. Alcohol, too, is a diuretic, causing the body to lose water. (For more information about alcohol and nutrition, see Chapter 21.)

11

Food Additives (Including Preservatives)

Victor Herbert, M.D., J.D.

∎

INTRODUCTION

There are few issues in nutrition that are more controversial and misunderstood than the question of food additives. Large numbers of Americans honestly believe that our foods are laced with poisons in the form of additives (including preservatives), and that we all would be healthier if we could eat nothing but so-called natural or organic foods. Overlooked is the fact that many of these additives are actually natural components of other foods (e.g., cornstarch). Others, such as sugar and salt, are added to make food tastier or as preservatives. Still others are preservatives that extend shelf life or make foods safer. In addition, some, such as food dyes, are added for cosmetic purposes to make food more attractive.

Sugar, salt, and corn sweeteners account for 93 percent, by weight, of all food additives consumed in the U.S. Another 6 percent is limited to 32 common substances, such as yeast, baking soda, vegetable colors, mustard, and pepper. The remaining commonly used additives, primarily flavoring substances, total only 1 percent of consumption, or 0.07 ounces of each additive per person per year. Some of these additives could be elimi-

nated without sacrificing flavor, nutritional quality, or safety. Food dyes are a classic example. The question is, Would consumers buy pale oranges, gray preserved meats, and so forth? In the public's mind, however, it is the safety of food additives that is of major concern. In recent years, food additives have been blamed—with little or no basis in fact—for a mind-boggling assortment of human physical and mental ills, everything from childhood hyperactivity to adult schizophrenia and cancer. Food manufacturers have hopped on the additive-free bandwagon by offering an assortment of all-natural foods—usually at a premium price.

The "chemical-sounding" names of additives increase the confusion. Most health professionals realize that all foods, even fruits and vegetables fresh off the vine, are mixtures of chemicals. The health food literature, however, misleads people into believing there are important differences between naturally occurring chemicals and the same chemicals produced synthetically and added to food.

Are concerns over the use of food additives justified? For the most part, no; in fact, food today is safer, more nutritious, and more plentiful than at any other time in human history, thanks largely to modern agriculture and the use of preservatives and other additives. Of course, there are some additives, such as dyes, artificial flavors, unnecessary (and often excessive) added vitamins, pesticide residues and other environmental contaminants that we could do without. In large amounts, some of these may be hazardous. On balance, most of these are not a valid threat to health, however. When they are hazardous, it is often due to individual circumstances. For example, a person with high blood pressure should avoid foods with large amounts of added salt, and people with sulfite-sensitive asthma should not eat foods treated with sulfiting agents. In this chapter, we will attempt to set the record straight by discussing the major categories of food additives, their use and misuse, benefits and hazards.

WHAT ARE FOOD ADDITIVES?

Broadly speaking, food additives are any substances that do not occur naturally in foods. They may be direct additives, also known as intentional additives, added to improve flavor, texture, or color or to prevent spoilage. According to the Food and Drug Administration, there are about 2,800 substances that fall into this category of intentional additives. In addition, there are more than 10,000 indirect additives (unintended additives); for example, environmental pollutants or substances that enter the foods during growing, processing, or packaging. Public confusion over additives is linked to the outpouring of misinformation and speculation on the effects of additives on nutrition. It is nutrition-cult dogma that the road to good health lies in the avoidance of additives. The spate of pop wisdom on additives has placed an increased burden on health professionals to separate fact from fiction and to communicate the scientific facts.

Some food additives, such as salt and various spices, have been used for thousands of years and it is hard to imagine food without them. Others, such as artificial flavor, colorings, and certain preservatives, are relatively new. Additives are carefully regulated for safety now, and must serve useful purposes. Preservatives, for example, help prevent food-borne disease, such as salmonellosis and botulism, and make possible the abundance and variety of foods upon which good nutrition depends. Tables 11.1 and 11.2 list some of the more common food additives. The different types of intentional (direct) food additives are generally categorized according to how they are used. Functions include:

Maintaining or improving nutritional value. Many of today's foods are enriched by adding nutrients to replace those lost in food processing. The B vitamins that are added to flour are examples of this. Others may not naturally appear in specific foods but are added to ensure against deficiencies. This is called food fortification. Examples include adding iodine to salt, vitamin A to margarine, or vitamin D to milk. *Enrichment* entails adding back a nutrient lost in processing. *Fortification* means adding a nutrient not naturally present in the product.

While these latter examples are laudable, adding vitamins and minerals to foods can be carried too far. A few years ago, for example, there were numerous media reports to the effect that some breakfast cereals, especially the sugar-coated varieties aimed at children, were "empty calories" (i.e., just calories, without containing vitamins and minerals). A number of manufacturers responded by adding vitamins and minerals, so that a serving would be equivalent to a multivitamin pill. A balanced diet, not cereal alone, provides all the needed vitamins and minerals. If regular cereal is part of a balanced and varied diet, added vitamins and minerals are not needed in it. What's more, millions of American adults and children already take unneeded vitamin pills, so turning a bowl of cereal into another dose is merely an expensive frivolity.

Often, fortification is to take advantage of current fads or public concerns. For example, calcium is now being added to cereals, fruit juices, and other foods to profit from increased public awareness of the mineral's role in promoting healthy bones. Breads, cereals, and a variety of other foods are fortified with extra fiber to take advantage of the current fiber fad. Vitamin C is being added to soft drinks or high-sugar drink mixes. Fortifying foods to replace lost nutrients is an acceptable strategy to maintain good nutrition. However, turning individual foods into vitamin and mineral supplements is quite another, and a trend that should be discouraged. It is unnatural, undercuts teaching good nutrition, is not accompanied by studies showing the added excess is desirable and does not produce adverse nutrient-nutrient interactions, while increasing selling prices.

Maintaining freshness or extending shelf life.
A number of food additives are intended to retard spoilage, prevent fats and oils from turning rancid, or maintain color and flavor (see Table 11.2). Some of the preservatives are natural food substances, such as salt, sugar, ascorbic acid (vitamin C), or vitamin E. Nitrites and nitrates are added to processed meats to retard spoilage and also help maintain the pink color characteristic of hot dogs, luncheon meats, ham, and other such products. United States law requires the addition of five parts of ascorbate to each part of nitrite or nitrate, thereby preventing nitrosamine (a carcinogen) formation. Sodium propionate (naturally present in Swiss cheese) is commonly added to bread and other baked goods to slow down the growth of molds. When

consumed in moderate amounts, these preservatives are not harmful; in fact, they actually make foods safer by preventing growth of disease-causing organisms. For example, botulism—a serious food poisoning resulting from a toxin produced by a bacterium—is now quite rare thanks to the use of preservatives such as nitrites and nitrates.

A good deal of the public suspicion regarding food preservatives stems from their unfamiliar chemical names. Many common food preservatives are chemicals that occur naturally in other foods. For example, sodium propionate helps give Swiss cheese its special taste, but it's not listed on the cheese label, because it's a natural ingredient in that product. Therefore, some natural-food advocates will eat Swiss cheese without giving sodium propionate a second thought but will decry the far smaller amounts that are added as a preservative to bread and other baked goods. An ounce of Swiss cheese naturally contains the same amount that is added to a pound of bread.

The safety of our food supply was emphasized in a 1989 report to Congress from 14 scientific societies with a total membership of more than 100,000 food scientists, microbiologists, toxicologists and veterinarians. This report, coming on the heels of the public furor over Alar—a growth regulator sprayed on apples—concluded that the major hazards in our food are not from additives and pesticide residues but, instead, from disease-causing microorganisms.

"The threat from pesticides is more calculated than real," the scientists maintained. Most food-borne illnesses are caused by preventable factors, such as mishandling, poor sanitation, and lack of hygiene, which promote the growth of salmonella and other organisms.

Why, then, do so many Americans believe that their food is unsafe? Why are they

Table 11.1. Common Food Additives

Additive	Foods Found in	Purpose
Acetic acid	Dressings, vinegar, sauces	Acidity control
Acetone peroxide	Fruit/gelatin desserts	Bleaching agent
Adiptic acid	Pie fillings, salad dressings, gelatins	Acidity control
Ammonium alginate	Processed foods	Thickening agent
Annato extract	Cheeses	Color
Arabinogalactan	Fillings, puddings	Thickening agent
Ascorbic acid	Fruit products	Nutrient
Aspartame	Low-calorie sweeteners	Sweetener
Azodicarbonamide	Baked goods	Bleaching agent
Benzoil peroxide	Flours, baked goods	Bleaching agent
Beta carotene	Margarine	Nutrient/color
Calcium alginate	Baked goods	Thickening agent
Calcium bromate	Baked goods	Bleaching agent
Calcium phosphate	Baked goods, mixes	Leavening
Calcium silicate	Powdered foods, table salt	Anticaking agent
Caramel	Baked goods, ice cream, puddings	Color, flavor
Carob-bean gum	Ice cream	Thickening agent
Carrageenan	Frozen desserts, puddings	Emulsifier
Carrot oil	Yellow foods	Color
Cellulose	Fiber products, "lite" breads	Thickening agent
Citric acid	Canned fruits, beverages	Acidity control preservatives
Citrus red no. 2	Red or yellow foods	Color
Corn syrup	Many foods	Sweetener
Dehydrated beets	Jellies, baked goods, other foods	Color
Dextrose	Fruit juices	Sweetener
Diglycerides	Ice cream, peanut butter	Emulsifier
Dioctyl sodium- sulfosuccinate	Mixes, processed foods	Emulsifier, flavor enhancer
Disodium guanylate	Canned meats, meat-based products	Flavor enhancer
FD & C colors:		
Blue no. 1	Foods, drugs, cosmetics	Color
Red no. 40	Foods, drugs, cosmetics	Color
Yellow no. 5	Foods, drugs, cosmetics	Color
Folic acid	Cereals, other foods	Nutrient
Fructose	Fruits, candies, other sweets	Sweetener
Gelatin	Desserts, canned products	Thickening agent
Glucose	Juices, sweets	Sweetener
Glycerine	Toaster foods, flaked coconut, marshmallows	Humectant
Glycerol monostearate	Cake mixes, baked goods	Humectant
Guar gum	Gravies, sauces, pet foods	Thickening agent
Gum arabic	Dry mixes, foods with butter and other fats	Emulsifier, stabilizer
Gum ghatti	Sauces, frozen desserts	Thickening agent
Hydrogen peroxide	White foods	Bleaching agent
Hydrolyzed vegetable protein	Processed meats, stock, dry mixes	Flavor enhancer

Table 11.1.   Common Food Additives *(cont.)*

Additive	Foods Found in	Purpose
Iodine	Salt	Nutrient
Iron	Grain products	Nutrient
Iron ammonium citrate		Anticaking agent
Karaya gum	Frozen desserts, puddings	Thickening agent
Lactic acid	Yogurt, cheese, other milk products	Acidity control
Larch gum	Fillings, desserts	Thickening agent
Lecithin	Mayonnaise	Emulsifier
Locust-bean gum	Ice cream	Thickening agent
Maltol	Strawberry, raspberry, soft drinks	Flavor enhancer
Mannitol	Baked goods, frozen desserts	Sweetener, antithickening agent
Modified food starch	Pie fillings, gravies, sauces	Thickening agent
Monocalcium phosphate	Baked goods	Leavening agent
Monoglycerides	Baked goods, ice cream	Emulsifier
Monosodium glutamate	Chinese cooking, frozen meat, vegetable dishes	Flavor enhancer
Niacinamide	Flour, rice, cereals	Nutrient
Pectin	Jams, jellies	Thickening agent
Phosphates	Tart beverages, gelatin desserts	Improves tartness
Phosphoric acid	Soft drinks, desserts	Improves tartness
Polysorbates	Many processed foods	Emulsifier
Potassium alginate	Frozen desserts	Thickening agent
Potassium bromide	Baked goods	Bleaching agent
Potassium iodide	Salt	Nutrient
Propylene glycol	Cake mixes, baked foods	Humectant
Riboflavin	Flour, rice, macaroni	Nutrient, color
Saccharin	Dietetic foods	Sweetener
Silicon dioxide	Dried foods	Anticaking agent
Sodium acetate	Tart foods	Acidity control
Sodium alginate	Chocolate products	Thickening agent, stabilizer
Sodium aluminum sulfate	Baked goods	Leavening
Sodium bicarbonate	Baking soda	Leavening
Sodium calcium alginate	Desserts, jellies	Thickening agent
Sodium citrate	Tart foods	Acidity control
Sodium stearyl fumarate	Baked goods	Bleaching agent
Sorbitan monostearate	Cake mixes	Emulsifier
Sorbitol	Sugar-free gum and candy	Humectant, sweetener
Tagetes	Yellow foods	Color
Tartaric acid	Pie fillings, tart foods	Acidity control
Thiamine	Breads, cereals, flour	Nutrient
Titanium dioxide	Frostings, other white foods	Color
Tocopherols (Vitamin E)	Baked goods, milk, cereal	Nutrient
Tragacanth gum	Puddings, sauces, mixes	Thickening agent
Ultramarine blue	Many foods	Color
Vitamin A	Milk, cereals	Nutrient
Vitamin D (D_2, D_3)	Milk	Nutrient
Yellow prussiate of soda	Baked goods, mixes	Anticaking agent

Source: Adapted from *FDA Consumer*, April 1979.

Table 11.2. Common Food Preservatives

Antimicrobials Type	Foods Found In
Ascorbic acid (vitamin C)	Fruit products, acidic foods
Benzoic acid	Fruit products, acidic foods, margarine
Butylparaben	Beverages, dressings, relishes
Calcium lactate	Olives, cheeses, frozen desserts
Calcium propionate	Breads and other baked goods
Calcium sorbate	Cheeses, syrups, mayonnaise, margarine
Citric acid	Acidic foods
Heptylparaben	Beverages, dressings, relishes
Lactic acid	Olives, cheeses, frozen desserts
Methylparaben	Beverages, dressings, relishes
Potassium propionate	Breads and other baked goods
Potassium sorbate	Cheeses, syrups, cakes, processed meats
Propionic acid	Breads and other baked goods
Propylparaben	Beverages, cakelike pastries, relishes
Sodium benzoate	Fruit products, margarine, acidic foods
Sodium diacetate	Baked goods
Sodium erythorbate	Cured meats
Sodium nitrate	Cured meats, fish, poultry
Sodium nitrite	Cured meats, fish, poultry
Sodium propionate	Breads and other baked goods
Sodium sorbate	Cheeses, mayonnaise, processed meats
Sorbic acid	Cheeses, fruit products, syrups
Antioxidants Type	**Foods Found In**
Ascorbic acid	Fruit products, acidic foods
BHA (butylated hydroxyanisole)	Bakery products, cereals, fats and oils
BHT (butylated hydroxytoluene)	Bakery products, cereals, fats and oils
Citric acid	Fruits, snack foods, instant potatoes
EDTA (ethylenediamine tetraacetic acid)	Dressings, margarine, canned vegetables
Propyl gallate	Cereals, snack foods, pastries
TBHQ (tertiary butyl hydroquinone)	Snack foods, fats and oils
Tocopherols (vitamin E)	Oils and shortenings
Vitamin C (ascorbic acid)	Fruit products, acidic foods

Source: Adapted from *FDA Consumer*, April 1979 and May 1979.

willing to pay premium prices for "organic" foods that, in fact, often harbor more disease-causing fungi, bacteria, and other organisms than foods not labeled "organic"? There are no simple answers, but a number of factors are involved:

1. *A general mistrust of big business.* Food production in this country is a major industry, with most of our produce grown on a large scale using high-tech or production-line methods rather than on family farms adhering to less economical, albeit "trusted" and nostalgic, methods. Chemical fertilizers have replaced barnyard manure (even on most family farms), and people have been led to believe that these artificial substances do not produce food that is as nutritious as that grown with organic fertilizers. Although there is no scientific basis for this belief, many "health-food" salespeople and self-styled nutritionists claim that foods grown with chemical fertilizers are lacking in nutrients. Unfortunately, large numbers of people believe them, even though the claims are false.

2. *A general mistrust of government.* In recent decades, the Food and Drug Administration and the Department of Agriculture have formulated more stringent regulations regarding food production, especially in the area of additives, pesticides, and food handling. As a result, hundreds of substances have been tested for safety, and those deemed unsafe have been banned. When new evidence is produced showing that a product is unsafe, it, too, is banned from the food supply. There may be shortcomings in the system, but there is no doubt that food produced and sold in the United States is among the world's safest. (See the section on Ensuring Food Safety on page 166.)

3. *Effective public-relations tactics of the "natural-food" industry and self-styled nutritionists.*

These basic facts are downplayed or distorted by the "natural-food" industry, self-proclaimed experts, and well-meaning but misinformed consumer advocates. For example, the terms "natural" and "organic" when used to distinguish grains, fruits, vegetables, and meats sold in health food stores from those sold elsewhere is misleading. No matter where one buys them, all grains, fruits, vegetables, and meats are inherently natural and organic. Similarly, all food is health food in moderation, and any food is junk food in excess.

The term "nutritional food" to distinguish what is sold in health food stores from what is sold elsewhere is merely consumer-deceiving hype. The health food industry actually set up a school run by a diploma-mill Ph.D. to sell "nutritionist" diplomas to "health food" promoters and salespeople so they can use their impressive-looking diplomas and initials after their names to lend credibility to their sales pitches, and health food stores sell literature written by diploma-mill Ph.D.s who regularly appear on talk shows as "nutrition experts." Some nutrition cult figures make a comfortable living and gain craved limelight by pandering to paranoia against "industry and government," and screaming "freedom of choice" when they mean "freedom to deceive."

Providing texture or consistency. Leavening agents, such as sodium bicarbonate or phosphates, are added to baked goods to make them rise or achieve a desired texture. Texture also is improved by various emulsifiers, such as carrageenan, gum arabic, or glycerine, which help hold in moisture or prevent the oils in foods such as peanut butter or mayonnaise from separating from the other ingredients. Thickening agents such as pectin or guar, both common and naturally occurring forms of soluble fiber, are added to ice cream, pudding, jellies, and other such foods to achieve and maintain their characteristic texture. Home cooks often use many of these same ingredients, but they know them under more familiar names, such as baking powder or Sure-Jell.

Enhancing flavor or appearance. Commercial foods contain many of the same natural spices, herbs, and other flavor enhancers used in home cooking. However, food manufacturers also may add a variety of artificial flavors, dyes, bleaching agents, and other ingredients to give a desired taste or color. Some of these coloring agents are natural food components, such as the carotene used to give margarine and some cheeses their yellow color. Others are artificial colors or vegetable dyes manufactured specifically for foods.

Food purists often argue that coloring agents are unnecessary cosmetic additions that none of us need, and, of course, these cosmetic additives are not needed to improve safety or nutritional values. Since some food dyes used in the past have since been banned as unsafe, an argument can be made for the removal of all dyes. However, the reality is that most people want their food to look and smell appealing, and when given a choice, they will select foods that have been doctored over less attractive, albeit all-natural and equally nutritious, counterparts. In the marketplace, people will invariably pick the "right"-looking (dyed) orange over a paler, all-natural one that may have come from the very same tree. Of course, a good deal of this is due to conditioning and food advertising that features picture-perfect produce. If a person wants to avoid food dyes, bleaches, and other mostly cosmetic additives, then he or she should be prepared to select foods that may not look as appealing as those that have been "improved."

Retaining moisture, preventing caking, and miscellaneous other functions. Certain additives, such as magnesium carbonate added to table salt, help keep it free-flowing by preventing caking. Humectants such as glycerine may be added to such foods as shredded coconut to prevent drying.

ENSURING FOOD SAFETY

Contrary to the popular notion that additives detract from the safety of our food, many of today's additives actually increase safety by retarding spoilage. This has not always been the case, however. In the post–Civil War era, for example, there was a major population shift from farms to industrialized cities, and consequently, changes in food production and distribution occurred. In 1870, New York newspapers carried alarming stories about cows cooped up in filthy stables and fed mostly city garbage, so "enfeebled from tuberculosis that they had to be raised on cranes to be milked." Food preservatives in those days included formaldehyde for milk, sulfurous acid for meat, and borax for butter. Eventually, in 1906, the Pure Food and Drug Act was passed, and from that time onward, various governmental agencies have been charged with ensuring the safety of our food supply.

The Pure Food and Drug Act has been amended a number of times since 1906, including 1958, when Congress passed the Food Additive Amendment and the Delaney Clause, which bars substances that have been shown to cause cancer in either animals or humans from being used as food additives. The Delaney Clause says in essence that even if it takes 10 pounds of a substance to produce a cancer in a rat, not a trace of that substance may be used as a food additive.

As noted earlier, there are some 2,800 substances that are intentionally added to foods. By far the most common of these are salt, sugar, and corn syrup, followed by citric acid, baking soda, vegetable colors, mustard, and pepper. According to a recent Food and Drug Administration report, these account for "more than 98 percent, by weight, of all food additives used in this country." Most other additives, including preservatives, are used in very small quantities as allowed by the FDA. For example, the FDA limits the amount of BHT (for butylated hydroxytoluene) or BHA (for butylated hydroxyanisole)—antioxidants that prevent fats from turning rancid—to less than 0.02 percent of the fat or oil content of a food. Health-food salespeople simultaneously condemn adding traces of BHT and BHA to foods, and sell concentrates of BHT and BHA as "life extension formula," presumably in the belief that since BHT and BHA are antioxidant food preservatives they are also antioxidant life preservatives. Some such concentrates are toxic.

New additives must be tested for safety and approved by the FDA before they can be added to foods. The extensive testing and ongoing reviews of aspartame, an artificial sweetener, is an example of the required process. Many older substances that have been used for years but were never formally tested are now undergoing safety evaluations. Others are generally regarded as safe (GRAS), even though they may not have been formally tested. The GRAS listing is limited to substances in use prior to 1961.

In discussing the issue of food safety, it should be noted that intentional (direct) additives rank far down on the list of potential hazards. In the late 1970s, Dr. Virgil Wodicka of the FDA ranked the hazards associated with foods in the following order:

1. *Disease-causing microorganisms.* A number of different bacteria, molds, viruses, and other microorganisms can contaminate foods. Some of these organisms produce toxins that can cause acute food poisoning; one of the most

familiar (albeit uncommon) examples is the *Clostridium botulinum* organism that produces a poison that causes botulism. This organism in "natural" (i.e., without added preservatives) honey has caused problems with infants in California. Others cause disease more rapidly; salmonella and shigella infections are relatively common examples. Most of the food-borne diseases reported to the Centers for Disease Control fall into this category. It is estimated that there are 1.4 to 3.4 million cases of food poisoning in the United States each year caused by food-borne bacteria or other microorganisms. Most of these cases are relatively mild and self-limiting, but there are exceptions, such as hepatitis caused by contaminated shellfish or other foods.

Some food-borne diseases may not show up for years. An example that is undergoing considerable study is liver cancer linked to aflatoxin, a poison produced by molds found on peanuts, cottonseed, and corn in some parts of the United States, particularly the Southeast. Crops produced in susceptible areas are now screened, and produce with an aflatoxin content of more than 20 parts per billion—the limit allowed by the FDA—is barred from the food supply.

According to Dr. Edwin M. Foster, director of the Food Research Institute at the University of Wisconsin, "virtually all food poisoning incidents in the United States are traceable to mishandling in the home or in food service operations. Rarely is a disease outbreak attributable to errors in commercial processing." (See Chapter 41.)

2. *Environmental contaminants.* There are a number of potentially harmful chemicals that can enter the food supply. These include pesticides used by food growers; residues of antibiotics, hormones (e.g., diethylstilbestrol), and other substances fed to animals; environmental pollutants such as heavy metals (e.g.,

mercury or arsenic), asbestos, PCBs, vinyl chloride, and other industrial waste products. Many people think that pesticide residues pose a major health hazard; in reality, however, the use of these agents is closely regulated in the United States and they are thought to be of very little hazard. When a hazard is demonstrated by scientific evidence, the substance is banned.

Industrial and other pollutants are a greater potential danger. Although foods are regularly tested for these substances and steps taken to eliminate the worst offenders (e.g., FDA efforts to reduce the lead content in cans used by food processors), it is almost impossible to eradicate them totally from the food supply, particularly when they contaminate waters with fish, groundwater, and animal feed. A commonsense approach that includes eating a variety of foods to ensure against overconsumption of one or two items that may have a particularly heavy load of contaminants is the wisest course.

When not covered by federal regulations, individual states and cities sometimes enact laws, regulations, and advisories to protect the public against the hazards of eating contaminated foods. For example, New York State recommends its citizens not eat fish caught in the Great Lakes more than twice a week, and it forbids clamming in areas heavily polluted with municipal sewage. Some midwestern states warn against eating game birds whose diet is polluted.

3. *Naturally occurring toxicants.* Since prehistoric times, humans have recognized that certain plants and animals are poisonous. By trial and error, these pretty much have been eliminated from the diet. Inadvertent food poisonings still occur from eating things such as toxic mushrooms and poisonous shellfish, plants, berries, and the like. Many of these accidental poisonings involve children who eat

toxic berries or plants. (See below for a listing of common toxic plants.)

4. *Reaction products.* These include substances that are formed during cooking or processing. Examples include the hydrocarbons (e.g., benzopyrene) that form in beefsteak when it is broiled over charcoal or the nitrosamines that can result when bacon or other cured meats are cooked at a high temperature. Although some of these reaction products in animal studies can promote cancer, their true impact on human health is unclear. While it is not necessary to eliminate these foods totally from your diet, the American Cancer Society advises a prudent approach and cooking techniques that minimize exposure. For example, the flavor of a char-broiled steak can be achieved by precooking the meat in a pan or under a broiler and then placing it on the grill for the last couple of minutes of cooking. Eighty-five percent of charcoal-flavored products sold in the United States have the flavor of grill cooking added, and thus don't contain the amounts of hydrocarbons and nitrosamines created in actual grilling.

5. *Food additives.* Although the general public perceives food additives to be a leading cause of diet-related illness, they actually are at the bottom of Dr. Wodicka's list. In recent years, several substances such as red dye no. 2 and cyclamates have been barred as food additives. The use of certain other substances is still under review by the FDA, but as noted earlier, most additives are used in such small quantities that they pose little or no danger to human health. Again, eating a varied diet can help minimize exposure to any particular ad-

Common Poisonous House and Garden Plants

The following plants are found in many homes and gardens in the United States. This does not include the many varieties of poisonous mushrooms and numerous poisonous plants found mostly in woods or wilderness areas.

Autumn crocus (bulbs)
Azalea
Belladonna (deadly nightshade)
Bird of paradise (seed pod)
Bittersweet (*Solanum dulcamara* variety, not the
   Celastrus scandens used in winter bouquets)
Castor bean
Delphinium
Dieffenbachia (dumb canes)
English ivy (berries and leaves)
Henbane
Holly (berries)
Hyacinth (bulbs)
Hydrangea
Iris
Jack-in-the-pulpit

Jasmine (flowers)
Jerusalem cherry
Jimson weed
Lily of the valley
Mistletoe (berries)
Narcissus (bulbs)
Oleander
Philodendron
Poinsettia
Poison hemlock
Potato (sprouts, stems, and leaves—only the
   tuber is edible)
Rhubarb (leaves)
Water hemlock
Yew

Note: Seeds from apples, apricots, cherries, peaches, plums, and other stone fruits contain cyanogenic glycosides. Cyanide poisoning has occurred from eating them.

ditive, and if a person knows he or she has problems with a particular additive (for example, sulfites may trigger a severe reaction in asthma sufferers), food labels should be carefully checked to avoid exposure and when eating out, reliable restaurant personnel should be asked whether the particular offending substance is in the food desired. A particularly tragic death occurred when a Brown University student who knew she was sensitive to peanuts ate the popular chili in a Providence restaurant—not knowing that the secret ingredient in the chili was peanuts.

A COMMONSENSE APPROACH

Despite public opinion to the contrary, our food supply today is the safest and most abundant that the world has ever known. The notion that somehow chemicals are bad for you ignores the simple fact that all foods (as well as human beings and other living matter) are made up of chemicals. Of course, some chemicals are harmful and even lethal. Some can

occur naturally in foods and others are added, usually in such small amounts that they pose no danger when consumed as part of a varied and balanced diet.

The consumer movement of the 1960s and 1970s raised public consciousness about food safety and the role of nutrition and health. Although much of this effort was misdirected "food terrorism," there have been positive results. Overconsumption has been recognized as the real problem. Large numbers of people today read food labels and have cut down on excess salt, sugar, fats, and calories. Wise consumers today know that catchwords for *healthy*, such as *natural* and *organic*, simply indicate higher prices and have little real meaning so far as either health or good nutrition is concerned. Some misconceptions persist, but increasingly, the public priorities are being shifted away from so-called unsafe processed foods and placed on more genuine health threats, such as alcohol and drug abuse, tobacco use, and obesity—all of which fit under the heading of overconsumption.

To quote Norman E. Borlaug, winner of the 1970 Nobel Peace Prize for pioneering the "Green Revolution," in his Foreword to Elizabeth Whelan's book *Toxic Terror* (Ottawa, IL: Jameson Books, 1985): "You have been told that as a result of your country's high state of technology and economic development, your environment is making you sick, when the exact opposite would be closer to the truth. . . . Life expectancy at birth continues to increase despite the doomsday predictions of the toxic terrorist. . . We have the luxury to worry about the "carcinogen of the week" and the "toxin of the month" . . . Banning chemical fertilizers and pesticides will inevitably lead to deadly serious food shortages. . . . Banning other industrial chemicals will likewise impoverish our nation."

Table 11.3.   Some Food Additives Whose Safety Has Been Questioned

1. Salt	16. Nitrate
2. Sugar	17. Phosphate
3. Xylitol	18. Cobalt salts
4. Mannitol	19. BHA-BHT
5. Aspartame	20. Caramel
6. Saccharin	21. Caffeine
7. Cyclamates*	22. Carrageenan
8. Red #2*	23. Monosodium glutamate
9. Red #3	24. Diethylpyrocarbonate*
10. Red #40	25. Modified starches
11. Yellow #5	26. Hydrogenated fats
12. Violet #1*	27. Brominated vegetable oil
13. Carbon black*	28. Synthetic colors and
14. Sulfite	flavors
15. Nitrite	

*Banned from U.S. food supply.

Adapted with permission from "Is There a Food Safety Crisis?" by Edwin M. Foster, Ph.D., in *Nutrition Today*, November/December, 1982. Most are safe as used.

Part III

Good Nutrition from Infancy to Old Age

■

12

Nutrition During Pregnancy and Breastfeeding

Richard Berkowitz, M.D., and Rosemary Wein, R.N.

■

INTRODUCTION

There are very few periods in a woman's life when eating properly is as important as when she is pregnant. The old saying that the mother-to-be eats for two is true in a sense. She doesn't need to eat twice as much food—after all, the fetus is only a fraction of the size of the mother—but what she eats is twice as important. The reason for this is that the growing fetus has significant nutritional needs as new bones, tissues, organs, and blood are formed.

Adequate nutrition is essential in order for a woman to give birth to a baby of normal weight, about seven and a half pounds. A baby with a low birth-weight, weighing under five and a half pounds, is at a distinct disadvantage. He or she is more likely to develop health problems and to reach adulthood with a smaller stature.

The necessity for good nutrition during pregnancy has been recognized since ancient times. Galen, Aristotle, and Hippocrates all believed good diet could prevent miscarriages and assure the delivery of a healthy infant.

Ideas shifted in the late eighteenth century, when the British doctor James Lucas proposed that pregnant women restrict their diet—particularly in the last weeks of pregnancy—in order to produce a smaller baby that would more easily pass through the pelvis during birth. Other leading European physicians of the day embraced and elaborated upon this erroneous concept. They regarded the baby as a parasite in the mother's body, taking whatever it needed to grow. There was little recognition of a link between maternal nutrition, the course of pregnancy, and the health of the baby. For almost two centuries, obstetrical thinking advocated a limit on protein intake and a weight gain of no more than 15 pounds during the course of a pregnancy.

The tide turned in the 1960s. A historic study of nearly 12,000 deliveries at Johns Hopkins Hospital in Baltimore showed that women who weighed more at the time they conceived, and who gained more weight when pregnant, gave birth to larger babies and fewer low-birth-weight babies. Today, there is no doubt that if the quantity and quality of a mother's diet are adequate—both at the time of conception and during pregnancy—fewer problems will arise and a larger, healthier baby will result. Obstetricians now favor greater weight gain, more protein and iron in the diet, and the abandonment of laxatives, diuretics, and sodium restrictions.

Old notions die hard, however. Some people continue to believe that dietary cravings in a pregnant woman are signals from the womb demanding specific missing nutrients. Others think the baby will get what it needs, regardless of what the mother eats. In truth, the baby and the mother compete for whatever nutrients reach the mother's bloodstream after digestion. If there is a nutritional shortage, both fetus and mother must turn to the mother's body reserves to meet the demand. When this occurs, both are shortchanged.

Modern medical research has left no doubt that cigarettes, alcohol, and what the ancients called unclean substances are bad for both mother and fetus. Many obstetricians now advise their patients not to drink any alcohol during pregnancy, and even when trying to conceive. Deformed, mentally retarded, or addicted babies born to mothers who abuse mind-altering drugs are dramatic evidence of the worst that can happen when toxic substances cross the placental barrier. While it is unlikely that caffeine in moderation adversely affects the fetus, moderation may stop at the equivalent of about two cups of coffee a day.

A nutritious diet is important not only *during* pregnancy but *after*, too, especially if the mother is breastfeeding. Just as during pregnancy, the mother is eating for the baby as well as herself. Only the specific requirements have changed. The postpartum period is also a time when paying special attention to diet—whether breastfeeding or not—can help the new mother shed extra pounds and regain her figure.

CONCEPTION AND DIET

Today, there is more and more emphasis on how good nutritional habits can set the stage for pregnancy, long before conception is con-templated. There is no doubt that a pregnant woman who is in poor nutritional shape will give birth to a baby of smaller size, and a smaller baby is at greater risk for a host of medical problems.

Moreover, if poor nutrition continues throughout that baby's life, it perpetuates a vicious cycle. Women who start life nutritionally compromised, and remain poorly nourished, are likely to have permanent physical damage, including reduced height and more narrow pelvic bones. Studies show that such women later have reproductive problems, including more difficulty during labor, babies smaller at birth, and more infant deaths from all causes.

Dieting—that great obsession of many young American women—often leaves a woman's nutritional status in jeopardy. If not corrected before conception, this threatens her ability to have a successful pregnancy. In fact, chronic dieting is the underlying cause of infertility in some women. Severe and prolonged caloric restrictions can cause the menstrual cycle to become irregular, even to the point of ceasing altogether. The lack of a menstrual period—called amenorrhea—signals that ovulation is so disturbed that conception is not possible.

By studying women on various diet regimes, researchers have found that fluctuating female hormones can lead to disturbances in the menstrual cycle within a few weeks of starting a calorie-restricted diet. A classic example of dieting-induced amenorrhea is seen in women with anorexia nervosa, an eating disorder in which the individual deliberately starves herself. Amenorrhea is also seen often in the dedicated female athlete, such as the marathon runner or long-distance swimmer.

Some methods of contraception can compromise a woman's overall nutritional status, causing problems if conception occurs just after use of the contraception stops. For example, some women experience increased menstrual-blood flow when using an intrauterine device (IUD). This puts them in negative iron balance, increasing their risk of developing iron-deficient tissues, and even iron-deficiency anemia. It is important to remember that only about half the women with iron-deficient tissues actually have anemia.

Oral contraceptives, particularly if used over a prolonged period, can alter the levels of various nutrients in the body. Iron and copper levels may increase, partly because the lessened menstrual flow means a lessened iron loss. Nutrient levels that may decrease moderately include: carotene, folic acid, vitamins B_6 and B_{12}, calcium, phosphorus, magnesium, zinc, and vitamins C and E. While such levels are usually still within the normal range, there could be significant losses in a woman whose diet is already poor.

Ideally, women who intend to become pregnant should take concrete steps to be ready before conceiving. The first weeks after conception are the most critical in the embryo's development. Frequently, a woman is not yet aware that she is pregnant. A woman who takes the attitude that she will change her diet and lifestyle *after* she is sure she is pregnant could be endangering the health of her baby.

The first step is to eat a balanced diet that meets all of the body's basic nutritional needs, including calories, protein, vitamins, and minerals. Women who are either underweight or overweight should modify their diets in an attempt to reach an ideal weight prior to conceiving. Desirable weight charts, such as the one in Chapter 17, can be used to determine what a woman's prepregnancy weight should be.

Women who are more than 15 percent under their desirable weight are particularly at risk for complications of pregnancy and childbirth. Research has found that underweight women are more likely to suffer cardiac and respiratory problems during pregnancy. Anemia also is more common among underweight women, a combination that increases a pregnant woman's chances of delivering a low-birth-weight baby. Indeed, compared to normal-weight women, underweight women give birth to smaller babies with lower Apgar scores (a measure of an infant's heart rate, respiration, muscle tone, reflexes, and color at birth, used to predict neonatal difficulties).

Upon the advice of a physician, women who are overweight should follow a reducing program to get down to a desirable weight before conceiving. Being overweight during pregnancy increases a woman's risk of developing gestational diabetes and high blood pressure. Furthermore, it increases the likelihood of her giving birth to a large baby, which can cause complications during delivery and may require her to have a cesarean section. Waiting to diet until after becoming pregnant is dangerous to the fetus, as it may be deprived of necessary nutrients.

Women who drink should cut back alcohol consumption, or even abstain completely, before conceiving. That is because a woman may not yet know she is pregnant when alcohol's worst effects are likely to occur—in the first weeks after conception, when the embryo is developing. Smoking also has a deleterious effect on the fetus, and every attempt should be made to reduce smoking or, ideally, to stop the habit before conception. The same advice applies to taking drugs—both prescription and nonprescription and even mild use of recreational drugs—and to taking over-the-counter food supplements, all of which should be stopped (except for those that will be prescribed in most prenatal clinics and by an obstetrician/gynecologist). This is especially important with respect to over-the-counter vitamin A supplements, including cod-liver oil. As little as 25,000 IU of vitamin A taken daily in the month before and during the first month of pregnancy (before a woman knows she is pregnant) may produce the same birth defects as does isotretinoin (Accutane), a molecule structurally similar to vitamin A. (See Planning for Pregnancy, below.)

HOW THE BODY CHANGES AFTER CONCEPTION

Pregnancy, from the moment of conception onward, is a period of intense growth for the fetus. Its weight increases from the nearly imperceptible weight of the egg and sperm to a seven-and-a-half-pound infant in a period of nine months. From a height of 1 inch seven weeks after conception, the fetus grows to almost 20 inches at birth.

Soon after conception, the growing mass of cells that will become the fetus implants it-

self in the uterine wall and the placenta begins to form. The placenta is the principal production site of several hormones that regulate fetal growth and development. It is also the means by which nutrients and oxygen reach the fetus and waste products are eliminated. The fetus's and the mother's blood vessels spread out and intertwine. Essential substances flow back and forth across the placenta. Surprisingly, the placenta acts more like a sieve than a filter. Many undesirable and even highly toxic substances, such as alcohol and drugs, readily pass across the placenta and can harm the fetus. In poorly nourished mothers, the placenta is smaller in size, weighs less, and has fewer villi, the structures through which the fetus receives nutrients and discharges wastes.

A good balance of all nutrients is needed

Figure 12.1.

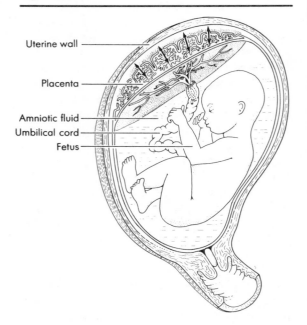

Uterine wall

Placenta

Amniotic fluid

Umbilical cord

Fetus

Planning for Pregnancy

Two to three months before a woman plans to become pregnant, it is recommended that she visit her obstetrician/gynecologist and discuss the following topics:

- Contraception (when to discontinue)
- Diet (weight gain/loss; intake of artificial sweeteners, caffeine, and alcohol; vitamin/mineral supplementation)
- Exercise
- Drugs (use of over-the-counter, prescription, and recreational drugs)
- Smoking
- Immunizations (especially rubella)
- Medical conditions (chronic diseases, sexually transmitted diseases, environmental or occupational hazards, family history)

Adapted from *Environmental Nutrition Newsletter*, January 1986, with permission of the publisher.

throughout pregnancy. The need for specific nutrients varies according to the stage of the pregnancy. Nutrition is particularly important in the first trimester, when cells differentiate and develop into the body's organs. If an organ's development is stymied by nutritional shortages, the full potential of that organ's growth cannot be made up later.

In the second trimester, the fetal demands for calcium are high because of intense bone and blood-cell formation. Good nutrition is vital in the third trimester, when the baby literally doubles in size. Adequate nutrients as well as calories are necessary to support the enormous demands of the fetus for energy. Adequate protein also is necessary to manufacture increasing amounts of new tissue during the last ten weeks of pregnancy.

A NUTRITIONAL PLAN FOR PREGNANCY

The overall goal of nutritional planning in pregnancy is for the mother to give birth to a healthy baby of normal size while remaining healthy herself. In the first weeks of life, low-birth-weight babies may suffer from what health professionals often describe as a failure to thrive. They also have a higher incidence of infant mortality. As they grow and develop, they are more likely to have physical handicaps, including hearing and visual disorders, lower I.Q.s or mental retardation, and serious illnesses during childhood. There is no question that a normal-size baby has a head start—both physically and mentally—over his or her smaller peers. (It should be noted, however, that very large babies—for example, nine pounds or more—also have an increased risk of serious problems.)

The precise amounts of nutrients required in pregnancy can vary widely from individual to individual. A woman's level of physical activity has a bearing, as does her overall size. Moreover, when pregnant, a woman's body apparently becomes more efficient in utilizing the nutrients she takes in. This plus other metabolic changes make interpretation of nutrient levels in the pregnant woman's blood difficult.

The Food and Nutrition Board of the National Research Council has formulated RDAs for a sample pregnant woman who is 23 to 50 years old, 5 feet, 4 inches, and weighs 120 pounds before conception. The RDA has built-in safety factors to assure that a woman is not receiving too little or too much of a nutrient. (See Chapter 7 for current RDAs.)

Table 12.1 provides a graphic illustration of the vitamins and minerals of most concern during pregnancy.

Table 12.1. Recommended Dietary Allowances for Adult Women (Ages 25 to 50 Years)

	Nonpregnant	Pregnant
Energy (kcal)	2200	+300
Protein (gm.)	46	+10
Vitamin A (RE)	800	same
Vitamin D (mg.)	5.0	+5.0
Vitamin E (mg.)	8.0	+2.0
Vitamin C (ascorbic acid) (mg.)	60	+10
Folic acid (mg.)	180	+220
Niacin (mg.)	13-15	+2.0
Riboflavin (mg.)	1.2-1.3	+0.3
Thiamine (mg.)	1.0	+0.4
Vitamin B_6 (mg.)	1.6	+0.6
Vitamin B_{12} (mg.)	2.0	+0.2
Calcium (mg.)	800	+400
Phosphorus (mg.)	800	+400
Iodine (mg.)	150	+25
Iron (mg.)	15	+15
Magnesium (mg.)	280	+40
Zinc (mg.)	12	+3.0

Adapted from *Recommended Dietary Allowances*, tenth edition, 1989, with permission of the National Academy Press, Washington, D.C.

Weight. Nutritional planning for an optimal pregnancy revolves around eating a balanced diet and gaining appropriate weight. The notions of a century ago about restricted weight gain have nearly vanished. There is general agreement that a woman who begins pregnancy at or near her desirable nonpregnant weight should gain between 24 and 28 pounds. Even among normal individuals, however, weight gain varies substantially. Younger women gain more than older women. Thin women gain more than fat women. First-time mothers gain more than women who already have had children.

Many obstetricians use 27 pounds as the magic number for weight gain. An underweight woman, however, should gain 27 pounds *plus* the additional pounds that she is under her desirable weight.

An overweight woman should not think of pregnancy as a time to lose weight. The fetus may be exposed to the ketones and other harmful substances that are stored in body fat and released when the fat is broken down. However, women who are very much overweight can gain a lesser amount—around 21 pounds—and still give birth to babies of normal weight.

It's easy to understand why nutrition is so important when you consider where all the 25 or so pounds of extra weight are distributed. Besides what is needed for the growth of the average seven-and-a-half-pound baby itself, there must be sufficient protein, calories, and nutrients to create about three pounds of additional maternal blood and five and a half pounds of tissue, fluid, and muscle to enlarge and support the uterus. One pound accounts for the increase in the size of the mother's breasts. The amniotic fluid weighs two pounds, while the placenta weighs one to two pounds. Only four of the 27 pounds are gained as fat, and it is needed to ensure adequate calories for breastfeeding. (See Table 12.2.)

For a woman whose prepregnancy weight is ideal for her height, a weight gain of two to three pounds during the first trimester, three to four per month during the second trimester, and three to four per month for the third trimester is desirable.

Calories. During the course of a pregnancy, the typical woman needs to consume 80,000 calories above and beyond what her body would need if she was not supporting a growing fetus. When spread over nine months, however, this represents only 300 extra calories a day. In contrast, protein, vitamin, and mineral needs are proportionately much higher, to create stores in a fetus starting with none. This means that the pregnant woman must choose her calories carefully so they are packed with nutrients. A candy bar, for example, would handily meet the 300 extra calories required but would not solve the pregnant woman's additional nutrient needs.

To calculate how many calories she needs, a woman should multiply her weight by the following number: 12 if she does little activity; 15 if she is moderately active; and 20 if she is very active. (If she is between the ages of 35 and 44, she should subtract 100 calories from the total). To this, a woman who is pregnant should add approximately 300 calories. During the first trimester, she will average about 150 extra calories; in the second and third trimesters, she will need an extra 350, to reach the average of an extra 300 calories daily during her pregnancy.

The empty calories of alcohol, sugar, and fats provide little that the growing fetus needs and serve only to increase the mother's fat stores. A pregnant woman's diet must emphasize nutrient-rich foods, such as skim milk, low-fat cottage cheese, lean meats, eggs, liver, and dark green vegetables.

The timing of the mother's weight gain is as important as the number of pounds gained.

Since most of the fetus's growth occurs in the last trimester, it is crucial for the mother not to cut down on calories in the last three months, even if she thinks she's already gained enough weight.

Protein. Within this 300 calories a day of extra food, there must be 10 grams of protein to meet the needs of the growing fetus. Most Americans, however, already eat far more protein than they need. A well-nourished woman may already be consuming 10 to 20 grams of protein a day more than her body requires. After becoming pregnant, she usually can easily meet her additional protein needs through one or two extra glasses of milk, an additional serving of lean meat, fish, or chicken, or through the protein contained in breads and cereals.

Vitamin A. The formation of skin and the linings of ducts in the gastrointestinal, urinary, and respiratory tracts of the fetus depend upon adequate amounts of vitamin A. Furthermore, a deficiency of the vitamin is known to cause eye abnormalities and impaired vision in some children.

The 1989 RDA for pregnant women calls for 800 RE of vitamin A per day (which is equivalent to 3,666 IU from animal sources), an amount easily met through consumption of a wide variety of vegetables, milk, cheese, and butter. There is no need for vitamin A supplements; in fact, they should be avoided during pregnancy and even during attempts to conceive.

Large doses of vitamin A—as little as five to ten times the RDA—can cause hypervitaminosis A in the mother, leading to headache, nausea, stiff neck, and other symptoms. Moreover, such excessive vitamin A intake during pregnancy may cause birth defects of the "Accutane baby" variety. Certain drugs that are derivatives of vitamin A—etretinate for psoriasis and isotretinoin (Accutane) for acne—can cause severe physical deformities if taken during the early part of or just prior to pregnancy, or at both times. The problems include misplaced ears, deformed or missing limbs, impaired kidney function, and central nervous system malformations. As of mid-1988, the FDA requires all packages of isotretinoin to include on the label a warning that there is an extremely high risk (one chance in four, or greater) of physical deformities in infants who are conceived while the mother is taking isotretinoin. Megadoses of vitamin A are dangerous, despite being recommended in some popular literature, and definitely should be avoided during pregnancy.

Thiamine, riboflavin, and niacin. These three B vitamins support the conversion of calories into energy. The 1989 RDA calls for pregnant women to get two milligrams of additional niacin a day and 0.3 and 0.4 milligrams more of riboflavin and thiamine, respectively.

Thiamine, riboflavin, and niacin are found in a wide variety of foods, making deficiencies unlikely. Thiamine is highest in pork, beef, nuts, whole grains, and wheat germ. Riboflavin is bountiful in milk and cheese, meats, wheat germ, and leafy green vegetables. Niacin is found in most foods—especially fish, meats, peanuts, and whole grains—and the body also can manufacture it from the amino acid tryptophan, which is found in high-quality protein.

Table 12.2.	Weight Gain During Pregnancy
Baby	7 to 8 lbs.
Placenta	1 to 2 lbs.
Uterus	2 lbs.
Amniotic fluid	1½ to 2 lbs.
Breasts	1 lb.
Blood volume	2½ to 3 lbs.
Fat	5 lbs. or more
Tissue, fluid	4 to 7 lbs.
Total	24 to 30 lbs.

A severe deficiency of thiamine can cause beriberi in the newborn, but mild deficiencies cause no known complications. Some studies of riboflavin deficiencies in pregnant women found an increased incidence of vomiting during pregnancy, premature births, and stillbirths, but the link is far from clear-cut. Deficiencies of niacin are not known to cause any difficulties. Likewise, excesses of all three vitamins are not known to have any effect.

Vitamin B_6. The metabolism of protein and fat requires vitamin B_6, which is widely available in meats and poultry, whole-grain cereals, nuts and seeds, peanut butter, and leafy green vegetables. Deficiencies of the vitamin have not been conclusively linked with problems during pregnancy or in the newborn. The RDA calls for an additional 0.6 milligrams per day of B_6 for pregnant women, an amount easily obtained from an adequate, mixed diet.

Folate and vitamin B_{12}. These two vitamins work closely together. The pregnant woman needs large quantities of folate, or folic acid, and vitamin B_{12} for the expanding blood volume required by the fetus and the placenta. The formation of new blood is important, because a blood volume that is too small can retard the fetus's growth. Moreover, the smaller the increase in a woman's blood volume, the more likely she is to have a spontaneous abortion, stillbirth, or low-birth-weight baby.

A pregnant woman should get more than twice as much folic acid as before, about 400 micrograms per day, as compared to about 180 micrograms ordinarily. Although folate-deficiency anemia can quickly develop in a pregnant woman whose folate intake is not sufficient, numerous studies in humans have failed to link a lack of folate to other problems in pregnancies. Limited evidence of such harm does exist, however. Women who are preg-

nant and receive anticancer drugs that destroy folate in the body often have spontaneous abortions. Low folate levels have also been linked by coincidental association with bleeding during the third trimester of pregnancy, low-birth-weight babies, and congenital malformations, particularly cleft palate and neural tube defects. Whether there is a cause-effect relationship is not yet clear.

Some doctors (including Dr. Victor Herbert) recommend low-dose (100 micrograms) folic-acid supplements for pregnant patients. Others advise meeting extra folate needs by eating more leafy green vegetables. There are no known ill effects from moderately increased dietary folic-acid intake. Large (350 microgram) supplements of folic acid (given with iron) may interfere with zinc absorption. Among vegetarians, for example, pregnancy supplements containing 100 milligrams of iron and 350 micrograms of folate may promote maternal zinc depletion, resulting in intrauterine growth retardation and low-birth-weight babies. Thus, pregnancy supplements should probably not exceed 150 micrograms of folic acid, when superimposed on the folic acid already in the diet.

Folate deficiency is almost as common in pregnant women as iron deficiency. A deficiency of vitamin B_{12} (rare in all but strictly vegetarian pregnant women), with or without a folic-acid deficiency, can also cause a condition called megaloblastic anemia, characterized by immature, large, oval red blood cells.

A serious vitamin B_{12} deficiency can cause damage to the nervous system, in addition to complicating folate-deficiency anemia. Providing folic acid alleviates the anemia, while allowing the nerve damage to progress. Therefore, it is essential to determine whether megaloblastic anemia is caused by a deficiency of folate, vitamin B_{12}, or both.

Low B_{12} levels are rare, however, because it takes years to use up the body's stores and because the vitamin is found in abundance in all foods of animal origin. It is usually a problem only in strict vegetarians—called vegans—who eat no meat, egg, or dairy products. It is also of concern to people who cannot absorb vitamin B_{12} because they lack intrinsic factor in their stomachs (a situation rare in premenopausal women) or have had part of their intestines surgically removed. Intrinsic factor is a substance found in gastric juice that facilitates the absorption of vitamin B_{12} in food.

Vitamin C. The 1989 RDA calls for a pregnant woman to get 10 milligrams of additional vitamin C per day. Her total RDA of 60 milligrams is an amount that is easily obtained by drinking an eight-ounce glass of orange juice. Women who smoke often have levels of vitamin C circulating in their blood 10 to 20 percent lower than those of nonsmokers. This is still about five times above deficiency levels, so they have no need for extra vitamin C. Pregnant women should not smoke.

There is no consensus about the effect of a vitamin C deficiency (almost never seen in the United States, except in alcoholics) on the pregnant woman. Some studies have suggested an association with premature births and spontaneous abortions, but other studies have found no such relationship.

Excessive consumption of vitamin C—a popular practice among some Americans in an attempt to prevent colds—can produce an infant that is conditioned to having large amounts of the vitamin in its blood. After birth, when breast milk or formula provides only normal amounts of vitamin C, the infant experiences discomfort. In fact, infants of mothers taking megadoses of vitamin C during pregnancy have been reported to have developed conditioned scurvy because of the sudden drop in vitamin C after birth. As a result, megadoses of vitamin C are definitely not advised during pregnancy.

Calcium, phosphorus, and vitamin D. Calcium is vital to the formation of the infant's bones and teeth. It also is needed for the proper functioning of blood, nerves, and muscles. Both phosphorus and vitamin D influence how well calcium is absorbed and utilized.

Calcium is most needed during the last trimester of pregnancy, when the fetus may draw as much as 13 milligrams of calcium each hour from the mother's blood. The mother should not delay calcium consumption until late in the pregnancy, however, because evidence suggests that her body begins storing calcium early on, in anticipation of the heavy demands later. Most physicians recommend a steady calcium intake throughout pregnancy.

A pregnant woman needs 50 percent more calcium and phosphorus per day, or a total of 1,200 milligrams of each. The easiest way to meet the extra calcium demands is to increase consumption of milk and other dairy products. Highly absorbable calcium also is found in sardines, mackerel, and salmon (only if eaten *with* the bones); calcium that is less well absorbed is found in broccoli and dark green leafy vegetables such as kale, collard, and turnip greens. The calcium in some other leafy vegetables—especially spinach, rhubarb, and beet greens—is poorly absorbed by the mother, and so therefore is unavailable to the fetus. (See Chapter 7 for a more detailed discussion.)

Since phosphorus is widely available in foods, dietary deficiencies are rare. In fact, phosphorus is so prevalent in meats, snack foods, and cola drinks that some pregnant women may consume too much of it. Calcium and phosphorus should be in a state of equilibrium in the body, but there are many misconceptions as to the real importance of this.

Many also believe that if a woman does not consume enough calcium during pregnancy, she will be at higher risk for osteoporosis (a debilitating condition in which the bones become porous and brittle) later in life. This belief is based on the presumption that calcium will be lost from her bones for the needs of the fetus. In fact, osteoporosis is more common among women who have never been pregnant. Some researchers speculate that because calcium absorption is enhanced during pregnancy, it may actually protect a woman from osteoporosis later in life.

Vitamin D has long been known to be essential for calcium absorption and balance. If vitamin D levels are adequate, then a high phosphorus-calcium ratio usually is not a problem. Low levels of vitamin D can lead to rickets in newborn infants. In a few cases, high vitamin D levels have been implicated in causing excessive calcium levels in newborns. If a pregnant woman is eating a balanced diet, her vitamin D level is probably adequate, particularly if she drinks fortified milk. Some doctors, however, prefer prescribing 10 micrograms (400 IU) of vitamin D per day during pregnancy.

Vitamin E. The importance of vitamin E has emerged over the years, although many of its functions are still poorly understood. For pregnant women, the RDA for vitamin E is two milligrams more per day. This is easily met with an ordinary diet that includes vegetable oil, nuts, seeds, and whole grains. Dietary vitamin E deficiency has never been seen on any average American diet. Supplements therefore have no value, and, in addition, a variety of problems have been alleged to occur from excesses of vitamin E, including headache, fatigue, vision problems, and muscle weakness.

Iron. Almost half the extra iron needed during pregnancy is used to manufacture hemoglobin for the mother's expanded blood supply. The placenta accounts for another quarter of the iron required. Demands for iron are greatest in the last trimester, when the fetus builds up its stores. The infant will need this iron in the first six months of life because breast milk contains little of its own.

Iron deficiency is unusual in a newborn, unless it is premature and therefore hasn't had time to build up adequate stores. A lack of iron in the mother's diet does not lead to iron deficiency in the fetus, because the baby draws iron from the mother to manufacture its own hemoglobin. As the pregnancy progresses, however, iron deficiency can affect the mother adversely. Insufficient iron causes a deficiency of hemoglobin, which is needed to carry oxygen to the fetus and the cells of the mother's body. Her heart must work harder to meet this need. The increased cardiac load leads to fatigue and physiological stress. Severe hemoglobin depletion increases the risk of cardiac arrest. Hemorrhaging during birth of the baby also can be life-threatening.

Although iron losses are reduced in a pregnant woman, because she is not menstruating, she still needs 20 to 30 milligrams a day of *added* iron. There simply is not enough iron in usual U.S. diets to meet this requirement, so pregnant women almost always are prescribed a daily iron supplement. Women who are iron-deficient when they become pregnant will need a still larger dose. Iron supplements are best taken with a citrus juice, since the ascorbic acid in the juice enhances iron absorption. Unfortunately, this can also enhance the chances of stomach upset, because greater gut irritability accompanies greater absorbability of inorganic iron.

Iodine. A deficiency of iodine can lead to cretinism in an infant, characterized by mental and physical retardation, potbelly, large tongue, and distinct facial features similar in appearance to Down's syndrome. On the other hand, women who consume excessive doses of iodine during pregnancy may give birth to infants with goiter and hypothyroidism; there also have been instances of mental retardation and deaths in such infants.

The 1989 RDA for a pregnant woman calls for 25 micrograms of additional iodine per day. Such needs can be met through the normal consumption of iodized salt (important for people living in noncoastal areas) and the iodine found naturally in seafood and other foods grown in coastal soil.

Zinc. In recent years, this trace metal has emerged as an important constituent of enzyme systems that regulate the major metabolic processes in the body. For example, zinc is essential to proper cell growth, such as is occurring in the fetus.

Various studies have statistically related low zinc levels in the mother to hypertension, abnormal deliveries, nervous-system malformations, and babies with lower birth-weight. Cause-and-effect relationships are now being evaluated. In the United States, zinc deficiency is unlikely except in vegetarian women who eat too much fiber.

Women who have taken zinc supplements in megadose levels during the third trimester of pregnancy reportedly have suffered premature births, stillbirths, and deformed babies.

The 1989 RDA calls for 3 extra milligrams of zinc per day during pregnancy, and 7 during the first 6 months of lactation. Zinc naturally present in foods can be lost during processing and cooking. Oysters, calves' liver, meat, poultry, seafood, spinach, dairy products, dry peas and beans, nuts, and wheat germ are all good sources of zinc. Whole grains are rich in zinc, but in a form that is not easily absorbed.

A PROFILE OF MATERNAL RISK FACTORS

Having a baby is not without the potential for complications, and nutrition plays a role in numerous risk factors in pregnancy.

Underweight and pregnancy. The underweight woman is defined as one who weighs 15 percent or more below her desirable weight. She is at risk for delivering a low-birth-weight baby if she is unable to gain enough weight during the pregnancy to account not only for the needs of the baby but to reach her own desirable weight, as well. For example, a woman whose desirable weight should be 120 pounds but who weighs only 100 pounds when she conceives should gain not only the 27 pounds required by the pregnancy itself but an additional 20 pounds to correct her underweight status.

Some women are deliberately underweight, suffering perhaps from mild forms of anorexia nervosa or merely being obsessed with having a model's figure. They may strongly resist gaining the extra weight needed to meet their ideal body weight. If such a woman limits weight gain, however, her own body will have to compete with the fetus for available nutrients in the blood, and both will suffer. The underweight pregnant woman is also more likely to develop toxemia.

Obesity and pregnancy. Women who are more than 20 percent over their desirable weight are defined as obese. When such women become pregnant, they are at increased risk of developing complications during pregnancy, particularly hypertension and diabetes.

Most doctors recommend that before becoming pregnant, an obese woman first reduce her weight to as near desirable as possible by following a nutritionally sound dietary regime. If conception occurs before the weight is lost, she needs to work closely with her doctor and a nutrition professional to design a dietary plan that will lead to the birth of a healthy baby. Dieting should not be attempted during pregnancy.

Obstetricians and nutrition professionals generally agree that some weight gain during pregnancy is necessary, even for an obese woman. How *much* weight is still being debated. Some experts advise, as a minimum, half the recommended gain for women of desirable weight, or about 12 to 15 pounds. Others feel the full weight gain of 24 to 28 pounds is safer.

The inherent danger in limiting weight gain is that to do so, the obese pregnant woman often must sharply curtail her dietary intake. If calories are too restricted, protein is diverted to meet the mother's and the fetus's energy needs rather than to manufacture new fetal tissue. Severe caloric restriction forces body fat to be converted into energy, releasing by-products called ketones. If too many ketones are produced, the body cannot rid itself of them fast enough, and a condition known as ketosis develops. This is especially harmful to the fetus, as it can impair brain development.

Two or more pregnancies in three years. A woman's body needs time between pregnancies to replenish its stores of essential nutrients. There are varying estimates of how much time this takes. Most likely, it is highly individual, depending on a variety of factors: the woman's overall health, whether she is underweight after recovering from the pregnancy, whether or not she breastfeeds, and of what her postpartum diet consists.

Many obstetricians recommend that at least a year pass between one child's birth and conception of the next child. During that period, the overweight woman should undertake a nutritionally sound weight-reduction program that includes adequate exercise. Most obstetricians and nutrition professionals recommend against

becoming pregnant while still breastfeeding, since the requirements of the growing fetus added to that of the nursing baby put excessive physical demands on the woman's body. Contrary to popular myth, conception *is* possible while a woman is breastfeeding.

Smoking. In a 1979 report and again in 1988, the U.S. Surgeon General estimated that one-third of American women in the childbearing ages of 15 to 44 years smoke cigarettes. Many of these women become pregnant without having kicked the habit. Yet smoking remains one of the most controllable risk factors in pregnancy. Moreover, smoking is dose-related. In other words, babies born to heavy smokers are more affected than babies born to light smokers. Smoking throughout the entire pregnancy is more harmful than smoking only during part of the pregnancy.

Numerous studies have shown that women who smoke are nearly twice as likely to deliver low-birth-weight babies. Other studies show that smokers are at greater risk for spontaneous abortions, premature deliveries, stillbirths, infant deaths, and complications involving the placenta.

Several explanations for the effects of smoking on pregnancy have been proposed. Carbon monoxide, a major constituent of cigarette smoke, binds to the hemoglobin in blood, leaving it unavailable to carry oxygen. As a result, the fetus is steadily deprived of oxygen, a condition known as hypoxia. The fetus tries to compensate by creating a larger placenta. In the mother, the carbon monoxide and associated hypoxia cause the heart to work harder and blood flow to be redistributed to more vital parts of the body than the uterus. Other researchers propose that smokers give birth to low-birth-weight babies simply due to the fact that smoking causes the mother to eat fewer calories and therefore gain less weight.

Various research groups have attempted to

discover whether children born to smokers suffer any long-term consequences. Results have been conflicting. In some studies of babies one year after birth, no difference could be found between those whose mothers smoked and those who had nonsmoking mothers. Other studies *have* found some differences at various ages. For example, one British study found that by age seven the children of smokers were shorter and had learned to read later. Such studies are criticized by the tobacco industry, however, for allegedly not adequately sorting out other lifestyle variables that could also account for the differences. Similar criticisms were raised against claims of harm from passive smoke (inhaling the smoke of others), until the U.S. Surgeon General's 1988 report, which affirmed that passive smoke is harmful.

Alcohol. Alcohol has long been suspected of causing harm to the fetus. The ancient Carthaginians had a wedding ritual that forbade the bridal couple from drinking wine on their wedding night, to prevent conception of a deformed child. Likewise, Roman mythology said that Vulcan was deformed because of the effects of strong drink on his mother.

Millennia later, it has been clearly established that heavy drinking can result in the birth of a baby suffering from a condition called Fetal Alcohol Syndrome (FAS). These babies are below normal in weight, height, and head circumference. They have a characteristic facial malformation in which the bridge of the nose is wider than normal. Frequently, they suffer from mental retardation and poor motor development. The combined occurrence of these characteristics is seen almost exclusively in babies born to alcoholic mothers.

Direct alcohol toxicity, rather than an indirect effect, is believed to be responsible for the damage. This means that *all* alcohol, including that in beer, wine, medicine, and even some foods, has the potential to be damaging.

How? Alcohol freely crosses the placental barrier, entering the amniotic fluid and the fetal blood and tissues. The fetus probably lacks sufficient quantities of the enzyme responsible for breaking down alcohol and the acetaldehyde and superoxide generated from it. As a result, the fetus is liberally exposed to the alcohol and its initial products.

Autopsies performed on some FAS babies have shown that their brain development had been severely affected early in the pregnancy. The first few weeks after conception are thought to be the most dangerous. What has not been definitely determined yet is how high alcohol levels must be and how long alcohol must be present to cause the damage. As a result, there is disagreement among health professionals about how much alcohol consumption during pregnancy is safe. Some allow a pregnant woman to have up to an ounce of alcohol a day. Others limit it to two or three ounces a week. Still others argue that a woman who drinks as little as one ounce of alcohol per week increases her chances of spontaneous abortion, and that one ounce per day increases the risk of giving birth to a low-birth-weight baby.

Although the issue remains controversial, many doctors advise their pregnant patients to avoid *all* alcohol, including that found in food and drugs. Binge drinking is definitely ill-advised.

Caffeine. There is only limited evidence that caffeine is deleterious to the fetus. Most of the warnings about caffeine are based on past animal studies that showed the stimulant caused birth defects. The most frequent problems seen were cleft palate, bone malformation, and problems in the development of toes and fingers. However, even if the effects on animals are directly applicable to humans, it would require drinking 25 to 30 cups of regular coffee each day or over 50 12-ounce cola drinks a day to receive comparable amounts of caffeine.

Caffeine is particularly difficult to study in humans because it is so hard to distinguish whether the observed effects are due to caffeine or to something else. Heavy users of caffeine—mostly coffee drinkers—are more likely than noncaffeine users to be heavy smokers, abusers of alcohol, and malnourished. Women whose lifestyles include these other risk factors are known to suffer more premature births, stillbirths, and babies with birth defects. It is possible that caffeine contributes to the problem, but evidence is lacking that it is the lone culprit.

Caffeine also acts as a diuretic, causing the kidneys to excrete more urine. High caffeine levels in the mother's blood, then, can lead to excessive loss of fluids and nutrients that are needed by both mother and fetus during pregnancy.

Several medical groups and the Food and Drug Administration have warned pregnant women to be prudent in their use of caffeine. For a normal, healthy woman, a caffeine consumption equivalent to two cups of coffee would be considered prudent. (See Chapter 40 for a discussion of caffeine.)

Drugs. A wide number of drugs easily cross the placental barrier and may affect the fetus just as they do the mother. It is well known that babies born to heroin addicts are themselves addicted at birth. There also is no doubt that use of cocaine and crack—a more potent form of cocaine that is smoked—are associated with both maternal and fetal complications. There is ample evidence that pregnant women should avoid the use of all mind-altering recreational drugs, including marijuana.

Cocaine constricts blood vessels, which decreases blood flow to the uterus. This contributes to several of the characteristic problems noted: rapid rise in blood pressure, premature delivery, growth retardation, and neurological impairment of the fetus. In addi-

tion, babies born to cocaine users suffer gastrointestinal and respiratory symptoms of withdrawal.

No drugs should be taken frivolously during pregnancy. However, there are medications that should be taken to treat certain disorders, even during pregnancy. Pregnant women should discuss with their obstetricians *all* medications they take, including over-the-counter drugs. In some instances, alternative medications or different dosages may be prescribed.

Natural and artificial substances in food. Pregnant women also need to be conscious of substances they ingest that may have a drug-like effect even though they are not thought of as such. Many herbal teas, for example, naturally contain medicinal substances that cross the placenta and affect the fetus. Few of these teas are labeled with their contents and none warns of the likely pharmacologic actions after they are brewed. Even chocolate has a chemical—theobromine—that acts similarly to caffeine and also crosses the placental barrier. (See also the discussion of herbal teas in Chapter 10.)

The use of low-calorie sweeteners has grown in the past decade, prompting questions of safety for pregnant women. Many soft drinks still contain saccharin, which has not been declared risk-free for humans despite considerable debate over the evidence. Although saccharin is known to cross the placenta, it is not known whether this is harmful. Nevertheless, the American Medical Association urges pregnant women to be cautious about its use.

Aspartame—the sweetener in NutraSweet—is now found in nearly all calorie-reduced products, and it generates similar controversy. Aspartame consists of two amino acids—aspartic acid and phenylalanine—both of which are essential to life but are toxic to the brain in large amounts. Aspartic acid poses no problem because it does not readily cross the placental barrier, but phenylalanine does.

Some scientists have expressed concern that aspartame may cause a subtle but distinct impairment in the brain function of the fetus. However, the FDA has found no evidence of this or other toxic effects at current levels of intake by mothers.

Another worry is over the methanol content of products containing aspartame. Over time, and hastened by heat, aspartame breaks down to yield methanol, which in turn yields formaldehyde, then formate—a known carcinogen. Fortunately, no significant levels of formate have been found in foods. Little is known about the effects of methanol itself on the fetus, or even how much crosses the placental barrier.

There is no clear evidence that any food additives presently in use and approved by the Food and Drug Administration cause harm to the fetus. However, pregnant women who are concerned about consuming high levels of additives can largely avoid them if they eat as many fresh, whole foods as possible and limit consumption of highly processed convenience foods and fast foods.

The pregnant vegetarian. The effects of a vegetarian diet on pregnancy depend largely on the type of vegetarianism practiced. Partial vegetarians—who merely avoid red meat—and lacto-ovo vegetarians—who avoid all meat, poultry, and fish but eat dairy products and eggs—should have no difficulty meeting the dietary requirements of pregnancy. The only exception may be iron, but even meat eaters usually require an iron supplement during pregnancy.

More serious are the nutritional deficits inherent in the diets of strict "vegans," who avoid all meat, egg, and milk products. They are likely to consume inadequate amounts of riboflavin, vitamin B_{12}, calcium, iron, zinc, and calories. It must be remembered that diet tables of the iron content of foods do not take into account the absorbability of iron. An average of only 2 to 10 percent of plant iron is absorbed, whereas an average of 10 to 30 percent of animal (meat, fish, poultry) iron is absorbed by normal people. Vegans must also be careful to eat a varied diet of vegetables, legumes, and nuts in order to consume an adequate mix of proteins that meets the amino-acid requirements of both the mother and fetus. Even then, the amount of protein may be inadequate. For these reasons, most nutrition professionals recommend that vegans supplement their diets with milk and eggs (and an iron supplement) during pregnancy and breastfeeding.

A special case is the pregnant adolescent who is also a strict vegetarian. It is nearly impossible for a diet devoid of dairy products to provide sufficient protein and calcium to meet the needs of her growing body as well as those of the fetus.

The pregnant adolescent. Girls begin their growth spurt between ages 10 and 11, reaching a peak at about 12. After they begin menstruating, the rate of growth slows dramatically, and energy needs slack off. But the needs for many other nutrients, such as calcium and iron, increase or remain the same.

Numerous studies have shown that at the very time when sound nutritional habits are essential for growth, teenage girls frequently skip meals and turn to snacks such as soft drinks, potato chips, French fries, candy, ice cream, and other sweets for a large proportion of their calories. Consumption of vegetables, milk, and other dairy products is low. The adolescent diet also tends to be low in calcium and iron. Moreover, teenage girls are often obsessed with their weight and may adopt bizarre diets that are severely restricted in calories as well as essential nutrients.

When a teenage girl becomes pregnant, these poor nutritional habits, coupled with the demands of her growing body and that of the developing fetus, place her at significant obstetrical risk. Complications of pregnancy can include toxemia, limited weight gain, and anemia. The risk of a low-birth-weight baby is high. Studies have found that the pregnant teenager does not suddenly improve her nutritional habits but, instead, continues to select a diet similar to her nonpregnant peers. A teenage girl who was obsessed with her figure before becoming pregnant may become even more concerned and attempt to limit the weight gain caused by the growing baby.

The total calories needed by pregnant adolescents vary widely, from 38 to 50 calories per kilogram (17 to 23 calories per pound) of body weight. Therefore, the best indicator that nutritional needs are being met is weight gain. Recommendations are that a pregnant teenager should gain between 24 and 30 pounds for the baby, *plus* the additional weight she would be expected to gain from normal adolescent growth. For example, a sedentary girl who is nearly grown might require only 1,800 calories per day, while a very active girl who is still growing rapidly might need 3,000 calories a day.

The protein requirement for pregnant teenagers, pound for pound of body weight, is higher than that for mature pregnant women. An adolescent between the ages of 15 and 18 needs 1.5 grams of protein for each kilogram of weight (compared to only 0.8 grams for grown women). If she weighs 100 pounds (45 kilograms), for example, she needs to eat about 68 grams of protein a day. Younger girls require 1.7 grams of protein per kilogram of weight.

Girls who avoid dairy products and meats, or allow less nutritious foods to account for the bulk of their diet, risk protein deficiency. Additional protein depletion can result if the young mother-to-be does not eat enough calories, because then her body is forced to use its protein reserves in muscle tissue to meet the combined energy needs of her and the fetus. This could place both the mother's and the fetus's health in jeopardy.

Dietary vitamin A is primarily supplied by fruits and vegetables, which are not staples in the typical teenage diet. Since maternal deficiency of vitamin A has been linked with vision problems in infants, eating dark green and deep orange vegetables and fruits should be encouraged, even though frank deficiencies of vitamin A are rare. Supplements are to be avoided because of the danger of birth defects from excessive doses.

Folate supplements are desirable for the pregnant teenager, since the leafy green vegetables that are rich in folate may be missing from her diet. Vitamin B_{12} supplements may also be necessary for the vegetarian teenager who is pregnant, since she may get only a trace of this vitamin in her diet.

A pregnant adolescent who is finished growing needs the same 1,200 milligrams of calcium daily that a mature pregnant woman requires. A pregnant adolescent who is still growing may need as much as 1,600 milligrams of calcium daily. Since it is difficult to obtain this much calcium from food alone, a supplement may be required to fill the gap.

An iron supplement of 30 to 60 milligrams per day is almost always required as well, since the typical teenage girl's diet is low in iron. Besides, it is practically impossible to meet this requirement even with a well-planned diet.

Zinc is also important for the growth of both the teenager and the fetus. However, foods that are rich in zinc—legumes and high-quality proteins, such as meat, poultry, and seafood—often are not included regularly in the diet of the typical teenage girl. She must choose foods carefully to meet the 1989 RDA of 15 milligrams per day.

Socioeconomic factors can complicate the nutritional picture for a pregnant adolescent. She may have limited funds with which to purchase food, particularly expensive protein sources, fresh produce, and dairy products. In addition, other stress factors—no husband, parental disapproval, peer pressure, denial of pregnancy—can aggravate the normal nausea of morning sickness, making proper eating even more difficult. Pregnant teenagers usually need considerable counseling about what foods to eat, how to spend limited money wisely, and how much to eat to gain the desired weight.

SPECIAL NUTRITIONAL PROBLEMS DURING PREGNANCY

Food cravings. Folklore is full of stories about the food cravings of pregnant women. For some, it is the first indication of pregnancy. Some women crave salty foods, such as pickles; others crave ice cream, cheese, or citrus fruits. While the cravings are real enough, in most cases little physiological basis for them can be found.

One exception is the increased need for salt in the pregnant woman. The doubling of the mother's blood volume requires extra sodium in order to maintain the body's balance of the mineral. Normally, the pregnant woman's salt needs can be met merely by salting her food to taste.

As a general rule, specific cravings can be indulged in moderation, depending upon the food that is craved.

Pica. Sometimes, pregnant women develop a craving for more bizarre substances, such things as clay, laundry starch, cornstarch, paint, ashes, ice, coffee grounds, paraffin, or baking soda. This phenomenon is known as pica and was written about as early as the sixth century.

The causes of pica are not known. Extensive research has uncovered an association between iron deficiency and pica, leading to the assumption that one causes the other. Studies have found both that iron deficiency causes ice pica, and starch pica causes iron deficiency. Other research suggests that some of the substances commonly consumed in pica, such as clay, bind to iron in the intestine, preventing its absorption and leading to a deficiency. Irrespective of which came first, when iron supplements are prescribed for patients with iron deficiency who experience pica, the pica usually disappears.

Pica has cultural links. The practice is more common in the southern United States, and it is surrounded by folk beliefs, such as that eating clay will ease delivery, relieve headaches, cure the swelling of edema, or assure handsome children. Some cultural beliefs include the idea that not giving in to the cravings of pica could cause a birthmark on the baby.

Pica is not without consequences, however. Intestinal obstructions and toxemia can result in the mother. Premature births and increased mortality among newborns also have been linked to pica. Hemolytic anemia has occurred in women who ate mothballs and toilet air fresheners. Babies have been born with lead poisoning after their mothers ate plaster and paint containing lead. Gastrointestinal parasites have been found after contaminated clay was eaten. Therefore, since pica can be harmful, such cravings should always be reported to a health professional, and a blood test for iron status should be sought.

COMMON MEDICAL PROBLEMS DURING PREGNANCY

Morning sickness. This condition is misnamed, since the nausea and vomiting that are typical of the first three months of pregnancy can occur any time of day or night. It's true, however, that it is experienced more often upon awakening. Some women go through pregnancy with very little morning sickness. Others experience the nausea and vomiting every day throughout the entire nine months.

The exact cause of the nausea and vomiting remains elusive. Clearly, the mother's changing hormones play a role. Levels of the hormone known as HCG—human chorionic gonadotropin—are high during the first trimester, helping the fertilized egg implant itself in the uterus and then readying the breasts for lactation. As HCG levels subside in the fourth month, nausea and vomiting usually also subside.

There are several steps the pregnant woman can take to reduce nausea and vomiting, but nothing is currently available to make it go away. The prescription drug Bendectin was voluntarily removed from the market in 1983, after controversy over whether it caused birth defects led to a rash of lawsuits. The weight of the evidence suggests Bendectin was not the culprit, but the issue was too emotional for Bendectin to survive.

Many women find that eating small and frequent meals helps relieve nausea and vomiting. Eating dry soda crackers is probably the most common folk remedy for morning sickness. Others benefit from popcorn, vanilla wafers, or dry cereal. It is best to eat one of these foods first thing in the morning, while still in bed. This removes excess acid from the stomach and can lessen the nausea upon arising.

It also is important for each individual to avoid any foods and beverages that she associates with nausea and vomiting. This varies widely from woman to woman. As a general rule, spicy or greasy foods that are richly laden with butter or other fats are absorbed more slowly and should be avoided. Foods with strong smells, particularly meat and fish, may trigger nausea in some women. If this is a problem, it may help to serve foods lukewarm or to prepare cold entrées. The diet should focus on carbohydrates, which are easier to digest and readily provide energy to the body. Substitutes for meat, such as milk, cheese, and eggs, can provide necessary protein during this uncomfortable phase.

If vomiting is frequent, the pregnant woman must be careful not to become dehydrated. Some doctors recommend taking soup or beverages between meals, instead of with food. Some women find that a small glass of fruit juice taken upon awakening helps relieve nausea. Substances that stimulate stomach-acid secretion, such as coffee and cigarettes, should be avoided. (See Tips to Relieve Morning Sickness on page 190.)

Tips to Relieve Morning Sickness

- Keep saltines or other plain crackers at your bedside. Eat them dry before getting out of bed. At other times of the day, try dry toast.

- Eat six small meals instead of three larger ones. Try not to go for long periods without eating.

- As soon as you feel nauseous, try to get a breath of fresh air. Relax and take deep breaths.

- Avoid greasy, fried, and rich, fat-laden foods.

- Avoid overly spicy foods.

- Eat foods at room temperature. Hot foods—particularly meats and fish—tend to have strong smells that may trigger nausea.

Heartburn. In the last months of pregnancy, the growing fetus puts pressure on the stomach and often interferes with the first stages of digestion. Food and gastric juices can be forced back into the lower part of the esophagus, a condition physicians call reflux. This causes pressure and the burning sensation that is commonly described as heartburn. Those who suffer nausea and vomiting in the first three months may also experience heartburn as a symptom of indigestion.

Typically, heartburn is worst after meals, particularly when lying down. It is best, then, not to eat within two hours of bedtime. The most effective self-help measure is to raise the head of the bed six inches by placing blocks under the legs. Using extra pillows doesn't work as well. Several small meals a day may further help to relieve the unpleasant sensation. Rich, spicy, and heavy foods should be avoided, as should any food that seems to particularly irritate the stomach. Such culprit foods vary with individuals.

Sodium bicarbonate, a common home remedy for heartburn, should not be taken by a pregnant woman, since it can interfere with the absorption of vitamins and minerals. Antacids should be taken only after consultation with a physician. (See Tips to Relieve Heartburn, below.)

Constipation and frequent urination. Many women experience the need for frequent urination, particularly during the first and last trimesters. In the first three months, the rising hormone levels cause an increased need to urinate. In the last three months, the growing uterus presses on the bladder, creating a full sensation more often.

Constipation also is caused by hormone changes and pressure on the bowel from the fetus. Bowel movements can be stimulated by drinking plenty of liquids, by exercise such as walking, and by eating a variety of foods high in fiber, such as whole grains, bran, dried and fresh fruits, and raw vegetables. Prunes, prune juice, and figs, which all contain the natural laxative isatin, also may help. Pregnant women with constipation are advised not to take over-the-counter laxatives without con-

Tips to Relieve Heartburn

- Raise the head of your bed with six-inch blocks or books. Don't rely on propping up your head with pillows; it's not as effective.

- Eat meals in a relaxed, unhurried atmosphere. Eat slowly, chewing your food well.

- Don't eat just before going to bed. It's best to wait two to four hours after eating to lie down.

- Avoid large meals. Eat six small meals instead of three large meals.

- Avoid alcohol, colas, tea, and coffee (regular *and* decaf), chocolate, peppermint, and spearmint. They can all relax the valve between the esophagus and stomach, allowing stom-

ach contents to flow back into the esophagus, creating the typical burning sensation.

- Also avoid any foods that seem consistently to give you problems. Common culprits include greasy or highly spiced foods, tomato products, and citrus fruits and juices.

- Drink liquids slowly, between meals if it helps. Limit what's taken at mealtimes to one cup. Avoid carbonated beverages.

- Chew gum or suck on lozenges (not mints) to stimulate saliva flow. This may help neutralize stomach acid.

- Consult your physician before using antacids.

sulting their doctor first. (See Chapter 9 for lists of high-fiber foods.)

Edema. Swelling of the extremities, particularly the ankles and feet, is called edema and is a normal part of pregnancy. The body retains water during the last months of pregnancy, partly because of the increase in blood volume. The edema gradually disappears in the first weeks after delivery. In some cases, before subsiding, it actually may become worse.

In the past, it was mistakenly thought that if such edema was not relieved, it might lead to toxemia. As a result, it was common practice for physicians to restrict a woman's salt intake and even prescribe diuretics to rid the body of excess fluid. Such thinking has now changed. In fact, it is now believed that such restrictions actually may be harmful.

Diuretics should not be taken unless prescribed by a doctor in the treatment of a special condition. Food should be salted to taste. Some relief of the edema can be found by resting frequently with the legs elevated; this will help the return flow of blood from the legs to the upper body.

Diabetes. A few years ago, it was not unusual for a doctor to advise a diabetic woman not to have children. Today, diabetic women routinely have healthy babies. It is essential, however, for them to receive proper medical management, with close attention paid to diet and blood-sugar levels. Women with diabetes should discuss the implications of pregnancy with their doctors before they stop using birth-control methods. If they decide to become pregnant, they should be prepared for a physically and emotionally demanding nine months.

Women who already have diabetes before becoming pregnant have a pancreas incapable of meeting their normal insulin needs for metabolizing glucose, or sugar, in the blood. They are under treatment either through diet alone or a combination of diet, drugs, and insulin injections. As the pregnancy progresses, shifting glucose levels and associated hormonal changes put an added strain on these women. Their condition must be routinely monitored to keep blood-sugar levels within an acceptable range.

Women in whom carbohydrate intolerance develops during pregnancy but returns to normal after delivery are said to have gestational diabetes. This occurs in about 5 percent of all pregnant women in the United States. Although the condition disappears, over half of these women will develop overt diabetes later in life.

Gestational diabetes is caused by the inability of the mother's pancreas to manufacture sufficient insulin to handle the fluctuating glucose levels that pregnancy induces. During the second trimester of pregnancy, other maternal hormone levels increase, partially blocking the action of insulin. The mother's pancreas must secrete more insulin to offset this hormonal effect so that blood sugar can be metabolized. If the pancreas cannot do this, the symptoms of diabetes appear, characterized by rising blood-sugar levels.

The goal of treatment in both types of diabetes is to keep blood-sugar levels within a narrow range in order to minimize the effects that a metabolic imbalance of glucose can have on both mother and fetus. Women who already have diabetes enter pregnancy knowing the potential complications. Diabetic women who become pregnant need to be emotionally and medically prepared to treat their diabetes carefully throughout the pregnancy. Women who develop gestational diabetes need to understand the potential seriousness of their condition if it is not treated properly.

Diabetes during pregnancy, if left untreated or treated poorly, can cause serious birth defects and even be life-threatening for both mother and infant. The first six to seven weeks after conception are especially important, since most diabetes-related congenital malformations occur in organs that are completely formed during this time. The most common defects are spinal-cord malformations, central nervous system defects, and congenital heart disease. Careful control of blood-glucose levels, particularly during the first eight weeks of pregnancy, can reduce the incidence of these birth defects.

Pregnant women with diabetes are also at increased risk for toxemia, excessive buildup of the fluid in the amniotic sac, and premature birth. Complications of diabetes can be worsened in the mother, including damage to the kidneys and retinas of the eyes.

Gestational diabetes does not usually occur until the middle of the pregnancy. For this reason, most obstetricians usually test their patients for it around the 26th week of their pregnancy.

Often, pregnant women are given a blood test early in pregnancy that measures the amount of glucose in the blood, particularly one hour after ingesting 50 grams of glucose. A glucose level is considered normal if it is 135 milligrams per deciliter or less. If normal, the test is repeated between the 24th and 28th weeks of pregnancy. If the initial screening reveals a blood-sugar level higher than 135, then a more rigorous blood-glucose determination or tolerance test is given. If this test also reveals high blood-glucose levels, a regime of diabetic care is begun, its exact nature depending upon the blood-glucose levels, medical history, and other factors. It is important for *all* pregnant women to undergo such screening, because over a third of those who test positive were not suspected of being at risk beforehand.

A pregnant woman with diabetes may be able to treat her condition by adhering to an individualized diet prescribed by her doctor

and a nutrition professional. This is particularly true of gestational diabetes. In more severe cases, she will need to take daily injections of insulin. (See sample diet in Table 12.3.) The pregnant diabetic must frequently perform tests on her blood (by finger-stick) to determine whether the level of glucose is within an acceptable range.

Toxemia. The term *toxemia* is a misnomer, because the condition does not involve toxins in the blood. A more correct name is pre-

Table 12.3. The Mount Sinai Medical Center Department of Clinical Nutrition Diabetic Diet

Sample Meal Plan: 2,000–2,200 Calories

Breakfast:	2 slices of bread or 1 cup of cereal
	2 eggs or 2 slices of cheese
	2 t of either margarine or butter
	1 cup of skim milk
Lunch:	3 oz. (3 slices) of meat, fish, chicken, or cheese
	2 slices of bread or 1 cup of cooked rice or 2 small potatoes
	Lettuce, if desired
	1 fresh fruit
	3 t of fat
	1 cup of skim milk
Dinner:	3 oz. of broiled lean meat, chicken, or fish
	1 cup of rice or noodles or 2 small potatoes
	½ cup of cooked vegetables
	1 fresh fruit
	3 t of fat
	1 cup of skim milk
Snack:	2 slices of bread or 6 crackers
	1 slice of cheese or meat
	1 cup of skim milk

Avoid these foods: Sugar, honey, jam, syrup, canned fruit in syrup, candy, cake, cookies, regular soda, chocolate, chocolate milk, hot chocolate, regular chewing gum (sugarless is okay), sweetened cereals (Frosted Flakes, etc.).

Serving Sizes: One 3-oz. serving of meat is a medium-size steak or chop, 1 chicken thigh or breast, 3 slices of roast beef, 3 slices of cheese.

One serving of potato or rice or spaghetti is ½ cup.

One serving of fruit is about the size of either a small orange or a large peach.

Calories should be distributed as follows: carbohydrate—40%; protein—25%; fat—35%.

eclampsia, a condition characterized by hypertension, headache, blurred vision, abdominal pain, edema, and excessive protein in the urine, which appear after the fifth month of pregnancy. If left untreated, pre-eclampsia can develop into eclampsia: the onset of convulsions and coma late in pregnancy.

Despite considerable research, the causes of toxemia are unknown. The illness has consistently been linked with poverty, leading to the supposition that poor quality of prenatal care may be a contributing factor. For example, early detection of high blood pressure or gestational diabetes may be important in preventing toxemia. Toxemia also strikes more often in very young pregnant women and women over 35. It has been reported in women who practice pica and in women with mineral deficiencies, such as zinc; but a definitive cause for this condition remains elusive.

Women with a little fluid retention late in pregnancy need not worry. The edema of toxemia occurs in addition to the normal swelling of the legs that accompanies most pregnancies. The treatment of toxemia demands careful medical management, often requiring hospitalization. A pregnant woman who experiences any of the above symptoms, together or progressively, should consult her doctor immediately.

BREASTFEEDING

Breastfeeding is on the increase, particularly among women with more education and higher incomes. By some estimates, more than 60 percent of new mothers in the United States are breastfeeding their babies when they leave the hospital. Some of these women discontinue breastfeeding within a few weeks, but a significant number continue for the next four to six months.

There also is a growing consensus among physicians and nutrition and other health professionals that breastfeeding is superior to feeding with commercial formulas because of the unique characteristics of human milk.

Breast Milk

- more closely meets the infant's nutritional needs during the first months of life

- is easier for the infant to digest

- contains the mother's antibodies and other immune components to aid the infant's developing immune system in fighting off outside infections.

- costs nothing

It is also true, however, that generations of healthy Americans were raised on the bottle. There is no concrete evidence that bottle-feeding a baby causes any long-term damage. Thus, currently, there is no strong reason to discourage new mothers from bottle-feeding.

Comparing Formula to Human Milk

Over the years, the manufacturers of baby formula have become increasingly sophisticated at duplicating the nutritional components in human milk. Although human milk still is considered superior, in many instances commercial formulas are quite similar.

Calories. Although it varies from woman to woman, breast milk provides about 20 calories per ounce: 40 percent as carbohydrate, 10 percent as protein, and 50 percent as fat. Formulas based on cow's milk are modified so that their caloric content is similar to human breast milk.

Carbohydrates. The high lactose content of breast milk has several benefits for the infant, increasing calcium and iron absorption while discouraging intestinal bacterial growth. Formula manufacturers add lactose to their products to imitate the carbohydrate content of human milk.

Protein. Cow's milk is harder to digest and utilize than human milk because it contains substantially more protein, as casein, which forms a curd in the infant's stomach. The extra protein also is difficult for the infant's immature kidneys to handle. To alleviate these problems, formula manufacturers alter the protein content of cow's milk to match more nearly human milk. Because the protein needs of premature babies are different from those of full-term babies, manufacturers market formulas to meet these special needs.

The amino-acid composition in cow's milk is vastly different from that in breast milk. Infants are thought to benefit from the larger amounts of the amino acids taurine and cystine found in human milk. The high levels of the amino acid phenylalanine in cow's milk have the potential to impair development of the central nervous system in premature babies.

Human milk also contains a variety of protein immune substances that strengthen the baby's developing immune system. Cow's milk and, therefore, formula lack these.

Fats. Human milk contains primarily unsaturated and polyunsaturated fats, although the mother's diet influences the exact composition of fatty acids in her milk. Many formulas that use cow's milk as a base replace its natural saturated fat content with polyunsaturated vegetable oils, to resemble human milk more closely. These vegetable fats seem to be well digested, even though human milk has an extra enzyme to aid its absorption.

Although the total fat content of formula is similar, on average, to human milk, the amount of fat in human milk varies considerably from mother to mother. In addition, the first milk produced by the breast at each feeding has a different fat content from the milk produced at the end of the feeding. The so-called hind milk has a higher fat content and gives the baby a full feeling, possibly to prevent overeating. It is not possible, of course, for formula to duplicate this.

Formulas contain almost no cholesterol, whereas human milk contains quite a bit. Whether this difference is harmful or beneficial is still unclear. Cholesterol is not needed in the diet because the body can make its own supply. It has been suggested, however, that the extra cholesterol in breast milk can improve the formation of nerve tissue and bile salts, particularly in premature infants. Moreover, animal research has suggested that cholesterol in the diet of an infant may trigger the body to manufacture enzymes that help control cholesterol levels later in life.

Vitamins. Human breast milk provides both water- and fat-soluble vitamins in sufficient amounts, with the possible exception of vitamin D. Infants who are not regularly exposed to sunlight may become deficient in this vitamin. Therefore, to prevent rickets, physicians often supplement the diet of a breastfed baby with vitamin D. Most formulas are fortified with vitamin D as well as other vitamins to ensure adequate nutrient intake.

The vitamin K content of human milk is low, and may even be missing in the milk secreted the first days after birth. Because low levels of this vitamin increase the risk of hemorrhage in infants, it is standard practice in most hospitals to administer vitamin K to newborns shortly after birth.

Although the fat-soluble vitamin content of breast milk remains fairly constant, the water-soluble vitamin content is particularly susceptible to daily variations in the mother's diet. This underscores how important it is that she eat a consistently nutritious diet.

Minerals. Research suggests that mineral levels in human milk are low because the infant's metabolic system is geared to such levels at first. Indeed, the higher mineral content of cow's milk is difficult for the infant's kidneys to handle, forcing formula manufacturers to lower it.

Sodium levels in human milk, for example, are substantially lower than those in cow's milk. Fluoride levels are also low in human milk, even when the mother drinks fluoridated water. Because fluoride has been proven to help prevent dental caries, some doctors prescribe fluoride supplements to breastfed infants. Others question the need, since breastfed babies usually develop fewer cavities, anyway. Concentrated formulas contain low levels of fluoride so that infants won't receive too much if the formula is mixed with fluoridated water. When formulas are mixed with unfluoridated water, fluoride supplements may be prescribed.

There is a high concentration of zinc in colostrum, the yellowish substance secreted by the breast during the first days after delivery. Later, breast milk's zinc levels decline but remain in an easily absorbable form. Formula manufacturers add zinc to their products, but if it is not absorbed well by the infant, a zinc supplement may be prescribed.

If the mother's iron supplies are adequate during pregnancy, the fetus is able to build up its own iron stores before birth. Thus, for most infants, the fact that breast milk contains little iron poses no problem for at least the first four months of life. Moreover, some studies have shown that the iron in human milk is ten times more efficiently absorbed by babies than the iron in commercial formulas. After four to six months of age, physicians agree that all infants, breastfed or bottle-fed, need a source of iron. Most doctors recommend introducing iron-rich foods at this point, beginning with an iron-fortified cereal. Some doctors prefer prescribing iron supplements. Formula-fed babies who up to this point were receiving formula without added iron are usually switched to an iron-containing formula.

Women who breastfeed need to take in extra calcium to meet the baby's demands. Otherwise, calcium will be drawn from the mother's bones to maintain the calcium content of her milk. Cow's milk contains significantly more calcium than human milk, so formula manufacturers reduce the calcium level in their products.

Diet for the Nursing Mother

It is a widely held belief among health-care professionals and advocates of breastfeeding that nursing a baby helps the mother lose weight faster. There is not enough data to substantiate this belief, although the sucking action of the infant does aid the uterus in contracting so it will decrease in size. However, some researchers who have carefully studied how much energy a woman needs to make milk question whether the mother requires as many extra calories as is commonly believed. The RDAs for lactating women may be too high, they argue.

Calories. Despite some controversy, current recommendations are that the mother who breastfeeds requires approximately 500 calories more each day—300 from food—compared to the nonlactating woman. These energy needs vary, depending upon the volume of milk produced, the woman's general health, and other factors. A woman who begins her pregnancy at desirable weight and gains the recommended 27 pounds will end up with 5 to 10 pounds of stored fat and these are used to produce milk. This provides about 200 to 300 calories per day during the first three months after delivery. That leaves at least 300 extra calories the lactating woman needs to consume each day to meet her requirements. If nursing continues beyond three months, her diet alone will have to provide the entire 500 extra calories a day.

A woman who begins pregnancy over her desirable weight obviously has fat stores that will assist with nursing beyond three months. However, a woman who begins her pregnancy underweight and does not make up the difference before delivery should eat a sufficiently robust diet to prevent further weight loss as nursing continues. Her goal should be to maintain desirable weight. The woman who deliberately uses nursing as a means to lose pounds runs the risk of draining her health and shortchanging her baby. Dieting while breastfeeding is likely to compromise the mother's ability to produce milk, particularly in the first weeks following delivery, before the lactation process is firmly established. Many doctors and nutrition professionals recommend that the mother's weight-loss goal be stretched over the first six months after the baby is born.

Protein. In the first six months of nursing, the woman who breastfeeds needs to eat 15 more grams of protein per day than the nonlactating woman, and 12 more grams thereafter. This amount—about 65 grams in the first six months and 62 as long as nursing continues— is somewhat more than the amount she needed during pregnancy. The additional protein can easily be obtained by drinking two extra glasses of milk a day. This also helps meet the extra calcium requirement.

Vitamins and minerals. In the first six months, the breastfeeding woman also needs 35 additional milligrams of vitamin C, 4 extra milligrams of vitamin E, and 1,100 additional

micrograms of folic acid. The total amounts are: 95 milligrams vitamin C; 12 milligrams of vitamin E; and 280 micrograms of folic acid. After the first six months, the requirements go down to: 90 milligrams of vitamin C; 11 milligrams of vitamin E; and 260 micrograms of folic acid.

The nursing mother who is a vegetarian will have little difficulty meeting her nutritional requirements if she follows a diet that includes milk and eggs. If she avoids these foods, however, she will need supplements of calcium and possibly vitamin B_{12}. She needs to consume high-quality protein by combining legumes, grains, nuts, and other protein sources. If her dietary practices do not permit supplements, then she must seek vegetables with a high available-calcium content. In such cases, careful diet planning is essential.

Foreign Substances Appearing in Breast Milk

A wide variety of substances that enter the mother's body appear in her milk and are passed on to the baby, including such common drugs as aspirin. Many medications, when used in moderation, do not bother the baby. Some drugs and other substances, though, are definitely contraindicated and should not be taken at all by a nursing mother.

Prescription and over-the-counter drugs. In 1979, the Food and Drug Administration ordered that all drugs developed and marketed after that date be labeled with whatever information is known about their excretion into human milk and the effect on the baby. The family pharmacist, as well as the physician prescribing a drug for a nursing mother, should be queried about such information. It can also be found in the *Physician's Desk Reference,* commonly known at the *PDR,* a book that describes all prescription drugs and their side effects. Most libraries have a copy in their reference section.

A nursing mother who is prescribed a drug should ask the doctor what effect, if any, it might have on her infant.

Birth-control pills. The estrogen and progestin in oral contraceptives can reduce both the quality and quantity of breast milk. So-called low-dosage or mini birth-control pills, which contain only progestin, are usually recommended as a substitute. The mother should not forsake birth control in the misguided notion that she cannot become pregnant while breastfeeding. Although the chances of this are reduced, it can happen.

Low-calorie sweeteners. Saccharin, like most substances, passes into breast milk. Its use is probably best avoided, or at least curtailed, since the effects on infants are unknown. Aspartame usage slightly changes the amino-acid content of the mother's milk, but this appears to have no significant effect on the infant's brain levels of phenylalanine. As during pregnancy, however, while there is no direct evidence of harm, cautious and moderate use is prudent.

Caffeine. Caffeine appears in the milk of mothers who breastfeed, so intake should be limited. Newborns lack the enzyme needed to metabolize caffeine, and even older infants are not as capable of handling it as adults.

Alcohol. Most physicians believe that a small amount of alcohol will not interfere with breastfeeding. In fact, some doctors even suggest the mother drink a glass of wine or beer to help her relax. Alcohol does pass into breast milk, however, and it is not known what amount might be harmful to the infant. In large amounts, alcohol depresses the milk-ejection reflex and can interfere with the mother's ability to provide milk. If any alcohol is taken, it is best done just *after* nursing, so that as much as possible will be metabolized out of the bloodstream by the next feeding.

Smoking. The mother's body excretes nicotine into breast milk. Moderate smoking probably has little effect on the infant, but milk production may be somewhat reduced. Heavy smoking is discouraged for nursing mothers.

Recreational drugs. The active ingredient in marijuana easily passes into human milk because it is fat soluble. Long-term effects of marijuana are not well understood, so nursing mothers should avoid its use. Cocaine and crack have more serious effects and definitely should always be avoided, especially by the breastfeeding mother.

CONCLUSION

In general, guidelines for nutrition during pregnancy include the following: Eat a wide variety of foods from all food groups; choose nutrient-dense foods rich in protein, vitamins, and minerals, especially calcium and iron; avoid drugs, smoking, alcohol, and excessive intake of caffeine. Early prenatal care is extremely important, including preconception counseling for women with known medical problems.

13

Nutrition in Infancy and Childhood

Neal LeLeiko, M.D., Ph.D., Denise Rollinson, M.S., R.D., and Robbyn E. Sockolow, M.D.

∎

INTRODUCTION

Few issues cause as much concern—and are as important—for parents as feeding the newborn. An infant doubles his weight in the first five to six months of life and triples it by one year of age. Good nutrition is essential to support this period of phenomenal growth, which is more rapid than at any other time in an individual's life.

To achieve normal growth, newborns must not only receive the proper quality and quantity of nutrients but also they must be nurtured, in a larger sense, in a supportive and caring home environment.

YOUR BABY: ONE TO SIX MONTHS

Breast Versus Bottle-Feeding

Most pediatricians and nutritionists concur that breastfeeding is best for infants. There are many advantages to breastfeeding, especially during the first four to six months.

It is true that companies that make formula for infants have recently made significant alterations in their formula. While the goal of these changes is to improve formula quality, there have been no scientifically vigorous studies of potential nutrient interactions. Since the scientific basis for changes in the infant formula given normal, healthy babies is lacking, the safest and most prudent course is to nurse—if this is feasible. If not, then parents need not be unduly alarmed about using commercial formula, but they should be certain that the growing baby receives regular checkups, which will include measuring the baby. (For tips, see Successful Breastfeeding from Hospital to Home on page 200, as well as Chapter 12.)

Vitamin and Mineral Supplements

While most physicians overwhelmingly agree that human milk is the best food for infants, much controversy surrounds the use of supplemental vitamins and minerals for the exclusively breastfed infant.

Vitamin K. Because the intestinal tract of an infant is sterile and free of natural flora that produce vitamin K at birth, infants are given a dose of vitamin K, either by injection (intramuscularly) or by mouth (orally). After receiving this initial dose, the infant is able to produce vitamin K through his or her own intestinal bacteria, thereby eliminating the danger of clotting and bleeding disorders caused by vitamin K deficiency.

Vitamin D. While the amount of vitamin D in human milk is greater than once recognized, current evidence suggests supplementation to ensure adequate intake, especially in areas with minimal sun exposure. Since rickets has been reported in some breastfed infants, many pediatricians advise supplementation of 400 IU daily as a preventative measure.

Iron. A term infant born to a mother with good iron supplies will have accumulated enough iron stores to last until four to six months of age. In addition, the small quantities of iron present in breast milk are more efficiently absorbed than the iron in other milk. Usually, additional iron is not required until the infant's stores have become depleted, roughly between four to six months. Ask your physician, since some physicians believe supplemental iron should be started before stores run low at four to six months.

Fluoride. Because human milk contains only traces of fluoride, and the breastfed infant consumes little if any water, the American Academy of Pediatrics has recommended fluoride supplementation for the breastfed infant. Fluoride supplementation, in an effort to reduce the prevalence of dental caries, is especially advisable if breastfeeding is to continue past six months.

Successful Breastfeeding from Hospital to Home

The following are tips to make the transition from breastfeeding in the hospital to the home smooth and successful.

- Arrange for rooming-in of the baby in advance of delivery, if it's available.

- Breastfeed as soon after delivery as possible.

- Be calm and comfortable in order to assist in the letdown reflex. Sit or lie down with the baby's head in the bend of your arm. Hold the breast between your fingers and touch the infant's lower lip with the nipple to stimulate the rooting reflex. Once the infant is latched on, the breast no longer needs to be held.

- Follow your pediatrician's advice about the frequency and technique for feeding.

- Don't hesitate to call your pediatrician for support.

- Nurse the baby from both breasts at each feeding.

- Don't give supplementary feedings of water or formula unless ordered by your pediatrician. Breast milk is 80 percent water and in most cases is sufficient for your baby's fluid needs.

- Learn how to express milk by use of a breast pump before being discharged from the hospital.

- Burp the baby frequently, both in the middle and at the end of a feeding to help release gas in the stomach.

Table 13.1. Basic Four Food Guide for Nursing Mothers (2,100 to 2,900 Calories a Day)

Food Group	Recommended Servings Each Day	Average Serving Size	Food Group	Recommended Servings Each Day	Average Serving Size
MILK GROUP			Apple, banana, most whole fruits		1 medium
(or equivalent)	4–5		**BREADS AND CEREALS**		
Milk, whole, low-fat, skim		1 cup	(whole-grain or enriched)	4	
Buttermilk		1 cup	Bread		1 slice
Powdered milk		4 T	Dry cereal (unsweetened)		¾ cup
Evaporated milk		3 oz.	Cooked cereal		½ cup
Ice cream		1¾ cup	Rice, noodles, pasta		½ cup
Cheese		1½ oz.	Roll		1 medium
Cottage cheese		2 cups	Bagel		½ medium
Yogurt		1 cup	Crackers		4 whole
Tofu		1 cup	Muffins		1 medium
Pudding		1 cup	**OTHER FOODS**		
MEAT, FISH, POULTRY			Fats and oils	6	
(or equivalent)	3–4	2–3 oz.	Butter, margarine, mayonnaise		1 t
Eggs		2 whole	Vegetable oil		1 t
Peanut butter		¼ cup	Salad dressing		1 t
Cooked dried peas or beans		¼ cup	Sour cream		1 t
Luncheon meat		2–3 slices	Olives		5 small
Tofu		1 cup	Nuts		6 medium
Nuts and seeds		½ cup	Avocado		⅛ medium
Cheese		2 oz.	Liquids (in addition to milk)	6 or more	
VEGETABLES AND FRUITS	4	½–¾ cup	Water		8 oz.
Citrus fruits (vitamin C source)	1 or more		Fruit juice		8 oz.
Orange, mango, guava		1 medium	Vegetable juice		8 oz.
Grapefruit, cantaloupe		½ medium	Seltzer water, club soda		8 oz.
Orange or grapefruit		1 whole	Caffeine-free soft drinks		8 oz.
Kiwi		1 whole	Coffee, tea		In moderation
Strawberries		1 cup			In moderation
Tomatoes or tomato juice		½ cup	**DESSERTS AND SNACKS**	As needed	
Yellow or green vegetable or fruit (vitamin A source)	1 or more		Pudding		½ cup
Broccoli		½ cup	Ice cream or ice milk		1 cup
Spinach		½ cup	Custard		1 cup
Carrots		½ cup	Dried fruits		3 oz.
Squash		½ cup	Cookies		2–3 medium
Cantaloupe		⅓ fruit	Cake		1 oz. (1/16 of a 9" layer cake)
Apricots		7 halves	Pie		1½ oz. (1/6 of a 9" pie
Other fruits and vegetables	2 or more				
Fresh, frozen, canned fruits and vegetables		½ cup	**SUGAR, HONEY, MOLASSES, JAM, JELLY, PRESERVES**		2 T
Potato, turnip, most whole vegetables		1 medium			

Adapted with permission from *The Parents' Guide to Nutrition,* Susan Baker (Reading, Mass.: Addison Wesley Publishers, 1986).

Food Guide for the Nursing Mother

Nutritional requirements for the lactating woman are higher than at any other stage of the life cycle. One must account not only for the nutrient and energy value of the milk itself but also for the demand placed on the body to produce it. (For more information, refer to the discussion of breastfeeding in the preceding chapter.) The guide in Table 13.1 is based on the Basic Four food groups and can be used to help plan daily meals.

Other tips for the nursing mother include:

- Drink plenty of fluids. In addition to four to five servings of milk, one and a half quarts of water and/or juice will help ensure adequate hydration for you, as well as furnishing the needed fluid to produce a good milk volume.

- Despite many old wives' tales, there are no specific foods that a woman should avoid while lactating. However, some women find that after they eat a highly spiced meal, or consume large amounts of strongly flavored foods such as onions, cabbage, and broccoli, their baby tends to shy away from the breast. The flavor of some foods can be transmitted through breast milk several hours after a woman eats. If the baby seems unusually fussy, the mother should look for any correlation to her consumption of a specific food. The effects of caffeine, alcohol, and other substances on breast milk are covered in the preceding chapter.

Breastfeeding for the Working Mother

Increasing numbers of mothers are returning to work after having their babies. For the woman who is breastfeeding, this choice presents some new challenges. Continuing to eat a high-quality diet is important for all mothers, but especially for those who have the additional demands and stresses of work. With a little planning and assistance, working mothers can continue to feed their babies. Ideally, a mother should allow two months of nursing at home to establish her milk supply and accustom the baby to a schedule. Table 13.2 can help in devising a nursing plan relative to the age of your baby.

In planning to nurse her baby, a working woman must first evaluate her job responsibilities, the kind of work she does, and the flexibility of her schedule in order to decide how nursing will best fit into her daily routine. Some options include:

- Going home for lunch, if it's convenient.

- Arranging for a baby-sitter near the workplace where you can also go to nurse the baby.

While it may not be possible for some mothers, others will find that they and their babies can adjust to novel schedules. The baby may be nursed early in the morning and then two or three times after the mother returns from work. During the day, the baby may be fed freshly expressed (within 24 hours and kept

Table 13.2. Breastfeeding Demands

The following are the approximate number of times a breastfed infant will want to nurse each day.

Age of Infant	Number of Feedings
Birth to 1 month	7 to 14
1 to 3 months	5 to 7
3 to 4 months	5 to 6
4 to 8 months	3 to 5
8 months to 1 year	3 to 4

refrigerated) mother's milk or infant formula. The key to success is a relaxed, positive attitude.

Weaning from the Breast

Weaning involves the gradual replacement of feedings at the breast with bottle or cup feedings, or with the initiation of solid foods. If the baby is under 12 months, one should use infant formula to wean the baby from the breast. The extent of the baby's neuromuscular development—namely, hand-eye and hand-mouth coordination—will determine whether a bottle or cup is most successful.

If breastfeeding is discontinued before four to six months, feedings should be provided by bottle. Parents of older infants may attempt to wean them directly to a cup, decreasing the number of breastfeedings as the baby begins to drink expressed breast milk or infant formula from the cup. While it may seem desirable to wean the breastfed infant directly to a cup and omit the bottle altogether, some pediatricians prefer a bottle. Strong beliefs are rarely warranted, and a relaxed, flexible attitude is always best.

Formula Feeding

Whenever breastfeeding is not chosen, is inappropriate, or is discontinued before one year of age, the baby should be fed a commercially prepared infant formula. Parents who decide to bottle-feed their baby can be practically assured of nutritious commercial formulas that are generally safe. Formulas have been modeled after human milk and contain the nutrients essential for growth.

When bottle-feeding, hold and support the baby in a semi-upright position, with the bottle held in the opposite hand. Neither the baby nor the bottle should be propped up by pillows. Propping a bottle and letting the baby feed without supervision could result in choking; moreover, it does not allow for the close interaction that is necessary to establish a trusting relationship between parent or other caregiver and the baby.

Estimates of the stomach capacity of an infant are meaningless, as babies tolerate varying amounts of formula. The only significant measure of the adequacy of formula intake is change in weight and length; that is, whether the baby is growing properly. The full-term infant rarely requires more than 32 ounces of formula per day, but be sure to address all questions about the adequacy of nutritional intake to your pediatrician.

Formulas are available with and without iron—in powdered, liquid concentrate, or ready-to-feed form. Since ready-to-feed formulas require no preparation, they are the most convenient but also the most expensive. Powders and liquid concentrates must be mixed with water. Assuming they are mixed properly, the various forms all provide equal caloric density, but it is vital to read labels on formula cans carefully and follow instructions accurately. This is especially true with the concentrates. Adding too much water will result in the baby not receiving adequate amounts of nutrients, and may lead to growth failure and/or specific vitamin or mineral deficiencies (as have been seen when parents overdiluted formula to save money). Adding less than the required amount of water may result in relatively acute dehydration, kidney disorders, and other serious medical conditions.

The need for sterilization of bottles and equipment in formula preparation receives less emphasis among pediatricians today. If you have questions about the safety of the water in your area, ask your pediatrician about sterilization of water. If there is still concern, then ready-to-feed liquids that are sterile in the can may be most appropriate. Whether or not a parent or caregiver chooses to sterilize the baby's water, good hygienic practices should always be followed prior to preparing formula: washing hands with soap and water, wiping the top of the can clean and free of dust, and rinsing the can opener under hot water after each use. For those who wish to sterilize bottles and/or equipment, refer to Sterilizing Baby Bottles on this page, which outlines three different methods.

Formula may be warmed or given at room temperature. Parents may assume that their infants prefer warm liquids, but many infants seem to prefer formula at room temperature, or slightly cooler. It is best to experiment and determine what your baby likes. One should never feed a baby extremely hot or cold liquids.

Many women today have become reliant on microwave ovens for fast heating of foods. Microwaving bottles can be dangerous and should be avoided. The bottle may feel cool while the formula inside is still hot. In addition, a bottle may explode if steam builds up in it. The safest methods of bottle warming remain the old-fashioned ones. (See page 205 for suggestions.)

If feeding a baby by bottle, be sure to remove the bottle when the baby appears to have had enough or has fallen asleep. Sucking on an empty bottle may lead to an uncomfortable buildup of gas in the stomach. In addition, pooling of milk or juice around the teeth can promote cavity formation; therefore, a baby should never be put to bed with a bottle. Whether bottle-fed or breastfed, a baby will usually swallow some air during feeding, which must be released by burping. At the middle and end of each feeding, a baby should be held upright and then lifted forward about 30 degrees and given gentle pats on the back until the air bubbles are released and a burp is heard.

Do not use sugar or honey in the bottle. The addition of honey or sugar to the formula can contribute to the formation of dental caries. (Honey can also cause infant botulism, see the discussion under Foods to Avoid in Infancy on page 208.)

Sterilizing Baby Bottles

Method 1:
- All the equipment is boiled for 20 minutes before the bottles are filled.
- The water to be used in the formula is boiled for five minutes.
- The bottles then are filled carefully and refrigerated. They must be used within 48 hours.

Method 2:
- The formulas are made up and placed in the bottles, the caps screwed on loosely, and the bottles placed in a large pot with three inches of water.
- The pot is covered and the water boiled for 25 minutes.
- The bottles, with the nipple rings screwed on tightly, are refrigerated and used within 48 hours.

Method 3:
- The bottles are filled with the required amount of water and sterilized as in Method 2.
- These bottles are stored at room temperature for no more than three days.
- When needed, the correct amount of concentrate or formula is added, shaken in, and fed to the infant.

Reprinted with permission from *Parents' Guide to Nutrition*, Susan Baker.

Weaning an Infant from the Bottle

Weaning from a bottle can start between the fifth to eighth month of age by first eliminating the mid-morning bottle. Regimens differ and the best one to use is that recommended by your pediatrician for your baby. We recommend starting fresh, ripe, crushed bananas for the noon meal. Baby cereals are an excellent first or second food, as well. Fruit juices are very popular but are really little more than flavored sugar water. Some juices may have too much indigestible sugar and this can lead to cramps, bloating, and/or diarrhea. If you must use fruit juice, dilute with an equal amount of water. Establishment of a three-meal-a-day pattern is the goal as the infant starts on solid foods. A cup with a spout may be used at mealtime but is not necessary. If the infant is fussy, offer a few swallows of the bottle to calm him or her down, and then offer the cup. An additional three or four ounces of milk can be given by bottle after the meal. More emphasis should be placed on learning the skill of holding and drinking from a cup than on the amount of fluid actually consumed. Between eight and twelve months, the amount in the afternoon bottle can be gradually decreased until it is eliminated. The bedtime bottle can be eliminated using the same procedure, although this may take longer to accomplish. Don't feel pressed to have the baby give up the bedtime bottle. Eventually, the baby becomes interested in other activities and may not finish the after-meal bottle or want one before bed. Once this has happened, the bottle should be put away and only the cup used.

Warming Infant Formulas or Expressed Breast Milk

1. Place the bottle in a pan of hot (not boiling) tap water or hold the bottle under hot running tap water for a few minutes.

2. When the bottle begins to feel warm, shake it gently.

3. Place the bottle back into the pan of hot water or under the hot tap water.

4. Test the temperature of the formula by shaking a few drops on the underside of the wrist. The liquid should feel lukewarm to slightly warm.

5. If the liquid feels too warm, let the bottle sit at room temperature for several minutes to cool. Always retest the temperature before feeding the infant.

Reprinted with permission from *The Parents' Guide to Nutrition*, Susan Baker.

The Premature Infant

Infants born before 38 weeks of gestation generally are referred to as premature, especially if they are smaller than normal. They usually weigh less than full-term infants and have special nutritional requirements because of their underdeveloped digestive systems. They have higher needs for fluid, calories, and protein and need extra amounts of calcium as well as other vitamins and minerals. Standard infant formula and breast milk lack sufficient amounts of many of these important nutrients. In addition, many premature infants have not developed the sucking reflex and are unable to take adequate volumes of formula or breast milk to meet caloric needs. Nevertheless, breast milk may offer advantages for these babies. Fortunately, special premature formulas as well as fortifiers for breast milk are available. Mothers who wish to give their babies breast milk may express their milk and add the special nutrient fortifier. Since premature infants often are born with a very poor sucking reflex, they may need to be fed by tube. (Such infants usually are not discharged from the hospital until they are able to feed from a bottle.) As they grow and become stronger, reflexive sucking occurs, and the special feedings, whether breast milk or special formula, can be fed by bottle. The proper nutrition of the premature infant is a highly specialized and individualized concern. Do not hesitate to discuss this with your doctor.

YOUR BABY: SIX TO TWELVE MONTHS

Introduction to Solids

Mothers are almost always encouraged to breastfeed past six months if they desire. At this point, however, the bottle or breastfed infant can no longer rely solely on formula or breast milk. There are several reasons for beginning the introduction of solid foods: Particularly for the breastfed baby, mother's milk is an inadequate source of iron. This usually doesn't pose a problem for the healthy, full-term infant, who is born with enough iron stores to last until between four to six months. When a source of iron needs to be provided, usually an iron-fortified cereal is chosen. Rice cereal is recommended at first because it is the least likely to trigger an allergy.

By six months of age, many babies need more calories than breast milk alone can provide. Some experts also suggest that the formula-fed infant taking one quart or more of infant formula is ready for additional calories and should also be started on solids.

It's helpful to get babies accustomed to spoon-feeding and the taste and texture of a variety of foods to set the stage for learning to chew.

The American Academy of Pediatrics points out that there are no known advantages to the introduction of solids before three to four months in formula-fed infants and even later in breastfed infants. Developmental readiness for feeding must be considered. An infant is born with certain reflexes, many of which are closely tied to feeding. The strong sucking and extrusion reflex make it very difficult for a baby to accept much besides a bottle or breast until four to six months. Any solid food will instinctively be pushed out of the mouth. Attempting to feed before this time may result in a frustrating and messy experience, with little food actually getting into the baby. Some parents perceive early feeding of solids as a landmark in their babies' maturity and development and will add cereal or other foods to the bottle, since spoon-feeding proves to be impossible. There also is a mistaken notion that cereal in the evening will prompt the baby to sleep through the night. Adding solids to the bottle is strongly discouraged for several reasons. It is a type of force-feeding; it prevents the baby from learning normal chewing and swallowing techniques; and it may increase the risk of choking.

At about six months, infants have lost their extrusion reflex and their lips have enough muscle control to seal the oral cavity, making spoon-feeding easier. They are usually able to sit with support; lean forward and open their mouths, indicating a desire for food; or lean back or turn away, indicating satiety or disinterest. These are important cues and they should be watched for to help prevent overfeeding. Feeding of any solid foods prior to the infant's being able to display these signs can also be considered force-feeding.

Sequence of Food Introduction

Four to six months. There are no hard-and-fast rules as to the order of introducing solid foods. However, an understanding of a baby's developmental, emotional, and physical growth can help explain some of the recommendations. A general rule of thumb is to offer one new food at a time at weekly intervals so that any food intolerance can be more easily identified. One should start by spoon-feeding a single-grain cereal to the baby. Rice cereal is usually recommended because, as mentioned earlier, it seems to be the least allergenic of the cereals. It is important to introduce single-grain cereals in order to simplify the identification of food intolerance.

Three to five tablespoons of cereal can be mixed with a little breast milk, formula, or tap water. This may be divided into two daily feedings by using a small plastic-coated infant feeding spoon. Do not add sugar, honey, butter, salt, or anything other than milk or water. Plain food tastes perfectly fine to the baby, even though curious parents who taste it find it bland.

Once the baby has demonstrated tolerance to cereal, pureed or strained fruits or vegetables can be introduced. Up-and-down jaw movements begin as the tongue also moves up and down to transfer food to the back of the mouth. Unsweetened fruit juice may be given by cup but should be diluted to half-strength with water at first.

Six to twelve months. By this age, swallowing is more controlled and the infant begins to munch and mash foods. Many mothers find commercial baby foods convenient to use, but by this age, most babies can eat mashed home-prepared foods, which also help develop the texture of the diet. As the year continues, the maturation of the intestines and kidneys allow the infant to handle foreign proteins and formulas with higher concentrations of solid foods and with less water. The diet may be broadened to include cottage cheese, egg yolk (avoid giving egg white, which is highly allergenic), and strained meats—starting with lamb at first, then adding chicken and beef. Meat alternatives such as pureed or mashed beans and lentils may also be offered. These foods help provide additional iron, protein, and energy needed for rapid growth, as well as encourage chewing.

It is absolutely essential to be wary of specific advice that suggests a step-by-step progression of feeding behavior. Maturation is continuous and proceeds at different rates in different babies.

The most important concern is that you and your baby feel good and also relaxed about meals. Stress and concern lead to maladaptive patterns of behavior. Just like you, your baby will have off days and days of interest and excitement. Your pediatrician should be able to reassure you about your infant's nutrition by checking his or her growth and development. Avoid fad books and magazine articles. Special diets may be a curiosity for you but are damaging for your infant.

Nine to twelve months. By now, rotary chewing movements have developed and the infant can bite off the correct amount of food. Whole cow's milk can be substituted for infant formula or breast milk at one year. The child should consume the equivalent of at least three cups of milk per day in order to meet his or her calcium requirements. Too much milk may exclude more nutrient-dense foods, and this can cause a decreased intake of iron and calories, resulting in iron-deficiency anemia and lack of weight gain. This is why pediatricians usually recommend limiting consumption of milk to one quart per day. (See Practical Tips for Infant Feeding on page 208.)

As your baby approaches one year of age, he or she will show increasing interest in the soft foods you eat, and this is a good point at which to start introducing them gradually.

Solids and Sleeping Through the Night

The widely held belief that a full stomach at bedtime helps a baby sleep through the night was recently tested in a large-scale study. One hundred and six babies were fed rice cereal at bedtime at either five or seven months of age. Researchers found no significant differences in the amount of time the two groups of babies spent awake, asleep, crying, or fussing.

Unacceptable Milk for the Infant

Milk is available in different forms for various consumer needs and tastes. All milk, however, is not suitable for infants; some, in fact, may even be dangerous for infant or child consumption.

Goat's milk. Goat's milk, often promoted as a health food, is sometimes used when a baby is allergic to cow's milk, but there is no documented advantage to using this type of milk. In fact, goat's milk is deficient in folic acid, and a folic-acid deficiency may lead to megaloblastic anemia.

Raw milk. Raw milk, which is unpasteurized, presents a great danger to the infant. It contains disease-causing organisms that have the potential to cause serious illness or even death. Pasteurization represents a great advance in human food technology. Feeding raw milk to your infant is abusing the child.

Imitation and substitute milks. Imitation and substitute milks may lack many of the nutrients recognized as essential components of commercial-formula milk. The American Academy of Pediatrics concluded that imitation milks are nutritionally inferior and inappropriate for feeding infants and young children. Consumers, especially parents, should be leery of marketing techniques that try to equate these low-priced white liquids with milk.

Foods to Avoid in Infancy

Certain foods should be avoided in the first year of life. These include foods that are tough or hard to chew, such as nuts (especially peanuts), popcorn, hard candy and carrots; foods with tough or resilient skins, such as grapes or hot dogs; and foods that are thick and sticky, such as peanut butter. Such foods can cause choking in infants who are still learning to coordinate chewing and swallowing. After age three, when coordination is improved, there is less danger in giving these foods to young children, but peanuts should be avoided at least until age five. (See the section on choking on page 212.)

Practical Tips for Infant Feeding

- Feed the baby at his or her own pace; don't rush because you have something to do.

- Allow the baby to touch and play with his or her food in order to develop self-feeding skills. Don't show your frustration or anger at any messes the baby makes, and try to wait until mealtime is over before cleaning up the mess. In this way, you will communicate your approval of the infant's attempt to feed himself.

- Pick a quiet, unrushed time. Avoid too many distractions, such as radio or TV, and engage in conversation with your baby.

- *Don't* get frantic if your baby gags a little. Learning how much food to put in the mouth is part of the process, but *do* be there to comfort him or her.

Honey is another food to avoid. The Centers for Disease Control report that honey can cause what is known as infant botulism, which arises when botulism spores, found in about 10 percent of sampled honey, are consumed by infants under one year of age. When ingested, these spores may go on to flourish and produce a toxin called *Clostridium botulinum*. Botulism-spore consumption doesn't pose a potential problem to older children and adults but can be dangerous to babies under one year of age.

It is best to postpone adding foods that are commonly not well tolerated in an infant's diet until after one year of age. Foods most likely to be associated with an adverse reaction are egg whites, wheat, buckwheat, corn, nuts, chocolate and cocoa, fish, citrus, pork, berries, and tomatoes. (For more information, see Chapter 33.)

Infantile Obesity and Parental Concerns

During the second to sixth month of life an infant is rapidly accumulating adipose (fat) tissue. In fact, the increase in fat tissue is more than twice as great as the increase in muscle. Many infants may take on a chubby appearance, which is normal, but which parents may mistake as an inclination toward obesity. Overconcern about weight and obesity compels some well-intentioned parents to select and provide low-fat, reduced-calorie diets to infants—similar to the prudent diet recommended for adults. The dangers of these parental misconceptions are exemplified in recent reports of retarded growth and delayed maturation among inadequately nourished infants.

Weight-for-age and weight-for-length percentiles are the most commonly used criteria for classifying underweight or overweight children. If an infant's weight-for-height falls below the 5th percentile or above the 90th or 95th percentile, or if there is a trend moving in that direction, a parent should seek nutritional guidance from a physician or registered dietitian. The physician or registered dietitian may request a three-day food diary in order to assess the child's caloric intake. The diary should include the number and volume of feedings, quantity of foods, dilution of formula, and any additional items such as margarine, gravy, sugar, honey, or corn syrup that may be added to foods. (See Table 13.3 for a sample food diary.)

The food diary is the first source of information determining whether caloric intake exceeds energy expenditure. The physician or nutritionist will also inquire about the child's level of physical activity. Additionally, the physician may request blood tests to rule out any endocrine abnormalities.

Treatment of the obese infant should focus on weight control rather than weight loss. Calories offered should match the requirements of the normal-weight infant, ap-

Table 13.3.   Sample Food Diary for Infants

The following record of an infant's food, formula, and beverage intake should be kept for at least three days.

Name of infant: _____

Age:_____

Kind of formula:_____
How formula is prepared:_____

Date	Time	Reason for Feeding	Solids/Liquids*	Amount
___	___	_____	_____	_____
___	___	_____	_____	_____
___	___	_____	_____	_____
___	___	_____	_____	_____
___	___	_____	_____	_____
___	___	_____	_____	_____
___	___	_____	_____	_____
___	___	_____	_____	_____
___	___	_____	_____	_____

*Solids include strained foods, teething biscuits, and table foods. Liquids include formula, juice, and other beverages.

proximately 40–60 calories/pound for the first six months, and a little less (35–55 calories/pound) for the second six months of life. Foods of high-caloric density should be omitted. However, skim and low-fat milk should never be fed to infants, whether obese or normal weight, unless specifically prescribed by a pediatrician. Above all, always seek and follow the advice of a physician in treating an overweight infant; do not try to place him or her on a diet of your own devising. (See the Suggestions for Avoiding Infant Obesity, below.)

Suggestions for Avoiding Infant Obesity

- Do not force-feed the infant: Watch for signals of satiety, and stop feeding when the infant leans away from the spoon, turns his head away from the spoon, or purses his lips shut.

- Avoid adding unnecessary ingredients, such as sweeteners or fats, to your baby's foods.

- Be sure that baby-sitters (including family members) have specific directions on what, how much, and how often to feed the baby.

- Do not equate food with love. Rather than showing affection for an infant or child by offering sweets, ice cream, or other high-fat, high-caloric foods, communicate your feelings by praising, holding, cuddling, and playing with an infant.

- Use simple strained fruits as a dessert instead of the custards or puddings of commercial infant desserts. The fruits are higher in vitamin C and lower in calories. If the infant is obese, do not allow unlimited quantities of fruit juices. The child should be able to receive adequate vitamin C from fruits in the diet.

THE TODDLER: AGES ONE TO THREE

In contrast to the smooth and accelerating growth curve of infancy, a child in the second year of life enters a rather long period of slow growth and irregular weight gain. It might take the entire preschool period (ages one to six) for the child to double his or her weight again, an event that took only five to six months during infancy.

The child's appetite may be poor, erratic, sometimes nonexistent; he or she may also demand the same food for days and then suddenly reject it. There are several reasons for this behavior. Primarily, the child has a less urgent demand for food and nutrients, due to the decline in growth rate. Secondly, greater mobility, independence, and sociability turn a child's attention from feeding and mealtime behavior toward toys, games, and other distractions. The new parent may fear that the child will starve, and out of despair will try any measure—to the point of bribing the child with sweet, nonnutritious treats. If this situation is improperly handled, the child may learn how to use food to manipulate the parent. The parent should realize that a child will not starve to death and should continue to offer a variety of small, frequent meals and nutritious snacks. Eventually, the child will eat.

Even though it can be frustrating and time-consuming to teach an infant to feed himself or herself, it is very important for the parent or caregiver to assist the infant in eating without hindering the learning process. By the toddler stage, a child is well into or making the transition to table foods. As his or her grasp develops, self-feeding and spoon-feeding improve. A child of this age will show interest in sitting with the rest of the family at the table. To make a child feel more secure, his or her feet should rest on a flat, stable surface. Feet that dangle are uncomfortable.

Toddlers may already have several teeth, but they still require foods that are easily chewed. For example, fibrous meats, such as steaks and roasts, are too tough to chew. Mashed, ground, or soft finger foods that don't require a lot of chewing are appropriate for this age group. If meat is rejected by a toddler, mild gravy or sauce will help moisten it and may make it more acceptable. Overly spiced and sharp-flavored foods may be overpowering to the sensitive taste preferences of a toddler. Therefore, it is best to give toddlers unseasoned food. Portion size should be age-appropriate. For example, a toddler will eat only one-third to one-half as much as an adult. See tables 13.4 and 13.5 for sample serving sizes.

The Picky Eater

Even though a child may be fussy, parents should offer foods from all four food groups; and if a child does not eat the entire portion, he or she should not be forced. It is a better idea to encourage the child to taste a food offered.

Snacks

Snacks are an important part of a young child's diet. A small stomach capacity makes it difficult for a toddler to fulfill his or her caloric needs in just three meals. Snacks should add important nutrients—not just fat or sugar. (See Snacks for Toddlers on page 214.) One should set times for snacks so that snacking doesn't interfere with food intake during meals. One and a half hours before the next meal should be enough time to satisfy hunger without decreasing mealtime appetite. Snacks

---

Guidelines for Feeding During the First Year of Life

The American Academy of Pediatrics advises the use of breast milk or iron-fortified infant formula for infants through the first year of life. The Academy recommends withholding the introduction of solids until the infant is developmentally ready for solid feeding (at least 3 months old or 13 to 15 pounds) in order to decrease the possibility of food allergies and of overfeeding. Some experts suggest delaying the introduction of solids until the infant is 5–6 months old, when there is better neuromuscular control of the head and neck, enabling the infant to communicate desire for food or satiety.

SUGGESTIONS FOR INTRODUCING SOLIDS

1. Start with small portions (1–2 teaspoons) and gradually increase volumes given at each feeding.

2. Introduce one single-ingredient food at a time and continue to feed each new item for three to five days before introducing new item.

3. Infant rice cereal is commonly introduced first, followed by other single-ingredient cereals, then strained fruits, vegetables, and meats. Juices should also be introduced one at a time, preferably from a cup, not a bottle.

4. Textures should be introduced according to the infant's ability to chew and swallow.

should be consumed in a designated place in order to establish good eating habits and develop the concept that food should be eaten consciously (i.e., at the table) rather than unconsciously (for example, while playing or watching TV).

Water

Children should be encouraged to drink water for normal body regulation. It is important that they learn to recognize thirst and satisfy that thirst with water rather than milk or juice. Depending on the local water supply, water also provides the important element fluoride. Fluoride has been found to be the most important nutrient involved in the prevention of cavities.

Choking

The risk of choking is greatest among toddlers, who are still learning how to chew and swallow. While it's important to know the correct way to treat a choking child, it's even better to prevent the situation from arising in the first place.

- Always supervise at meal and snack time.

- Children should eat while sitting in an upright position, never lying down or running.

- Avoid foods that are hard or tough to chew, foods that are small and round, sticky foods, and foods with resilient skins. These include frankfurters, pea-

Table 13.4. Guidelines for Suggested Daily Servings for Infants from Birth Through 8 Months to Meet the Recommended Dietary Allowances

Age	Foods	Portions
Birth to 2 months	Breast milk with supplemental vitamin D and iron after 4 months or commercially prepared iron-fortified formula	6–8 bottles (2–3 oz. each)
3 months	Breast milk or commercially prepared iron-fortified formula	5–6 bottles (4–6 oz. each)
4 months	Breast milk or commercially prepared iron-fortified formula	5 bottles (6–7 oz. each)
	Iron-fortified infant cereal	Start with ½ teaspoon mixed with formula. Increase to 4 tablespoons
5 months	Breast milk or commercially prepared iron-fortified formula	5 bottles (6–8 oz. each)
	Iron-fortified infant cereal	4–5 tablespoons
	Strained fruit and vegetable	½–1 jar of each
6 months	Breast milk and/or commercially prepared iron-fortified formula	4–5 bottles (6–7 oz. each)
	Iron-fortified infant cereal	4–5 tablespoons
	Strained fruit and vegetable	1 jar of each
	Strained meat	½ jar
7–8 months	Breast milk and/or commercially prepared iron-fortified formula	4 bottles (7–8 oz. each)
	Iron-fortified infant cereal	¼ cup
	Junior or soft-cooked fruit and vegetable	1 jar each
	Junior meat or finely chopped table food	1 jar

nut butter, grapes, raw carrots, nuts, whole-kernel corn, popcorn, and hard candy.

Some of these childhood favorites can still be enjoyed by modifying their size and texture. For example, a frankfurter can be cut lengthwise into four sections; carrots and corn can be cooked and mashed; grapes can be cut in quarters; and peanut butter can be served with jelly, not by itself from a spoon.

If a child does choke, the American Academy of Pediatrics, the American Red Cross, the American Heart Association, and the Surgeon General all recommend the abdominal thrust—commonly known as the Heimlich maneuver—to treat all children over one year of age and adults who are choking. For the infant under one, deliver a series of four back blows between the shoulder blades with the heel of the hand. Hold the child's body upside down to make use of the force of gravity to dislodge the food item.

THE PRESCHOOL CHILD

The preschool child, ages three through five years, is refining skills and learning new ones. Height increases relative to weight, and the chubby toddler now takes on a leaner appearance. With luck, by the time a child has turned three or four years of age, most of the dietary problems common to the toddler years have been resolved. The preschool child may still be finicky when making food selections, but parents should always see to it that a wide variety of food is offered at mealtime.

Table 13.5. Suggested Daily Servings for Infants and Children (Ages 8 Months +) to Meet the Recommended Dietary Allowances

Food Group	Infant I 8–12 months	Infant II 1–2 years	Toddler 2–4 years	Reg. Pediatric 5 years +
Milk	2½–3 cups (iron-fortified infant formula)	2 cups	3 cups	3 or more cups
Meat, Protein	2–4 ounces, strained or finely chopped	4–5 ounces, finely chopped	5–6 ounces, chopped or whole	6 ounces or more
Vegetables (at least one good source of vitamin A)	2 servings (⅛ cup)	2 servings (⅛ cup)	2 servings (¼ cup)	2 servings (½ cup)
Fruit (at least one good source of vitamin C)	3 servings (⅛ cup)	3 servings (¼ cup)	3 servings (¼ cup)	3 servings (½ cup)
Bread, Cereal, Starch	4 servings (½ slice bread; ¼ cup cereal)	4 servings (½ slice bread; ½ cup cereal)	4 servings (1 slice bread; ½ cup cereal)	5 servings (1 slice bread; ¾ cup cereal)
Fat	2 teaspoons or to meet caloric needs	1 teaspoon or to meet caloric needs	1 tablespoon or to meet caloric needs	1 tablespoon or to meet caloric needs
Sweets	To meet caloric needs	To meet caloric needs	To meet caloric needs	To meet caloric needs

Common Nutritional Concerns

Childhood Obesity

Obesity is one of the most common nutritional disorders affecting Americans today. The most widely accepted method of classifying an individual as obese is if weight is 20 percent greater than desirable for age and height, and sex. Many pediatricians classify an obese child as one who falls above the 95th percentile in weight for height. A study by the U.S. Department of Health and Human Services revealed that children in the 1980s are significantly fatter and less physically fit than children were in the 1960s.

Most experts believe the reason children are fatter today than they were 20 years ago is because they consume more calories than they expend. Although individuals can have a genetic predisposition to obesity, for the most part, overeating and underactivity are still believed to be responsible.

Lack of activity. Children today have access to and enjoy watching television, video games, and playing on computers. Unfortunately, these are sedentary activities requiring little energy expenditure above that required for basal metabolism. The time spent watching television or playing on the computer may also take the place of activities that burn more energy. Furthermore, recent studies suggest that TV viewing encourages snacking on heavily advertised, calorically dense foods such as cookies, ice cream, candy, and high-calorie fast foods. If these sedentary activities are combined with an increased caloric intake, the scale can easily be tipped in the direction of obesity.

Overconsumption of calories. Several scenarios in childhood result in the consumption of more calories than the child can use for normal growth. All result in overweight, obesity if severe.

Sometimes parents or baby-sitters are not aware of the portion size a young child needs to eat. Parents frequently serve adult-size portions to children, then urge the child to clean his or her plate. This can develop the habit of overeating in children.

Some parents or baby-sitters use food as a reward or punishment. Food should never be offered as a reward for good behavior, nor should it ever be withheld as a punishment, as in the boy who brings home a poor report card and is sent to bed without dinner. These behaviors may later lead a child to eat, or more likely overeat, for reasons other than hunger. It is especially important that parents give explicit instructions about feeding to baby-sitters or other caregivers.

Dental Caries

Dental caries, one of the most common nutrition-related diseases, affects children of all ages. By following some basic rules, par-

Snacks for Toddlers

Appropriate Snacks (easy to chew and swallow)	Inappropriate Snacks (difficult to chew or may cause choking)
Dry, unsweetened cereal	Grapes (fruit with skin or peel)
Cut-up soft fruit (skin removed)	Coconut
Banana slices	Hot dogs
Graham crackers	Nuts, including peanuts
Yogurt	Peanut butter
Pudding	Popcorn
	Potato, corn, tortilla chips

ents can help children prevent decay and fight cavity formation:

1. *Take care of primary (baby) teeth.* As soon as teeth erupt, usually between 6 and 10 months of age, they should be cleaned daily. At first, teeth can be wiped with a piece of gauze or damp washcloth. A soft-bristled children's toothbrush can be tried later.

2. *Set a good example: Teach toddlers how to brush.* Children can begin brushing their own teeth as early as age two or three. Let them watch and imitate you.

3. *Make sure the child snacks wisely.* When a child does snack, try to limit sugar- and starch-containing foods. These act as food for decay-causing bacteria. Snacks that do not have this effect and are safe for teeth are cheese, milk, yogurt, raw vegetables, plain popcorn, nuts, and pizza. (Remember, however, that children under three should not be given foods that can cause choking.)

4. *Avoid snacks at bedtime.* Saliva flow is lowest at night, so any food or drink (except water) will stay in the mouth longer and feed cavity-producing bacteria.

5. *Avoid nursing-bottle syndrome.* Nursing bottle syndrome is one of the biggest dangers to a baby's teeth. It is caused by giving a baby a bottle of juice or milk for prolonged periods during the day or night. This causes a pooling of milk or juice in the mouth, thus promoting growth of cavity-causing bacteria. (For more information, see Chapter 37.)

Iron Deficiency

Nutrient-deficiency diseases are rare in the United States today, with the exception of iron deficiency, which is especially common among growing children.

During the growth process, blood supply must keep up with the expansion of tissues and cells. This blood supply is dependent on the element iron. Young infants are born with an iron supply acquired in utero. Toddlers and preschool children, who have used up their infant stores, are at greater risk for deficiency. Certain foods are better sources of iron than others. The iron present in meats is known as heme iron, and it is better absorbed by the body than the iron found in plants. Remember that a young child who has not yet mastered chewing will often refuse roasts and steaks. Try offering moist and tender meats that are easy to chew. Eating a vitamin C source at the same meal enhances iron absorption. See page 216 for a list of iron-rich foods.

Suggestions for Preventing Childhood Obesity

- Limit sedentary activities.
- Encourage energy-expending activities.
- Include the entire family, not just the child, in a healthier way of eating.
- Offer the child food from the four basic food groups daily.
- Never skip meals, especially breakfast, and limit snacking.
- Pack a nutritious and yet appealing lunch using lean meats, poultry, and fish rather than high-fat choices such as bologna and salami.
- Pack fresh fruits and raw vegetables instead of potato chips or cookies.
- Keep nutritious snacks on hand and don't bring low-nutrient, high-calorie, junk foods into the house.

Nutritious Snacks for Preschoolers

The preschool child is full of energy and consequently needs to snack frequently, sometimes up to four times a day. Snacks should be nutritious yet small enough so mealtime appetite is not curtailed. Here are some ideas:

- 1 to 2 oatmeal cookies or graham cracker squares with ½ cup low-fat milk
- ½ English muffin with 1 slice cheese
- ½ cup dry cereal with ½ cup low-fat milk
- 1 small or ½ large piece of fresh fruit
- 2 to 4 pieces of dried fruit, with no pits
- 1 piece string cheese with low-fat crackers or breadstick
- ½ cup low-fat yogurt

School-age children can add snacks such as popcorn, nuts, individual juices, and fresh or dried fruits that are easy to carry to school and after-school activities. After school, easy-to-prepare items such as English muffin pizza, frozen French toast, waffles, or pancakes can be made with a toaster or microwave oven. Instead of sugar-laden syrup, try applesauce, low-sugar jam, low-fat ricotta cheese with cinnamon, or peanut butter as fillings or toppings.

Concern over Cholesterol

Renewed interest in elevated blood cholesterol and dietary recommendations for adults has caused concern, controversy, and confusion over what and how to feed children. Two conclusions drawn from a forum of experts of the American Heart Association assembled to discuss this issue were:

1. Although pediatricians could not agree on the precise age that children should begin eating a diet low in saturated fat, they did agree that it shouldn't be before the age of two. Many believe that the ideal time to begin making the change to low-fat foods is during the preschool years, ages two to five.

2. When dietary changes are instituted, they should not be drastic. Recent reports have described cases of "failure to thrive"—a condition characterized by slowed growth and development—among children who ate extremely low-fat diets that lacked sufficient energy and nutrients for growth.

The best approach for children seems to be variety and choice. Although red meat and dairy products should not be cut out completely, leaner cuts of meat with visible fat trimmed, then baked or broiled instead of fried, and lower-fat cheese, milk, and frozen desserts should be offered. (See Table 13.6.)

Diet and Behavior

When discussing childhood nutrition, the question of sugar and behavior inevitably comes up. As noted in Chapter 8, many Americans have long held the notion that hyperactivity and other behavioral problems are in some way related to the diet, and food ad-

Iron-Rich Foods

Liver	Raisins
Lean meats and poultry	Lima beans
	Minestrone soup
Sardines and mackerel, drained and without bones	Bean soup
	Prune juice
	Dried, pitted prunes
Kidney beans	Iron-fortified cereals

ditives and sugar have been labeled the leading culprits. The 1988 Surgeon General's Report on Nutrition and Health acknowledges the fact "that diet influences behavior is an ancient human belief. Primitive people attributed friendly and unfriendly feelings to plants and animals and expected these feelings to be transferred to anyone who ate such foods. . . ." However, the report also stresses that there is little or no scientific evidence to support contentions that diet has a marked effect on behavior.

In 1975, the late Dr. Benjamin Feingold published an article maintaining that food additives, especially artificial colors and dyes, caused childhood hyperactivity. The article was followed by a flood of stories in the popular press in which Dr. Feingold's theories, which were supported by anecdotal accounts, were indeed said to be established fact. Researchers set about to establish whether these claims were, in fact, true, and a number of controlled double-blind studies were carried out. As recounted in the 1988 Surgeon General's report, "A statistical analysis of the results of 23 of these studies concluded that artificial colors have, at most, a negligible effect on the behavior of children. . . . At most, a few predisposed preschool and school-aged children may be adversely affected by artificial colors." The report also notes that because there is a possibility that a few children may benefit from diets that eliminate food dyes, and that such diets are not harmful, there is "no reason to advise against therapeutic trials of food additive avoidance in individual cases." If, however, no improvement is noted after a few months, it is safe to assume that these substances have no effect on behavior.

Similarly, scientific studies have failed to document an adverse effect of sugar on behavior. Indeed, since sugar elevates the levels of serotonin—a natural body chemical that has a mild sedative effect—in the brain, it would seem logical that sugar would have a calming effect rather than inducing aggression and hyperactivity. Short-term challenge studies, in which children are given a sugar drink and their behavior compared with those receiving a placebo, have failed to show that sugar affects hyperactive behavior. In fact, a major study conducted by researchers at the National Institute of Mental Health found that giving sugar to children considered by their parents to be hyperactive had no effect on their behavior, and in some, it seemed to produce drowsiness. (See Chapter 8 for a more detailed discussion of this study.)

Even though sugar may not have any documented effect on behavior, this does not mean that it should have a major part in a child's diet. Sugar and other sweeteners, including honey, do not provide nutrients, and thus are referred to as empty calories. Many sugary foods such as candy bars, cookies, ice cream, and pastries also contain large amounts of fat, making them high-calorie, low-nutrient items. Sugar also is a factor in dental disease. In fact, the Surgeon General's report recommends that "those who are particularly vulnerable to dental caries (cavities), especially children, should limit their consumption and frequency of use of foods high in sugars."

THE SCHOOL-AGE CHILD: AGES SIX THROUGH TEN

The school-age child tends to be relatively stable in terms of physical growth. Height may increase in increments of five to six centimeters, or about two to almost two and a half inches per year. While weight gain averages two kilograms, or nearly four and a half pounds, per year in early childhood, it increases to four to four and a half kilograms, or approximately nine to ten pounds, per year as puberty approaches. A child begins to make food choices independently, with more peer influence and less parental supervision. It is a period of few apparent feeding problems. Appetite and food intake will naturally increase with the added activities of school and play.

Breakfast

Breakfast can be an important meal for adults and children alike. A child who is accustomed to sitting down to eat in the morning will probably be more likely to retain this habit as he or she grows older.

Breakfast doesn't have to be the time-

Table 13.6. Healthy Eating Tips for Children

Choose:	Instead of:
Fresh fruit	Ice cream
Fruit-juice bars	
Sorbet	
Sherbet	
Ice milk	
Frozen low-fat yogurt	
Homemade cookies, fruit muffins (made with recipes that call for minimal amounts of fat and sugar)	High-fat, store-bought cookies
Low-fat cottage cheese	Regular cottage cheese
Part-skim mozzarella	Whole-milk mozzarella
Other low-fat cheeses	Higher-fat varieties
Peanut butter on whole-wheat bread	Bologna and mayonnaise sandwich on white bread
Leaner cuts of meat such as:	Meats with higher fat content such as:
Ground round of beef	Ground beef
Brisket of beef	Hot dogs
Center loin of pork	Sausage
Chuck pot roast	Bacon
Short loin of beef	Liverwurst
Flank steak	Heavily marbleized steaks
Chicken, baked without skin	Chicken, fried with skin
Margarine made with an unsaturated vegetable oil	Butter
Products made with monosaturated or polyunsaturated vegetable oils such as olive, safflower, peanut, et al.	Products made with coconut or palm kernel oils

The following are suggestions for nutritious meals and snacks for young children:

For Breakfast Serve:
Fresh fruit on unsweetened whole-grain cereal with skim or low-fat milk
Hot oatmeal with raisins and skim or low-fat milk
Fresh fruit with low-fat yogurt
Whole-wheat raisin toast with margarine made with an unsaturated vegetable oil and sprinkled with cinnamon or low-fat cottage cheese

For Lunch Serve:
Peanut butter on whole-wheat bread
Whipped low-fat cottage cheese on whole-wheat bagel
Low-fat Swiss cheese and tomato sandwich on whole-wheat bread
Whole-wheat pita with tuna salad
Homemade vegetable or broth-based soups

For Snacks Serve:
Fresh fruit
Raw vegetables
Celery stuffed with low-fat cottage cheese
Carrots or apple slices with peanut butter
Popcorn (dry or with margarine made with an unsaturated vegetable oil), can be sprinkled with cinnamon
Unsweetened fruit juices
Raisins

For Desserts Serve:
Low-fat yogurt, unsweetened with fresh fruit added
Custards made with skim milk
Bananas
Puddings made with skim milk (brown rice or whole-wheat bread can be used)
Warm apple cider sprinkled with nutmeg and cinnamon
Homemade oatmeal or ginger cookies, made with margarine consisting of an unsaturated vegetable oil, instead of butter or shortening
Fresh fruit
Ice cream

consuming and high-fat meal of bacon and eggs. A breakfast of cereal, milk, and fruit requires little or no preparation. An egg simply prepared can be given to a child several times per week.

Healthy breakfasts include:

- Homemade muffin, such as corn, fruit, oatmeal, and raisin-nut, with milk and fruit or fruit juice

- Cereal, lightly sweetened or unsweetened, with low-fat milk and fruit

- Low-fat cottage cheese or ricotta on toast with fruit or juice

- Yogurt with fresh fruit and muffin or whole-grain bread

Do Children Instinctively Choose the Right Foods?

A researcher named Clara Davis conducted a study in the 1920s allowing children to choose their own foods without adult intervention. The foods presented to them, from which they made their choices, were all fresh, unprocessed, unseasoned, and simply prepared. No sweets, sugars, corn syrups, or processed foods were offered. Ms. Davis found that the children selected an adequate combination of foods that allowed for sufficient weight gain. The children in the study would often go on food jags, eating only one particular item. Over time, however, they ate a balanced selection of foods.

In interpreting the data, many people overlooked the fact that Ms. Davis offered only nutritious, unsweetened foods and concluded that children instinctively know what to eat. The environment in this study was artificial, because the children were not exposed to foods of dubious nutritional value. The reality is that most children leading normal lives are exposed to foods with little nutritional value and may choose them over a well-balanced diet.

School Lunch

The federally subsidized school lunch program was established to provide a third of the recommended dietary allowance. Budgetary considerations frequently preclude the inclusion of fresh fruits and vegetables or a variety of foods. Home-prepared lunches allow for increased variety.

In recent years, parental concern over the nutritional quality and variety of school lunches has led many schools to publish their school-lunch menus in advance. Parents can go over these menus with their children and suggest the best selections. If a school-lunch program falls short of your nutritional goals, persuade your parents' organization to press for change. Alternatively, you can pack a home lunch for your child.

Regardless of its source, a good, well-balanced lunch should include selections from the Basic Four food groups:

- A source of protein such as lean beef, poultry, fish, eggs, cheese, dried beans, or peanut butter

- A grain product, preferably whole grain, such as bread or crackers (breadsticks or unsweetened cereals as a welcome change)

- A fruit or vegetable, preferably one of each, fresh whenever possible (small cans or containers of tomato, vegetable, or unsweetened fruit juice as a change of pace)

- A dairy product such as milk, cheese, or yogurt

Several measures can be taken to ensure against spoilage:

1. Wash hands and utensils. Never use the same knife or cutting board for raw meats and ready-to-eat foods.

2. Pack foods and sandwich fillings with an ice pack.

3. Freeze some items, such as yogurt, some sandwiches such as sliced meat, poultry, and fish (don't freeze with lettuce and tomato) overnight. They will defrost by lunchtime.

4. Avoid using leftovers that have been in the refrigerator for days.

For more information on safe food preparation, see Chapter 41.

TEACHING GOOD EATING HABITS

It's never too early to instill good eating habits in a child. Start by setting a good example yourself. Take stock of your own refrigerator and pantry shelves. Are the foods you find there the ones you really want your child to eat? Remember, children learn by imitating those around them, and there is no time that you are going to have greater influence or control over your child's diet than during these early years.

When introducing new foods, pick those that are healthful alternatives, and show that you yourself prefer these foods to less healthful ones. For example, serve whole-grain breads instead of the soft white varieties. Pick low-sugar, whole-grain cereals and offer them as finger foods to a toddler. Offer snacks of fresh fruits or vegetables or real dried fruits such as apple slices instead of fabricated foods such as fruit snacks or high-sugar breakfast bars. Real unsweetened fruit juice has more nutrition than fruit drinks or fabricated powdered drinks. Young children who develop a taste for these products will be more likely to stay with them in later years.

Take care, however, not to become a food dictator. Respect your child's likes and dislikes. If, for example, a toddler absolutely

Well-Balanced Lunch-Box Meals

For well-balanced lunches, select an item from each group.

Dairy
Thermos of milk
Container of yogurt
Swiss cheese slices
Cheese cubes
Cottage-cheese

Protein
Tuna (water-packed)
Sliced turkey
Peanut butter with raisins, banana, or apple
   slices for variety
Sliced or chopped egg
Sliced or cubed ham
Thermos of chili with beans

Fruit/Vegetables
Fresh apple or orange
Fruit bars or roll
Carrot and celery sticks
Broccoli florets
Thermos of vegetable soup
Fresh tomato slices
Sliced green pepper
Carrot/raisin slaw

Grain
Whole-wheat crackers
Rye bread
Breadsticks
Pita bread
Bran or whole-grain fruit muffin
Sesame crackers

hates broccoli, don't fight it. Offer an alternative vegetable and try the broccoli again in a few months. Remember, too, that your child's friends may have different eating habits. When your youngster comes home from a birthday party, for example, with glowing accounts of all the candy, cake, cookies, soft drinks, and other items you may consider junk food, don't try to belittle what was served. Be noncommittal and stick to your own food preferences at home. Chances are your child's friends will be equally glowing about what they sample when they come to visit. A child will not fall into bad eating habits by occasionally tasting something different out of the home. A commonsense, low-key approach is likely to be more successful and lasting than a dogmatic one.

14

Adolescent Nutrition

Neal LeLeiko, M.D., Ph.D., and Denise Rollinson, M.S., R.D.

■

INTRODUCTION

Adolescence, generally defined as ages 10 to 20, is a time of significant physical and psychological maturation. The rapid growth occurring during adolescence dramatically increases nutrient needs. Yet adolescents do not necessarily consume nutritionally adequate diets. For example, diets are often low in iron and calcium and may contain an excess of fat and calories. Adolescents who are misinformed about their nutritional needs and who make independent food choices are at risk for developing nutritional deficiencies.

GROWTH

Adolescents have increased nutrient needs because of the growth spurt that occurs during this life stage. The adolescent growth spurt occurs at a different time for boys than for girls. The male growth spurt usually begins around the ages of 12½ to 15½ years, with the highest rate between ages 14 and 15. The female growth spurt usually occurs from the ages of 10½ to 13½ years, peaking around 12 to 13.

Hormonal changes and the later onset of the growth spurt in males contribute to greater muscle and skeletal growth, requiring a higher intake of protein, iron, calcium, and zinc. In contrast, the growth spurt in females is characterized by a smaller increase in muscle mass and a greater increase in fatty (adipose) tissue. The nutrient needs for girls are therefore somewhat lower than those for boys, except girls require more iron because of the onset of menstruation.

THE RECOMMENDED DIETARY ALLOWANCES

The recommended dietary allowances for adolescents are not based on experimental data from adolescents; instead, most of the RDAs are either extrapolations from studies of younger children or adults, derived from results of animal experiments, or based on the intakes that have been found to be associated with good health and optimal growth. The RDAs do, however, serve as useful general guidelines. (See Table 14.1.)

Energy requirements are based on the median intake of adolescents engaged in light activities. An individual teenager's actual caloric (energy) requirement will vary depending on his or her growth rate, degree of physical maturation or body composition, and activity level. In general, males have higher energy requirements than females because males have a higher proportion of lean body mass to adipose tissue than do females. Also, adolescents who are sedentary have lower energy requirements than those adolescents who are more active.

Iron. Iron requirements increase in adolescence because of the greater muscle mass and blood volume associated with the growth spurt. In addition, the onset of menstruation slightly increases the iron requirements for females. The recommendations for iron are based on the assumption that iron is not well absorbed. Iron found in foods containing heme iron (such as red meats) is absorbed best. Iron from nonheme sources (such as

Table 14.1. Recommended Dietary Allowances for Adolescents, Ages 11 to 18[a]

	Age and Size			
	BOYS		GIRLS	
Nutrient	11–14 Years (99 lb. 62 in.)	15–18 Years (145 lb. 69 in.)	11–14 Years (101 lb. 62 in.)	15–18 Years (120 lb. 64 in.)
Calories	2500	3000	2200	2200
Protein (gm.)	45	9	46	44
Vitamin A activity (RE)[b]	1000	1000	800	800
Vitamin D (μg.)[c]	10	10	10	10
Vitamin E (mg. α = TE)[d]	10	10	8	8
Vitamin C (mg.)	50	60	50	60
Thiamine (mg.)	1.3	1.5	1.1	1.1
Riboflavin (mg.)	1.5	1.8	1.3	1.3
Niacin (mg. NE)[e]	17	20	15	15
Vitamin B$_6$ (mg.)	1.7	2.0	1.4	1.5
Folacin (μg.)[f]	100	150	150	180
Vitamin B$_{12}$ (μg.)	2.0	2.0	2.0	2.0
Calcium (mg.)	1200	1200	1200	1200
Phosphorus (mg.) (mg.)	1200	1200	1200	1200
Magnesium (mg.)	270	400	280	300
Iron (mg.)	12	12	15	15
Zinc (mg.)	15	15	12	12
Iodide (μg.)	150	150	150	150

[a]The allowances are intended to provide for individual variations among most normal persons as they live in the United States under usual environmental stresses. Diets should be based on a variety of common foods to provide other nutrients for which human requirements have been less well defined.
[b]Retinol equivalents; 1 RE = 1 μg. retinol or 6 μg. β carotene. From animal source, 1 RE = 3⅓ IU; from plant sources, 1 RE = 10 IU.
[c]As cholecalciferol; 10 μg. cholecalciferol = 4000 IU of vitamin D.
[d]α-tocopherol equivalents; 1 mg. *d-α* tocopherol = 1 α-TE.
[e]Niacin equivalent; 1 NE = 1 mg. of niacin or 60 mg. of dietary tryptophan.
[f]The folacin allowances refer to dietary sources as determined by *Lactobacillus casei* assay after treatment with enzymes (conjugates) to make polyglutamyl forms of the vitamin available to the test organism.

Adapted from *Recommended Dietary Allowances*, ninth edition, 1980, with 1989 RDA numbers.

grains and vegetables) is not absorbed as well as heme iron, but consumption of vitamin C along with nonheme iron enhances its usefulness to the body.

Teenagers may have difficulty obtaining the recommended 15 milligrams of iron a day from food sources alone, particularly if their calorie intake is low. Therefore, adolescents need to consume foods with a high availability of iron, such as red meats, or eat combinations of good nonheme sources of iron along with foods rich in vitamin C. They may even need an iron supplement in order to avoid iron-deficiency anemia.

Calcium. The increase in skeletal mass that is part of the adolescent growth spurt increases calcium requirements. If calcium intake is very low, the body maintains normal blood-calcium levels by drawing calcium from the bones. This can have serious consequences: Adolescents may not develop optimal bone density, which may increase their susceptibility to osteoporosis later in life.

The RDA for calcium of 1,200 milligrams a day is designed to cover the needs of adolescents at the height of their growth spurt; those who are not growing as fast may not need so much. Nevertheless, girls typically have too low an intake of calcium throughout adolescence, largely because milk—the food that is our single best source of calcium—is so often shunned as fattening. Another reason for this low calcium intake is the substitution of soft drinks for milk. Adolescents who do not drink milk should be encouraged to include other good sources of calcium in their diet. For example, low-fat yogurt is an excellent source of calcium and contains less fat than other snack foods.

Protein. Many boys in later adolescence (ages 15 to 18) eat twice the recommended allowance of protein, or more, in the belief that a diet high in protein will give them a competitive advantage in sports (see Nutrition and the Young Athlete on page 232). Unfortunately, once the body's requirements for protein have been met, excess protein is processed just like any other excess form of calories; it is deposited as fat, not muscle.

Vitamins. The recommended vitamin allowances for adolescents are extrapolated from data from children and adults, but they can be comfortably met by a well-balanced diet.

FOOD HABITS

With adolescence, children no longer eat what they are given but increasingly make their own decisions about what to eat—and when, where, and with whom. As a group, adolescents have food habits that differ markedly from those of any other, often to the dismay of parents and nutritionists. Among the factors that appear to influence these idiosyncratic eating habits are:

- Desire for independence. Adolescents commonly defy parental edicts and reject traditional family eating patterns.

- Need for acceptance by peers. Peers' food preferences often determine food choices; peer activities have priority over family mealtimes. Socializing with peers, whatever the setting, almost always involves snacking.

- Increased mobility. Fast-food restaurants and other eating places that cater to teenage preferences are readily accessible.

- School and work schedules. An adolescent may be away from home from early morning until well after dinner hour. Time for sit-down meals may be hard to find, leading to badly planned meals consumed on the run, or missed meals.

- Concern with self-image. Looking good and feeling good about oneself are of overwhelming concern in adolescence. Girls are commonly worried about being overweight, boys about being skinny. While most teenagers understand that diet contributes to good looks and energy, misperceptions and superstitions are common.

Skipping meals. Adolescents have a well-deserved reputation for skipping meals. Breakfast and lunch are the meals most often missed, with older adolescents (those 15 to 18) twice as likely to skip breakfast as the younger group, and girls more than boys. In one survey, almost half of the high school students questioned had no breakfast.

Those who skip breakfast often plead lack of time, early school activities, or a poor appetite first thing in the morning. It seems probable, however, that many, especially girls, skip breakfast to save calories. The calories that are skipped are potentially high-calcium (milk) and iron-fortified (cereal.) However, the calories "saved" are often made up for by a nutrient-poor snack, or by overeating at the next meal. Adolescents should be advised to consume nutritious snacks, especially if meals are skipped.

Snacking. Casual eating—as opposed to a sit-down meal—is an important part of adolescents' eating and socialization patterns. One study showed that boys have an average of 6.4 daytime snacks and 2.9 evening snacks a week; girls have even more: 7.7 snacks in the day, and 3.8 in the evening. Consequently, teenagers need to be taught how to improve the overall quality of their diets with nutritious snacks. For example, instead of selecting high-calorie, high-fat, nutrient-poor snacks (such as candy bars and foods fried in saturated fats), teenagers should select foods with lower fat contents and more nutrients (fresh fruit, low-fat yogurt, vegetarian pizza).

Parents commonly worry that empty-calorie snacks will displace real food in their teenagers' diets. A poorly timed snack may indeed blunt an adolescent's mealtime appetite, and a poorly chosen one may make an inappropriate contribution to the daily nutrient intake. However, while snacks typically provide 20 percent or more of adolescents' daily calorie needs, they may also deliver 12 percent of the protein, 20 percent of the calcium, 11 percent of the iron, 14 percent of the vitamin A, 13 percent of the thiamine, 17 percent of the riboflavin, and 18 percent of the vitamin C needed. This proportion of nutrients to calories is similar to that contributed by the rest of the diet. Moreover, it is yet to be shown that it is healthier to eat only three times a day, and heavily on those occasions, than to break up the intake of food into smaller, more frequent meals.

Fast food. Adolescents are big consumers of fast food. The food is inexpensive, familiar, safe, and available without delay at almost any hour of the day or night. Many adolescents also go to fast-food restaurants to socialize with their peers. What's more, consuming a meal away from home and from the school environment is an expression of freedom and independence.

According to the restaurant's analysis, a teenager who lunches at McDonald's on a Big Mac, a serving of French fries, and a chocolate shake will be getting 40 percent of his or her energy (calorie) needs and more than 40 percent of the needed protein, vitamin C, thiamine, riboflavin, calcium, and iron, but only 10 percent of his or her vitamin A requirement. With good food choices at breakfast and dinner, a teenager easily should be able to meet the remaining 60 percent of his or her daily needs, perhaps with the exception of vitamin A. Unless a teenager eats at a fast-food restaurant many times a week, nutritional disorders are not likely. (On the minus side, it should be noted that this meal is high in saturated fats and cholesterol.)

However, in calculating the contribution of a fast-food meal to a teenager's daily requirements, it is the combination of foods chosen that is important. If, for example, the chocolate shake is passed up in favor of a diet soft drink, the meal will have fewer calories and less fat but significantly less calcium. In fact, both calcium and vitamin C are notably low in most fast-food meals actually eaten, despite the fact that milk is on the standard menu in most restaurants and that salad bars have become more prominent. However, even if calcium requirements are met, it is difficult to choose a meal that is not high in calories, fat, and salt.

A nutrition-conscious teenager may want to decrease the salt and fat eaten at other meals and, at the restaurant, make choices that will keep these ingredients to a minimum. For example, he or she could order a hamburger instead of a cheeseburger and omit items with special (high-fat) sauces, and skip fried fruit-pie desserts. Teenagers should avoid pickles and relishes to reduce sodium, and, if a salad is chosen, use dressing sparingly or not at all. (See Chapter 39 for more information on how to eat healthfully at fast-food restaurants.)

Unconventional meals. It can be disconcerting to watch a teenager breakfast on a slice of pizza, start dinner with dessert, or fix a large lunch at 10 A.M. Meals that are unconventional in timing, composition, or in the order eaten often represent either a rebellion against the customs that parents have established in their home or an experiment in eating habits. It is custom—not nutritional dogma—that dictates that certain foods be eaten at certain meals, or that a particular meal is always con-

---

Table 14.2. Nutritious Snacks for Teenagers

High in Vitamin A (needed for healthy skin and eyes)	High in Vitamin C (needed for healthy gums and skin)	High in Calcium (needed for strong, healthy bones and muscle function)	High in Iron (needed for healthy blood and muscles)
Apricots	Broccoli	Beans, baked	Apricots, dried
Broccoli	Cantaloupe	Broccoli	Avocado
Cantaloupe	Coleslaw	Cheese*	Beans, baked
Carrots	Grapefruit	Custard	Iron-fortified breads
Mangoes	Green pepper	Ice cream*	Iron-fortified cereals
Milk, low-fat	Oranges	Milk, low-fat	Chicken
Nectarines	Papayas	Pudding (made with low-fat milk)	Chili
Papayas	Potatoes	Sardines	Eggs*
Peaches	Strawberries	Shrimp	Hamburgers*
Red pepper	Tangerines	Tofu	Nuts
Tomatoes	Tomatoes	Yogurt	Prunes
Watermelon	Watermelon		Sunflower seeds

*These foods should be eaten in moderation, as they are high in fat and cholesterol.

sumed at a particular time of day. The teenager's rearrangements are usually short-lived and nutrition is not likely to suffer.

Dieting. Few teenagers are satisfied with their weight or their shape and their self-criticism is harsh. Concern with body image is a completely normal part of adolescence; that the perception may be distorted or the goals unrealistic does not make the concern any less important. It is reinforced by advertisements, magazines, movies, by society's emphasis on sexual attractiveness, and most strongly by the desire to fit in with the group.

Girls typically consider themselves too fat. One study of teenage girls found that 70 percent wanted to lose weight, although only 15 percent could be considered obese. Boys, on the other hand, generally think of themselves as too light, though the same study found that only 25 percent were below average weight. Their goal is to put on weight in the form of muscle, especially upper-body muscle—biceps, shoulder muscles, pectorals.

For teenage girls, the most usual method of dieting is to cut out certain fattening foods. Unfortunately, milk and other dairy products are generally consigned to this category. The result is a diet low in several major nutrients, most notably calcium. (Skim and 1%-fat milk are low in calories and slightly higher in calcium than whole milk.) More immediately hazardous approaches to weight loss are not uncommon among adolescent girls, including liquid-formula diets, fasting or starving, self-induced vomiting, and the use of laxatives and diuretics. Severe restriction of calorie intake can lead to a decrease in lean body mass and to a less than optimum growth in height. Moreover, the weight lost by fad or crash dieting is usually quickly regained. This is the notorious yo-yo pattern of weight control that is dangerous to the cardiovascular system and can, in fact, increase the percentage of weight

attributable to fat. All diets that are highly restricted in calories, and all plans that unbalance the diet, should be avoided at any time, but especially during adolescence, when a girl needs energy and nutrients for growth.

Boys generally view exercise, rather than diet alone, as the solution to a more attractive appearance. A frequent tactic is to undertake a program to build muscles along with a diet that stresses protein and eliminates carbohydrates. However, most American boys already eat more than enough protein and need extra carbohydrates to meet their calorie needs. The unbalanced diet can actually end up being high in fat and low in carbohydrates, depriving muscle of needed fuel. This might make the adolescent male feel tired and weak instead of stronger and more muscular.

It does little good to tell dieting adolescents, male or female, that they look fine the way they are, because that is not what they see when they look in the mirror. Instead, parents can try to point out the ill effects of unbalanced diets on energy and growth, while providing low-calorie, nutrient-dense foods such as skim-milk products and fresh fruits for the teenager to include in his or her diet.

Vegetarianism. Many older teenagers eat vegetarian diets, some out of concern for animal life, some for ecological reasons, others to avoid the contaminants in animal products. A vegetarian diet may be a radical departure from the family's eating patterns. If the teenager's diet is to support normal growth, both the adolescent and the parents have to become knowledgeable and sophisticated about nutrition requirements and which foods can meet these needs.

Vegan diets, which contain absolutely no animal products, are very low in vitamin B_{12} and, unless carefully planned, may be deficient in vitamin B_6, riboflavin, calcium, iron, and zinc. Strict macrobiotic diets, which exclude everything except grains, are, to be frank, hazardous. More moderate vegetarian diets that include milk and eggs and perhaps fish and/or poultry, meet the nutritional needs of growing teenagers if carefully planned. Adolescents consuming vegetarian diets must still be careful to consume a wide variety of foods and limit intake of fat. (See also Chapter 25).

ACNE

It may be as mild as a couple of pimples or so severe as to leave the skin scarred for life, but some degree of acne is almost inevitable in adolescence. Acne is the direct result of the rapid acceleration in the production of hormones, mainly androgens, that occurs in puberty. Studies have failed to find any connection between skin outbreaks and the consumption of specific food items such as chocolate, cola drinks, nuts, pizza, or French fries—foods that are popularly blamed for skin outbreaks. However, in perhaps one teenager in a hundred, these or other foods seem to aggravate the condition. It is therefore worth a try to eliminate the suspect food from the diet for a week or so to see whether the skin condition improves.

A derivative of vitamin A (retinoic acid) is sometimes prescribed for the topical treatment of difficult cases of acne. This does not mean that ingestion of large amounts of this vitamin (or any other) as a supplement will clear the skin. In fact, large doses of fat-soluble vitamins can be toxic. (See also Chapter 7.)

OBESITY

Mild obesity is usually defined as 10 to 20 percent above the ideal weight-for-height. Frank obesity is defined as a weight of more than 20 percent above ideal weight. By this definition, an estimated 3 to 20 percent of American adolescents are obese—about 10 million teenagers.

Many obese adolescents were overweight as children, maturing earlier than those of normal weight and achieving greater skeletal growth. Many others, however, were slim children and began to accumulate excess fat only in puberty. Some accumulation of fat in existing adipocytes (fat cells) is normal in adolescence, especially in girls. But, in addition to this normal accumulation, the obese adolescent produces increasing numbers of new adipocytes. Once adulthood is reached, the number of fat cells cannot be appreciably decreased (or increased). Excess adipocytes may be shrunk by dieting, but they always remain present, ready at any time throughout the individual's life to fill with fat again. Thus, adolescent obesity presages adult obesity, or at least poses a very substantial risk of obesity. In fact, the odds against an obese adolescent becoming a normal-weight adult are 28 to 1.

The desirability of having a slim body— even an excessively slim body—is relentlessly stressed by all the media and is reinforced as a social norm. In the teen years, when appearance and acceptance by peers are of overriding importance, obesity is a greater psychological burden than at any other age. Studies have shown that obese teenage girls show traits typical of other minority groups: passivity, withdrawal, and a self-image so poor as to verge on self-contempt. In addition to being mercilessly teased by their contemporaries, obese teenagers may suffer actual discrimination: They may be excluded from social and athletic events, have trouble getting a job, or—all other things being equal—be passed over for a place at the college of their choice. It is not surprising that many find an outlet for their frustration and depression in further eating and thus set up a vicious cycle that leads to even greater obesity.

Boys have fewer problems with their weight in adolescence than do girls, partly because their hormones encourage muscle development rather than the accumulation of fat, and partly because they tend to be far more active. Obese teenagers may have a caloric intake similar to or even lower than their peers, but their activity level is often significantly lower. This is not hard to understand: Sports make them feel awkward and embarrassed and their extra weight makes them tire easily. However, it is difficult to say whether these adolescents are obese because they are inactive or inactive because they are obese.

Treatment of obesity. Weight control is a more complicated undertaking in adolescence than in adulthood. Calories are needed for growth just as much in the obese adolescent as in an adolescent of normal weight, and the necessary balance of carbohydrates, proteins, and fats must be maintained. A rigidly restrictive diet is not recommended: At an intake of 1,800 calories or less, it is difficult to meet teenagers' requirements for nutrients such as calcium, iron, zinc, and vitamins A and C.

The most successful approach to dieting is one that combines a modest restriction in calorie intake (smaller portions at meal and snack time rather than total deprivation), dietary guidance, supportive counseling, especially if there are accompanying social or emotional problems, and—most important—exercise. Exercise improves body composition by reducing fat while sparing lean body tissue; it benefits the cardiovascular system; and it is associated with a lowered food intake. The benefits of exercise can be seen quickly in

weight and fat loss, greater shapeliness, and a feeling of accomplishment. Since most obese adolescents will have lifelong weight problems, the best activities are those that can be easily continued on a regular basis in adulthood: for example, tennis, swimming, walking, hiking, or skating.

Goals for weight loss must be realistic and short-term; a new goal should be set only after the previous one has been reached. In setting goals, the individual adolescent's physiological age should be taken into account. Those who are still in their growth spurt can grow into their weight, reducing fatness rather than losing pounds. Those whose growth spurt is over, however, must aim for an actual reduction in weight. Joining a support group of peers may be very helpful, since adolescents' concerns are different from adults' and are best discussed with contemporaries. (See How to Help an Adolescent with a Weight Problem on page 231.)

ANOREXIA NERVOSA

At the opposite extreme of obesity is the anorexic adolescent, emaciated and hyperactive. Anorexia nervosa is complex, serious, and potentially fatal. Although adolescent girls are by far the most frequent sufferers, the disorder may also affect women in their twenties and thirties and, occasionally, adolescent boys.

The problem usually begins in the mid-teens, at the time when a girl begins to be concerned about her sexual maturation. Convinced that she is fat—and denying all arguments and evidence to the contrary—she drastically restricts her eating. Success in losing weight leads to the setting of unreasonable and even lower goals and also, in most cases, failure to menstruate (amenorrhea). Dieting becomes a primary focus of her life. It may alternate with binge eating, a binge being followed by self-induced vomiting or heavy doses of laxatives or both. (This "gorge and purge" phenomenon—bulimia—can occur independently, as well.)

Compulsive exercise is part of the drive for thinness and the adolescent usually exercises alone, denying fatigue or the need to rest. Another behavioral pattern is preoccupation with food. The anorexic adolescent collects recipes, cooks elaborate meals for the family, and is usually far better informed about nutrition than her contemporaries. Efforts to persuade or tempt her to eat almost invariably fail, however.

The emotional factors that seem to contribute to adolescent anorexia nervosa include a fear of growing up, especially a fear of sexual maturation, and strong dependence/independence conflicts. Some experts believe that a disturbance of the hypothalamus triggers the weight loss and menstrual problems and may even be responsible for some of the typical behavior patterns. However, most think that the syndrome stems from a combination of circumstances: a youngster whose expectations of herself are unreasonably high; a family that puts great emphasis on social, academic, and financial success and attempts to maintain strict control of the children; and the arrival of adolescence.

Semistarved and often with fluid and electrolyte imbalances from vomiting and purging, an adolescent with this disorder is in dire shape nutritionally. In a small percentage of cases, the disorder is fatal.

Mild cases of anorexia nervosa can be treated by the family doctor, but if the disorder is severe, hospitalization and specialized care are needed. Treatment is usually a combined nutritional-medical-psychiatric approach. Therapy focusing on family relationships and functioning is often very successful, if started early (that is, within a year of the first signs of trouble), although relapses do occur. (For more information, see Chapter 19.)

PREGNANCY

Teenage pregnancy continues in epidemic proportions in the United States. About 600,000 live infants are born each year to girls in their teens. Fully 10 percent of these young mothers are 15 years old or younger. Young teenagers, in particular, tend to have more babies and to have them closer together than women in other age groups. A pregnant teenage girl is a poor obstetrical risk if she has not finished her own growth spurt, and/or if she had an inadequate diet before she became pregnant. Pregnant teenagers tend to seek prenatal care later than older women and even then tend to see the doctor less often. They have a higher proportion of stillborn and low-birth-weight babies, and the babies have a higher risk of severe problems or even death in infancy.

Pregnancy by itself increases a woman's caloric and nutrient requirements. The nutritional demands of pregnancy superimposed on the requirements of a growing adolescent place the pregnant adolescent at risk for developing nutritional deficiencies such as anemia and place the growing fetus at risk for less than optimal outcomes, especially low birth weight. The usual rule of thumb is to add the recommended dietary allowances for a pregnant woman who is not a growing adolescent to those for 15-to-18-year-old girls. This should help meet the nutrient requirements of pregnancy and adolescent growth.

ALCOHOL

Automobile accidents are the leading cause of death among adolescents, and in a very large percentage, alcohol is a factor: The drivers are teenagers who have had too much to drink. The legal drinking age in most states is now 21, but it is estimated that more than half of all teenagers (aged 12 to 17) have at least one drink monthly and that nearly 3 percent drink daily. (Given the fact that it is illegal for them to drink at all, these figures are almost certainly underestimated.) Adolescents do not drink as frequently as adults do, but when they drink, they drink more and, since their bodies still have not build up a tolerance to alcohol, they are more likely to become drunk. Peer pressure accounts for much adolescent drinking: It may be hard to say no when all your friends use alcohol (or say they do).

The effects of alcohol on adult body metabolism are well known, but it is not known how much of this applies directly to teenagers. However, it is clear that with their high nutrition needs, adolescents are particularly vulnerable to the nutritional effects of alcohol use and abuse. The degree of risk depends, of course, on how much is consumed.

Alcohol has plenty of calories but almost no nutrients; it depresses the appetite; and it takes money that might otherwise be used for nutritious food. Moreover, the steady consumption of alcohol has a toxic effect on the mucosal lining of the gastrointestinal tract, interfering with the digestion and absorption of food. Pyrodoxine, folic acid, thiamine, and vitamin B_{12} are the nutrients most likely to be lacking.

Teenage myths about alcohol center on beer. Many believe, for example, that beer drinkers do not become alcoholics, because there is so little alcohol in beer (as compared to hard liquor). However, it is susceptibility to alcohol in any concentration that predisposes a person to alcoholism. Another myth is that

---

How to Help an Adolescent with a Weight Problem

The following are tips for families and friends of adolescents with a weight problem.

Do:

- Comment favorably on constructive changes in the teenager's eating habits.

- Compliment the teenager for avoiding situations that trigger overeating.

- Keep problem foods (high-calorie, high-fat foods) out of sight, and preferably out of the house.

- Stock tasty low-calorie foods such as skim-milk products, fresh fruits, and raw vegetables in the cupboard and refrigerator.

- Encourage the teenager to plan meals and to choose healthful, low-fat cooking methods.

Don't:

- Be pessimistic.

- Scold or nag if the teenager fails to keep to the diet plan; negotiation is the better approach.

- Tell other people about any failure or backsliding on the teenager's part.

- Offer food that is forbidden. ("A little won't hurt you.")

- Offer food as a sign of affection. ("But I prepared it especially for you.")

beer is nutritious. Although beer does contain a little niacin and a trace of protein, an adult male would have to drink a six-pack to meet his niacin needs, and nine six-packs to meet the requirement for protein. Given the nutritional and social consequences of alcohol, teenage drinking should be discouraged.

NUTRITION AND THE YOUNG ATHLETE

Misconceptions about the role of diet are rife in the competitive world of sports. However, the basic facts are simple: Fitness and good performance require an adequate intake of calories and nutrients; with a few minor exceptions, eating enough from the four food groups provides this intake; supplements and special preparations are generally unnecessary and may be harmful.

Calories. All other things being equal, it is calorie intake that determines how well an athlete performs. The RDAs for calories for adolescents provide for light to moderate physical activity, so athletes may have to add extra calories—roughly between 600 and 1,200, depending on weight and the sport they are engaged in—to the daily allowance. (See Chapter 24.)

Protein. Many people, including many coaches and professional athletes, believe that large amounts of protein are needed by athletes in training. A small increase in protein intake may be warranted in order to support increased blood volume and muscle mass, but large amounts are not. If an athlete eats a balanced diet, the extra 600 to 1,200 calories will add more than enough protein. Excess protein, rather than building muscle mass, will be stored as fat, and many protein sources such as meats, cheeses, and peanut butter are high in fat, as well.

Vitamins and minerals. Athletes do not need special vitamin and mineral supplements to give them a competitive edge. A balanced diet will generally provide what is needed, with the possible exceptions of iron and calcium.

Iron deficiency is often a problem for girls and boys experiencing the growth spurt and not consuming adequate amounts of iron. It can lead to loss of strength and endurance and cause the athlete to tire easily. Because it may be difficult to consume adequate amounts of iron in food sources alone, a low-dose iron supplement may be necessary.

For girls and women who exercise strenuously, weight loss and thinness may go along with menstrual dysfunction: Some 20 percent have irregular periods or none at all. Athletes who do not menstruate should discuss calcium supplementation with their physicians. Recently, osteoporosis, the bone-loss disorder usually thought of as affecting postmenopausal women, has been implicated in bone problems (curvature of the spine and fractures of the bones in the foot) in young professional dancers. These young women typically began their periods very late and thereafter menstruated infrequently. Although exercise normally strengthens the bones, it does not seem to offset the lack of estrogen. Here again, calcium supplementation, after consulting with a physician, may help offset bone loss of calcium due to estrogen levels.

Fluids. When heavy exercise in hot weather causes profuse sweating, body stores of sodium and potassium may be depleted. Usually, it is not so much the loss of electrolytes but the dehydration that gives athletes problems. When exercising, dehydration often starts before the desire to drink becomes apparent. Therefore, it is important to keep well hydrated by drinking adequate water during training and athletic events.

Weight. Low levels of body fat are desirable for optimal performance in many sports such as dance, gymnastics, and long-distance running. Lower-than-average levels of body fat are desirable for cycling, swimming, skiing, and track. Hormonal changes in adolescent girls result in the accumulation of body fat and this is in opposition to the desire to attain a leaner body mass. This almost unattainable goal leads many young female athletes to skimp excessively on calories—especially during the competition season—in an effort to keep their weight down and improve their performances. It is safe to reduce fat to about 5 to 7 percent of body weight, but less than that results in the loss of lean muscle tissue— the last thing an athlete wants—and compromised growth and development. After the season is over, the athlete may gain considerable weight (sometimes as much as 20 pounds), only to lose it again the following year in another bout of drastic calorie restriction. The added nutrients consumed in the process of gaining weight in the off-season do not make up for the nutrient deprivation during the peak athletic season. Optimal nutrients need to be consumed on a regular basis, not just sporadically.

In wrestling and some other sports, a lower weight classification may give an athlete an advantage. Before a competition, athletes sometimes restrict their water intake, induce sweating, or go on a fast to achieve a quick weight loss. These drastic methods may produce a transient reduction in weight, but they also bring dehydration and electrolyte imbalance and a performance that is less than optimal, and this should be avoided.

Weight gain. Weight and strength are important considerations in basketball, football, hockey, and heavyweight crew. High school athletes, often with the encouragement of their coaches or in imitation of older players, may try to take a shortcut to greater weight by using special diets, protein supplements, or steroid drugs. However, increased weight is an advantage only when it comes from an increase in muscle mass; increased fatness merely slows an athlete down and makes the individual more susceptible to injuries. In addition, increased muscle size and strength come only from months of weight training, along with an appropriate addition of energy. This extra energy requirement may be met with the addition of an extra meal or large snacks each day.

With a well-planned weight-training program and the diet to complement it, male high school athletes can put on about one pound a week, *if* they have reached the stage of development at which their muscles can respond to the work and their musculoskeletal system can safely withstand the stress. Unfortunately, it is often the skinny, late-maturing boy who most wants to develop muscle and strength. However, young men grow first in height, then develop muscle mass, and finally increase in strength and endurance. The sequence of events is controlled by the hormonal changes of adolescence and correlates directly with sexual maturation. Boys simply do not have the potential for developing larger muscles until about a year after the peak of their growth spurt, at which time their testes will be nearly adult-size and genital hair will have begun to appear on the inner thigh. Coaches (and parents) tend to base their expectations on a boy's size, not on his stage of maturity. It is important that a boy not be enrolled in demanding weight-training and regulated-diet programs before his maturation is such that he can benefit from them. (See also Chapter 24.)

15

Nutrition in the Adult Years

S. Robert Levine, M.D.

■

INTRODUCTION

Of the many books and articles on diet and nutrition, most discuss adult nutrition in the context of a popular goal: for example, losing weight or excelling at sports. Much of this "pop" information is pseudoscientific gibberish, often stating a literal truth for caged rats as if it were also true for free-living humans, which it is not. The up side is presented and the down side concealed. The typical down side is that the proposed "nutrition" regimen has never been shown in humans to be both effective and safe. Few popular books provide balanced information based on responsible evidence regarding desirable nutrition for the healthy adult, which is the goal of this text. Overall, popular advice to the public is varied, often contradictory or confusing, sometimes inappropriate, and occasionally downright dangerous. In the past, the medical profession tended to look at the minority of the population who were overtly ill and ask how and why they got that way, and to focus more on disease treatment rather than health promotion and disease prevention. However, most people are "apparently healthy" even though they may harbor or have a predisposition to develop illnesses that modification of current behavior might forestall or prevent.

It is clear that a good diet, including appropriate weight control, appropriate exercise, adequate sleep, and a stable social and physical environment are all important to good health. It is not, however, entirely understood to what degree each of these factors protects against chronic diseases, or retards their progression, and whether it is possible or appropriate to study them separately when evaluating health promotion and disease prevention strategies. It is also unclear to what extent diets that have been proven beneficial for those genetically predisposed to certain disorders are helpful to those not at risk.

Adult nutrition must be discussed, therefore, in the context of healthy behaviors in general as well as with respect to environmental influences. Nutrition is inextricably linked with emotional and physical health; exercise; sleep; alcohol and drug use; economic, social, and marital status; cultural background; level of education; and type of employment.

This chapter will review healthful behaviors—which are popularly called "health enhancing"—and discuss the eating patterns and nutritional needs of adults, as well as highlight the most common nutrition problem of adulthood: overweight. We will emphasize the "how-to's" of a healthy eating style, appropriate physical activity, and effective emotional stress management. In addition, we will suggest some strategies for overcoming common environmental obstacles to practicing healthful behaviors.

HEALTHFUL BEHAVIORS

Americans increasingly recognize that factors such as cigarette use, excess weight, lack of exercise, high blood cholesterol, poor emotional stress management, alcohol and drug use/abuse, and untreated high blood pressure constitute serious threats to their well-being. Although there is a genetic component to many of these factors, they remain, for the most part, within our control. Many of us are making appropriate changes in some of our health-threatening behaviors. Specifically, the number of smokers has declined, overconsumption of fat is down, more individuals are exercising regularly, and more people know their blood pressure and their serum cholesterol level and seek proper treatment when indicated. Nevertheless, there is still much room for improvement in the public's health awareness and in individuals' willingness to participate in their own and others' health enhancement through the practice of these healthful behaviors. Of particular concern is the current level of drug and alcohol use/abuse, particularly among children, adolescents, and young adults (see Chapter 21).

While encouraging lifestyle changes where desirable, we acknowledge that the initiation of health behavior change may not be terribly difficult, but sustaining these changes over time presents the greater challenge. As you contemplate making some of the behavioral changes recommended in this and other chapters, keep in mind the following points:

1. The factors involved in the initiation of a behavior change differ from those involved in maintaining it.

2. Changing a health habit consists of three stages:

    The first stage involves motivation and commitment to change and the realization that rewards are long-range rather than instantaneous. It is difficult for otherwise healthy young adults to imagine that they will eventually be old and suffer a debilitating disease as a result of current habits that presently don't make them feel bad (or even make them feel quite good). Others make compulsive decisions to change a particular behavior pattern without considering that instituting healthful habits is a lifetime commitment. This frequently results in only a short-lived commitment.

    The second stage is the actual implementation of the change itself. Mistakenly, many people focus only on this aspect of behavior change—sloughing off the need for long-term motivation and commitment, and therefore not planning for the final, most important stage of behavior change: maintenance.

    The third stage is maintenance of behavior change, which requires finding new ways to respond to old cues and cravings. It involves learning new behavioral approaches and testing their effectiveness, often by trial and error, until new health behaviors become established as normal and routine.

3. Slips or relapses are the norm. No one is capable of sustaining perfect health behavior every minute of every hour of every day. Making flawless adherence an essential goal is almost a guarantee of failure. How one deals with slips is the important

factor in the success of long-term behavior change.

4. Failed attempts to change health behavior will help highlight obstacles and possibly increase the likelihood of future successful change, and therefore will serve some purpose. However, short-lived diet or exercise regimes are probably of no help, medically. It is important, therefore, to plan for healthful behavior maintenance strategies to give yourself the best shot at long-term success (see Strategies for Health Behavior Change, page 237).

The essentials of changing health behaviors lie first in the use of positive, personal motivators, rather than fear or pressure from others—a constant bombardment of don'ts, shoulds, and have-tos can cause many to throw up their hands in despair and ignore the good as well as the bad advice; second, in the setting of modest goals and the implementation of behavior changes that recognize the highly individual and valuable nature of and need for pleasure and satisfaction—a healthy lifestyle need not be equated with deprivation; third, in the planning of strategies to deal effectively and appropriately with the inevitable slip, and therefore enhance the likelihood of long-term success; and finally, in the strength gained through acceptance of and cooperating with the unique needs of family members or significant others—getting support from them while supporting their responsible choices as well.

EATING PATTERNS IN ADULTHOOD

Some people enter adulthood with a background of prolonged overnutrition; obesity that originated in childhood is notoriously difficult to overcome. Others are chronically undernourished, lacking adequate stores of nutrients (iron and calcium are the two most common examples) they will need to be healthy throughout adulthood and into old age. If good eating habits are not established in childhood and adolescence, early adulthood is the time to make appropriate changes. Even those who are well nourished in childhood and who keep their good eating patterns in adolescence, however, will find those patterns challenged when they enter the adult years. Environmental, biological, and psychological factors directly or subtly affect the quality of the adult diet.

Adults' choices of living arrangements, whether they live alone, with friends or companions, or in a traditional family, do much to determine their eating patterns. Moreover, patterns are not static; they change along with the changing and conflicting schedules of family or group members. With marriage, two sets of eating traditions and food preferences must be blended into one menu. Educational background, cooking skills, cultural factors, and available time also have enormous influence over food choices.

Occupation has a major impact on the timing, frequency, and type of meals eaten. Income directly affects the amount and type of food that can be purchased. A job may demand frequent travel, numerous business lunches and cocktail parties, or the work schedule may be so heavy that it is hard during working hours to find time to eat at all. On the other hand, increased free time from a shortened work week tends to increase food consumption. Finally, unemployment, with its feelings of defeat and frustration, often leads to a change in eating or drinking patterns.

Physical changes in adulthood may lead to the elimination of specific foods from the diet. Many adults, for example, have a decreasing tolerance for milk; eliminating it from the diet, rather than just reducing intake quantity to tolerance levels, can lead to inadequate intake of calcium, and consequently increase the chances for developing osteoporosis in later life.

Psychological factors also have a role in determining eating patterns in adulthood. Depression, for example, is often reflected by changes in eating patterns. Emotional stress may manifest itself in the development of physical disorders such as irritable bowel syndrome and peptic ulcers, which in turn can force unchosen changes in the diet. In addition, psychological factors can lead to specific eating disorders, such as binge eating (with or without purging) and anorexia (see Chapter 19). In these cases, the amount and type of food that is eaten has less to do with physical needs than with some emotional imperative.

NUTRITIONAL NEEDS

A significant obstacle to good nutrition in adulthood is the belief that since growth has stopped, quality nutrition is no longer important. While this is obviously not true, nutritional needs do change. There is no one specific ideal diet that everyone can follow for a lifetime, but there are general rules for desirable diet to guide your diet choices (see Diet Pointers).

As adulthood progresses to middle age and later, it is associated with gradual physiological changes that ultimately result in a reduced overall energy (calorie) requirement. Starting in early adulthood, the basal metabolic rate (BMR)—the metabolic rate of the body when it's at rest—slowly drops. This is, in large part, due to a reduction in our lean body mass (muscle). Since it is our muscles that account for the bulk of our energy needs, less muscle means less need for calories.

Strategies for Change in Health Behavior

- Give careful thought to your motivation and reasons for wanting to make particular changes. Make a conscious effort to think about them every day. Consider the long- and short-term advantages and disadvantages of changing.

- Prepare for expected difficulties. Identify potential triggers for slips (i.e., an uncomfortable social engagement or physical illness). Avoid high-risk situations when possible.

- Formulate a list of coping methods that can be used when the "old urge" arises (see other boxes in this chapter).

- Don't be overly compulsive or controlled in your new habits. Go with the 80 percent rule (if you can do so honestly). For example, 20 percent of the time, allow yourself to eat taboo foods in limited quantities.

- Develop and read a list of coping self-statements for times when you experience urges to slip, or following a slip. For instance: "Just because I don't feel like jogging doesn't mean I shouldn't," or "Having that piece of cake wasn't great, but it did taste good. I'm only human, so let me just go back to eating right and have no more cake today." Practice and rehearse these types of statements, particularly while visualizing yourself in high-risk situations.

- Practice deep breathing exercises and other relaxation skills (see Tactics for Coping with Stress on page 253) when an acute craving episode occurs.

- Develop a network of people who practice healthy behaviors to serve as good models and to provide support.

The BMR deceleration is slow: 2 percent a decade after age 30. It does result in a correspondingly slow but steady reduction in the number of calories needed to maintain desired weight, however. For example: A woman of average height and weight whose overall energy need is 2,100 calories a day at age 20 will need 2,000 or fewer at age 35 and fewer than 1,800 when she is 50. If she were to ignore this biological reality and continue to eat like a 20-year-old does until she was 35 (without compensating through increased activity) she might gain up to 50 pounds over the 15-year span. For men of average height and weight, the reduction is larger, from a recommended average of 2,900 calories at age 20 to about 2,400 at age 50.

While the recommended calorie (energy) intake decreases with age, the recommended intake of most nutrients (vitamins and minerals) remains much as it was in early adulthood. (There are a few exceptions: For women, protein needs decrease slightly during adulthood and the recommended intake of iron drops after menopause.) Constant nutrient requirements in combination with reduced calorie needs mean that foods consumed must be more nutrient-dense. There is less room in the diet for large quantities of extras such as the milk shakes, triple ice cream cones, and other high-calorie foods that the young seem to eat with little effect on their waistlines. Such foods still may be enjoyed now and then, but in smaller quantities. Overall, adults must pay more attention to portion size than children and adolescents (see tables 15.1 and 15.2).

Diet Pointers

- Avoid calorie-dense, low-nutrient foods (see Table 15.1).

- Broil, steam, or bake, using small amounts of oil or margarine and seasonings such as lemon, garlic, and herbs and spices. Avoid frying and sautéing in butter.

- Include at least eight portions daily of foods high in fiber and complex carbohydrates (see Table 15.2), including four portions of fruits and vegetables, especially a variety of different colored fresh and frozen vegetables (yellows, reds, deep green leafy, etc.; raw or lightly cooked is best), and four portions of grains (breads, cereals, pastas).

- Reduce salt intake modestly. Remember, however, that when you are very active and when the weather is hot and humid you will need to consume more salt than usual.

- Keep yourself well hydrated by drinking daily eight glasses of liquids such as water, mineral water, club soda, fruit juices, lowfat milk, etc.

- Avoid alcohol. Drinking a glass of wine (4 oz.), a glass of beer (6 oz.), or single drink (1½ oz. hard liquor) occasionally (or even nightly), is almost certainly not harmful (except for pregnant women), but the physical health benefit of this practice is debatable, and regularly drinking any more than this amount has substantial negative physical, emotional, and social health consequences.

- Limit foods from the "fifth food group" (fats, sweets, alcohol).

- Use low-fat and nonfat (skimmed) dairy products when possible.

- Keep fish, poultry, and meat portion sizes modest, and trim away obvious fat.

- Include whole-grain cereals and breads.

WEIGHT CONTROL

As noted earlier, with age our lean body (muscle) mass generally decreases, and the ratio of percent body fat to lean body mass increases. Simply put, we get fatter even if we remain at the same weight. This process occurs to some degree even among people who are physically active, but it is far less pronounced than among those who are sedentary. It is important to remember that muscle burns calories and fat does not, so the fatter we are (by percentage body weight), the easier it is to get even fatter through dietary indiscretion. In addition, throughout adulthood, women tend to have a higher ratio of percentage of body fat to lean body mass than men, and with age the women's ratio increases more than men's. Thus, a woman's effort to maintain her figure, even at constant weight, may be more difficult than that of her male counterpart.

Therefore, without changes in diet and/or exercise behavior the scene is set for automatic weight gain in the adult years. This is reflected in national statistics: According to a recent National Institutes of Health survey, as well as the old 1980 census figures, some 32 million American adults are overweight, and of these, 11.7 million are obese (defined as 20 percent or more above desirable weight). Chapter 17 deals with obesity; here we will concentrate on those who are overweight but not yet obese. Overfat would be the more accurate term, since a very muscular professional athlete may weigh more than a sedentary office worker of the same age and body type and still not be fat. Muscle weighs far more than fat, so you can't always tell by total pounds alone whether a person is overfat. In this example, physical appearance will likely reveal which one is actually overweight. The athlete will look lean and fit, while the more sedentary person of the same weight will look plump and pudgy. In other circumstances, fatness can be assessed by determining the percent of body fat through underwater weighing, use of special fat calipers, or with the new simple-to-use electronic devices, and by comparing results to established

Table 15.1. Calorie-Dense Foods

Highly Sweetened Foods	High-Fat Foods
Soft drinks	Untrimmed, well marbled red meats, lunch meats, and sausage
Desserts	
Candy	
Jams and jellies	Fried foods
Alcoholic Beverages	Salad dressing and mayonnaise
All types	Butter and margarine
High-Fat and Sugar Foods	Nut butters
Pastries	Shortening, lard
Ice cream, whipped cream	Oils
Granola cereals	Most cheeses and cream

Table 15.2. Low-Calorie, High-Fiber, High-Nutrient-Value Foods

Cereals and Grains	Legumes
Shredded wheat	Peas
Wheat and corn cereals	Kidney, pinto, lima beans
Bran cereals	Lentils
Unsweetened whole-grain cereals	**Vegetables**
Whole-grain breads	Asparagus
Brown rice	Broccoli
Whole wheat pasta	Brussels sprouts
Rolled oats (oatmeal)	Cabbage
Buckwheat groats	Cauliflower
Cracked wheat	Corn
Fruits	Winter squash
	Spinach, kale, collards
Apples	Lettuce (dark green varieties)
Apricots	Carrots
Oranges, grapefruit	Potatoes
Bananas	Green beans
Berries	Bean sprouts
Peaches	Tomatoes
Kiwi fruit	Sweet peppers

norms (acceptable body fat for men is less than 15 percent; acceptable body fat for women is less than 25 percent).

Consequences of Being Overweight

Maintaining a desirable body weight/ percentage of body fat and eating a balanced diet is an essential challenge for the health-conscious adult. Failure to do either may contribute to the onset or worsening of a host of disorders. Failure to maintain desirable weight has a direct relationship to longevity: the greater the excess weight, the shorter the life expectancy.

Most of the chronic health problems that plague Western society result from an interplay of hereditary, environmental, and behavioral factors. One specific factor alone often can predispose to disease, with the other factors then bringing it out.

Overweight plays a role in bringing out all the following conditions, and in some cases, reducing to normal weight can cause the condition to recede completely:

High blood pressure (hypertension). This is often associated with weight gain and becomes less severe on losing weight. Overweight people with mild hypertension can sometimes cure their high blood pressure with weight loss alone or with a combination of weight reduction and restricted salt intake (see Chapter 26).

Changes in cardiovascular function. Such changes can result from being overweight. Heart rate increases, as does blood volume, forcing the heart to work harder to meet increased demand for oxygen. Weight loss reduces these changes. Overweight can precipitate or complicate many heart problems, thus weight loss may be an essential adjunct to medical care (see Chapter 17).

Type II diabetes. This kind occurs in adults and is strongly linked with excess weight. It appears that excessive fat tissue interferes with the body's ability to utilize insulin, and this insulin insensitivity can lead to Type II diabetes. The majority of Type II diabetics do not require insulin. Weight reduction alone frequently eliminates the need for medical treatment of Type II diabetes (see Chapter 28).

Certain cancers. Particular cancers seem to occur more frequently in the overweight. These include cancers of the prostate, breast, and uterus. The relationship is not fully understood, but it appears in part related to the altered hormonal status associated with excess fatty tissue. The stromal (supporting) tissue in body fat contains a hormone called aromatase which converts male hormones to female hormones. This may largely explain why women with more body fat have more breast cancer. Similarly, men with more body fat have more testosterone, which may explain their higher rate of progressing prostate cancer (see Chapter 27).

Achieving and Maintaining Desirable Weight

Many overweight people complain that even when they cut down on food consumption, they still fail to lose weight. Recent studies do indicate that there is a genetic basis for some types of weight problems, and that people who have inherited so-called fat genes may indeed require fewer calories than their normal-weight counterparts to sustain normal weight. However, regardless of heredity, weight problems still stem from individuals consuming more calories than their body's machinery needs or is able to expend. Being overweight often becomes self-perpetuating because when one is overweight, one is generally less physically active than those of normal weight, and, as discussed subsequently, physical activity is an essential component in the struggle to achieve and maintain ideal body weight. In addition, thanks to insulation from extra body fat, the overweight do not need to consume as much energy in order to maintain normal body temperature when the weather is cold.

To bring caloric intake and energy expenditure into balance, there are three alternatives, of which only the third is recommended:

1. *Significantly reduce the amount of food consumed.* This is the basis of modified fast programs. Done independently, severely restricted–calorie diets are dangerous. For the morbidly obese, a medically supervised program may be a first step in dealing with a life-threatening problem; however, even in this circumstance such an approach is not a long-term solution, and uniformly fails (sometimes making the problem worse) if not followed up with a less spartan approach. Fasts are not appropriate for individuals who are only 10 to 20 percent overweight, and create more problems (from gallstones to death) than they solve.

2. *Greatly increase exercise.* No practical amount of exercise can compensate for extremes of dietary indiscretion. It is a failing attitude to assume you'll be able to, as a general practice, work off excess food. Because of the realities of life's other responsibilities most people cannot commit the hours of additional

Table 15.3. Calories Used in Exercise

Moderate Activities (150 to 350)	Energy Costs calories/hour	Moderate Activities (150 to 350)	Energy Costs calories/hour
Bicycling (5 mph)	174	Golf (pulling cart)	270
(6 mph)	270	Bowling	270
(8 mph)	330	Rowboating (2½ mph)	300
Walking (1 mph)	136	Swimming (¼ mph)	300
(2 mph)	210	Badminton	350
(3 mph)	270	Horseback riding (trotting)	350
Gardening	220	Square dancing	350
Canoeing (2½ mph)	230	Volleyball	350
Golf (using power cart)	200	Roller skating	350
Light housework, cleaning, etc.	246		
Vigorous Activities (more than 350)		**Vigorous Activities (more than 350)**	
Table tennis	360	Football (touch, vigorous)	498
Bicycling (10 mph)	390	Swimming (crawl, 45 yards/minute)	522
(11 mph)	450	Aerobic dancing	546
(13 mph)	612	Racquetball	588
Walking (4 mph)	390	Skiing (10 mph)	600
(5 mph)	440	Squash and handball	600
Ice Skating (9 mph)	384	Jogging (6 mph)	654
Rollerskating (9 mph)	384	Cross-country skiing (5 mph)	690
Scrubbing floors	440	Circuit weight training	756
Basketball (recreational)	450	Scull rowing (race)	840
Tennis (recreational singles)	450	Running (5 mph)	620
Water skiing	480	(8 mph)	720
Hill climbing (100 ft. per hour)	490	(10 mph)	900

Adapted from the President's Council on Physical Fitness and Sports, Washington, D.C.

activity needed to counterbalance the excesses associated with many routinely available goodies. In addition, as you mature, there are likely to be greater limits to the intensity, duration, and frequency of exercise you perform without injury.

3. *Combine a moderate reduction in calories with a moderate increase in exercise.* This is the preferred and most successful approach to achieving and maintaining desirable or near desirable body weight. Weight lost through a program of combined calorie reduction and increased exercise is based on improvement in body composition: Fat tissue is reduced and muscle is spared or increased. Adopting some of the Diet Pointers and other tips included in this chapter is all that is generally necessary to reduce calorie intake adequately. Along with a modest increase in physical activity, such a diet should promote a weight loss of one to

Finding Your Training Heart Rate

Exercise that increases the heart rate for sustained periods of time makes the heart and skeletal muscles more efficient and has been shown among other things to lower blood pressure and blood cholesterol. Current recommendations for physical activity include being as active as possible during your daily routine and exercising at what is known as a training heart rate at least three to five times a week (five is preferred) for 30 to 60 minutes, depending on the intensity of the exercise, to improve cardiovascular fitness. Always consult your physician before beginning an exercise program, especially if you are over 35 and have not been physically active throughout adulthood, or if you are taking medications or are under treatment for any medical condition.

To find your training heart rate, subtract your age from 220, which gives you your maximum predicted heart rate (MPHR). For persons 35 or under, multiply this figure by 0.70 and 0.85 to arrive at your training heart rate range, the range or target zone to be sustained during exercise. As an example, a 35-year-old woman would have a MPHR of 185 (220-35) with a target zone of 125 to 153 beats per minute. If you're over 35, and as noted above especially if you are out of shape and have not been very active in your life, it is recommended that you multiply your MPHR by only 0.60 and 0.75 and use this lower target zone for your training until you have gained confidence and an improved level of fitness, or your doctor indicates that it is safe for you to exercise more vigorously.

To determine that you reach and don't exceed your target zone, learn how to take your own pulse. The best place is at the wrist. Either during or immediately after exercise (during cool-down), find your wrist pulse (with palm up, run three fingers down your thumb to the wrist and press lightly). Count the beats for ten seconds and multiply by six (see Table 15.4).

Important rules by which to exercise include always feeling well beforehand, preparing yourself with a proper light warmup, sustaining a level of exertion at which you feel invigorated (not exhausted) and are able to carry on reasonable conversation without gasping for breath during activity (regardless of heart rate), consuming adequate fluids throughout exercise, properly cooling down before stopping activity ("walking it off"), and resting for at least ten minutes following exercise. If you feel extreme fatigue, shortness of breath, dizziness, chest or jaw discomfort, nausea, or any other ill feelings during or immediately after exercise, it's best that you consult your doctor before continuing your exercise program.

To combine conditioning with weight loss, exercise physiologists recommend daily low-intensity exercise (walking, swimming, casual bicycling, stretching) for 40 to 60 minutes, in addition to more vigorous, preferably low-impact (cycling, race walking, cross-country skiing, rowing, low-impact aerobics, etc.) activity for 30 to 40 minutes a minimum of three times a week.

two pounds per week, the recommended level to ensure success in long-term weight control.

Any amount of increase in activity helps better balance the consumption/expenditure equation, and therefore, over the long term favors weight control. If possible, activity should be sustained, at modest or greater intensity (see Table 15.3), for 40 or more minutes. It is this length of activity, done five to seven days per week (depending on intensity), that is most effective in promoting more substantial weight loss and body reshaping (see Finding Your Training Heart Rate on page 242).

On dietary restriction, the body slows its basal metabolic rate to compensate for the reduced calorie intake, which the body perceives as starvation. Thus, increased exercise is almost mandatory to lose weight.

Exercise has many benefits in addition to burning calories. To name but a few, it keeps bones healthy; improves cardiovascular function, digestion, sleep, muscle, and skin tone; and enhances emotional well-being.

Combating the Sedentary Lifestyle

Today, approximately 55 percent of all adult Americans are considered sedentary. There are many reasons for this: labor-saving devices, the automobile, and mass transit all reduce much of the activity of normal daily life. City dwellers tend to walk more than suburbanites or those living in small towns or rural areas, but otherwise activity levels do not differ widely among groups, with the exception of those people engaged in the small number of occupations that still require intense activity.

Although technological innovation has gone a long way toward fostering a sedentary lifestyle, a significant role is also played by personal preference, often dating to child-

hood. For instance, children who do poorly in school athletics tend to grow up with an aversion to exercise. As adults, they may plead a dislike for sports, clumsiness or boredom with solitary activities such as running, and balk at undertaking a formal exercise program. Nevertheless, it is possible to get adequate exercise, often without radically changing daily patterns, even for those out of condition. For example, instead of taking the elevator all the way to your floor, get off two or three stops before and walk up, or get off the bus or subway earlier than usual and walk the last few blocks. Park the car at the far end of the supermarket lot; substitute hand tools for some of the electronically operated ones.

For those who do better with an established exercise regimen, there are a large number of suitable activities: brisk walking, bicycling, jogging, playing tennis, swimming, aerobic dancing, and using a variety of exercise machines are but a few of the more popular ones. In recent years, walking has enjoyed increasing popularity. In fact, brisk walking for at least 30 to 45 minutes at a stretch a minimum of five times a week is considered

Table 15.4. 10-Second Pulse/Heart Rate Conversion Table

10-second count	Heart Rate	10-second count	Heart Rate
8	48	21	126
9	54	22	132
10	60	23	138
11	66	24	144
12	72	25	150
13	78	26	156
14	84	27	162
15	90	28	168
16	96	29	174
17	102	30	180
18	108	31	186
19	114	32	192
20	120	33	198

by many to be the most beneficial and versatile exercise. Walking for exercise can be incorporated into almost everyone's daily routine, requires no special equipment other than appropriate shoes, rarely results in injury, and is suitable even for older adults whose health does not allow for more vigorous sports. Acknowledging the increased interest in walking, a number of shopping malls now have special early-morning hours to accommodate walkers, which is particularly useful when the weather outside is inclement.

For those who enjoy exercising with others, there are now many exercise clubs and organized programs, ranging from fancy exercise parlors for the rich and famous to more modest offerings at the local Y, church or synagogue, senior citizen center, and adult education programs, among others. There are so many, in fact, that almost everyone can find a program that suits his or her interests and needs.

The type of physical activity selected is not as important as making it a routine part of your day. To achieve the desired results, a person should be as active as possible while meeting his or her daily obligations (climbing stairs, walking, standing at your desk, etc.) and should exercise more vigorously at least three to five times a week.

RISKY BEHAVIORS AND CIRCUMSTANCES

There are many habits or situations that work against good nutrition, usually by creating conditions conducive to overeating. Among the most common are skipping breakfast, eating alone, eating while working, snacking, and dining out (including traveling). Learning to change, control, or compensate for these behaviors can go a long way toward remedying the chief problem in this country, overeating.

Skipping Breakfast

After eight to twelve hours without food, the body needs refueling. Most people agree with this reasoning but many fail to act on it. Some people say they don't feel like eating early in the morning, or that they enjoy a leisurely breakfast on the weekend but haven't time on weekdays. Others avoid breakfast because they dislike the traditional breakfast choices. Still others would rather save the calories for another meal or eliminate them entirely.

Of the time-honored adages regarding food and eating habits, perhaps the wisest is, Eat breakfast like a king, lunch like a prince, and dinner like a pauper. For those who can and will, eating a sit-down breakfast at home is the best way to take in nutrient-rich foods and provide sufficient energy for the entire morning without need for additional boosts from snacks or caffeine.

Many people leave the house in the morning thinking they'll get breakfast at some later point. However, this usually goes awry; people who do not eat before starting their daily activities are likely to miss breakfast altogether. Unanticipated events, transportation snags, an unexpected phone call or an unscheduled meeting can cancel out the postponed meal. However, even those under time pressures can prepare and eat a nutritious, if untraditional, breakfast in less than ten minutes (see Breakfast Suggestions on page 245).

Some avoid breakfast in the mistaken notion that they are saving calories. By skipping breakfast, however, a person is likely to be so hungry come midmorning that he or she will gorge on candy, doughnuts, pastries, or other typical offerings from the office coffee wagon or from whatever is in the refrigerator. As a general rule, those who skip breakfast for whatever reason more than make up for the omitted calories through mid-morning high-calorie snacks or overly generous meals later in the day.

Breakfast Suggestions

For most of us, breakfast means cereal, milk, juice or fruit, toast, and an egg about two to three times per week (egg whites can be used more often; it's the yolk that contains fat and cholesterol). These are time-honored, perfectly acceptable ways to start the day. For those who want something a bit more interesting and varied, however, breakfasts are limited only by your imagination. Here are a few suggestions.

- *Consider making breakfast the day's main meal.* By reversing your normal schedule and leaving time enough to prepare and eat a full evening-type meal in the morning (for example, a piece of fish or chicken, rice and a vegetable or pasta with a sauce and salad) you would be provided with both wholesome nutrients and energy for a full morning. In this regimen, you would have a regular lunch and a light supper instead of the usual full dinner.

- *Save leftovers from a previous dinner for breakfast.* If there isn't time to cook in the morning, substitute with a leftover chicken sandwich and a glass of tomato juice, a dish of pasta and an orange, or a low-fat peanut butter sandwich stuffed with sliced apple.

- *Make a breakfast shake.* If you haven't the time or appetite for a full meal at breakfast, try making a nutritious all-in-one blender shake. Using low-fat or nonfat milk, yogurt, or fruit juice as a base, add berries, melon, or other fresh fruits to provide a meal in a glass. When the salmonella scare is over, we can go back to also tossing in a raw egg for a good old-fashioned eggnog.

- *Prepare hot cereal overnight.* Measure the dry cereal (quick-cooking oats, wheat, etc.) into a preheated wide-mouth thermos. Add the boiling water or hot skim milk and close tightly. The cereal will be fully cooked and piping hot in the morning. For a different taste, garnish with fresh sliced peaches, berries, or other fruit and a sprinkling of cinnamon.

- *For a different hot breakfast, try a bowl of soup or stew.* The soup can be left over or made quickly by using an envelope of instant broth mix (use the low-sodium kind if you're watching your salt intake) and leftover diced vegetables, noodles, or pasta. Always skim the fat off the top of refrigerated leftover soups *before* reheating.

- *Make a breakfast salad.* Fill half a cantaloupe with low-fat cottage cheese, ice milk, berries, or crunchy cereal mixed with low or nonfat yogurt for a filling yet low-calorie meal.

- *Try a breakfast sandwich.* Keep a variety of whole-grain breads in the freezer and have pumpernickel one day, wheat another, and so forth. Instead of margarine and jelly, top the toasted slice with Muenster or farmer's cheese mixed with dried fruit, or a spread made with salmon, chives, and a teaspoon of reduced-calorie French dressing.

- *Plan ahead to allow more time for eating and less for preparation.* Set the table the night before. Make extra pancakes or French toast on the weekend and freeze the leftovers for quick toasting during the week.

- NOTE: Traditional large breakfasts of eggs and a meat such as sausage or bacon can be reduced in fat and calories by substituting Canadian bacon, fish, chicken, or turkey for the meat, making scrambled eggs with half the yolks, and using vegetable cooking spray instead of butter. Remember, if you do have a big breakfast, reduce calories at lunch and dinner proportionally.

Eating Alone

In virtually every society, mealtimes are also social gatherings of family members, friends, colleagues, and others. But there are indications that this is changing and large numbers of us are increasingly likely to eat many meals alone. For most, however, this is more often due to circumstance or necessity rather than preference.

Family members with busy schedules often eat apart and on the run, a practice that can lead to eating without sitting down, eating too fast, or consuming only those items that can be eaten as is or, at the most, warmed up. Single people who work may find it easier to eat out or to pick up prepared food than to cook; frequently, they rely on snack items as a substitute for a meal, and thus reduce the variety of foods eaten.

Tips for Eating Alone

- Make frequent trips to the supermarket, buying small amounts each time. The smaller quantities are more likely to stay fresh. The additional trips also provide an opportunity for socializing.

- If finances permit, patronize specialty shops rather than supermarkets. Although buying a single fish fillet at the fish market or two apples and a half-pound of green beans at a fruit and vegetable store may cost more than at a supermarket, the reduced waste makes up for the initial expense.

- Put together a healthful meal at one of the salad bars that have become increasingly popular in supermarkets and fruit markets. Avoid selections that look as if they are prepared with large amounts of oil or mayonnaise, choosing instead steamed or raw vegetables, legumes, or grains.

- Make ordering out more heart-healthy by specifying toppings of vegetables (broccoli, pepper, mushrooms, etc.) instead of sausage or ground beef on a pizza, and steamed or lightly stir-fried rather than sweet-and-sour or fried Chinese food.

- Double recipes and freeze the extra servings to use over the next few months in varying combinations.

- With commercially prepared frozen foods, select a baked or broiled entrée. Entire frozen meals often include high-calorie side dishes. You can put together the meal yourself by adding a salad or vegetables.

- Take the time to set the table. When dining on take-out foods or frozen dinners, transfer them to dinnerware for a more appetizing and leisurely meal.

- Try for variety not only in the food, but the setting. Make mealtimes leisurely, not hurried. If you can, use your dining room (rather than kitchen counter, bar, or breakfast table), or eat on the terrace or in your backyard. If you have only limited space, spread a tablecloth on the living room floor or on a coffee table; challenge habits of convenience.

- Try to avoid reading or watching television while eating. If you can't, prepare a tray beforehand with the appropriate amounts of food in order to prevent overeating while you are distracted with another activity. Avoid rushing through the meal.

- Invite two or three friends over for a potluck dinner on a regular basis. This breaks the monotony of dining alone and offers the chance to sample others' cooking.

- If eating out is required or preferred, become a regular at at least one restaurant. The kitchen will then be more likely and willing to prepare food as you request, for example, steaming vegetables and broiling entrées with a little olive oil and garlic instead of butter. Getting to know waiters and waitresses, as well as the other regulars, also makes for a more social meal.

Those who live alone and stay or work at home, especially widows and widowers, may have the greatest difficulties of all. Eating alone is a reminder of lost companionship. What's more, many foods come in family-size quantities, and cooking for one means eating the same food for several meals, dividing and freezing for future use, throwing away spoiled produce, stale bread, and so forth. (This is changing somewhat as manufacturers respond to the increase in solo dining by providing single-portion entrées.) Eating out alone is an unattractive prospect for most of us, but particularly for older women for whom dining out has generally been a social occasion.

In spite of the potential problems, dining alone need not lead to poor nutrition. For ways to enhance the meal, avoid the pitfalls, and assure good nutrition, see Tips for Eating Alone, page 246. For older people, see Chapter 16.

Eating While Working

Eating while on the job has become another very common practice. Too much work, deadline pressures, the need to prove one's dedication or the importance of one's work are a few of the reasons. Lunch may be ordered from a delicatessen, fast-food restaurant, or the mobile canteen that is now standard in many larger office buildings. Even workers who take their own lunch often end up eating at their desks, especially if there is no communal lunchroom. Since they are at their desks, work continues. Such desktop meals are typically hurried, interrupted, or consumed under stress, conditions that can lead to indigestion as well as inadequate nutrition.

The at-home equivalent of eating at the desk is eating at the kitchen counter; here, in addition to eating too fast, there is an added danger of overeating because of the easy access to large amounts of food. Since it takes about 20 minutes for the brain to register satiety, it is easy to overeat when rapidly gulping down food. The work/lunch pattern, whether in the home or the office, is one behavior that can usually be changed by simply deciding to do so (see Breaking the Work/Lunch Habit, below).

Breaking the Work/Lunch Habit

- If you take lunch from home, take a 20-minute walk (at a relaxed pace) before eating to provide a break in the schedule. This will help relieve tension, aid in digestion, and burn up some calories. In bad weather, alternatives to walking outside can include walking through the corridors or climbing stairs rather than taking the elevator.

- Try eating lunch out rather than working through the hour. You don't need to go to an expensive restaurant, a simple lunch room or salad bar will do fine. Studies have shown that those who stop working and take a true lunch are more efficient and productive than those who combine lunch and work. Formally sitting down to eat often means that the meal will be better digested than if eaten while in the midst of another activity.

- Plan more vigorous exercise during your lunch break. Start by simply having something to drink (water, fruit juice) and a fruit (orange, peach, plum, banana) before your activity. Follow exercise with a ten-minute rest and a light meal (green salad, fruit, whole-grain bread, nonfat yogurt, etc.)

- Those who have the habit of eating while standing at the kitchen counter or other worksite should try to prepare a tray and sit down somewhere away from the kitchen and the project at hand. This limits the food available and puts work out of sight for the moment.

Snacking

According to the teachings of our mothers or grandmothers, we all should eat three square meals a day and nothing in between. In reality, most people do at least some between-meal eating. Snacking has gotten a bad reputation and is often associated with junk food and poor weight control. While it is certainly true that snacking on candy, cookies, potato chips, nuts, and other high-calorie foods in addition to eating two or three full meals can result in weight gain for most people, judicious between-meal snacks can actually be part of an effective weight-loss program. Properly timed, snacking can prevent overeating at regular or postponed meals, resulting in fewer total calories. Although

---

Sensible Snacking

Snacking in itself is not harmful. Even an occasional high-calorie, relatively low-nutrient snack such as an ice cream cone or a cookie is acceptable, provided the day's nutrient needs have been met and the calories are within the day's limits. By and large, however, eating healthful snacks that are an integral part of the daily diet is the wisest policy. Here are some tips on snacks and snacking.

- Designate a part of a meal, such as a glass of juice, a salad, or a piece of fruit, to be eaten later as a snack.

- Choose snacks that fulfill part of your nutritional needs rather than empty-calorie foods: Select a beverage with a base of low- or nonfat milk instead of a soda, a bran muffin instead of a doughnut, carrot sticks in place of potato chips.

- Vary fruit snacks by wrapping ripe bananas in foil and freezing. Frozen seedless grapes or berries also are good snacks. A blenderized frozen banana is as creamy and satisfying as a dish of ice cream, with no added sugar or fat. (Make sure you have a heavy-duty blender or food processor and secure the lid for safety).

- Reduce calories by making your own flavored yogurt. Start with plain nonfat yogurt and add a favorite chopped fruit, a few spoons of a crunchy cereal, vanilla extract, cinnamon, or other flavorings.

- At work, keep snack foods in the office refrigerator rather than in a desk drawer so that they will be a little less accessible. Acknowledge that there are times when you will feel hungry, and keep a supply of healthful snacks on hand to avoid being tempted by the vending machine or coffee cart.

- To cut down on excess snacking at home, plan in advance the time and type of snack for the evening. Then take time out from your other activities and savor your snack; appreciate it. This is safer than having a bowl of nuts, chocolate, chips, or what have you within reach while reading or watching TV. Easy access and distraction make automatic, even unconscious, excess snacking the rule.

- Since a high percentage of snacks include both food and drink, be sure that the beverages are either low-calorie, such as tea or club soda, or nutritious, such as a fruit or vegetable juice or low-fat milk.

- Never eat from the original container or bag. Snack food placed on a plate rather than hidden in wrapping looks bulkier; this helps cut the risk of eating a whole package.

- Unbuttered air-popped popcorn at only 23 calories a cup makes a filling, high-fiber snack and takes a long time to eat. For those who can't avoid snacking while watching television, this is one of the few relatively safe items.

- Follow a basic behavior-modification technique: Never eat while moving. The amount of food eaten unconsciously while focusing on riding or driving in a car, for example, can add up dramatically.

many convenience snacks, for example vending machine selections, are high in calories and low in nutrients, there are numerous alternatives for those willing to exercise some forethought and imagination. In fact, the recent trend to "grazing," i.e., six or seven mini-meals a day instead of three maxi-meals, has led to several studies suggesting that sensible grazing is a healthy alternative to three square meals a day (see Sensible Snacking, page 248).

Traveling

Traveling usually means eating out three times a day, often alone and sometimes in different time zones. The usual problems associated with dining out tend to be compounded by fatigue, unfamiliarity with the restaurant, and either the necessity of eating alone or the requirement of entertaining business associates or being entertained (see Tips for Travelers, below, and also Chapter 39).

WORK-SITE WELLNESS PROGRAMS

In recent years, increasing numbers of business and industry organizations have started programs in the workplace designed to improve employees' health and wellness. Millions of workers and their families are now involved in a range of health-oriented activities: classes in weight control, nutrition, and stress management; efforts to quit smok-

Tips for Travelers

- Don't settle for the usual airline food. Most airlines offer a large variety of special meals, available by calling the company at least 24 hours before departure. Choices include meals for the diabetic, vegetarian, or individual on a low-sodium or low-calorie diet.

- Don't skip lunch and make supper a huge meal, as many travelers do. Also, many of the better restaurants offer the same food for lunch as for dinner, but at substantially lower prices.

- When dining out, select restaurants that offer a large variety and are more likely to include nutritious low-calorie choices (see Chapter 39). If necessary, ask whether the kitchen will prepare a dish with a small amount of olive oil rather than butter, skim or low-fat milk rather than whole, and so forth. Make note of restaurants that fulfill these criteria for future reference. When one city is a regular stop, it is worth the time to do some research. Ask hotel personnel, clients, or other guests for recommendations and read restaurant menus when walking around the hotel neighborhood.

- When you are a guest, either in a restaurant or someone's home, remember there is *no* insult in steering clear of alcohol or food offerings that you would not ordinarily select for yourself. A true friend will not take offense at your desire to preserve your health and may even benefit by your example. If the circumstances of choice are completely out of your control, relax, eat smaller portions, and "fake it" like you did when you were a child and got more food than you wanted—spread it around the plate.

- Don't forget about exercise. Walking briskly, using the stairs instead of the elevator, and swimming in the hotel's pool all help burn calories, aid in assuring restful sleep, and give you an opportunity to release some of the pressures of the day that might otherwise contribute to excess eating and drinking.

ing and deal with drug abuse and alcoholism; counseling for family problems; screening for cancer and cardiovascular disease, among others. Some companies claim that decreased incidence of absenteeism, sickness, and accidents have resulted from these programs and saved them millions of dollars.

Classes in nutrition (usually coupled with weight control) typically cover such topics as vitamins and minerals, the role of dietary fiber, the body's requirements for fat and protein, food labeling, and the importance of exercise. The need for such employee programs is evident: Some 40 percent of all employees are estimated to be overweight and 70 percent practice poor nutritional habits, at least at work. However, things appear to be changing and the concern with good nutrition is increasingly reflected in the food offered and the food choices made in company cafeterias, executive dining rooms, mobile canteens, and vending machines.

EMOTIONAL STRESS, NUTRITION, AND HEALTH

Emotional stress is omnipresent in our lives. Emotional stress, or "stress" for short, defined as bodily or mental tension, actually is an essential element in human existence, and it often goes unnoticed unless it is increased significantly above usual "background" levels. It is distinct from physical stress, i.e., the stress from an athletic endeavor, with which it is often confused. Stress may result from unpleasant events, such as the death of a relative or a job loss, or pleasant ones, such as marriage or the birth of a baby. Besides the actual event, how much control the individual feels he or she has over the situation plays an important part: Those who feel helpless experience more stress, often accompanied by

depression, than those who feel they have some control of the situation. However, whether we deem the source of the stress good or bad, our behavioral and physiological responses to stress are essentially the same.

Behavioral Response

The most typical and apparent short-term effect of stress upon nutrition is a disruption in eating behavior. During periods of stress, people often skip meals, consume high-calorie/low-nutrient snacks, and increase their intake of coffee (or other sources of caffeine) and/or intake of alcohol or other mood-altering substances such as nicotine from tobacco. Depending upon the individual response to anxiety, overeating or loss of appetite may result. For the well-nourished, well-rested, well-adjusted person, an occasional period of such stress-induced behavior will have no harmful long-term effects. In general, as soon as tension is decreased, the well-adjusted individual regains a feeling of control and returns to previous healthful habits. Of course, the situation is different for people who experience persistent, stressful situations where unhealthful patterns become habitual.

Physiological Response

The physiological response to stressful situations, in particular, novel ones, and those over which we have no control, has a more subtle effect on overall nutritional status and the way in which the body utilizes specific nutrients.

In response to a perceived threat (classically physical but in the modern era equally likely psychological), a variety of neural (nervous system) and biochemical (hormonal) reactions occur to prepare us to cope better.

The hypothalamus (the brain's relay station) releases a hormone called CRF. CRF, in turn, triggers both sympathetic nervous system and pituitary gland responses.

The sympathetic nervous system prepares us for this so-called fight-flight reaction by stimulating the release of epinephrine (adrenaline) and norepinephrine (noradrenaline) from the adrenal glands. These stress hormones cause the heart rate to speed up, the blood pressure to increase, and the rate and depth of breathing to increase in order to help the heart and lungs to deliver more nutrients and oxygen to the working muscles. At the same time, blood is diverted from the digestive system, thus favoring support of the muscles needed for fleeing or fighting, but limiting nutrient absorption capacity. Norepinephrine also increases the stickiness of blood and can assist in causing arteries to spasm in order to cause clotting and prevent excessive bleeding in the event of injury.

The pituitary gland, in response to CRF, releases its own hormone, ACTH (adrenocorticotrophic hormone). ACTH stimulates another area of the adrenal gland, which, in turn, releases a different stress hormone, cortisol. Cortisol, through a series of mechanisms including breakdown of muscle and other vital body proteins, increases the level and availability of glucose (blood sugar) in order to provide energy (fuel) for the working muscle, brain, and heart.

Health Consequences of Chronic Stress

The "fight or flight" reaction evolved as a response to the physically dangerous environment of early humans. The changes were temporary, as were the challenges. With the conflict resolved (either the challenge was met and one survived or it wasn't and one didn't), bodily functions essentially returned to normal.

As noted above, however, in the modern era our stresses are more likely psychological and the challenges to our sense of well-being and conflicts regarding day-to-day life, relationships, work, money, and the like, are numerous, often persistent, and without easy or simply defined resolution. There is, therefore, growing concern over the long-term health consequences of repeated stress and/or poor techniques of coping with it.

Studies link stress with an increased risk of high blood pressure, elevated blood cholesterol, stroke, heart attacks and sudden death, immune-system dysfunction and therefore susceptibility to infection and autoimmune diseases, certain cancers, diabetes, some stomach and intestinal disorders, the "chronic fatigue syndrome" (which usually turns out to be a form of depression, but is sometimes organic), muscle and joint problems (in particular, low back syndrome), and other chronic medical problems. The precise roles or exact biological mechanisms by which stress contributes to these problems are yet to be fully identified. Enough is known, however, to encourage most individuals to seek appropriate psychological and/or family counseling and learn and practice stress-management/reduction techniques (see Tactics for Coping with Stress on page 253). These techniques include abdominal breathing, deep relaxation, self-hypnosis, and biofeedback, and adoption of a more physically active lifestyle, free of alcohol, tobacco, and drug use, and the extremes of dietary indiscretion, with enough activity to keep one from ruminating on things one can't control.

Stress and Nutrient Requirements

Physical stress resulting from trauma, surgery, a severe burn, prolonged fever, serious infection, extremes of temperature, poor air quality, and even exercise variably increases the need for calories, fluids, salt, and a variety of nutrients.

Deficiencies of certain B vitamins (B_6, B_{12}, thiamine) can produce depression, confusion, and other mental disorders, but such deficiencies have no connection to the psychological tensions that make up much of modern-day stress, which has no effect on our nutritional needs, including need for so-called stress vitamins. In fact, the New York State Attorney General recently forced a major seller to stop advertising that vitamins help overcome emotional stress.

Maintaining a varied diet and appropriate calorie intake (described in Chapter 1) will generally provide all of the dietary vitamins and other nutrients needed to help see a person through a psychologically stressful period.

Overall, it appears that healthy people can withstand short periods of severe stress quite well. Prolonged stress, however, can compromise health by contributing to the onset and/or worsening of many diseases. Through proper diet, a balance of exercise and rest, and the practice of effective coping skills one can substantially reduce the deleterious effects of stress on health.

The 1988 U.S. Surgeon General's *Report on Nutrition and Health*, the 1989 U.S. National Research Council's *Diet and Health*, and the U.S. Government's 1990 *Dietary Guidelines for Americans* all agree that consumption of vitamins, minerals, and other supplements is not a necessary part of a healthy adult's diet (except for some pregnant women, and elderly people who are eating little food).

SUMMING UP

The routine practice of healthful behaviors such as eating regular balanced meals, getting adequate exercise, getting enough sleep (at least seven hours a night for most people), and employing effective coping strategies cannot guarantee perfect health. They are, however, our best bets in slowing the gradual deterioration of a number of physiological functions that occur with aging, and slowing development and progression of many chronic or degenerative diseases. Indeed, they make possible many of the better things in life: greater energy, higher productivity, fewer illnesses, and an overall sense of well-being. That seems a fair enough bargain for the investment in time and energy required to learn about our bodies and to pay attention to the basics of good nutrition throughout the adult years. For peace of mind, many find useful the silent prayer: Grant me *serenity* to accept the things I cannot change/*Courage* to change the things I can/And *wisdom* to know the difference.

RESOURCES

For more information on nutrition resources, menus, recipes, and nutrient information, see the following:

Books

Brody, Jane. *Jane Brody's Good Food Book.* New York: Bantam, 1987.

Brown M. L. (ed). *Present Knowledge in Nutrition.* Washington, D.C.: International Life Sciences Institute, 1990.

Brownell, Kelly. *LEARN Program for Weight Control* (available through Dr. Kelly D. Brownell, Dept. of Psychiatry, University of PA, 133 S. 36th St., Phila. PA 19104-3246).

Debakey, Michael, et al. *The Living Heart Diet.* New York: Simon and Schuster, 1987.

Editors of Consumer Reports Books. *The New Medicine Show.* Consumers Union, 1989.
Katch, Frank I., and McArdle, William D. *Nutrition, Weight Control, Exercise.* Second edition. Philadelphia: Lea and Febiger, 1988.

Tactics for Coping with Stress

Studies show that those who are unable to express their emotions are at greatest risk of stress-related disorders. The following steps promote constructive emotional expression and ways of minimizing daily stresses. They should in no way be considered a substitute for appropriate psychiatric, psychological, or family counseling to help deal with situations in which depression is a significant factor.

- Learn to bring out into the open hidden or suppressed feelings of anger. For example, a headache that almost immediately follows an event may be a sign of suppressed anger.

- Try to deal with anger as soon as possible by helping the person involved understand why and when you feel angry.

- If the anger stems from a situation or person who cannot be confronted, or is out of your control, try to acknowledge this fact. You might try to blow off steam through physical activity. Exercise is one of the best stress reducers, whether the cause is anger, frustration, anxiety, or another emotion. In addition to sports, physical activity such as gardening, dancing, or even cleaning the house may also help diffuse negative emotions.

- Recognize other manifestations of stress, particularly those which may suggest significant depression—insomnia, irritability, nervous eating or skipping meals, withdrawal from friends, loss of interest in sex. If the source of the stress is difficult to define, or seemingly overwhelming, get help; share your concerns, feelings, and anxieties with your spouse, family, a close friend, clergy, or family or psychiatric counselor, if necessary. Sharing feelings allows for ventilation, better perspective, and reassurance. Sharing enlarges the spirit, whereas withholding feelings and internalizing serves only to isolate and thereby magnify the impact of the problem beyond reasonable bounds.

- Avoid particularly exasperating situations: If long lines produce stress, choose nonrush periods, or transact business by mail or telephone.

- Some like to learn a relaxation technique such as yoga, meditation, biofeedback, relaxation exercises, or deep breathing. Taking a warm bath, reading a good book, listening to music, or going for a massage can also be relaxing. Use what works best for *you* as a daily stress-reducing strategy.

- Avoid becoming upset over events that you cannot change and, instead, focus efforts on those within your control. Be honest about acknowledging the difference. As the late Reinhold Niebuhr so aptly put it: "God grant us grace to accept with serenity the things that cannot be changed, courage to change the things which should be changed, and the wisdom to distinguish the one from the other."

- Finding the humor in events or your reaction to them (when possible) is a very effective tension releaser.

- Learn to recognize and modify, if possible, attitudes that may promote stress, for example, extreme perfectionism, preoccupation with time, sensitivity to criticism, and lack of flexibility, among others. Have faith and confidence in yourself without relying on external factors such as material success, good looks, and status to determine your self-worth.

- Remember, get professional counseling if other methods are ineffective in coping with stress.

Kavanagh, Terence. *The Healthy Heart Program*. Toronto: University of Toronto Press, 1987.

Metropolitan Life Insurance Company. *Eat Well Be Well Cookbook*. New York: Simon and Schuster, 1986.

Committee on Diet and Health, National Research Counsel. *Diet and Health: Implications for Reducing Chronic Disease Risk*. National Academy Press, 1989.

Report of the Dietary Guidelines Advisory Committee on the Dietary Guidelines for Americans, 1990. U.S. Department of Agriculture and U.S. Department of Health and Human Services.

Shepard, R. J. *Fitness and Health in Industry*. Farmington, Connecticut: S. Karger, 1986.

Stare, F. J., Olson, R. E., and Whelan, E. M. *Balanced Nutrition*. Bob Adams Inc., 1989.

The Surgeon General's Report on Nutrition and Health. U.S. Department of Health and Human Services, 1988.

Organizations

The Walking Association
P.O. Box 37228
Tucson, AZ 85740
1-602-742-9589
Coordinates small walking clubs, publishes a quarterly newsletter, plus guides and manuals.

Walkways Center
733 15th Street, N.W., Suite 427
Washington, D.C. 20005
1-202-737-9555
Provides information on organized walking activities, competitions, products, and trends.

For information on stress control, see the following:

Benson, Herbert, and Klipper, Miriam Z. *The Relaxation Response*. New York: Avon, 1976.

Brownell, K. D., and Rodin, J. *The Weight Maintenance Survival Guide*. Dallas: Brownell and Hager Publishers, 1990.

16

Nutrition and the Elderly

David T. Lowenthal, M.D., Ph.D.

■

INTRODUCTION

Today, over 26 million Americans are 65 or older, placing the percentage of people in this age bracket at an all-time high (11 percent). By the year 2030, it is projected that 30 percent of all Americans—more than 33 million people—will be over 65. Moreover, the elderly are getting older and boundaries are shifting. For example, the typical 65-year-old of today is considered to be in the upper range of middle age, rather than elderly. Increasingly, people are putting off retirement until their seventies, and it's not uncommon for people in this age range to start new businesses or careers. The numbers of the so-called old-old also are growing, as reflected by the fact that the over-75 segment is increasing at a faster rate than the elderly population as a whole.

NUTRIENT NEEDS OF THE ELDERLY

There is a fairly good amount of solid knowledge about the nutrient needs of the elderly, as these are affected by age-related phys-

iological and lifestyle changes. Evidence is accumulating that the elderly may have unique requirements for certain nutrients. For example, some experts feel that the current RDA for calcium (800 milligrams) should be increased to 1,000 to 1,500 milligrams to achieve calcium balance and good skeletal health in older people. (See below for general recommendations.)

Calories

With age, lean body mass (muscle and bone) decreases, while the proportion of fat increases. (The weight may stay the same, but the composition of that weight is different.) With a larger proportion of fat, and with the decrease in activity typical of the aging, the body needs fewer calories. Daily calorie needs drop by about 10 percent each decade after age 50, but there does not appear to be any significant decrease in the need for other nutrients. Thus, foods must be chosen for their nutrition density since there is no room in a calorie-restricted diet for empty calories. Many older people spontaneously lower their calorie intake, but even so, fat may accumulate.

Some elderly people overeat as a way of

255

coping with loneliness and feelings of helplessness. Such people are often both overweight and undernourished, since comforting foods such as cake and candy are high in calories but not in nutrients. Overweight puts the elderly at special risk for adult-onset diabetes and cardiovascular disease, and may be an indirect cause of falls. Moderate overweight, however, is not a proven risk factor.

According to some gerontologists, a modest weight increase in middle age, continued into the later years, is associated with the lowest death rates. On the other hand, animal studies show that a severely calorie-restricted diet results in longer life in caged animals.

Desirable body weight is far more variable among the diverse elderly population than it is among younger people. The rule of thumb in younger people (for men: 106 pounds for the first 60 inches, plus 6 pounds for each additional inch; for women: 100 pounds for the first 60 inches, plus 5 pounds for each additional inch) may be applicable

Dietary Recommendations

As is the case with all other age groups, the elderly are best served by a varied diet drawn from the four basic food groups. The National Institute on Aging advises that a daily diet for elderly people should include:

- At least two servings of milk (or dairy products low in lactose, such as aged hard cheeses and yogurt)
- Two servings of high-protein foods (lean meat, poultry, fish, eggs, legumes, nuts, peanut butter)
- Four servings of fruit and vegetables, which should include a citrus fruit (or juice) and a dark green leafy vegetable
- Four servings of bread or cereal products, whole-grain or enriched

for a vigorous elderly person who has kept a relatively high percentage of lean body mass. For a more sedentary person with a higher percentage of fat, however, the calculation produces too heavy a weight. Daily calorie intake for a moderately active elderly man or woman who is neither obese nor malnourished should be in the range of 10 to 14 calories per pound (for someone of 150 pounds, 1,500 to 2,100 calories).

Protein

Protein needs remain steady (about one-third gram daily per pound of body weight). Eleven to 12 percent of the total caloric intake should be from protein.

Difficulties in chewing, a limited food budget, and digestive problems may provide obstacles to adequate protein intake. Protein can be supplied by soups, small portions of lean meat or fish, eggs, cottage cheese, and vegetable proteins. (Supplements of amino acids such as cysteine and glycine do nothing to protect from aging or disease.)

Carbohydrates

Carbohydrates are easily digested and contain valuable fiber and nutrients. Whole-grain breads, cereals, enriched pasta, green and root vegetables are all good choices. Carbohydrates should supply 55 to 60 percent of daily calories.

Fats

As for younger adults, generally no more than 30 percent of total daily calories should come from fats, although the danger of atherosclerosis, linked to cholesterol-rich foods and a high fat intake, does not seem to be as critical for the elderly as for the middle-aged.

Vitamins and Minerals

It is widely assumed that the elderly do not need the full adult RDAs for vitamins and minerals, but this is not the case. The need for calcium actually may increase: As mentioned previously, a daily intake of 1,000 to 1,500 milligrams has recently been suggested, especially for postmenopausal women. Intolerance of dairy products and decreased calcium absorption may make calcium supplementation necessary. For the body to utilize calcium, there must be sufficient vitamin D. Older people who do not get much sunshine (especially those in nursing homes) and who avoid vitamin D–enriched dairy foods may need a vitamin D supplement, with a doctor's approval.

Iron supplementation may also be necessary because of poor diet. With poor intake of meats and other sources of iron, elderly people may suffer from iron-deficiency anemia. Studies suggest that some older people also do not get enough zinc, a mineral needed for proper wound healing, metabolism, and immune response. Here responsible professional advice is needed, because iron supplements can interfere with zinc and calcium absorption; zinc supplements can hinder folic-acid absorption, and so on.

The poor-eating elderly may have inadequate dietary sources of vitamin K (needed for blood clotting), folic acid (needed for the production of red blood cells), and vitamin B_2 (needed for metabolism and healthy mucous membranes). On the other hand, older people frequently consume excessive amounts of vitamin C (in the mistaken belief that it prevents colds) and vitamin E (popularly alleged to prevent aging) in the form of vitamin supplements. They may do harm.

THEORIES OF AGING

Improved medical care, sanitation, and nutrition have dramatically increased average life expectancy, from about 45 years in 1900 to approximately 75 years today. However, the maximum human life span—the greatest age obtainable by the species—has remained very much the same for centuries—approximately 110 years. A number of theories have been advanced to explain why this seems to be the maximum life span and why, even in the absence of disease, the human body inevitably ages and dies. The theories include the following.

Progressive damage to DNA. DNA (deoxyribonucleic acid) is found in the nuclei of cells and is the fundamental component of all living matter, controlling and transmitting the genetic code. Environmental influences (solar radiation, X rays, chemical mutagens and carcinogens, for example) can damage DNA, so that it fails to duplicate itself perfectly. Although DNA damage is repaired, the rate of damage slightly exceeds the rate of repair. According to this theory, aging is the result of cumulative DNA damage, exceeding the recuperative ability of the cells.

Limit to number of cell divisions. This theory stems in part from the work of Leonard Hayflick in the 1950s. He found that a population of connective-tissue cells would divide only about 50 times before dying out. Before that point, moreover, cell division resulted in an increasing number of mutations. This hypothesis holds that aging and death occur as the maximum number of cell divisions—as determined by the genetic blueprint of DNA—is approached.

An internal "aging clock." According to this theory, our bodies are programmed to age and die (thus removing from the population those who have served their primary evolutionary purpose: reproduction). It is thought that release of hormones from the hypothalamus is responsible for the deterioration of organs, the slowing down of metabolism, and the decline in function of the immune system that characterize aging. Aging is seen as part of a species-specific, chronologically organized progression: growth, maturation, aging, death.

Free-radical damage. Free radicals are a by-product of oxygen metabolism. Oxygen is essential to life, but, as it passes through the cells of the body, it breaks down and substances called free radicals are formed. Free radicals attack cell membranes, affecting their normal functioning and producing an accumulation of lipofuscin, a brown pigment. Commonly referred to as age pigment, lipofuscin in brain tissue has been related to senility; in the skin, it appears as liver spots. Damage to the cells by free radicals appears to be irreversible. However, substances known as free-radical scavengers, among them intracellular enzymes such as superoxide dismutase and antioxidant chemicals such as vitamin E, vitamin C, and selenium, which in excess can deprive tissue of needed oxygen, are able to deactivate the free radicals to some extent. Longer-living species (such as man) manufacture more free-radical scavengers than shorter-living species (such as mice).

It is probable that several of these mechanisms and a number of others, all working together, are responsible for the aging of the cells. An organism is only as long-lived as the weakest of its vital cells. The ability of the cells to replenish essential substances, or to duplicate themselves exactly after maturity, determines their life spans—and so ultimately the life span of the whole organism.

THE OLDER POPULATION

Older Americans form a very diverse group. They include the healthy and the infirm, the active and the sedentary, the rich and the poor. The majority of people in their later years are still in fairly good health and enjoy a good quality of life, but significant numbers are lonely, depressed, and ill.

As a group, they also have very diverse lifestyle arrangements: Some live alone, others with a spouse, companion, or younger family members. A relatively small number (about 5 percent) live in nursing homes or other institutions.

Nutritional knowledge, needs, and habits are probably as diverse as the group itself. It has been estimated that one-third to one-half of the health problems experienced by the elderly are related, directly or indirectly, to nutritional problems. Nutritional problems, in turn, are often related to the physiological changes associated with aging, and to the psychosocial problems that are shared by many elderly people.

PHYSIOLOGICAL CHANGES

In general, as bodily functions begin to slow, as energy expenditure decreases, caloric needs diminish. The processing or metabolism of ingested foods, that is, salivary, gastric, and intestinal enzyme secretions, are reduced, as is the hepatic (liver) handling of these products through enzymatic activity. No enzyme or liver supplements have been shown to be capable of totally rectifying these age- and/or disease-related changes.

Recent research suggesting growth hormone may help elderly people applies only to that minority of the elderly who make almost no growth hormone of their own, so have your blood serum growth hormone level measured before you consider taking this product, which can have serious side effects.

Changes in the Mouth

Although tooth loss is not an inevitable consequence of aging, many elderly people face this prospect. The American Dental Association estimates that as many as half of those aged 65 have lost all their teeth. Of these, 50 percent have no dentures, have incomplete or poorly fitted sets, or for one reason or another have dentures that are not used. Those with well-fitting dentures often find it hard to chew properly, because even properly fitted dentures exert only about a quarter of the chewing force provided by a good set of natural teeth.

The elderly also experience a marked increase in periodontal disease, which attacks the supportive tissues of the teeth and accounts for more than half the tooth loss in this group; an increase in cavities in the tooth roots; a decrease in saliva flow and salivary enzymes; and impaired circulation. With lessened salivation, the lining of the mouth becomes thin, friable, and easily bruised; and chewing and swallowing become more difficult. Oral cuts and sores may be slow to heal because of impaired blood circulation.

Problems such as these cause an obvious decline in the ability to chew, together with a decreased enjoyment of food. For many elderly people, these problems lead to a sharp limitation in food selection. Older people with no teeth or poorly fitting dentures tend to choose foods because of their texture rather than their nutritional value, preferring soft, easy-to-chew foods over crisp, crunchy ones. This means a dietary decrease in meats, raw fruits, and vegetables, and an increase in processed foods. When dietary fiber is reduced, intestinal problems such as constipation often result; when the intake of meat is low, there may eventually be an iron deficiency; when food is swallowed without being properly chewed, gastrointestinal distress may follow.

These problems are generally surmountable. Fruits and vegetables can be cooked and mashed, diced, or grated. Protein can be found in legumes, cottage cheese, soft cheeses, and tender, thinly sliced or ground meats. (For more on nutritious "soft" diets and for information on replacements for missing teeth, see Chapter 37.)

Diminished Sense of Taste and Smell

The number and sensitivity of taste buds decreases with age. The taste buds that detect sweet and salt deteriorate first, leaving those that are responsible for bitter and sour tastes. Taste sensitivity may also be affected by decreased salivation and by many of the drugs prescribed for the treatment of health problems common among the elderly. In addition, the ability to recognize and discriminate among various odors and flavors is lessened. It is not surprising, then, that many elderly people lose their interest in food.

A common problem associated with the lessened ability to taste salt is the liberal salting of food, which is inadvisable for older people, who have an increased incidence of high blood pressure or other problems requiring low-sodium diets. Herbs, lemon juice, garlic, and spices can be used instead to enhance flavor.

A diminished sense of smell may make it

difficult for an elderly person to detect burned food or soured milk. Cooking should be done by the clock. Dates stamped on perishables should be carefully noted.

Impaired Hearing and Vision

Aging is often associated with a decrease in the ability to hear and see clearly. These, too, have implications for nutritional status, making it harder to choose, prepare, and enjoy foods. Those who have difficulty reading labels or identifying packages displayed above or below eye level will have trouble in shopping for food and in taking advantage of store specials. They will have little interest in trying new products if the packet directions cannot be deciphered. People with diminished hearing may be reluctant to ask for information in food stores, for fear of embarrassment, and may be uncomfortable eating in public places or sharing a meal with others. (See Tips for More Enjoyable Eating, opposite.)

Gastrointestinal Discomfort

The elderly often report discomfort associated with eating certain foods. These discomforts include heartburn, gas, constipation, and diarrhea. Food selection will often be limited as a result of these associations that may be real but whose origins sometimes are psychological rather than physical.

With age, secretions of hydrochloric acid and digestive enzymes decrease, sometimes significantly, and the body has difficulty absorbing certain nutrients. (Nutrient uptake by the cells may diminish to the point of malnutrition, even when adequate nutrients are available.) In particular, it becomes more difficult to digest milk sugar (lactose) because of decreased production of lactase in the small intestine. Undigested milk ferments in the intestine, causing gas, bloating, or sometimes diarrhea. To circumvent this problem, low-lactose dairy products such as yogurt and aged cheese are recommended. However, many elderly people can tolerate milk if it is in cooked foods, such as cream sauces or puddings, or taken in small amounts, spread throughout the day.

The intestines become more sluggish with age and a tendency to constipation is common. A high-fiber diet and an adequate intake of water can usually alleviate the problem. So-called bulk expanders—for example, Met-

---

Tips for More Enjoyable Eating

To perk up appetites, consider the following.

- Plan regular meals and resist eating out of containers or saucepans. Instead, set an attractive table and eat from real dishes.

- For those living alone, a pet can provide needed companionship.

- Try to get some exercise daily, even if it's only a walk to the corner and back.

- Look into local group meals programs; these not only provide a source of nourishing foods but also companionship, making meals a social event.

- Try to organize cooking exchanges or potluck meals with neighbors in a similar situation.

- Turn on a radio, TV, or play some favorite music at mealtime to make eating more enjoyable.

If chewing is a problem, do the following.

- Use fish, ground meat, baked beans, nourishing soups, cottage cheese, eggs, and other soft but nourishing foods.

- Cook stews, soups, and casseroles, and freeze leftovers for future use.

amucil—are made from ground psyllium seed (a soluble fiber that may also help lower high cholesterol) and can be helpful. It should be noted, however, that some elderly people have an overanxious approach to their bodily functions and *may* consider themselves to be constipated when, in fact, they are not. Daily bowel movements are not the norm for everyone; every other day is fine. Laxative abuse may become a chronic problem and may cause actual deficiencies of certain nutrients.

Decreased Sensitivity to Thirst

Frequently, elderly people just don't feel thirsty, even when their bodies need water. In addition, studies have shown that young and elderly bodies may fail to conserve water in the face of a physiologic need for fluid. Six to eight cups of fluid a day are recommended and will help prevent kidney problems and constipation.

Loss of Appetite

Lack of appetite may be associated with many of the changes discussed previously, as well as with chronic illness. It may reflect a deficiency of thiamine, niacin, vitamin B_6, or zinc; more often it is a manifestation of loneliness, unhappiness, or anxiety.

It is important that the elderly maintain the quantity as well as the quality of their food intake. Eating in pleasant surroundings—at a table set with dishes instead of eating out of containers, or with the accompaniment of music or a radio if eating alone—helps. A little wine with a meal or a light soup to begin also may help to stimulate the appetite. (Care should be taken, however, not to substitute alcohol for food.) More frequent

and smaller meals are helpful. Finally, the underlying problem (or problems) should be sought out and dealt with.

Limitation of Activity

Even though large numbers of older people enjoy a variety of activities, including vigorous exercise, advancing age often does take its toll. The likelihoods of illness and physical impairment increase with age, bringing with them disability and a limitation of physical activity. Eighty-five percent of the elderly living in the community have at least one chronic disease; half have to limit their activity because of health problems. Arthritis, Parkinson's disease, and the partial paralysis resulting from a stroke are three of the many conditions that can limit activities.

Even those who are not so limited become increasingly less active with age. It should be emphasized, however, that most people—including those with physical disabilities—can manage some sort of exercise. Physical activity benefits the elderly just as much, or perhaps even more, as it does younger people. Regular exercise improves the appetite, helps retain muscle and joint function, increases lean body mass while decreasing fat, helps alleviate gastrointestinal problems, increases the sense of well-being, and may help relieve depression.

Weight-bearing exercise has been shown to increase the mineral content of bone, while immobilization results in accelerated bone loss. Postmenopausal women who have remained physically active have less osteoporosis than those who are sedentary. Exercise, in fact, is an important part of the overall treatment of osteoporosis.

Exercise in a group setting is highly recommended for elderly people. In addition to the physical and emotional benefits it offers, group exercise provides an excellent social outlet.

Reduced Muscular Coordination

With age, there is frequently a decline in fine muscle coordination. It becomes harder, for example, to handle eating utensils. (See below for a list of utensils that are easier to handle.) Rather than risk the embarrassment of spilled soup or the humiliation of having to ask for help in cutting meat, many elderly people avoid foods that present such problems. This may lead to significant changes in the diet, with accompanying nutritional deficiencies.

General debilitation and declining ability to coordinate movements may also make it difficult for the elderly to cook for themselves, get to food stores, or carry shopping bags. As a result, they may rely increasingly on food sources that minimize these tasks—and that are likely to be poor nutritional choices. (See Tips for Easier Food Preparation on page 263.)

Useful Utensils

- A plate with a raised rim
- A suction cup or sponge cloth under the plate to prevent slipping
- A two-handled drinking cup, or one with a spout, or one with a built-in straw
- Terry-cloth or foam covers for glasses
- A spork—part fork, part spoon, and part knife

PSYCHOSOCIAL PROBLEMS

Poor nutritional status is the direct result of poor food selection, but poor selection may be due to social rather than to health reasons. Reduced income, loss of spouse and friends, isolation, depression, all are factors that can contribute to poor selection of foods and, occasionally, to malnutrition. Families (and some doctors) have a tendency to accept physical and mental deterioration as being the inevitable consequence of aging, but much may be avoidable.

Reduced Income

For many Americans, aging goes hand in hand with reduced income. About one out of seven elderly people, especially black women, have incomes below the poverty line. Another large fraction is near poor, living just on the poverty line. Together, the poor and the near poor constitute one-quarter of the elderly population.

The effects of reduced income on nutritional status are often compounded by the circumstances and conditions of living. Housing may be substandard, lacking adequate cooking and refrigeration facilities. Changes in the neighborhood—especially in urban neighborhoods—may mean that familiar merchants close shop, customary foods are no longer available, and the streets seem unsafe. Lack of transportation may force a reliance on small neighborhood stores where prices are generally higher and selection more limited than at a supermarket.

The net result may be that the elderly person eliminates fresh meat, fruits, and vegetables from the shopping list and buys instead prepackaged or convenience foods. Such foods (as well as being expensive) are typically high in sodium, potassium, and sugar, which don't help chronic diseases such as hypertension, heart disease, and diabetes, all of which are more common with aging.

Isolation

The loss of spouse or companion, the death of friends, the breakdown of family ties, a neighborhood in transition, these events may add up to bleak isolation for an elderly person. The isolation of elderly people living alone or with few social ties is all too often reflected in the diet, resulting in deficiencies of iron, calcium, folic acid, and vitamins A and D. It is important to remember that isolation cuts across social and economic boundaries: The affluent can be as lonely (and as mal-

---

Tips for Easier Food Preparation

If it's hard to get around, try the following suggestions.

- Sit while working in the kitchen if it's tiring to stand. Choose a chair appropriate to the height of the countertop and stove.

- To move dishes and other items from one place to another, use a serving cart with wheels. Everything can be placed on the cart and then wheeled to the table, sink, and so forth.

- Place a rubber mat in front of the sink to ease strain on feet and legs and also to prevent slips on wet spots.

- Wear flat, well-fitting shoes to reduce fatigue and ensure better balance.

- Arrange the kitchen to keep things handy and organized. Pots and pans can be kept on hooks. Move items you use the most often to low, easy-to-reach shelves and cabinets. Use a sturdy step stool (instead of a chair) to reach high shelves.

- Consider forming a shopping and cooking cooperative, with people taking turns for the group so that no one person has to cook or shop all the time.

- When cooking, double or quadruple recipes for time-consuming dishes such as stews or soups. Freeze individual portions to be reheated later on.

- If you can afford it, buy a microwave or a toaster oven, which is easier to use for small meals than a conventional oven.

If you're on a budget, consider these options.

- Family-size packages are generally less expensive than individual or small portions. Share them with a friend or repackage and freeze in individual portions. Even the large economy-size loaves of bread can be divided, with smaller portions frozen for future use.

- Check newspaper ads and store circulars for specials. Use coupons, but only for items you really use and need.

- Look for unbranded or store-brand items. Many stores also have bins of generic products, such as dried legumes, pasta, and so forth, which are less expensive than name-brand goods.

- Buy fresh fruits and vegetables that are in season.

- Avoid health or organic foods, which tend to be more expensive yet no more healthful than regular foods.

If you lack a refrigerator, stock up on the following items.

- Nonfat dried milk

- Peanut butter

- Enriched or whole-grain cereals and breads

- Canned fish, stew, chunky soups, pork and beans

- Dried fruits and nuts

- Dried peas and beans

- Shelf-stable entrées and dinners

nourished) as those living below the poverty line.

A meal is a cultural and social event as much as it is a physiological necessity. Those living alone are often simply not motivated to shop and prepare food for just themselves. A downward spiral may set in as isolation leads to depression, depression leads to appetite loss, which in turn produces undernutrition because of inadequate food intake or poor food selection or both. Undernutrition aggravates depression and the cycle may continue through mental confusion (resembling senility) to death.

It is important that this cycle be broken. Elderly individuals may themselves be able to make an effort to shop and prepare meals, given help and encouragement. If there are friends in the area, exchange cooking may stimulate interest and appetite. If family members live close by, they can help with invitations to meals in their homes. However, it is very often the lack of friends and the absence of family that is at the root of the trouble.

Some Solutions

Government nutrition projects, such as those funded under Title IIIc, can help meet the social as well as the nutritional needs of some of the elderly. The target groups for these projects are people 60 years old or older who may not eat well because they cannot afford to, because their mobility is limited, or because they do not have the skills or motivation to purchase food and prepare nourishing meals. For those who are housebound—among the elderly who live in the community (as opposed to nursing homes or institutions), 5 percent are housebound and 1 percent are bedridden—meals can be delivered, which means that the shut-in has both hot food and a visitor five days a week. (Meals-on-Wheels,

a program under the auspices of local volunteer groups, provides the same service and the same beneficial social interaction.) For those living in the community, meals are served in such settings as church halls, senior centers, and schools. No charge is made but contributions are welcome.

The meals, whether home-delivered or served in congregate settings, include a minimum of one-third of the RDAs, and efforts are made to provide special menus to meet dietary needs related to health problems or religious beliefs. The opportunity to eat with others may be the most valuable feature of the program: studies show that the major positive effects are the participants' increased socialization and greater satisfaction with their lives. It is unfortunate that Title IIIc food programs are underfunded at present.

For those who qualify, food stamps help extend the budget. Volunteer drivers from churches, synagogues, and senior centers may be available to take an elderly person to the market and help with carrying shopping bags. Home health aides can help with the purchase and preparation of food for shut-ins. To learn about a local program, contact the nearest health department, Family Services agency, county extension office, or Area Agency on Aging. Other good sources of information include churches or synagogues; many local newspapers also carry listings of local programs and services.

OTHER FACTORS

Food Preferences

The choice of foods—what should be eaten and when, how it should be prepared, what accompaniments should go along with it—is greatly influenced by family patterns, ethnicity, traditional and religious beliefs. Preferences and habits are formed early in life and are very resistant to change. For the elderly, familiar foods and patterns of eating represent security and a comforting link with the past. Even though the foods may have no nutritional value (and may even cause gastrointestinal distress), elderly people generally prefer the foods they have been familiar with since childhood: regional or ethnic foods, down-home cooking.

Food choice may also be influenced by religion (kosher foods, fish during Lent) or the season of the year (for example, soup in the winter months). Some foods may be considered prestigious and be chosen for that reason (white bread rather than whole-wheat or rye). Food suitable for invalids may be chosen on the basis of tradition or folklore (that chicken broth is strengthening, or that illnesses such as arthritis should be treated with hot medications and foods).

Those elderly people who have a knowledge of the caloric value and nutrition composition of food often will make good choices of foods that have a high nutrient-to-calorie ratio. Unfortunately, nutrition science was in its infancy when today's elderly people were in theirs. Most of their information has been gleaned from newspapers, magazines, and quack food experts who have paid $50 for a certificate proclaiming them to be knowledgeable as nutritionists—all often unreliable sources. Consequently, these people may select foods they think are nutritious but that in fact are not.

Special Diets

Ironically, special diets are a major cause of malnutrition in the elderly. Chronic diseases affecting different organ systems and requiring different special diets are common. An elderly person may be on a low-protein diet for renal failure and a low-sodium diet for congestive heart failure, for example. The superimposition of diets—either on the advice of different doctors, who don't know about each other, or as the result of a friend's suggestions, or because of an individual's own ideas of what is needed—commonly causes low food intake and dietary inadequacy. The adverse effects of the diets may be compounded by nutritional deficiencies due to disease or drugs or both.

Fad Diets and Supplements

Elderly people are often attracted to fad diets by claims that adherence to a particular diet will protect them from acute or chronic disease, or increase their vitality, or fend off the aging process, or relieve the many health complaints associated with aging. Fad diet books may also advocate health foods (which are no more healthful than foods not so labeled and are almost always more expensive), or megadoses of amino acids such as lysine, sugars such as fructose, vitamins, minerals, and trace elements. As stressed in Chapter 3, fad diets can be dangerous. For example, high-protein, high-fat diets are not recommended for those whose liver, kidney, or digestive function is impaired. Weight-reducing diets that stress soup or bouillon (high in sodium) can precipitate congestive heart failure in an elderly person with heart disease or worsen high blood pressure.

It is not enough simply to point out the dangers. Persuading an elderly person to abandon a fad diet involves providing a rational alternative diet that will ameliorate the health problems from which the person is seeking relief.

Elderly persons spend more than $2 billion a year on anti-aging products. The Select

Committee on Aging of the House of Representatives has reviewed several hundred products that allegedly prevent or reverse aging. Not surprisingly, none performed as advertised; some were even found to be dangerous.

Among these products were numerous dietary supplements. An example is the intracellular enzyme superoxide dismutase (SOD). The basis for the claim that SOD has anti-aging properties is the fact that animals with longer life spans produce in their cells more of this free-radical scavenger. But any SOD that is eaten is digested in the intestine and does not reach the cells. Similar claims are made for ribonucleic acid (RNA), which is also digested in the intestine and does not affect the cells. Selenium is dangerous and can be lethal when taken in excess.

Gerovital (also known as GH3) has had a 30-year run as a remedy for almost all the illnesses and physical changes associated with aging. The main ingredient—procaine hydrochloride, found also in the local anesthetic Novocain—allegedly acts as an antidepressant, but it can be harmful and there is no foundation for any other claims of value. Vitamin "B$_{15}$" ("pangamic acid") is promoted for the treatment of heart disease, diabetes, and glaucoma, among other conditions. "B$_{15}$" has no medical usefulness, is not a vitamin, and has no nutritional value. Neither is PABA (para-aminobenzoic acid), although it is often shelved with the vitamins in health-food stores. PABA does not reverse any aspect of the aging process and can cause blood disorders and vomiting when taken in excess. Ginseng root is sold as an aphrodisiac. In large quantities, it can cause insomnia, hypertension, and gastrointestinal problems, as well as swollen, painful breasts in men. Another herbal mixture, Gotu Kola, is promoted to cure senility, again without real evidence.

Not only are supplements and preparations of this kind ineffective and sometimes dangerous, they are expensive. The elderly, of all people, can ill afford them.

Medications

Most elderly people take at least one prescription drug every day; many take five or more. For this reason, the elderly are more at risk than the general population for adverse food/drug interactions. In addition, drugs may affect food intake by depressing the appetite, altering sensitivity to taste or smell, changing the secretion of saliva, irritating the stomach, or causing nausea. Both the diseases themselves and the drugs taken to alleviate them can limit food choices and interfere with good nutrition.

Certain drugs contribute directly to dietary deficiencies. For example, aspirin, which may be taken in large doses by elderly people with arthritis, can cause bleeding in the gastrointestinal tract, leading to an iron deficiency. Aspirin also appears to increase the amount of folic acid that is excreted in the urine. Chronic use of certain antacids can interfere with the absorption of folic acid and calcium. Some laxatives (e.g., mineral oil) can affect the absorption of the fat-soluble vitamins D, A, K, and E. Drugs used for different pharmacological purposes can have additive effects. For example, certain laxatives and many diuretics produce potassium depletion, but taken together they can bring about a definite potassium deficiency.

Clearly, elderly people, who use 20 to 25 percent of all prescribed and over-the-counter drugs, should be well informed about their medications: what their side effects and their effects on nutrients are, how they may interact with other substances (alcohol, for example), what the proper dosage is, and when they should be taken (with meals or between meals, for example). (See Chapter 20 for a more detailed discussion of food/drug interactions.)

Alcohol

Alcohol abuse is a serious problem, both personal and social, for 2 to 10 percent of elderly people. It also is a problem that may easily be overlooked. The signs that suggest alcoholism in a younger person—impaired driving, for example, or absence from work—are likely to be missing in the elderly; denial is as prevalent in the old as in the young; and the effects of alcohol on mental acuity may be attributed to the aging process.

Due to depressed liver function, the elderly are less well able to tolerate large amounts of alcohol than are younger people. Moreover, alcohol consumption increases the body's requirements for folic acid, thiamine, vitamin B_6, zinc, and magnesium—nutrients that may be in short supply in the diets of the elderly, in any event. Research at Mount Sinai has shown that alcohol may actually destroy folic acid.

Because of their use of medication, elderly people are particularly at risk for drug/alcohol interactions. Tranquilizers, antihistamines, barbiturates, and painkillers depress the central nervous system; alcohol compounds the effect. Anticonvulsants and anticoagulants are metabolized more quickly when there is alcohol in the bloodstream, resulting in loss of antiseizure or anticoagulant responses. Taken with diuretics, alcohol may produce a drop in blood pressure and cause dizziness; with antibiotics, it may cause nausea and vomiting, stomach cramps, and headache; with monoamine-oxidase (MAO) inhibitors, used for depression, or tyramine in certain wines (Chianti) it may provoke a sharp rise in blood pressure.

Small amounts of alcohol, such as an occasional glass of wine or a light beer, may stimulate the appetite and make meals more enjoyable. Large amounts, or repeated small amounts taken throughout the day, are dangerous. (For a more detailed discussion on the nutritional effects of alcohol use, see Chapter 21.)

Institutional Food

The diets of elderly people in nursing homes are often even less well balanced and nutritious than those of old people living in the community. Interest in food—and in socialization at mealtimes—is typically low.

When a nursing home is being considered, questions about the diet are as much in order as questions about activities and the provision of care. Families should get satisfactory answers to such queries as:

Is there a dietitian on staff at the home?

Does the staff keep track of each person's weight?

Is the dining room attractive?

Does someone help those who have trouble feeding themselves?

Does the patient get a choice of foods at meals?

How often are fresh fruits and vegetables offered?

Does anyone monitor what and how much the patient eats?

Is the patient encouraged (or helped) to get to the dining room, or are the meals often given in the patient's room?

Are minced or finely chopped foods offered to those who have trouble chewing?

Can dietary restrictions due to religion be honored?

Part IV

Special Nutritional
Needs and Problems

■

17

Weight Control

Jerome L. Knittle, M.D., and David P. Katz, Ph.D.

■

INTRODUCTION

To say that Americans are preoccupied with weight and weight control is something of an understatement. Each year, some 70 million Americans spend a total of about $30 billion on thousands of methods of weight control, including diet books, diet pills, weight-loss clubs, low-calorie foods, health spas, and other reducing aids. One out of six Americans maintains that he or she is on a diet all the time, and at any given moment, as many as 75 percent of high school girls are trying to lose weight. Indeed, weight consciousness begins well before adolescence, according to a study indicating that some children start dieting as early as the fourth grade.

Although many Americans may think their diets are nutritionally lacking, most of us are actually overnourished, or at least overfed, as evidenced by the fact that roughly half of all American adults aged 20 to 74 are either overweight (up to 19 percent above desirable weight) or obese (20 percent or more above desirable weight). A small fraction of the population, about 4 percent, is considered morbidly or malignantly obese: defined as 100 pounds overweight or twice their desirable weight (see Table 17.1). Even more discourag-

ing is the fact that the prevalence of obesity has grown over the past 25 years, according to recent studies by the National Center of Health Statistics. In 1988, the Surgeon General of the United States formally declared overweight the most significant nutrition problem in the country.

For both physicians and their overweight patients, few medical conditions are as complex, frustrating, and difficult to treat as obesity. Of all the people who go on diets and lose weight, only some five percent maintain the weight loss beyond the first year. Being overweight can have detrimental psychological effects; it also carries a social stigma. Heavy people are frequently viewed as less competent, less attractive, and less likable than their slim counterparts. While the prevalence of obesity seems to be growing, current standards of beauty, especially for women, emphasize a lean, athletic physique. The widespread promotion of this ideal not only adds to the anguish of those who are truly fat, it encourages unrealistic expectations among women whose weight falls within a safe, normal range. This is reflected by the marked increase in bulimia and other eating disorders stemming from a morbid fear of obesity.

To be comprehensive, a discussion of

obesity and overweight should address certain key questions:

- What causes obesity?
- What is the difference between being obese and overweight?
- How can people determine whether they are too fat?
- What are the social and psychological consequences of these conditions?
- How can obesity be prevented and treated?

This chapter will address each of these questions in turn.

THE ORIGINS OF OBESITY

Obesity is a problem that is both simple and complex: simple because it is well known that people get fat because they consume more food than their bodies can use, and complex because it is not known why some people chronically overeat. Nor is it known why some people get fat and others stay slim despite consuming comparable amounts of food. Research indicates that obesity is linked to a combination of factors that include genetics, metabolic and/or hormonal differences, levels of physical activity, and a host of cultural and environmental influences.

In the evolution of human beings and other animal life, the ability to store fuel for future use in the form of fat has been crucial to survival through periods when food was not readily available. Indeed, our prehistoric ancestors devoted most of their waking hours to the quest for enough food to ensure survival. This is still true in many Third World countries where food is in short supply—and

Table 17.1. Body Mass Index

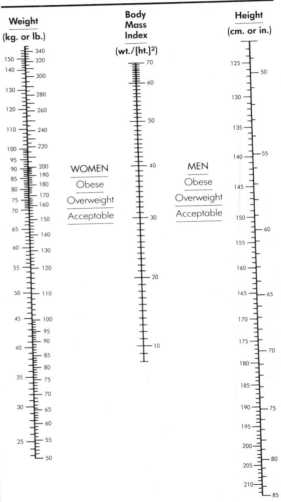

A nomogram for determining body mass index (BMI). To use this nomogram, place a ruler or other straightedge between the column for height and the column for weight, connecting an individual's numbers for those two variables. Read the BMI in kg./m² where the straight line crosses the middle lines when the height and weight are connected. Overweight: BMI of 25-30 kg./m²; obesity: BMI above 30 kg./m². Heights and weights are without shoes or clothes.

Source: The Medical Journal of Australia, copyright 1985, reprinted with permission.

obesity is unknown except among the very rich. In the United States and other industrialized Western countries, however, we are blessed by an unprecedented variety and abundance of food. Dr. Jean Mayer, the noted nutrition scientist/writer, observed in his 1968 book, *Overweight: Causes, Cost and Control*, that "we are the fat of the land: never in history, nowhere else in the world have such huge numbers of human beings eaten so much, exerted themselves so little, and become and remained so fat. . . . And we suffer because of it." In the intervening 20 years, Americans have become even fatter. Still, obesity is not simply a problem of supply and demand; if it were, even more of us would be overweight. Self-control may be a factor for some, but there are large numbers of people who maintain a desirable weight, even though they eat whenever they feel hungry. Almost unconsciously, they simply stop eating when they have consumed enough to maintain their weight. Also, there are many degrees of obesity. Many people who are overweight gain until they reach a certain point; after that, their weight remains constant, even though their food intake is unchanged.

Much of what is known—or speculated—about human obesity comes from studies on animals. Animals can be made obese in three ways: They can be bred for metabolic traits that make them obese; their brains can be damaged in certain parts to cause them to eat voraciously; or they can be fed fattening, highly palatable diets that induce them to ignore whatever prior restraints governed their eating.

Genetics

Several strains of rats and mice can be bred for their ability to get fat. Their body weight appears to be set at a higher level, so that genetically obese animals "defend" their weight and, when deprived of food, their metabolism slows to preserve as much of their body weight as possible.

Table 17.2. Body Mass Index (kg./m²) Used to Define Desirable Weight and Overweight According to Three Different "Ideal" Reference Populations

| Study[a] | "Ideal" Reference Population | BMI for "Ideal" Reference Population | | | | | |
| | | MEAN | | OVERWEIGHT | | SEVERE OVERWEIGHT | |
		Men	Women	Men	Women	Men	Women
NHANES II	20- to 29-year-olds	24.3	23.1	27.8	27.3	31.1	32.3
Metropolitan 1959	Desirable weight insured	22.0	21.5	26.4	25.8	30.8	30.1
Metropolitan 1983	Desirable weight insured	22.7	22.4	27.2	26.9	31.8	31.4

[a]The NHANES II data define overweight as the 85th percentile or more of the distribution of BMI for men and women ages 20 to 29, and severely overweight as the 95th percentile for that reference population (NCHS 1987). The Metropolitan 1959 data are taken from the 1959 Metropolitan Life Insurance tables. Weights and heights were adjusted to approximate those without shoes or clothing (Simopoulos and Van Itallie, 1984; NIH, 1985). The Metropolitan 1983 data are taken from the 1983 Metropolitan tables. Height and weight were with shoes and light clothes (Van Itallie, 1985; NIH, 1985). For both the 1959 and the 1983 Metropolitan data, the weights for midpoint of medium-frame persons were used, and for both studies overweight and severe overweight were defined as 20 percent and 40 percent, respectively, over desirable weight.

With humans, it has long been observed that obesity seems to run in some families. At one time, it was generally assumed that the problem was environmental: The family members tended to have similar food habits and, consequently, a shared weight problem. According to one popular formula, if one parent is obese, the child has a 40 percent chance of becoming obese; if both parents are obese, the child's risk doubles to 80 percent. While food habits are important, recent research indicates that there is also a hereditary basis for obesity: People who are markedly overweight have a genetic tendency to use food more efficiently, leaving more to be stored as body fat.

A number of traits seem to distinguish genetically obese people from their normal-weight peers. As noted, their metabolism is more efficient, so they don't require as much food as normal-weight people. They also have an increased tendency to convert food into body fat quickly and have more difficulty in converting it back into a form that can be used for energy. Some have a tendency to produce large amounts of a substance called lipoprotein lipase—an enzyme that cells use to absorb lipids carried in the blood.

At an early age, obese children seem to develop a larger number of fat cells (adipocytes). Most of the cells in the body can hold up to 20 percent fat, but adipocytes hold up to 62 percent fat and they store the excess fat left when other types of cells reach their limit. The Fat Cell Hypothesis states that the more fat cells a person has, the fatter he or she will become and the harder it will be to lose weight and maintain the loss.

There are certain times in life when humans are particularly prone to develop adipocytes. Researchers have found that people who gain excessive amounts of weight (defined as above the 95th percentile on standard growth charts) during these periods— from birth to age 2, around age 10 to 11, and during adolescence—will develop more fat cells than those who stay slim during these periods. New evidence suggests that fat cells may proliferate in adulthood as well, perhaps explaining why some people who have been thin all their lives become fat in middle age.

People with a large number of fat cells find it more difficult to lose weight for several reasons. Once adipocytes are formed, their numbers remain fairly constant; they can shrink, but for the most part, fat-cell number does not decrease. It has been speculated that after a person loses a certain amount of weight, it is difficult to lose more because of some control exerted by the stored body fat.

In summary, a person who is obese from childhood may store fat more easily than someone who is thin. A lean person who eats more than is needed will, up to a point, burn off the excess calories by becoming more active or generating more body heat. It is possible that fat cells that are larger, more numerous, and more enzymatically active may be more efficient at storing excess calories. Observations of genetically obese rats, who get fat even on a near-starvation regimen, support the theory of increased "feed efficiency." The rats weigh less, to be sure, but they retain the same percentage of body fat. Despite this, the fact is that the majority of obese people can lose weight by following a commonsense regimen aimed at achieving a gradual but steady reduction. This entails eating less and increasing physical activity. (Sample regimens are provided in later sections in this chapter.)

Set Point for Weight

The set-point theory maintains that each person has a specific biologic set point for his or her "ideal" weight, and that the body will strive to achieve and maintain this set point. According to this theory, metabolism will change to make more efficient use of food (and thus prevent weight loss) during periods of weight-reduction dieting. If weight is lost, the body will alter its metabolism and increase the hunger drive in an effort to regain it. That 95 percent of overweight people who lose excess pounds regain them within a year—and that once they achieve their former weight, or perhaps a few pounds more, they stop gaining—supports the theory.

Assuming that the set-point theory is valid, it still does not mean that an overweight person is powerless to change it. Research indicates that the set point can be reset at a lower level by gradual weight loss and increased physical activity. This suggests that set point is just a description of what actually happens and not an unchangeable fact built into the body's blueprint.

Physical Activity

A number of studies have found that overweight people are not as physically active as their normal-weight counterparts who may eat even more but burn up the extra calories in various kinds of activities. It also is well documented that the most successful weight-reduction programs are those that combine increased physical activity with reduced food intake, plus support for the necessary willpower to continue the program for life.

Many people have the mistaken notion that unless a person engages in very vigorous or sustained exercise, such as long-distance running, insufficient energy is used to make much difference as far as weight is concerned. This is not true; regular moderate exercise—for example, a half hour of brisk walking (three and a half miles per hour) every day—will burn up the equivalent of about 15 pounds of fat in the course of a year. A half hour of heavy housework, gardening, cycling at eight miles per hour, or playing doubles

tennis will produce comparable results. Even people who insist they cannot spare a half hour for a daily walk can work a comparable amount of exercise into their daily schedules; for example, climbing up two or three flights of stairs a few times each day instead of taking the elevator, walking the last few blocks to work, doing a few chores with hand devices rather than laborsaving devices (e.g., a hand lawn mower or old-fashioned garden spade). Turning down the thermostat a few degrees not only saves fuel but also requires the body to use more energy to maintain body temperature. Resisting having a telephone in every room requires more walking around the house. (See Table 24.1 on page 00 for a list of activities and calories consumed.)

Food Availability

In the 1970s, researchers found that normal-weight laboratory rats who ate a highly palatable supermarket diet of salami, candy, peanuts, sweetened condensed milk, and other high-calorie foods became obese. At first, animals placed on this regimen responded with an increased metabolic rate and greater body-heat production, which kept their weight down. After time, however, they adapted to the fattening diet and gained weight. Like the genetically obese animals, rats with so-called supermarket obesity seem to defend their new, higher weight. Thus, even when switched to a low-calorie diet, they attempt to retain their fat.

Such laboratory studies have enabled scientists to develop new theories about human obesity. In this instance, the persistent obesity of the overfed rats is similar to the plight of so many Americans who enjoy a calorie-rich diet of sweet, fatty foods.

This is a prime environmental factor behind the growing prevalence of overweight in the United States. As stressed in Chapter 2,

Americans today have easy access to the best food from every part of the globe and at a cost that most people can afford. Even the smallest American towns are apt to have fast-food outlets offering burgers, hot dogs, French fries, pizza, ice cream, and other low-cost, high-calorie favorites. Food companies spend millions of dollars advertising high-calorie snacks, sweets, and treats. The same magazines that tout the latest diets also carry pages of food advertising and recipes for high-calorie desserts and other dishes that only a stoic could resist.

Not surprisingly, Americans have become more sophisticated and knowledgeable about food. Even in small towns, supermarkets have gourmet sections and restaurants offer dishes once associated with gourmet capitals such as Paris, San Francisco, New Orleans, and New York. In such a climate, it is not surprising that obesity is on the rise. If anything, it is surprising that even more people are not markedly overweight.

Unlike heredity, however, environment can be controlled. Many people head for a gym instead of a bar to unwind after work; still more stock their kitchens with low-calorie foods and concentrate on preparing good-tasting gourmet dishes that are not loaded with butter and other fattening ingredients. With knowledge and some careful planning, even people who are genetically predisposed to gain weight can prevent themselves from doing so and, at the same time, enjoy good food. Gourmets need not be gourmands.

Eating Behavior, Habits, and Cultural Factors

We eat for many reasons other than simply to provide the body with essential energy. For example, food is important for most social and many business occasions. The terms *power breakfast* and *power lunch* have become part of our national vocabulary. It's hard to imagine a wedding, party, or other gala occasion that does not offer an array of tempting foods. Business is conducted over meals; employees regularly gather around a food canteen to share break time—and to fill up on doughnuts, candy, and other snack foods. People who keep accurate food diaries are often surprised to learn just how much food is consumed in nonmeal situations.

Obese people often exhibit certain eating patterns that promote weight gain. In fact, a number of studies have found that overweight people are particularly likely to eat for reasons other than to satisfy hunger. For example, the mere presence of food is enough to prompt some people to eat even if they aren't hungry. Early eating habits often contribute to their weight problems. They have been taught from an early age to clean their plates and that asking for second or even third helpings is an expected compliment to the cook. Parents often respond to a baby's cries for attention by offering food. That baby may grow up to have a tendency to eat when frustrated, lonely, depressed, or upset.

Observations of overweight people have found that many eat very fast. Since it takes about 20 minutes for the appetite center in the brain to register satiety, eating too fast is likely to result in overeating. Behaviorists recommend that overweight people put down their utensils after each mouthful and then pick them up before the next mouthful in order to slow the eating pattern.

Meal patterns also may contribute to obesity. Many overweight people contend that they eat very little: "I starve myself all day" is a common refrain. Many do just that—skipping breakfast and eating very little lunch. By dinnertime, these people are more likely to overeat to make up for the rest of the day.

Finally, not all ethnic groups regard

obesity as undesirable. In some cultures, over-weight women are considered more attractive and fertile than thin women; and for men, being fat is a sign of success. Americans from these ethnic backgrounds may want to be thin, but from an early age, they are encouraged to overeat. A fat baby (above the 95th percentile in the growth tables) is considered healthy and happy, while a lean one is regarded as less healthy and a reflection of parental stinginess or neglect. The fact that fat babies are more likely to grow into fat adults is well documented.

Endocrine and Other Abnormalities

Although glands (i.e., hormonal imbalances) are often blamed for obesity, they actually account for less than 2 percent of obesity. Even so, endocrine disorders should not be ruled out when determining the cause of obesity. Specific disorders that can lead to weight gain include hypothyroidism (reduced production of thyroid hormones, which lowers the metabolic rate and also causes fluid retention) and Cushing's syndrome, a disease characterized by overproduction of adrenal hormones.

Medications

A number of medications can result in weight gain. Examples include steroids (used to treat asthma, inflammatory disorders, and other conditions), some drugs used to treat anxiety and depression, sex hormones, and certain antidiabetes medications. Generally, the weight gain is minor or due to fluid retention, but there are instances in which the drugs can alter metabolism and/or promote fat storage enough to cause considerable gain.

Other Miscellaneous Causes

Animal studies have found that when a portion of the brain called the ventromedial hypothalamus, or VMH, is damaged, the animals respond by eating voraciously until they reach a new, higher weight. In humans, abnormalities in the brain's appetite-control center may result in overeating. There also are rare genetic disorders in which a person has faulty appetite control and therefore will eat uncontrollably unless restrained from doing so. These disorders usually are accompanied by mental retardation and other genetic abnormalities.

OBESITY VERSUS OVERWEIGHT

Terms such as *being fat, chubby, overweight,* or *obese* mean different things to different people. A normal-weight teenaged girl may describe herself as huge if she gains two or three pounds before her menstrual period, while a middle-aged man may not notice his spare tire until the scale hits 200 pounds. A laboratory researcher may think in terms of percentage of body fat and body water, while a physician may express concern over health risks incurred at a certain level of weight.

What Is Meant by Desirable Weight?

Desirable weight, or more accurately, the desirable weight range for any given height and body build, is the range in which death and disease are lowest. There are a number of standard height and weight tables, with the ones developed by the Metropolitan Life Insurance Company the most-used among physicians. (See Table 17.3.) All of the standard tables have problems; some are overly generous, others too stringent. Still others do not take into account differences in age, frame, body type, and other variables, such as muscularity.

Someone of average bone structure and muscularity can estimate his or her desirable weight with a simple formula. Men should allow 106 pounds for the first five feet of height, and then add 6 pounds for every inch over that. Using this formula, the desirable weight for a man six feet tall would be 178 pounds. A man who stands less than five feet tall should figure 106 pounds minus 4 pounds for every inch under five feet. Women should allow 100 pounds for the first five feet and add 5 pounds for every inch above or subtract 4 pounds for every inch below five feet. Thus, the desirable weight for a woman of average bone structure who is five feet four inches tall is 120 pounds.

In general, someone who is 20 percent or more above "desirable" weight is considered obese. Thus, a six-foot man of average bone structure would be obese at 214 pounds or more; a five-foot-four-inch woman would be considered obese starting at 144 pounds.

These formulas do not account for differences in frame size and type. Bones and muscle tissue weigh more than fat. Thus, someone with light, slender bones should probably weigh less than someone of the same height with a heavier, sturdier frame. Similarly, a person who is very muscular—a professional football player, for example—may tip the scales in the obese range, but, in fact, have a very low percentage of body fat. (See Table 17.4, which tells how to determine body-frame size.)

Table 17.3. "Desirable" Weight*

Height	Metropolitan Life Ages 25–29		Gerontology Research Center Men and Women by Age (Years)				
	MEN	WOMEN	25	35	45	55	65
Feet/Inches	Pounds				Pounds		
4-10	——	100–131	84–111	92–119	99–127	107–135	115–142
4-11	——	101–134	87–115	95–123	103–131	111–139	119–147
5-0	——	103–137	90–119	98–127	106–135	114–143	123–152
5-1	123–145	105–140	93–123	101–131	110–140	118–148	127–157
5-2	125–148	108–144	96–127	105–136	113–144	122–153	131–163
5-3	127–151	111–148	99–131	108–140	117–149	126–158	135–168
5-4	129–155	114–152	102–135	112–145	121–154	130–163	140–173
5-5	131–159	117–156	106–140	115–149	125–159	134–168	144–179
5-6	133–163	120–160	109–144	119–154	129–164	138–174	148–184
5-7	135–167	123–164	112–148	122–159	133–169	143–179	153–190
5-8	137–171	126–167	116–153	126–163	137–174	147–184	158–196
5-9	139–175	129–170	119–157	130–168	141–179	151–190	162–201
5-10	141–179	132–173	122–162	134–173	145–184	156–195	167–207
5-11	144–183	135–176	126–167	137–178	149–190	160–201	172–213
6-0	147–187	——	129–171	141–183	153–195	165–207	177–219
6-1	150–192	——	133–176	145–188	157–200	169–213	182–225
6-2	153–197	——	137–181	149–194	162–206	174–219	187–232
6-3	157–202	——	141–186	153–199	166–212	179–225	192–238
6-4	——	——	144–191	157–205	171–218	184–231	197–244

*Heights and weights are given for people without shoes or clothing.

Courtesy *Statistical Bulletin*, 1983, Metropolitan Life Insurance Company.

Matching weight and frame size is not always indicative of whether a person is actually overweight; one must also consider body composition. A muscular, athletic person may weigh considerably more than a sedentary person of the same height and frame size and still be considered trim, while the sedentary counterpart may be overweight. If the athlete's extra weight comes from muscle, he or she may technically fall into the overweight column on a standard scale yet not appear fat and probably not run the same health risk as someone whose extra pounds come from excess adipose. In general, however, as one approaches 20 percent or more above desirable weight, the excess weight usually comes from fat. It has been observed that aging athletes who become sedentary have a higher frequency of heart attacks than those who remain active.

Conversely, there are people who may not be overweight according to standard charts but who still may be carrying more body fat than is good for them. In short, body weight does not always indicate whether someone is, indeed, too fat. Because of this, scientists have devised other methods of determining body fat. (See Indirect Methods of Determining Body Composition on page 281.)

Table 17.4. How to Determine Body Frame Size

The Metropolitan Life Insurance Company, which periodically determines the weight at which mortality is lowest among its subscribers, offers this method for determining frame size:

- Extend one arm and bend the forearm upward at a 90-degree angle.
- Keep fingers straight and turn the inside of the wrist toward the body.
- If a caliper is available, use it to measure the space between the two prominent bones on either side of the elbow.
- Alternatively, place the thumb and index finger of the other hand on these two bones. Measure the space between the fingers against a ruler or a tape measure. Compare it with the figures below, which list elbow measurements for medium-framed men and women. Measurements less than those listed indicate a small frame; greater measurements indicate a large frame.

Medium Frame	
HEIGHT IN 1-INCH HEELS	ELBOW BREADTH
Men	
5′2″–5′7″	2½ ″–2⅞″
5′8″–6′3″	2¾ ″–3⅛″
6′4″	2⅞″–3¼ ″
Women	
4′10″–5′3″	2¼″–2½″
5′4″–6′0″	2⅜″–2⅝″

Courtesy *Statistical Bulletin*, 1983, Metropolitan Life Insurance Company.

HEALTH IMPLICATIONS OF OBESITY

Obesity and overweight do present real risks to health, including an increased incidence of early death. In one long-term study involving several thousand people, every pound of excess weight in men aged 30 to 49 increased death rates by 1 percent. Among men aged 50 to 62, each pound increased the death rate by 2 percent. Other studies involving several million people have shown that mortality is lowest in healthy, nonsmoking men aged 20 to 69 who range from 25 percent underweight to 5 percent overweight, and among women aged 30 to 69 who range from 15 percent underweight to 15 percent overweight.

As the United States Surgeon General formally reported in 1988, the more overweight a person is, the greater the risk of premature death. In addition, obesity carries an increased risk of a number of diseases. These include:

Certain forms of cancer. Specific cancers that have been linked to obesity include cancers of the breast, uterus, ovaries, and gallbladder in women and cancers of the colon, rectum, and prostate in men. Several studies have suggested that cancer risk may be related either to the excessive number of calories consumed or to proportion of body fat. (See Chapter 27 for a more detailed discussion of diet and cancer.)

Diabetes. Type II or adult-onset diabetes—the form characterized by a resistance to, rather than lack of, insulin—is much more common among overweight adults. This is believed to be due to reduced insulin sensitivity of the fat cells. Very often, weight loss alone is all that is needed to treat this form of diabetes. (See Chapter 28.)

Cardiovascular diseases. Several forms of heart and blood-vessel disease are more common among obese individuals. High blood pressure and atherosclerosis (the blocking of coronary and other arteries with fatty deposits) are two major cardiovascular disorders that increase the risk of heart attacks and strokes; both are associated with obesity. Overweight people may tend to have high blood-cholesterol levels—another major risk factor for a heart attack. (See Chapter 26.)

Respiratory disorders. The burden of excess weight on the chest and in the abdomen often taxes the lungs. Extremely obese people may develop a condition known as the Pickwickian syndrome, named after an obese character in Charles Dickens' novel *The Pickwick Papers* who was always falling asleep. This condition, which is also referred to as cardiovascular-pulmonary obesity syndrome, is characterized by twitching, drowsiness, lethargy due to the inability to breathe properly. It can lead to life-threatening congestive heart failure.

Arthritis and other musculoskeletal problems. Excess weight places a strain on the muscles and joints and may hasten or exacerbate the onset of osteoarthritis and other joint problems, particularly in the weight-bearing joints of the hips and legs. Men who have a genetic predisposition to gout are more likely to develop the disease if they are overweight. Back and foot problems also are worsened by being overweight. (See Chapter 35.)

Gallbladder disease. As weight rises, so does the risk of gallstones and other forms of gallbladder disease. According to one study, people who were at least 20 percent above the median weight for the population as a whole had twice the risk of developing gallbladder disease as people who were less than 90 percent of the median weight for their height.

Menstrual irregularities and other gynecologic or obstetrical problems. The relationship between body fat and the menstrual cycle is not fully understood, but it is well known that overweight girls experience an earlier menarche (onset of menstruation) than normal-weight or thin girls. Obese women may experience irregular periods or stop menstruating altogether, indicating ovarian dysfunction. Markedly overweight women have an increased incidence of fertility problems, and those who do conceive have a higher risk of complications, such as high blood pressure during pregnancy, toxemia, gestational diabetes, and spontaneous abortion. (See Chapter 12.) An enzyme in fat tissues makes hormones.

Miscellaneous. Obese people have an increased likelihood of developing abdominal hernias, backaches, and other problems related to weight-related muscle problems.

Role of Fat Distribution

In addition to total weight, the way in which fat cells are distributed throughout the body may have important implications for health, although this concept is not yet fully accepted. People who are apple-shaped or who have a spare tire, with most of their excess fat concentrated around the upper abdomen, seem to be more susceptible to obesity-related diseases such as high blood cholesterol and an increased risk of stroke, heart disease, and diabetes, compared to pear-shaped people, whose fat is concentrated in the hips, buttocks, and thighs. This is believed to be due to the fact that fat in the abdomen is more active metabolically than fat elsewhere in the body. This more active fat increases the level of blood lipids, and because of the proximity of the abdomen to the blood supply entering the liver, this increase may help raise blood cholesterol.

Men tend to fall into the apple-shaped category, whereas women tend to be more pear-shaped. The reasons for this are believed to be hormonal: Men store fat in places where it can be metabolized more readily, whereas women store fat in areas where it is not metabolized as readily but is available if needed during pregnancy and lactation. Interestingly, after menopause, women accumulate more abdominal fat, and their incidence of heart attacks and other obesity-related problems rises.

Overweight Versus Underweight

Of course, not all overweight people encounter health problems. It also has been argued that leanness entails certain health hazards, and workers at Johns Hopkins in Baltimore suggest that people who are of average or slightly above-average weight when they are age 50 or older live longer than

---

Indirect Methods of Determining Body Composition

Underwater weighing. This method (called densimetric) is based on the fact that fat tissue is lighter than other body tissue—bones, muscle, blood, and water. The person is weighed while submerged underwater, with as much air as possible exhaled from the lungs. He or she is then weighed normally on the ground. By using a formula based on the two weights, the percentage of body fat can be determined.

Skinfold thickness. About 50 percent of body fat is situated just below the skin, and by measuring folds of skin on certain parts of the body, the percentage of body fat can be estimated. The most accurate measurements are obtained by using calipers; indicative body sites include the triceps (the skinfold on the back of the arm midway between the shoulder and elbow), the subscapular area below the shoulder blades, and the area just above the hip bone.

Total body water (hydrometry). Most fat-free tissue (muscle) contains water, while fat tissue has very little. Therefore, measurement of total body water provides an estimate of Fat Free Mass (FFM). One approach to this measurement is taken by injecting a known amount of a substance that distributes itself throughout the body's water compartments. A blood sample, taken after enough time has elapsed for the substance to reach a stable concentration in the body, reveals the substance's distribution in body water, allowing the tester to measure total body water and from that to calculate the amount of FFM. The result obtained by subtracting FFM from total body weight is the body-fat content. Another approach is by putting two electrodes on a limb and measuring resistance to an electric current. The amount of electric impedence measures body water.

Whole body potassium. Almost all of the body's potassium is contained in cells other than adipose tissue. A naturally occurring isotope of potassium exists as a fixed proportion to all potassium found in the body. The radioactive portion can be measured by counting the gamma rays it emits, and this can be used to estimate the total potassium. The greater the amount of potassium in relation to body size, the smaller the percentage of body fat.

those who are underweight. Researchers at the Harvard School of Public Health analyzed 25 studies that linked low body weight to health problems, however, and found that some were seriously biased. For example, cigarette smokers, who tend to be thin, had not been excluded, nor had people who were underweight due to illness. In contrast, the studies had excluded people suffering from diseases caused by obesity, such as hypertension. Since smoking and wasting illnesses are clearly associated with a higher death rate, including these people while excluding from the studies those with high blood pressure or diabetes would make it appear that being underweight is more hazardous than being overweight. The Harvard researchers found that when the results were adjusted to resolve these biases, longevity favored the lean.

PSYCHOSOCIAL CONSEQUENCES

Obese people are constantly reminded that they have a weight problem. Turnstiles are too small, theater, airplane, or bus seats too narrow. They may be unable to fasten seat belts; clothing and shoes are difficult to find and may be available only in limited sizes or styles.

Social and professional opportunities are curtailed: Surveys have found that the obese are less likely to be admitted to the prestigious colleges and the best jobs are likely to go to a slimmer candidate, even if he or she is less qualified. According to one estimate, for every pound of excess weight, an executive may lose $1,000 a year in pay. Health and life insurance may be more difficult to obtain, and rates are apt to be higher than for normal-weight people. In a recent, highly publicized court decision, an obese couple was denied permission to adopt a child. There are laws

against discrimination on the basis of physical disabilities, and to many, being obese is a disability. These laws are difficult to enforce, however, especially when it comes to hiring and other job practices.

One of the most dramatic examples of the prejudice obese people face was revealed in a study involving a wide variety of children and adults. Some were obese, others were not. The participants were asked to look at drawings of children with different kinds of handicaps: One was in a wheelchair, another on crutches with a leg brace. A third had a facial disfigurement; a fourth child was missing a hand. The fifth child was markedly obese. When asked which child they liked least, most of the participants—including those who were overweight—pointed to the obese child, justifying their selection on the grounds that he could control his handicap, while the others could not. Even physicians tend to view fat people as unattractive, awkward, and weak-willed. At a time when obesity is increasing, tolerance of the obese appears to be decreasing.

Psychological Problems of the Obese

Contrary to popular belief, there is no compelling evidence that overweight people suffer more from serious psychological problems such as depression than the general population. At one time, it was thought that psychological disorders were a major cause of obesity; it is now recognized that when emotional disorders occur among the obese, they are more likely to be a consequence than a cause of the weight problem.

Of course, the fact that obese people are not disproportionally afflicted by serious mental illness does not negate the fact that there are emotional consequences associated with being overweight. Not all emotional problems can be measured by psychiatric tests, and many obese people describe emotional handicaps resulting from their excessive weight. For example, repeated diet failures can shatter self-confidence, and a lack of sympathy from others can instill feelings of inferiority, frustration, and isolation.

According to Dr. Albert Stunkard, a psychiatrist at the University of Pennsylvania who with various colleagues has written extensively about the psychological disorders of the obese, "disparagement of body image" is perhaps the most common problem among the overweight. For example, in an article coauthored with Dr. Thomas Wadden, Dr. Stunkard observed: "Obese persons characteristically feel that their bodies are grotesque and loathsome, and that others view them with hostility and contempt." In another article, this time in the *Journal of the American Dietetic Association*, Dr. Stunkard wrote: "It makes no difference whether the (obese) person be also talented, wealthy, or intelligent; his weight is his only concern, and he sees the whole world in terms of his weight."

THE PREVENTION AND TREATMENT OF OBESITY

The effective prevention and treatment of obesity hinges on bringing caloric intake and energy expenditure into balance. Even people with a genetic predisposition to obesity are unlikely to become fat if, from an early age, they achieve this nutritional balance. A first step in bringing a diet into balance entails determining how many calories are required to meet the body's basic, or basal metabolic needs—the energy required to carry on vital processes such as circulation, respiration, digestion, metabolism, and other functions that continue even when a person is resting

quietly or asleep. This is referred to as the basal metabolic rate, or BMR. (See How to Determine Your Daily Caloric Needs, below.) To this number of calories are added those burned up in day-to-day activities. As would be expected, this depends upon an individual's level of physical activity. Clearly, a person who drives to and from the office, spends most of her day behind a desk, and her evenings watching TV will need fewer calories than a person who has a more physically demanding job or who does housework and cares for small children. Similarly, a person who earns his living farming and harvesting crops probably burns more calories than the president of the company that buys the food.

How to Determine Your Daily Caloric Needs

The following formula applies to the average rather sedentary American adult:

Basal metabolic needs: 10 calories for each pound of body weight. For example, a 150-pound man would need about 1,500 calories a day to maintain a normal BMR.

Normal daily activities: 3 calories for each pound of body weight. For example: a 150-pound man would need about 450 calories in addition to the 1,500 for his BMR, or a total of 1,950.

Adjustments for Age

Subtract about 2 percent for each decade after age 30. Thus, if the 150-pound man cited above is 55 years old, his average daily caloric needs would be 6 percent less, or 1,833.

Extra calories can be added to cover additional physical activity. For example, if this 150-pound man starts walking briskly for a half hour each day, and burns up 150 calories doing so, he can consume 1,983 calories a day without gaining weight.

Other determinants of caloric need include age; for example, rapidly growing children need more calories than their parents. The state of health is also important; a person recovering from surgery or an injury, for example, will have greater caloric needs. Even climate seems to play a role; caloric need rises slightly in cold weather in order to maintain body temperature.

Since very few of us follow the same routine day after day, energy expenditure also varies. Five days at a desk job, for example, may be followed by a day or two of intense physical activity. The body adjusts for these variances; eating a bit more or less than is needed on one day will not necessarily mean a weight change so long as a balance is maintained over the course of a week or two. Body weight reflects one's average daily intake over a period of time. In short, weight gain results when caloric intake *consistently* exceeds caloric needs.

GENERAL GUIDELINES TO REDUCE WEIGHT

Medical Consultation

Before a person embarks on any major dietary change, it's a good idea to check with a doctor, especially if the dieter is markedly obese. A medical checkup may reveal an underlying cause of the obesity or, more likely, concomitant disorders such as high blood pressure, high blood cholesterol, or diabetes, all of which should be treated. It also may reveal reasons why weight loss must be slow to avoid serious harm.

Success is more likely if the diet is followed under professional guidance. A responsible, registered dietitian (R.D.), a physician with training in sound nutrition practices, or a qualified state-licensed nutrition professional can be helpful in structuring a sensible weight-loss diet. A word of caution here, however: As stressed in Chapter 3, most states have no regulations over who can set up practice as nutritionists. Diploma-mill nutritionists and irresponsible ones outnumber the responsible ones. Always check out the qualifications of the promoter before embarking on a weight-loss program; billions of dollars are wasted each year on worthless and even dangerous schemes. (Chapter 3 outlines questions you should ask.) Any responsible weight-loss program will follow the general principles outlined here. (See also Group Dieting and Diet Clinics on page 290.)

Start with a Food Diary

Most dieters are unaware of just how much they eat during the course of a day. An accurate food diary (see Sample Food Diary on page 285) can help pinpoint faulty eating habits. For example, many people find it difficult to dispose of small leftovers, and rather than waste perfectly good food, they will eat those last dabs that are not suitable to store for a future meal. Such people end up storing them in their bodies as fat. Letting someone else clean up after a meal removes the temptation to eat the leftovers.

A food diary also can identify overlooked sources of calories. When trying to remember what they eat, for instance, many people forget that numerous beverages contain calories. Few realize that 22 percent of America's calories come from beverages. Thus, a person who has two or three sodas, a glass of juice, a beer or cocktail, and a couple of glasses of milk during the course of a day can almost unconsciously consume an extra 1,000 calories or so. (See Table 17.5 for a food diary that illustrates this and Table 17.6 for a sample food diary under a weight-loss program.)

Sample Food Diary

In keeping a food diary, write down what you eat or drink immediately; it's almost impossible to accurately recall everything that you've consumed if you wait until the end of the day to do so. You can use a small pocket diary, copies of the form below, or another convenient format. In any instance, the information you record should include the headings listed below:

Date_____ Day of the Week_____

Food Eaten	Time	Circumstance	Amount	Calories
_____	_____	_____	_____	_____
_____	_____	_____	_____	_____
_____	_____	_____	_____	_____
_____	_____	_____	_____	_____
_____	_____	_____	_____	_____
_____	_____	_____	_____	_____
_____	_____	_____	_____	_____
_____	_____	_____	_____	_____
_____	_____	_____	_____	_____
_____	_____	_____	_____	_____
_____	_____	_____	_____	_____
_____	_____	_____	_____	_____
_____	_____	_____	_____	_____

Examine Eating Patterns and Food Habits

These almost unconscious food habits can contribute to weight gain:

- Eating too fast

- Frequent snacking on high-calorie foods

- Skimping on food early in the day, then overeating in the evening

- Substituting juice, soft drinks, beer, and other high-calorie beverages for water

- Adding high-calorie (usually fat-laden) sauces, dressings, and gravies to otherwise low-calorie salads, vegetables, and other dishes

- Use of high-calorie convenience foods (e.g., breaded frozen chicken or fish, take-out fast foods, etc.) instead of plain or homemade

- Eating for reasons other than satisfying hunger, such as to be sociable, ease boredom or frustration, or at the bidding of a parent, spouse, or other well-meaning person who urges overeating

Table 17.5. Examples of One Day's Diary

Food Eaten	Time	Circumstance	Amount	Calories
Cereal	7:30 A.M.	Breakfast	1 cup	150
Low-fat milk	"	"	½ cup	50
Orange juice	"	"	1 glass	110
Coffee with sugar	"	"	1 cup/t	16
Danish roll	11 A.M.	Coffee break	1 medium	350
Cola	"	"	1 can	145
Cheeseburger	12:30 P.M.	Lunch	1 large	305
French fries	"	"	Medium serving	220
Cola	"	"	1 can	145
Potato chips	3 P.M.	Snack	2-oz. pkg.	300
Milk (whole)	"	"	8 oz.	150
Beer	5:30 P.M.	After work	12 oz.	145
Peanuts	"	"	3-oz. pkg.	500
Frozen fried chicken	7:00 P.M.	Dinner	2 pieces	554
French fries	"	"	Medium serving	220
Salad	"	"	1 cup	50
French dressing	"	"	2 T	115
Peas (frozen in sauce)	"	"	½ cup	150
Cola	"	"	1 can	145
Ice cream	"	"	1 cup	300
Coffee/sugar	"	"	1 cup	16
Corn chips	10 P.M.	Watching TV	3-oz. pkg.	450
Cola	"	"	1 can	145
Milk (whole)	11 P.M.	Before bed	1 cup	150
				Total 4886

A glance at this food diary, which is typical of the eating habits of millions of Americans, shows why the person has a weight problem: He simply eats too much. Yet, until keeping a food diary, this person was unaware of just how much high-calorie food he managed to consume during the course of a day. In this particular instance, it was determined that the person—a 43-year-old accountant who weighed 195 pounds and stood 5'9"—would gradually lose weight if he cut his daily food consumption to 1,200 to 1,500 calories a day and, at the same time, started walking a half hour each day. He decided to walk home from work rather than stop in at a pub with his coworkers. Table 17.6 shows a typical day's food intake under his new eating program. Note that except for the afterwork beer and peanuts, it allows the same number of meals and snacks. The low-calorie substitutes are not so different from his usual food choices that he feels deprived, and the meals and snacks are timed to prevent his becoming overly hungry.

- Feeling obligated to take large portions (or even seconds) and to eat everything on the plate

These are but a few common food habits that can result in overeating. A careful examination of a food diary and assessment of personal eating habits can reveal such patterns. Changing these faulty eating patterns—for example, making a conscious effort to eat slowly by taking small bites, chewing thoroughly, and counting to 10 before taking another bite—can both help lose weight during a

food-reduction period and also prevent regaining the lost weight. Simple tricks such as switching to a smaller luncheon plate to make portions look larger and reversing meal patterns—eating a large meal in the morning and a light dinner—also help promote weight loss. (For a list of low-calorie substitutes for high-calorie foods, see Table 17.7.)

Menu Planning

There are hundreds, even thousands, of different weight-loss schemes. These all have

Table 17.6. Examples of One Day's Diary Under Weight-Loss Program

Food Eaten	Time	Circumstance	Amount	Calories
Cereal	7:30 A.M.	Breakfast	1 cup	150
1%-fat milk	"	"	½ cup	50
Orange slices	"	"	1 medium	75
Coffee with sugar	"	"	1 cup/t	16
Wheat crackers	11 A.M.	Coffee break	4 small	35
Seltzer	"	"	1 glass	0
Chicken salad	12:30 P.M.	Lunch	½ cup	125
Rye bread	"	"	2 slices	80
Apple	"	"	1 medium	85
Iced tea/ lemon/ sugar	"	"	Large glass	25
Bagel	3 P.M.	Snack	½	80
Grape jelly (low calorie)	"	"	1 T	25
1%-fat milk	"	"	1 cup	100
Vegetable soup	7 P.M.	Dinner	1 cup	50
Soda crackers	"	"	2	25
Green salad	"	"	1 cup	30
Lemon juice/herbs	"	"	2 T	10
Macaroni, tender	"	"	1 cup	150
Tomato sauce	"	"	½ cup	35
Parmesan, grated	"	"	1 T	25
Steamed broccoli/ lemon	"	"	⅗ cup	40
Sorbet	"	"	½ cup	40
Seltzer	"	"	1 glass	0
Coffee/sugar	"	"	1 cup	16
Popcorn, spicy	10 P.M.	Watching TV	1 cup	50
Diet cola	"	"	1 can	3
1%-fat milk	11 P.M.	Before bed	1 cup	50
				Total 1370

This diet is nutritionally balanced, with food intake timed to prevent hunger. The foods are varied and include enough regular or nearly regular choices (e.g., sorbet instead of ice cream, seltzer or diet cola instead of regular cola, bagel and jelly instead of Danish) so that the person does not feel deprived or on a diet. The above is actually under the allowed 1,500 calories. This regimen, coupled with the increased exercise, should result in a steady weight loss of two to three pounds a week. Once the desired weight of 160 pounds is achieved, the daily caloric intake can be increased to about 2,000 calories to maintain that weight.

Table 17.7. Low-Calorie Substitutes for High-Calorie Foods

As the following examples prove, one can lower the calorie content of many meat dishes simply by trimming away excess fat, removing skin, or slightly altering preparation.

High-Calorie Choice	Serving Size	Calories	Lower-Calorie Choice	Serving Size	Calories
MEATS AND FISH					
Beef brisket, with separable fat, braised	3 oz.	330	Beef brisket, trimmed of separable fat, braised	3 oz.	205
Ground beef	3 oz.	225	Ground round	3 oz.	165
Lamb chop, loin, with separable fat	1 medium	318	Lamb chop, loin trimmed of separable fat	1 medium	116
Lamb chop, shoulder, with separable fat	1 medium	427	Lamb chop, shoulder, trimmed of separable fat	1 medium	185
Pork chop, loin, with separable fat	1 medium	275	Pork chop, loin, trimmed of separable fat	1 medium	165
Chicken, batter-dipped and fried	¼ chicken	673	Chicken, dipped in flour and fried	¼ chicken	422
			Chicken, light and dark meat, with skin, roasted	¼ chicken	358
Breast, meat and skin, roasted	½ breast	195	Breast, without skin, roasted	½ breast	140
Drumstick, meat and skin, roasted	1 medium	110	Drumstick, meat only, roasted	1 medium	75
Duck, meat and skin, roasted	¼ duck	643	Duck, meat only, roasted	¼ duck	222
Oil-packed tuna	3 oz.	280	Water-packed tuna	3 oz.	135
SAUCES AND DRESSINGS					
Béarnaise sauce	1 T	44	Mock béarnaise sauce made with cornstarch and chicken stock	1 T	15
Blue-cheese dressing	1 T	75	Oil & herbed vinegar (⅔ vinegar, ⅓ oil)	1 T	17
French dressing	1 T	85			
Italian dressing	1 T	80			
Russian dressing	1 T	75			
Thousand Island dressing	1 T	60			
MILK AND MILK PRODUCTS					
Whole milk	1 cup	150	Low-fat (1%-fat)	1 cup	100
			Skim (no fat)	1 cup	85
Mayonnaise	1 T	60	Mayonnaise, low-calorie	1 T	20
Sour cream	1 T	25	Mock sour cream	1 T	10
Chocolate milk	1 cup	210	Low-fat chocolate milk (1%-fat)	1 cup	158

Table 17.7. Low-Calorie Substitutes for High-Calorie Foods *(cont.)*

Fresh fruit or fruit packed in water, which is naturally sweet, contains many fewer calories than artificially sweet fruit packed in juice or syrup.

High-Calorie Choice	Serving Size	Calories	Lower-Calorie Choice	Serving Size	Calories
MILK AND MILK PRODUCTS *(CONT.)*					
Ice cream, vanilla	1 cup	350	Ice milk, vanilla	1 cup	180
			Fruit sorbet	½ cup	123
Commercial yogurt with fruit preserves	1 cup	230	Nonfat yogurt with fresh fruit topping	1 cup	125
FRUITS					
Apples, dried	20 slices	310	Apple, fresh	1 8-oz.	125
Applesauce, canned and sweetened	½ cup	97	Applesauce, canned, unsweetened	½ cup	53
Blackberries, canned and in heavy syrup	½ cup	118	Blackberries, fresh	½ cup	35
Blueberries, frozen and sweetened	1 cup	187	Blueberries, frozen and unsweetened	1 cup	80
CAKES AND PIES					
Chocolate devil's food cake with icing	1/12 of 2-layer 9" diameter	378	Chocolate cupcake with icing	1 cupcake	157
Spice cake with icing	1 medium slice	374	Spice cake with brushing of powdered sugar instead of icing	1 medium slice	155
Pound cake	1/10 of a loaf	204	Angel food cake, plain or chocolate	1/12 of 10" diameter	125
Apple pie	1/6 of 9" diameter	405	Deep-dish apple pie	1/8 of 8" diameter	170
Berry pie	1/6 of 9" diameter	380	Meringue	large shell, 9" diameter	60
SNACKS					
Corn chips	10	97	Popcorn, plain	1 cup popped	30
Caramel-coated popcorn	1 cup	134			
Hard pretzels	1 cup	175	Bread sticks	1	43
Peanuts	1 oz.	165			
Dry-roasted pistachio nuts	1 oz.	165	Soy nuts, roasted	⅓ cup	127
Walnuts	1 oz.	180			
Chocolate-covered nuts	1 oz.	155			
Chocolate-covered raisins	28	115	Cucumber and low-fat yogurt dip or low-fat curry-yogurt dip with fresh raw vegetables	1 T	25
			Broccoli or cauliflower florets	½ cup	15
			Carrot sticks	½ cup	24
			Green pepper	1	20

one thing in common: reduced caloric intake. Some weight-reduction diets are rigid and restricted, allowing only a few foods. The Kempner fruit and rice diet—named for the Duke Medical Center physician who originally developed it as a treatment for high blood pressure before antihypertensive drugs were available—is a good example. This diet emphasizes low-calorie foods and is limited to rice, fruit, and perhaps some vegetables. It is boring and nutritionally unsafe, but following it does produce weight loss. A major problem with this diet—and thousands of others that emphasize a restricted regimen—is that it does little to change basic food habits, and as soon as the desired weight loss is attained, the dieter is likely to celebrate by resuming the eating patterns that produced the obesity in the first place. In a few months, the dieter may well be back to his or her original weight.

It is far more sensible to follow a basic food plan, such as the one outlined in Table 17.8, or to adapt your own using the guidelines in Chapter 1. Table 17.9 lists sample menus; see also recipes on pages 292–95.

Group Dieting and Diet Clinics

Many overweight people find they do better when dieting with the support of others who share their problem. In recent years, a number of self-help support groups have gained popularity. Examples include Weight Watchers, Overeaters Anonymous, and TOPS (for Take Off Pounds Sensibly). Some of these use the same principles as Alcoholics Anonymous, others employ a buddy system, and still others offer combinations of diet and exercise programs. The dietary regimens of most of these programs are sensible and have been developed under the guidance of physicians and/or registered dietitians.

Table 17.8. Basic Menu Planner

Following are numbers of servings from different food groups that should be consumed in the course of a day for three different calorie levels.

Food	Typical Portions	Servings per Calorie Level		
		1,200	1,500	1,800
Vegetables	½ cup cooked or 1 cup raw	2	3	3
Fruits	Serving of 75–100 calories	3	3	3
Starches	1 slice bread; ½ cup cooked cereal; ⅔–1 cup dry cereal; ½ cup cooked beans or other starchy vegetable	5	6	8
Protein	3 oz. lean meat, fish or poultry; ½ cup cottage cheese; 1 oz. cheese; 1 T peanut butter; 1 egg	2	2	3
Milk/milk products	1 cup skim or 1%-fat; 2¾ cup nonfat yogurt (See protein group for other foods that can be shifted to this group.)	2	2	3
Fats	1 t margarine, butter, oil; 6–10 nuts; 1 t mayonnaise; 2 t French or other salad dressings made with oil	2	3	3

Free foods: Unlimited amounts of certain low-calorie foods (lettuce, escarole, radishes, watercress, etc.), flavorings (spices, herbs, lime or lemon juices), low- or noncalorie beverages (seltzer, tea, coffee, bouillon or broth) are permitted as desired in all categories.

Refer to calorie-content charts in the appendix to accurately fill in the numbers of calories per serving. Also see sample menus in Table 17.9.

Their major disadvantage is their cost, but there are people who are more likely to stick with something for which they pay.

In addition to organized or franchise weight-loss groups like Weight Watchers or TOPS, there also are many weight-loss clinics. Many of these are affiliated with hospitals, medical schools, and research centers; others are operated by private physicians, registered dietitians, and self-styled nutritionists. When enrolling in a diet clinic, it is important to check out the program in advance and to make sure that it is medically sound. Any program that promises fast, painless weight loss should be suspect.

THINGS TO AVOID

Fad Diets and Repeated Crash Dieting

As noted in the beginning of this chapter, the diet business is a $70-billion-a-year industry, and a large portion of this money is spent on fad or crash diets. By now, it is well known that fad diets simply do not work in the long run; the dieter may lose weight, but there's a 95-percent chance that he or she will regain it all within a year or so. However, more than money is lost on these fad diets; they also are detrimental to health.

Table 17.9.   Sample Menus

1,200 Calories	1,500 Calories	1,800 Calories
BREAKFAST	**BREAKFAST**	**BREAKFAST**
¼ cantaloupe	1 medium orange	½ mango
½ cup oatmeal with sprinkling of cinnamon and sugar	1 poached egg	1 cup puffed cereal with ½ banana
½ cup skim milk	1 English muffin/1 t margarine	½ cup skim milk
Tea/coffee	Tea/coffee	Tea/coffee
MID-MORNING SNACK	**MID-MORNING SNACK**	**MID-MORNING SNACK**
1 cup bouillon	1 cup nonfat yogurt	½ bagel with 1 t margarine
Up to 25 oyster crackers	½ cup fresh berries	½ cup raw vegetable sticks
LUNCH	**LUNCH**	**LUNCH**
1 cup pasta	1 cup lentil soup	Mixed green salad with oil/vinegar dressing
½ cup tomato sauce	2–3 soda crackers	1 cup chili with ½ cup rice
Lettuce/endive salad with French dressing	Lettuce salad with French dressing	Poached pear
1 cup skim milk	Noncalorie strawberry gelatin dessert (a free food)	**MID-AFTERNOON**
MID-AFTERNOON SNACK	**MID-AFTERNOON SNACK**	3–4 graham crackers
4–5 wheat crackers with ¼ cup herbed cottage cheese	1 cup skim milk	1 T peanut butter
Diet cola or tea	Small corn muffin	1 cup skim milk
DINNER	**DINNER**	**DINNER**
Fruit cup	Mixed green salad with Italian dressing	1 cup vegetable soup
3 oz. lean roast beef	1 cup pasta with zucchini/tomato sauce	3 oz. turkey breast
½ cup saffron rice	Angel food cake with ½ cup sliced strawberries	1 medium baked potato with chives
½ cup gingered carrots	**BEFORE BED**	½ cup broccoli spears
Lettuce/endive salad with herbed vinegar	½ cup fresh vegetables	Sherbert
Lemon ice	1 oz. slice Muenster cheese	Tea/coffee
Tea/coffee		**BEFORE BED**
BEFORE BED		English muffin with 2 T tuna salad made with mayonnaise
1 cup skim milk		1 cup skim milk

Recent studies suggest that a yo-yo pattern of going on a very low-calorie diet—less than 1,200 calories a day for men, 1,000 calories for women—then resuming former eating patterns and repeat dieting may actually result in an upward spiral of ever-increasing weight. During a period of semistarvation—which is what a very low-calorie diet represents—the body responds by lowering its metabolic rate. This is actually a survival mechanism, because someone who requires fewer calories to survive during a famine or other extreme food shortage is likely to live longer.

When the dieter resumes his or her usual eating habits, the metabolism does not return to its former level. As a result, the dieter will gain weight even more quickly than before, even if the food intake would normally maintain the desired weight instead of providing excess calories. Each successive crash diet may

SAMPLE RECIPES

Gazpacho

½ green pepper, chopped
1 cucumber, peeled and chopped
1 large stalk of celery, with or without the leaves
1 medium yellow onion
5 large ripe tomatoes, chopped
3 cloves garlic, crushed

Dash cayenne or 2 drops hot sauce
¼ cup vinegar
Water
Accompaniments: croutons made without oil or butter, chopped cucumber, red or green peppers, chopped onions

1. Place ingredients in a blender. Add water to fill. Blend well.

2. Place in refrigerator until chilled (several hours).

3. Serve with the accompaniments.

Serves 6.

Stuffed Tomatoes

4 large ripe tomatoes
1 6½ oz. can water-packed tuna or chicken
1 T low-fat yogurt
1 T low-calorie mayonnaise

1 small stalk celery, diced
Pepper
Lettuce

1. Cut tops off tomatoes and scoop out center.

2. Combine tuna or chicken and the other ingredients (except the lettuce) in a bowl.

3. Fill tomatoes with tuna or chicken mixture. Place on lettuce leaves.

Serves 4.

result in decreased metabolic needs. Studies have found that some people who engage in repeated bouts of crash dieting reach a point where they gain weight if they eat more than 800 or 900 calories a day.

In addition to resetting the BMR at lower levels, crash dieting can result in serious nutritional imbalances; excessive loss of lean muscle tissue, including heart muscle; and with some regimens, biochemical imbalances. In short, any weight-loss diet requires reduced food intake, but it should provide enough va-

---

Broiled Fish

4 filets of fish
  (halibut, sole,
  cod, blue, etc.)
Juice from 2
  lemons
Juice from 3
  limes or 1
  orange
Grated rind from
  1 lemon, 1
  lime, or ½
  orange
3 garlic cloves,
  finely chopped

4 scallions, finely
  chopped
½ green pepper,
  diced
⅔ cup
  mushrooms,
  diced
1 t of fresh basil,
  chopped
1 t of fresh
  parsley,
  chopped
Pepper

1. Marinate the fish for ½ to 1 hour in the juice and rinds from the lemons and limes or oranges.

2. Combine remaining ingredients with the marinade in a small bowl.

3. Place fish on broiler. Pour mixture over fish.

4. Broil for 7 to 10 minutes. Do not overcook.

Serves 4.

Stir-Simmered Chicken

2 cloves of
  minced garlic,
  or a 2-inch
  piece of fresh
  ginger, peeled
  and chopped
½ cup
  mushrooms,
  diced
4 scallions,
  chopped
¼ cup water
  chestnuts,
  chopped
2 chicken breasts,
  without skin,
  cut into 1-inch
  by ½-inch
  pieces

¾ cup broccoli
  florets, chopped
¾ cup zucchini,
  cut in small
  pieces
½ cup orange
  juice
1 T cornstarch
1 T low-salt soy
  sauce

1. Place garlic or ginger, mushrooms, scallions, and water chestnuts in a small amount of water in a nonstick pan and cook for 4 minutes.

2. Add chicken pieces and continue to cook, adding water as needed to prevent scorching. Cook 10 to 15 minutes until chicken is cooked.

3. Add broccoli and zucchini. Dissolve cornstarch in a small amount of orange juice. Add mixture to remaining juice and soy sauce. Pour this mixture into pan. Simmer until the colors of the broccoli and zucchini have brightened, about 3 minutes.

Serves 4 to 6.

Mock Béarnaise Sauce

⅓ cup egg
   substitute (or 4
   egg whites, 1
   egg yolk, and 2
   T corn oil)
2 T lemon juice
   with ½ t
   gelatin
   dissolved in it
2 T reduced-
   calorie
   margarine

½ cup mock sour
   cream
Dash of cayenne
1 T chopped
   parsley
2 t chopped fresh
   tarragon
2 t chopped
   chives

1. Place the egg substitute and lemon juice with gelatin in the top of a double boiler over simmering water. Blend until thickened.
2. Add margarine and stir.
3. Add mock sour cream and stir.
4. Add cayenne and fresh herbs.

Serves 5 to 6.

Steamed Carrots with Mint

Carrots, peeled
   and cut into
   rings

Fresh mint

Place carrots in 1 inch of water with mint. Cook until tender.

Mock Oriental Green Beans

2 cups green
   beans, trimmed
4 scallions,
   chopped
2 cloves of garlic,
   minced

3 t low-salt soy
   sauce
4 to 6 drops hot
   oil

1. Place beans, scallions, garlic, and soy sauce in saucepan with ¾ inch of water.
2. Cook over medium-high heat until bright green and tender enough to eat.
3. Drain and add hot oil.

Serves 4.

Spicy Tofu

3 T low-salt soy
   sauce
2 t peanut oil
6 to 8 drops of
   hot oil

2 cakes tofu, cut
   into 1-inch
   squares
6 scallions,
   chopped

1. Combine soy sauce and oils.
2. Marinate tofu and scallions in mixture for several hours.
3. Serve cold or at room temperature.

Serves 4.

riety and calories for the individual to maintain nutritional status while *gradually* losing weight.

Diet Pills and Formulas

Although there are a number of medications that suppress appetite, they should not be used except under strict medical supervision. Some appetite suppressants are habit-forming. Even those that have been approved by the FDA for nonprescription use carry hazards. Both phenylpropanolamine and benzocaine—ingredients in most over-the-counter diet pills—can raise blood pressure or cause irregular heartbeat. Their appetite suppressant effects are temporary, requiring increased dosage (and risk of side effects).

Some of the newer "diet pills" are nothing more than fiber. While replacing some foods high in calories with foods high in fiber is a legitimate weight-loss strategy, fiber supplements are inappropriate and should be

---

Stuffed Zucchini

4 large zucchini
3 cloves of garlic, minced
1 large onion, chopped
2 large fresh tomatoes, chopped

2 t fresh thyme, chopped
Cayenne
Black pepper
1½ cups cooked brown rice
¾ cup grated low-fat cheddar or Swiss cheese

1. Parboil zucchini until just tender. Remove from heat and pour cold water on them to prevent further cooking. When cool, cut in half lengthwise. Scoop out centers.

2. Place zucchini pulp in a skillet with garlic, onion, tomatoes, thyme and seasonings. Simmer until most of the moisture is removed. Add rice and stir well.

3. Place zucchini in shallow oiled pan. Fill centers with the vegetable mixture. Top with grated cheese. Any remaining mixture can be heated separately.

4. Bake at 350° F. for 30 minutes.

Serve 4.

Brown Rice or Bread Pudding

2 cups skim milk
1½ cups cooked brown rice or 1 cup whole-wheat bread (preferably a little stale) broken into small pieces

1 t cinnamon
½ t nutmeg
1 t vanilla extract
2 eggs, beaten
2 cooking apples, chopped, with skins left on

1. Heat skim milk to just under boiling. Add all ingredients except eggs and apples. Stir well and cook for 2 minutes. Remove from heat.

2. Add beaten eggs and stir well. Add apples.

3. Place in oiled glass dish. Place dish in pan with water. Bake in preheated 350° F. oven until custard is set—about 30 minutes.

Serves 4.

avoided, since they can produce gastrointestinal upsets, nutritional imbalances, and have even produced digestive tract obstruction. Diet candies are of little value in dieting; they have little or no effect in controlling hunger pangs, and sweets generally stimulate rather than kill appetite. Finally, the abuse of laxatives or medications to induce vomiting—both hallmarks of serious eating disorders—have no place in weight control. (See Chapter 19.)

OTHER MEDICAL AND SURGICAL TREATMENTS OF OBESITY

There are instances of extreme obesity in which the excess weight becomes life-threatening. Most of these morbidly obese people have tried dieting without success; for such people, more drastic obesity treatments may be required. Approaches include the following methods.

Liquid Protein Diets

These diets, which allow little or no food other than 300 to 800 calories of a poor-quality protein (collagen or cowhide, for example) are based on the theory that the protein supplements will reduce the loss of muscle (lean body tissue) while fasting. These diets were first introduced in the 1970s and initially generated considerable interest among both the general public and physicians. The FDA tried to forbid direct sale to the public of one low-calorie powder, but the food-supplement industry's Council for Responsible Nutrition got a federal court judge to stop the FDA. By 1978, however, more than 50 deaths had occurred among women who had been on the liquid protein diets for two to three months.

Some of these deaths were attributed to disturbances in heart rhythm, but the precise causes of the fatal results have not been established, although in a number of cases autopsies showed cardiac atrophy. Such a diet should not be confused with the newer protein-sparing regimens that are low in calories but contain higher-quality protein. Although these are safer than the previous liquid-diet formulations, they should be used *only* under careful medical supervision and in conjunction with behavior-modification programs to alter faulty eating habits. These newer formulas, which carry an FDA-mandated warning, can result in rapid weight loss when taken under a physician's guidance. Possible side effects with any extreme weight loss over a short period of time include hair loss, intolerance to the cold, dry skin, and gallstones.

Surgery

Several operations can result in weight loss. These include the following procedures.

Intestinal bypass. In this operation, a portion of the small intestine is removed or bypassed. At first, it was assumed that the resulting weight loss was due to the lack of absorption of digested food. Subsequent studies have found that most of the weight loss is actually due to diarrhea. After 12 to 24 months, the weight loss levels off, and some patients even begin to gain weight, but usually not as much as before the operation. The operation, however, has serious side effects, including fluid and electrolyte imbalances, diarrhea, severe itching, and anal sores. There also have been deaths resulting from the operation, and it is now rarely done.

Gastric bypass or reduction. In this operation, a small pouch is created in the upper part of the stomach so that it cannot hold so much food. Special surgical staples are used. There are not as many complications as with the intestinal bypass, but even so, it is a drastic procedure that can cause numerous serious GI problems, including vomiting, chronic reflux (heartburn), ulceration, perforation of the stapled area, and severe internal bleeding. Follow-up studies have found that some patients lose about 60 percent of their excess weight within two years, but others begin eating more often to make up for the smaller stomach volume, thus defeating the purpose of the operation. Mount Sinai does this operation.

Gastric balloon. This is yet another obesity treatment that failed to live up to its initial enthusiastic promotion. A tube with a deflated balloon was inserted into the stomach, the balloon was released and inflated, and the inserting tube was removed. The idea was that the inflated balloon would give a feeling of fullness and also take up space, thus preventing overeating. Problems with the device included gastrointestinal obstruction and sometimes fatal destruction of bowel tissue.

Surgical fat removal and liposuction. Surgical fat removal is a plastic-surgery procedure in which layers of fat are removed, usually from the abdomen. The operation is complicated and carries the potential for serious side effects, including bleeding, infection, and nerve damage. Among people who are moderately overweight, the so-called tummy tuck has become a popular cosmetic operation. For a markedly obese person, it is not an effective method of weight loss, however.

Liposuction is also more appropriate for cosmetic purposes than for weight loss. This procedure entails injecting a saline solution into fatty tissue and, using small suctioning tubes, vacuuming out the fat. The procedure is used mostly among people under the age of 40 or 50 who want to rid themselves of fatty tissue in their thighs, abdomen, or throat area. Although it is now one of the most popular plastic surgery procedures, it is not without complications, including lumpiness and infection.

SUMMING UP

Obesity is an increasingly common problem among Americans. Despite considerable research, there is still much to learn about why so many people gain weight and have so much difficulty losing it and then keeping it off. Although there are thousands of different weight-loss schemes, devices, and regimens, the surest and safest is still the old-fashioned combination of eating less, exercising more, and having the determination to make a sensible eating and exercise program a lifelong pattern.

Overeaters Anonymous*

For those who compulsively overeat, Overeaters Anonymous may be helpful. Unlike other programs, this program is cost-free. They use the same 12-step recovery program as does Alcoholics Anonymous, have over 11,000 meeting groups around the world, and can be reached at: Overeaters Anonymous, World Service Office, 4025 Spencer Street, #203, Torrance, CA 90503, tel: 213–542–8363.

This section written by Victor Herbert, M.D., F.A.C.P.

18

Genetic Considerations

Artemis P. Simopoulos, M.D.

■

INTRODUCTION

"You are what you eat" is an old saying. This might be more accurately stated, you are what your body absorbs and metabolizes. Although these two processes are affected by what we eat, the efficiency of each is genetically determined. The nutrients absorbed from food are broken down inside the body cells (metabolized) to produce energy and essential substances for cell growth. The performance of particular cells in metabolizing specific nutrients can vary from one person to another, and it is this variation that is frequently due to an individual's genetic inheritance.

Genes control many physiologic components, including digestion, absorption, and metabolism. That genetic factors can affect the ability of a person's cells to function chemically is less apparent but just as important as the more obvious hereditary traits, such as eye color.

Over 140 years ago, scientists began to deduce the existence of genes, which are blueprints for specific traits, and to study patterns of inheritance. Today, advances in biomedical research are enabling us to understand more about genetic processes and disorders, including those involving nutrients.

To date, more than 2,000 diseases and disorders have been linked to specific genetic abnormalities. Five percent of the American population—about 12 million people—suffer from such disorders. Researchers believe that many more illnesses will be shown to have ties to inheritance, and numerous recent scientific advances stress the role of genetics in health and illness.

The role of genetics in human disease can be seen most clearly in the so-called single-gene disorders, which range from relatively minor conditions, such as color blindness, to devastating illnesses, such as Tay-Sachs or sickle-cell disease. However, there is evidence now that many common diseases such as atherosclerosis, hypertension, diabetes, and cancer involve not only changes in genes or a genetic predisposition to the illness but also dietary factors that may enhance or inhibit the expression of genetic predispositions.

Genetic predispositions to arthritis, allergies, and digestive diseases such as colitis and ileitis have been well documented. Heredity seems to play an important role in increasing the susceptibility to several common forms of cancer, asthma (but not bronchitis and emphysema), polycystic kidney disease, depression and schizophrenia, and alcoholism. To some degree, every illness—from a mild cold to life-threatening cancer—may be affected by a person's inherited ability to combat it. Questions are raised as scientists make discoveries in this wide and complex field. It may seem that genetics is a subject overly complex for a book on the practical aspects of nutrition. However, because it is basic to many of the fundamentals of nutrition, it is important to provide an overview of the science and its relationship to nutrition.

HEREDITY

Heredity is the means by which parents transmit characteristics to their offspring; genetics is the study of heredity. The study of genetics at the level of the molecule is a twentieth-century science, but humankind has been involved in the application of this knowledge for at least 10,000 years, from the beginnings of agriculture. Wild plants were selectively bred for desirable characteristics; for example, various kinds of wheat were developed from wild grasses. The domestic pig is a cousin to the wild boar. Even though the theory behind the experiments on crops and animals remained largely uninvestigated, succeeding generations of farmers developed relatively sophisticated breeding techniques.

In early nineteenth-century Europe, theories regarding evolution, based on observations of fossils, were being formulated. For example, Lamarck believed that an organism's changing biological needs promoted a change in its habits, which, in turn, resulted in acquired characteristics that could be passed on to its offspring. Thus, an animal that ate tree leaves would constantly stretch its neck to reach higher leaves and, over generations, would improve its ability to do this, eventually ending up as a giraffe.

Darwin's concept of natural selection supplanted Lamarck's ideas about heritable acquired characteristics. According to natural selection, there are individual variations within a species. In competition with others, those best fitted to their environment are the most likely to survive and thus pass on their individual characteristics.

Although Darwin described relationships and probable genealogies, he did not know what the mechanisms of inheritance and change were. It is unlikely that he read the obscure scientific papers of an Austrian monk named Gregor Mendel, who lived at the same time as he did. In 1865, Mendel discovered the principles of heredity, but his work was not recognized until the turn of the century, well after his death. Although Mendel did not uncover the actual mechanisms of inheritance and change, modern genetics is based on his work.

Figure 18.1 shows the result of a Mendelian experiment with the inheritance of flower color in pea plants. Mendel crossed a red-flowered (*RR*) plant with a white-flowered (*rr*) plant. (The traits are represented by double letters because each plant has a maternal and paternal component.) All the offspring from the *RR* by *rr* cross had red (*Rr*) flowers. In this case, the color red overwhelmed white; thus red may be said to be the dominant trait, and white the recessive trait. This usage later gave rise to the terms *dominant* and *recessive* with regard to genes; however, it should be noted that a trait, such as flower color, is not necessarily equivalent to a gene, since a trait may be the result of the interaction of several genes.

Mendel noted that it did not matter whether the red plant was male or female; the results were the same, independent of sex. (Later, of course, some genetic conditions were shown to be sex-linked.)

When he backcrossed the first generation

(*Rr*) with the red parent (*RR*), only red flowers resulted (*RR* and *Rr* in a 1:1 ratio). However, backcrossing the first generation (*Rr*) with the white parent (*rr*) produced equal amounts of red-flowered plants and white-flowered plants (*Rr* and *rr* in a 1:1 ratio).

Crossing the first-generation plants (*Rr*) with one another produced *RR*, *Rr*, *Rr*, and *rr* in equal proportions; in terms of color, this meant three red for every one white. These second-generation white-flowered (*rr*) plants fit the description of genetic throwbacks.

GENES

In the early twentieth century, the gene was recognized as the fundamental unit in the transmission of hereditary characteristics. Genes occur on chromosomes, which are paired structures that appear in the cell nucleus prior to cell division. Each human body cell has 23 pairs of chromosomes. Damaged or otherwise abnormal chromosomes and missing or extra chromosomes can influence inheritance through their effect on the genes that they carry. Most genetic change or muta-

Figure 18.1. Mendelian Experiment with Inheritance of Flower Color in Pea Plants

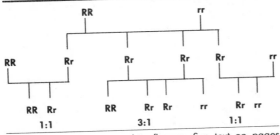

RR = red flowers; rr = white flowers. See text on pages 299–300 for commentary.

tion is restricted to the actual genes, however, and the changes are mostly minor rather than drastic.

For the most part, the actual mutations involve a gene passing on a message different from the one it transmits normally. The chromosomes, in which genes are located, consist of strands of DNA (deoxyribonucleic acid), which is the basic genetic material of all cells. Each DNA molecule usually consists of paired chains of nucleotides in the form of a double helix. The gene is the actual part of the DNA molecule that specifies the code for a particular function. The function of many genes is to specify the structure of polypeptides, which are precursors of amino acids, the building blocks of proteins. Any change in such a gene's message results in a somewhat different polypeptide. This altered polypeptide may or may not result in an amino acid or protein that is impaired in its chemical functioning.

Genetic change usually results from a very small variation in an individual gene. The changed gene most often performs its function in a faultless way but with a slightly different result. This mutation may or may not be beneficial or it may be neutral. When such a changed gene establishes itself in a population, it can no longer be regarded as abnormal in the strict sense, although it may be highly undesirable. The various versions of a particular gene are known as alleles. Often it is not possible to decide which allele was the original one; in fact, the original version may have become extinct in competition with later improved models.

The presence of a genetic variation does not necessarily always produce a change, since the variation may be recessive rather than dominant or may require interaction with other genes or factors. The first-generation plants in Figure 18.1 provide a simple example. When these red-flowered (*Rr*) plants are bred with one another, they produce three unchanged red-flowered plants (one *RR* and two *Rr*) for every changed white-flowered (*rr*) plant. Because of the dominance of red over white, the real frequency of genetic variation is not reflected by the frequency of change evident in the offspring.

Rr genes are a dissimilar pair, and are called heterozygous. Similar pairs, such as *RR* and *rr*, are termed homozygous. Some genetically transmitted human diseases are latent in the heterozygous (*Rr*) condition; some only manifest themselves as a homozygous recessive (*rr*).

In 1902, the first genetic disorder (alcaptonuria, a hereditary metabolic disorder characterized by dark-colored urine) was reported by Sir Archibald Garrod, who coined the term *Inborn Errors of Metabolism* for the inherited metabolic diseases due to single-gene defects (described on page 306). With Darwin's cousin Francis Galton, Garrod ranks as a founder of medical genetics. He postulated a genetic basis for all human biochemical individuality, which is the basis of our understanding of health and disease in man. In 1941, Beadle and Tatum developed the "one gene-one enzyme" hypothesis and thus formulated the crucial role of genes in life processes.

In the 1950s, the scientific study of human chromosomes led to the understanding of chromosomal defects in causing congenital anomalies, retardation, and reproductive failure. The study of chromosomal anomalies led to the assignment and mapping of the location of certain genes on certain chromosomes.

In the 1970s, the development of a powerful new technology for the manipulation and analysis of DNA expanded the field of molecular genetics and research into the human genome (the complete set of hereditary factors contained in the arrangement of genes on our 23 chromosomes) for application to the prevention of disease. Further investigation into this area should also clarify the interactions of genetics with environmental factors, including diet. It is expected that many of the common conditions, such as coronary heart disease, hypertension, and diabetes mellitus, that have genetic components will be more precisely diagnosed and treated.

HUMAN VARIABILITY

Human populations represent storehouses of genetic variability. Advances in genetic studies over the past 30 years have pinpointed significant variability in biochemical and immunologic characteristics for individuals; these involve many enzymes, proteins, blood groups, HLA systems, and so on. By using DNA probes (DNA probes are single-stranded DNA fragments that are given radioactive labels to permit their mapping when they bind to specific genes or to DNA sequences), researchers can analyze mutations or track the inheritance of genes through families. This method detects important differences in the DNA sequence of a normal gene and a changed or mutant gene.

Individual humans vary widely genetically, even within apparent uniform subgroups. One study compared many different proteins from hundreds of individuals; for a third of the proteins, variant forms existed in 2 percent of the individuals.

Every healthy person carries four to eight harmful genes. The great majority of genetic variations seem to have no detectable advantages or disadvantages, however. Of course, with a sudden change in environment, some of these previously neutral variations may become advantageous and ensure the survival of those who possess them.

Just as predisposition to disease is much

harder to observe than a heritable characteristic, so, too, are the structure and quantity of enzymes a person possesses, even though these characteristics may be just as familially typical, and perhaps a lot more important, for the individual as is eye color.

Genetic variability underlies many of the nutritional factors. It appears that the first people to show signs of disease in the face of dietary excess or deficiency are people who have genetic predispositions to these diseases.

The Nature/Nurture Issue

Diseases that run in families need not always have a genetic component. A family's lifestyle can at times have powerful influence on the development of certain diseases among family members.

Understanding how much of an individual's characteristics are determined by nature (genes) and how much by nurture (environment) is crucial for preventing and treating disorders resulting from the interaction of genes and environment. Methods of computer analysis are being developed to study the relationships between many human characteristics—both genetic and nongenetic, such as food preferences, specific lifestyles, and cultural and other environmental variables—in order to determine how these affect family-related traits. For example, susceptibility to heart disease may be influenced by the interaction of cultural factors such as food choices *and* genetic factors related to metabolism.

It is now possible to identify predisposition to heart disease, hypertension, colon cancer, and breast cancer for predictive medicine and health care by studying "candidate" genes. A candidate gene is one that causes a disorder. Already 4,300 such genes have been mapped. (The total human genome, however, contains 50,000 to 100,000 genes.)

Using molecular genetics, which combines family genetic studies with the new recombinant DNA techniques, it is possible to develop diagnostic tests for specific inherited diseases. Predictive tests called RFLPs have been developed. These use genetic markers referred to as Restriction Fragment Length Polymorphisms. RFLPs have great potential for human gene mapping, and they have already been used with considerable success in the analysis of certain genetic diseases. RFLPs, inherited as simple Mendelian codominant markers, can be used as markers of a gene even when the gene itself has not been isolated or even mapped and without any knowledge of its biochemical product. It has been estimated that 150 RFLPs spaced throughout the genome would, in principle, be enough to allow any human gene to be mapped.

Figure 18.2. Diagnostic Process Using Genetic Markers

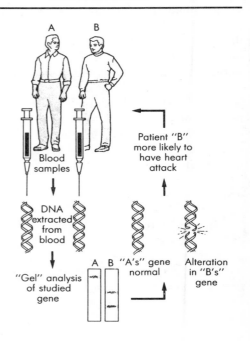

Some of these genetic markers are indicative of an individual's susceptibility to cardiovascular disease and others are indicative of decreased susceptibility to the disease (see figures 18.2 and 18.3). These markers are specific for susceptibility to cardiovascular disease, whereas cholesterol levels are not. Several significant diseases are already known to be linked to RFLPs. If the pace of discovery continues, it soon should be possible to show linkage of almost any disease locus to an RFLP, map it, and use the information in genetic medicine both for prevention and prediction of disease susceptibility. This concept of using genetic markers as diagnostic tools is being applied to other diseases such as hypertension and mental illness.

The genetic approach for the prevention of disease and promotion of health is based on the analysis of each individual's genetic blueprint, or genotype. Such a carefully targeted approach is different from the current preventive medicine shotgun approach in which universal rules of avoidance or moderation are recommended for everyone. The genetic approach, which clearly indicates that not everyone is equally vulnerable to all threats, spares those who are not susceptible from the unnecessary fears of health problems that will never materialize for them, as well as from onerous dietary prescriptions that are not relevant for them. For those whose individual genetic endowment may fail to protect them from a particular condition, knowing so may encourage them to modify their diets.

However, in the underdeveloped areas of the world where there is a lack of basic nutrients and the chance of exposure to disease-causing organisms and parasites, universal rules of preventive medicine make more sense (and save on medical costs).

Assessing individual nutritional needs may be most important in single-gene defects (discussed later on page 306); however, an assessment of an individual's genetic profile is also applicable to multifactorial diseases and can help to identify persons at specific risk so that they can benefit from dietary management. For example, about one-third of the adult population has hyperlipidemia (high blood levels of lipids), particularly in the form of high blood cholesterol. Because hyperlipidemia may predispose an individual to coronary heart disease, it has been recommended that the whole population be treated by dietary modification. However, the hyperlipidemia and the resulting artherosclerosis relate mainly to specific gene defects in some cases and to dietary factors in others. These different forms of hyperlipidemia do not re-

Figure 18.3. An Example of Genetic Markers Associated with Cardiovascular Disease

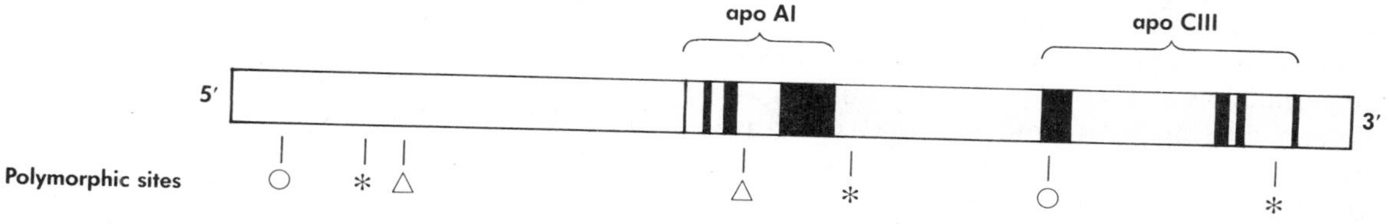

*Markers associated with a high risk of cardiovascular disease
△Markers associated with a reduced risk of cardiovascular disease
○Markers showing no association with cardiovascular disease

spond equally to a universal dietary prescription. The preferred approach is tailored to the individual: diagnosis before treatment, identification of the individual who has a genetic form of hyperlipidemia that may require drug therapy, or a form where specific dietary management is needed to reduce the risk.

In the genetic form, despite normal or low amounts of cholesterol and saturated fats in the diet, severe high blood cholesterol will still be present because of a genetic defect in the metabolism of cholesterol. This form responds to drug treatment. In the nongenetic variety of hypercholesterolemia, the genotype of the individual is normal, but excessive cholesterol and saturated fats in the diet raise the individual's serum-cholesterol level. This environmentally or diet-induced form of hypercholesterolemia may respond to changes in the diet—such as decreasing saturated fats and cholesterol, eating more fish—and to weight loss and exercise.

GENES, RISK FACTORS, AND HEART DISEASE

As early as 1897, Sir William Osler, the famed Canadian physician, recognized the importance of genetic factors in heart disease. Since then, hypercholesterolemia and hypertriglyceridemia have been recognized as significant predisposing factors in heart disease. An estimated 0.6 to 1 percent of the population carries any one of three genes that cause hyperlipidemia. The evidence for single-gene defects causing hyperlipidemia was obtained by examining the survivors of heart attacks and their relatives who had high blood lipids. There are three types of hyperlipidemic trait: isolated hypercholesterolemia, isolated hypertriglyceridemia, and combined hyperlipidemia. One allele (alternative forms of a gene occupying corresponding sites on chromosomes) is responsible for familial hypercholesterolemia. It is carried by 0.1 to 0.2 percent of the general population. A second allele is responsible for familial hypertriglyceridemia in 0.2 to 0.5 percent of the general population. A third allele is responsible for familial combined hyperlipidemia in 0.3 to 0.5 percent of the people.

In total, these hyperlipidemia genes occur in about 1 percent of Americans, or more than 2 million people. Early recognition and identification of such persons could offer an opportunity to direct preventive measures toward those at high risk for coronary heart disease.

Epidemiologic studies have identified risk factors that contribute to the development of coronary heart disease, such as smoking, hypertension, serum cholesterol, diabetes, and obesity. The emphasis has been to control these risk factors through lifestyle changes, predominantly through antismoking campaigns, the education program on high blood pressure, and more recently through the cholesterol education program.

In parallel with these efforts research has identified coronary heart disease risk factors with *genetic* determinants, such as early onset of coronary disease in a first-degree relative (parent or sibling), familial hypercholesterolemia, familial hypertriglyceridemia and combined hyperlipidemia, LDL receptor activity, HDL cholesterol, clotting factors, blood pressure, insulin level and insulin response, and many other genetically determined factors. In fact, it has been estimated that heritability accounts for 63 percent toward the development of coronary disease (single-gene defects 15 to 20 percent; remaining genetic factors 43 percent, most likely explained by multifactorial inheritance [gene-environmental interaction]). Some feel that more single-gene defects will be identified as predisposing to coronary heart disease.

The percentage of dietary cholesterol that is absorbed by the body and the level of serum cholesterol are controlled by genes that determine the nature of the protein parts of lipoproteins, producing higher rates of coronary heart disease in Finns (who absorb more cholesterol) than in Japanese (who absorb less), and an intermediate frequency in Minnesotans. Genetic screening early in life will identify those at risk for increased absorption of cholesterol from foods, who ought to avoid foods high in cholesterol (for example, eggs and organ meats).

Genetically determined lipoprotein Lp(a) promotes clotting and atherosclerosis. Omega 3 fatty acids decrease elevated serum Lp(a) levels when they are above 20 mg/dl. Since omega 3 fatty acids appear to lower serum Lp(a), it is important to carry out clinical trials to see if lowering the Lp(a) by diet—using fish or fish oils—will decrease the risk for coronary disease with mild familial hypercholesterolemia. Similarly, all drugs used to lower serum cholesterol level should be examined to make sure that they do not *raise* serum Lp(a) levels.

These recent findings emphasize the interaction of our genetic blueprints and what we eat. Dietary cholesterol intake should be low in patients with genetic blueprints for high cholesterol absorptions, and omega 3 fatty acid intake should be high in patients with genetic blueprints for elevated serum Lp(a) levels.

Present knowledge is still limited on the combined effect of the various risk factors. It is becoming clear that markers that are genetically linked to disease loci will also be useful in the study of cardiovascular-risk-factor profiles. Future research should lead to the recovering of major genes influencing risk factors and to the recognition of specific gene-environmental interactions in patients and their relatives with or without coronary dis-ease. New information will improve the ability to identify at an early stage (childhood and early adult) persons susceptible to the disease. In this way, individuals at high risk will be able to take full advantage of all available preventive measures.

High Blood Pressure

High blood pressure, or hypertension, is another example of multifactorial disease, involving both environmental and genetic factors. Genetic factors have long been assumed to be most important in the development of hypertension, a view supported by both animal and human studies. For example, in families where there are both natural and adopted children, the blood pressures of the latter do not fall into the same close grouping as those of the natural children and parents, thus supporting the importance of genetic rather than environmental factors. Genetic markers based on RFLPs have also been developed as a diagnostic test for an individual's susceptibility to hypertension.

The genetic link is also supported by evidence that patients with similar degrees of high blood pressure vary considerably in the course and prognosis of their disease, response to salt restriction, calcium intake, and to treatment with different antihypertensive drugs.

There are about 60 million Americans diagnosed as having hypertension; less than half respond to salt restriction. It is important to distinguish between the patients who respond to salt restriction and those who do not. Salt restriction, like other forms of therapy, should be applied only to those patients in whom its effectiveness has been established.

Patients who respond to salt restriction also respond to diuretics. Therefore, diuretic treatment has provided a convenient alternative to the lack of palatability of a strict low-salt diet. As with salt restriction, only 25 to 50 percent of hypertensives respond to diuretics by demonstrating a significant fall in blood pressure.

Sodium balance, blood volume, and blood pressure are all regulated simultaneously by the renin-aldosterone system, which controls the rate of sodium excretion. In the normal person, there is a relationship between secretion of renin—an enzyme produced by the kidneys—and the rate of sodium excreted in the urine. When salt intake is low, plasma-renin activity rises, and when sodium intake is high, plasma-renin activity falls (or is suppressed). Aldosterone, an adrenal hormone, triggers renin release.

Some patients with hypertension, however, have an abnormally low plasma-renin activity or an abnormally high renin activity regardless of their salt intake. With low plasma-renin activity, the kidneys perceive the blood as containing too much sodium and the body responds with a rise in blood pressure. As expected, this type of patient responds best to a reduction in salt, either by dietary restriction or diuretic treatment. In patients with a high renin value, known as high-renin essential hypertension, the kidneys inappropriately perceive a shortage of sodium and the renin excess is a basis for the hypertension. In these patients, salt restriction is not likely to be helpful because the patient will respond by producing more renin and aldosterone. The plasma-renin level based on the rate of sodium excretion provides a marker that helps identify the hypertensive patient that could be helped by a low-sodium diet. A patient with low renin will respond to low salt intake by showing a decrease in blood pressure.

The national public-health policy for limiting sodium intake is not warranted by current evidence and is not likely to be successful in the prevention or treatment of hypertension. The genetic approach of early identification through genetic markers of the individual prone to hypertension; the management through nutritional means (salt restriction), based on the individual's response to salt; and the identification of low renin combine to offer a more sensible approach.

INBORN ERRORS OF METABOLISM

An inborn error of metabolism is due to a heritable gene mutation affecting the breakdown of nutrients in the body cells. Such disorders are caused primarily by the mutation of a single gene or a small number of related genes, rather than by mutations of multiple genes interacting with the environment, or by chromosome abnormalities. Not all these genetic mutations involving cell metabolism result in disorders. As with other mutations, many seem to have no detectable effects. For obvious reasons, mutations that cause metabolic disorders are the ones most closely studied. Many types of inborn errors of metabolism occur. Only those conditions that respond to nutritional therapy are considered here.

Inborn errors of metabolism have been shown to be caused by defects in structural proteins, functioning proteins, transport proteins, and gene-regulating proteins. Most of the disorders considered here result from a block in a metabolic pathway caused by the mutation of one particular gene.

ENZYME DEFECTS

Many inborn errors of metabolism are caused by enzyme defects, the enzyme being the protein affected by the gene mutation. An enzyme is a catalyst; that is, it brings about or accelerates chemical reactions without becoming greatly consumed itself. An inborn error of metabolism is usually caused by abnormal enzyme function in major metabolic pathways. (A metabolic pathway is a sequence of chemical steps normally followed.) Four types of inborn errors of metabolism are caused by enzyme defects.

1. *Accumulation of a precursor to toxic levels.* This is the most common inborn error of metabolism. Here, a substance that is normally changed to something else in a reaction builds up in the body tissues because the reaction is not functioning properly.

2. *Deficiency of end product.* A poorly functioning reaction can be responsible for the absence or insufficiency of a particular end product, thereby affecting health.

3. *Production of toxic by-products from a normally minor metabolic pathway.* When a major metabolic pathway is blocked, a minor pathway that has its own characteristic products may be utilized. This can result in production of large quantities of substances usually present in only small amounts.

4. *Overproduction of intermediate products through loss of feedback control.* A reaction that is governed by feedback from a particular end product that is manufactured may go out of control in the absence or insufficiency of that end product due to faulty enzyme action.

OTHER DISORDERS

Defective plasma-membrane transport. Here the cell membranes do not function properly in permitting substances to pass through them into or out of the cells. These disorders mostly concern the kidney tubules and intestinal absorptive cells.

Reduced coenzyme production or binding. These are known as vitamin-dependent inborn errors or vitamin-dependency syndromes. A large number of these disorders occur, but few are understood.

Deficiency or abnormality of circulating proteins. Nutritional therapy is effective with very few disorders of proteins in the blood circulation.

Abnormality of structural protein. Disorders of collagen-related proteins do not respond well to nutritional therapy.

Abnormalities of enzymes that regulate drug metabolism. Avoidance of the drugs, rather than diet therapy, is usually recommended for these disorders.

NUTRITIONAL THERAPY

Although comparatively few inborn errors of metabolism respond to nutritional therapy, such treatment when effective can save lives and avoid mental retardation. In the future, genetic engineering may do much to repair or replace the destructive mutations that cause the disorders. At present, however, so little is known about these conditions that genetic engineering techniques alone would not be the solution. Today, five general nutritional therapeutic approaches are in use. Each approach is geared to a particular type of disorder.

1. *For accumulation of precursor to toxic levels:* The nutritional source of the precursor is restricted. If this source occurs widely in food, dietary counseling and menu planning may be necessary. When an essential nutrient must be restricted, close attention must be paid to en-

sure that the minimum daily requirement of the nutrient is consumed. For example, when a particular amino acid essential to a child's growth must be restricted, there may be very little difference between excess quantity—causing illness—and insufficient quantity—resulting in inadequate growth.

2. *For deficiency of end product:* Missing or insufficient reaction end products are replaced.

3. *For production of toxic by-product:* The nutritional source of the by-product's precursor in the reaction is restricted.

4. *For sensitivity to drugs and environmental factors:* Exposure to these nonnutritional factors is avoided as much as possible.

5. *For deficient coenzymes:* Increased amounts of the vitamins lacking are administered.

Nutritional therapy often proves to be a challenge for both the family and physician. The patient, usually a child, has biochemical needs that change with growth, and these needs must be met, in some cases with great accuracy. The child's progress and medication, which may need frequent adjustment, must be closely monitored by the physician. The family can help ensure that the child stays on the diet by providing encouragement, variety in foods, and attractive menus.

EFFECTS OF METABOLIC DISORDERS

The effects of metabolic disorders vary widely. Some impose no serious limitations, whereas others quickly cause changes in the central nervous system, which can result in mental retardation. The most severe disorders can cause death shortly after birth. In some conditions, the effects appear in the first few days of life, while other conditions, such as gout, may take years to develop.

If some disorders are not diagnosed and treated quickly, they typically cause severe mental retardation. An infant's brain develops at such a fast rate that any impediment to its progress may result in irreversible damage.

Table 18.1 shows some genetic disorders that respond to nutritional therapy. For conditions discussed elsewhere (such as hypertension, atherosclerosis, hypercholesterolemia, hyperlipidemia, and diabetes), see the relevant chapters.

HEMOCHROMATOSIS (IRON OVERLOAD)

Hemochromatosis or iron overload is an inborn error of metabolism that causes the intestine to absorb more iron from food than the body needs. Since no iron-excretion system exists, the excess iron is stored in body tissues. The iron-loading gene responsible for this condition is recessive and perhaps the most common abnormal gene among Americans. Approximately 10 percent of Americans inherit one iron-loading gene (heterozygous), and about 1 in every 250 is born with two such genes (homozygous).

An individual with one iron-loading gene absorbs just a little more iron than normal, and therefore is less likely to develop an iron deficiency during the three times in life when this is common: the first four years, the onset of puberty, and, for women, the childbearing years. The fact that the heterozygous (single-gene) individual shows some clinical symptoms is interesting, because it is often assumed that such recessive genes give rise to detectable abnormalities only when homozygous.

A person with two iron-loading genes

has such a sharply increased absorption of iron from food that if not treated, he or she eventually dies from iron overload. The iron gradually piles up in the pancreas, destroying insulin-secreting cells and causing the onset of diabetes. Some people are treated for conventional diabetes for years instead of for iron overload, which can be prevented by a chelating agent, a drug that draws iron out of the food in the intestine, and out of the body tissues.

Some people with homozygous genes develop liver damage with symptoms similar to those of hepatitis. Others develop what looks like rheumatoid arthritis because of iron buildup in the joints. Iron accumulation in the heart causes cardiac arrythmias. Excess iron may also cause fatigue, impotence, early menopause, sterility, or cancer.

No method of detecting the abnormal gene has yet been devised. However, it is a mistake to believe that hemochromatosis can be diagnosed only when the disease is fully developed and organs have been damaged. A blood test yielding a serum iron greater than 160 milligrams per milliliter and an iron-binding capacity greater than 60 percent suggests the possibility of hemochromatosis.

Most affected people do not know they are accumulating iron at dangerous levels. Although iron overload is twice as common as iron deficiency in men, large numbers of people are convinced that deficiency is actually a more common problem. Indeed, many take iron supplements in the mistaken notion that these are in their best interest, when in reality, they worsen the situation. (Further information may be obtained from Iron Overload Diseases, Inc., 224 Datura Street, Suite 912, West Palm Beach, Florida 33401; telephone 305–659–5616.)

HOMOCYSTINURIA (HCU)

Three forms of homocystinuria (HCU) are recognized. All three are inborn errors in the metabolism of the essential amino acid methionine. (Essential in this sense means it is not manufactured by the body and therefore must be obtained from the diet.) In one form, the blood levels of methionine are high; in the other two forms, the blood levels are low. The form with high levels is caused by the lack of the enzyme cystathionine synthetase, due to a recessive trait. This is one of the most common genetic abnormalities among Americans. One of the remaining forms is caused by deranged vitamin B_{12} metabolism, and the other by insufficient levels of reductase enzyme.

Homocystinuria is nearly as common as phenylketonuria (PKU), and about one-half the cases are associated with mental retardation. (See page 312 for a discussion of PKU.) Other symptoms include ectopia lentis (dislocation of the eye's lens) and a number of skeletal deformities. In the classic form of the disorder, lack of the enzyme cystathionine synthetase causes increased blood levels of methionine and the intermediate product homocystine; the latter is excreted in the urine in large quantities. Premature blood clots in arteries and veins are frequent occurrences and are responsible for sudden death, which can occur as early as childhood.

The main goal of nutritional therapy is to lower the intake of precursors of homocystine while at the same time supplying the essentials for growth and development. Diagnosis at birth and treatment in early infancy allow normal physical and mental growth.

Pyridoxine therapy is effective in some cases; in this therapy, a normal but not excessive intake of proteins is permitted. For those who do not respond to this therapy, diets low in methionine and adequate in cysteine are

Table 18.1. Genetic Disorders for Which Nutrient Intake Should Be Modified

Disorder	Therapy
Abetalipoproteinemia	Medium-chain triglycerides and vitamins A, E supplements
Acrodermatitis enteropathica	Zinc sulfate supplement
Alkaptonuria (ochronosis)	Ascorbic acid supplement; phenylalanine, tyrosine restriction
Anemia: hypochromic, sideroblastic	Pyridoxine supplement
Argininemia	Protein restriction; essential amino acids supplement; ornithine supplement
Argininosuccinic aciduria	Arginine, benzoic acid supplements; protein restriction
Beta-methylcrotonylglycinuria	Leucine restriction
β-sitosterolemia	Plant sterol restriction
Biotinidase deficiency	Biotin supplement
Branched-chain α-ketoaciduria	Branched-chain amino acid restriction; thiamine supplement
Carbamylphosphate synthetase deficiency	Arginine, benzoic acid supplements; protein restriction; essential amino acids
Chédiak-Higashi syndrome	Ascorbic acid supplement
Chloride diarrhea	Sodium chloride supplement
Citrullinemia	Protein restriction; essential amino acids; arginine and benzoic acid supplements
Combined hyperlipidemia	Calorie, carbohydrate, saturated fatty acid restriction; nicotinic acid and lovastatin and compactin therapy; cholestyramine
Cystathioninuria	Pyridoxine supplements
Cystic fibrosis	Enteric enzyme supplements (trypsin, lipase, chymotrypsin)
Cystinosis	Alkali; cysteamine, phosphate; vitamin D supplements
Diabasic aminoaciduria	Arginine supplement; protein restriction
Diabetes insipidus	Water; low-solute diets; vasopressin
Diabetes mellitus	Insulin; controlled diet
Ehlers-Danlos syndrome; lysyl hydroxylase defect	Ascorbic acid supplement
Folic acid reductase deficiency	N^5-formyltetrahydrofolic acid supplement
Folic acid transport defect	Parenteral folate supplement
Fructose intolerance	Fructose-free diet
Fructose-1,6-diphosphatase deficiency	Frequent glucose; folate supplement; reduced fructose intake
Galactokinase deficiency	Galactose-restricted diet
Galactosemia	Galactose-restricted diet
Glucose-galactose malabsorption	Glucose, galactose restrictions; fructose supplement
Glucose-6-phosphate dehydrogenase deficiency	Avoidance of fava bean and drugs that cause erythrocyte hemolysis
Glutamate-aspartate transport defect	Glutamine supplement
Glutaric acidemia	Protein restriction
Glycogen storage	
type I (glucose-6-phosphatase deficiency)	Frequent feeding; complex starch supplement
type III (amylo-1,6 glucosidase deficiency)	Frequent feeding; high-protein diet
type VI (phosphorylase deficiency)	Frequent feeding
type VIII (phosphorylase kinase deficiency)	Avoid fasting, high-protein diet
Gout	Purine restriction; allopurinol
Hartnup disease	Nicotinamide supplement
Homocystinuria	
cystathionine β-synthase deficiency	Methionine restriction; cysteine supplement; pyridoxine and betaine supplements

Table 18.1. Genetic Disorders for Which Nutrient Intake Should Be Modified *(cont.)*

Disorder	Therapy
N^5,N^{10}-methylenetetrahydrofolate reductase deficiency	Folic acid supplement
CH_3-cobalamin deficiency	Parenteral B_{12}
Hydroxykynureninuria	Nicotinic acid supplement
Hyperbeta-alaninemia	Pyridoxine supplement
Hypercholesterolemia	Restriction of saturated fatty acids and cholesterol; lovastatin and compactin, nicotinamide, cholestyramine supplementation
Hyperlipoproteinemia I	Fat-free diet; medium-chain triglyceride and essential fatty acid supplements
Hyperphenylalaninemia	
dihydropteridine reductase deficiency	Phenylalanine restriction; carbidopa; 5-hydroxytryptophan; BH_4
biopterin biosynthetic blocks	Tetrahydrobiopterin carbidopa; 5-OH-tryptophan
Hypertriglyceridemia	Weight reduction; carbohydrate restriction
Hypophosphatemia	Vitamin D, phosphorus supplements
Isovaleric acidemia	Leucine restriction; glycine supplements; L-carnatine supplements
Ketoacidosis of infancy	Alkali, glucose supplements
Lactic acidosis, intermittent	
(pyruvate decarboxylase deficiency)	High-fat, low-carbohydrate diet; thiamine supplement; alkali
(pyruvate carboxylase deficiency)	Frequent feeds; alkali, thiamine and biotin supplements
Lactose intolerance	Lactose restriction
Lysine intolerance (hyperlysinemia)	Protein restriction
Methionine malabsorption	Methionine restriction; cysteine supplement
Methylmalonic aciduria	
defective reduction or transport of cobalamin	B_{12} supplement, megadoses parenterally
impaired synthesis of 5'-deoxyadenosylcobalamin	Parenteral B_{12}, megadoses
methylmalonyl-CoA mutase deficiency	Isoleucine, methionine, threonine, valine restriction, B_{12}
methylmalonyl-CoA racemase deficiency	Biotin supplement
Multiple carboxylase deficiency	Biotin supplement
Nonketotic hyperglycinemia	Protein restriction, calorie supplements; strychnine
Ornithine transcarbamylase deficiency	Arginine, benzoic acid supplements; protein restriction; essential amino acids
Orotic aciduria	Uridine supplements
Oxalosis	Pyridoxine, magnesium, orthophosphate, water supplements
Periodic paralysis	
hypokalemic	Carbohydrate restriction, potassium salts, sodium chloride
hyperkalemic	Increased carbohydrates
normokalemic	Sodium chloride
Phenylketonuria	Phenylalanine restriction, tyrosine supplement
Porphyria, acute intermittent	High glucose, hematin infusions
Propionicacidemia	Isoleucine, methionine, threonine, valine restriction; biotin supplement
Pyridoxine dependency with seizures	Pyridoxine, parenterally
Pyroglutamic aciduria	Alkali, protein restriction
Pyruvate dehydrogenase deficiency, partial	Thiamine supplement, carbohydrate restriction; energy supplement (lipids)

recommended. Low-methionine commercial products are available.

Approximately 2 percent of Americans are heterozygous (have one gene) for homocystinuria. It has recently been shown that such people may be at risk for premature arteriosclerosis and premature thromboembolic events such as strokes. Although results have not been consistent, some studies of the diets of people heterozygous for homocystinuria show that methionine loading can bring on pathological homocystinemia—the blood disorder associated with premature peripheral and cerebral occlusive disease, often in the form of strokes occurring from the early forties through the sixties. As with hemochromatosis, this reveals that people with one recessive gene are not always simply unaffected carriers. Research on the health of people heterozygous for other inborn errors of metabolism may yield valuable advances in medical knowledge.

PHENYLKETONURIA (PKU)

Phenylketonuria (PKU) is the most common genetic defect involving the metabolism of an amino acid, in this case, phenylalanine. The primary defect is the inability to convert excess phenylalanine from food to tyrosine, resulting in an accumulation of phenylalanine in the blood and cerebrospinal fluid. An enzyme defect produced by a recessive gene is responsible. The primary clinical manifestation of the disorder is mental retardation, which is usually severe. Seizures may occur, and muscular hypertonicity, exaggerated tendon reflexes, tremors, and hyperactivity may be present. A dermatitis resembling eczema occurs in 15 to 20 percent of the untreated patients. Skin, hair, and eye pigments are often affected: patients with more darkly pigmented parents often have blond hair, blue eyes, and fair skin.

The recessive gene causes the disorder only in the homozygous (two-gene) state. About 1 person in 12,000 (estimates vary from 10,000 to 14,000) are homozygous.

Table 18.1. Genetic Disorders for Which Nutrient Intake Should Be Modified *(cont.)*

Disorder	Therapy
Refsum's disease	Phytanic acid restriction (diet low in dairy and ruminant fats)
Renal tubular acidosis	Alkali supplements
Sucrose-isomaltose malabsorption	Sucrose restriction
Tryptophanuria with dwarfism	Nicotinic acid
Tyrosinemia, type I	Phenylalanine-tyrosine restriction, high calorie; hematin infusions if porphyric symptoms persist
Tyrosinemia with keratosis and corneal dystrophy	Phenylalanine and tyrosine restriction
Valinemia	Valine restriction
Vitamin A defect (beta-carotene 15, 15'-dioxygenase)	Vitamin A
Vitamin B_{12} defect (conversion of B_{12} to precursor of 5'-deoxyadenosyl-B_{12} and methyl-B_{12})	Vitamin B_{12}
Vitamin D-dependent rickets	1,25 dehydroxy D
Vitamin K-dependent coagulation defect	Vitamin K
Xanthinuria	Purine restriction; allopurinol, fluids, alkali supplements
Xanthurenic aciduria	Pyridoxine

Reprinted with permission from "Nutrition Support in Inherited Metabolic Diseases" in *Modern Nutrition in Health and Disease,* Maurice E. Shils, M.D., S.D., and Vernon R. Young, Ph.D., editors (Philadelphia: Lea & Febiger, 1988).

About 1 in 44 people of Western European origin are heterozygous; they seem to show no ill effects. PKU is most common among Northern Europeans and Italians, and most rare among blacks and Ashkenazi Jews.

Since the early 1960s, screening of newborns for the disease has been widespread; today all hospitals in nearly every state are required by law to test newborns. The infants are fed protein in the form of breast milk or formula and the phenylketone concentration in the urine or blood is measured. (Massachusetts, for example, has detected PKU in about 1 out of every 14,000 babies screened.)

Adults are not routinely screened for PKU for a number of reasons. PKU is a rare disease that can be controlled by continued dietary vigilance. Those who are homozygous have the disorder and are very much aware of it. PKU can be passed along unwittingly only if both parents are heterozygous (carry one defective gene) for the disorder and they each pass it to the child. If both parents are carriers (with one defective gene), there is a 25-percent chance that their child will inherit PKU. There also is a 50-percent chance the child will be a carrier, and a 25-percent chance the child will be normal.

Newborns are routinely screened for PKU before the phenylalanine can accumulate and damage the brain. These babies then can be given the proper dietary therapy to prevent the deleterious effects of unmanaged PKU. However, unafflicted adult siblings of those with PKU may want to have carrier testing done on themselves and on their spouses before having children.

Nutritional therapy must begin in the first weeks of life for mental development to be normal. Differences of opinion exist as to whether or not the diet treatment can ever be safely discontinued. Treatment consists of controlling the amount of phenylalanine in the diet. This essential amino acid contributes to the manufacture of body proteins and therefore cannot be totally excluded from the diet. Since all food proteins contain about the same quantity of phenylalanine, none can be selectively chosen for a low-phenylalanine diet. Thus, the child is fed special foods in which the natural proteins are treated to remove some of the phenylalanine or are replaced by synthetic amino-acid mixtures.

With therapy, mental development and body growth are normal and the other manifestations of PKU are eased. For example, the dermatitis usually clears, normal hair and skin pigmentation are restored, neurological impairments improve, hyperactivity is eased, and seizures often disappear. It is essential that treatment continue until at least the age of five or six if mental retardation is to be prevented. Even when the treatment is phased out after this age, however, a subsequent buildup of phenylalanine may cause learning difficulties, speech defects, behavioral problems, and, in some cases, small but significant losses in I.Q. A major issue is the fact that the diet of the pregnant PKU patient needs to be monitored and the phenylalanine kept low in order to prevent mental retardation and other abnormalities in the fetus. Unfortunately, most insurance programs and Medicaid do not cover the special foods the pregnant woman should eat; thus, low-income PKU mothers are more likely to have babies damaged by the disease.

Because it contains phenylalanine, the safety of aspartame, the nutritive sweetener in some carbonated beverages and diet foods, has been questioned, especially for pregnant women. The Food and Drug Administration continues to maintain that aspartame consumed during pregnancy is not harmful. After evaluating data, the Council on Scientific Affairs of the American Medical Association concluded that aspartame was safe for consumption except by those who have phenylketonuria or by other individuals who need to curtail their intake of phenylalanine.

The amount of phenylalanine in aspartame is a fraction of that contained in other foods. For example, the amount of phenylalanine in aspartame-sweetened soda is only one-twelfth that which is found in one four-ounce hamburger. A woman who avoided aspartame during her pregnancy but not other foods that contain phenylalanine would not be reducing her intake of phenylalanine by any significant amount. However, as with all foods, the best recommendation during pregnancy is for moderation. Pregnant women with a history of phenylketonuria in their families should be particularly careful with their phenylalanine intake.

GALACTOSEMIA

Defects in all or any of three enzymes that help convert milk sugar in the body can cause galactosemia. Each molecule of milk sugar (lactose) contains one unit of galactose, which is normally converted to glucose in the liver. When infants with galactosemia are fed milk, galactose and two related compounds accumulate in the blood and tissues. (Mother's milk is particularly rich in galactose.) The infant may suffer from loss of appetite, vomiting, occasional diarrhea, drowsiness, jaundice, puffiness of the face, swelling of the hands and feet, and weight loss. The liver and spleen enlarge; liver failure may occur, with lethal results. Mental retardation is noticeable at an early stage. Cataracts develop before the child is a year old.

A recessive gene is responsible for the enzyme defects. Homozygous genes (inheriting both genes) cause the full disorder. However, heterozygous carriers (people with one gene mutant) do not convert galactose as well as normal individuals, although they can consume milk and dairy products. During pregnancy, heterozygous women—known as such because they gave birth to a child with the disease or have it in the family history—are advised to avoid galactose.

Nutritional therapy simply involves avoidance of galactose; that is, eliminating from the diet milk and dairy products, as well as organ meats, such as liver, that also contain galactose. Unlike phenylalanine in PKU, galactose is not a nutrient that the body must have, so there are no nutritional problems with eliminating it from the diet. A number of commercial nonmilk formulas are available. Milk and other dairy products must be avoided throughout life, although sometimes products containing small amounts of milk, such as bread, may be acceptable later in life.

With treatment, symptoms of nausea, vomiting, and diarrhea disappear, an enlarged or cirrhotic liver may return to normal, and cataracts diminish. However, the damage to the brain and central nervous system is irreversible, emphasizing the importance of early diagnosis and treatment.

HEREDITARY FRUCTOSE INTOLERANCE (FRUCTOSEMIA)

This condition is similar to galactosemia, except that the symptoms are milder. Treatment consists of avoiding fructose, which is present in fruits as well as many other plant foods and from the digestion of sucrose (sugarcane and sugar-beet sugar). Therefore, all fruits, some vegetables, some grain products, and all foods and drinks sweetened with sucrose, fructose, or sorbitol (a sugar alcohol) must be eliminated from the diet. Other plant foods are allowed only in limited quantities. Glucose is a safe substitute for fructose.

MAPLE SUGAR URINE DISEASE

Known also as branched-chain ketoaciduria, maple sugar urine disease is so named because the patient's urine smells like maple syrup. Because of a recessive gene, the person lacks an enzyme in white blood cells; this, in turn, interferes with the breakdown of three amino acids. The amino acids and their ketoacids accumulate in the blood and are excreted in large amounts in the urine, accounting for the unusual odor.

Newborns appear normal but symptoms develop within a few days. These babies are unable to suck and swallow properly, their breathing is irregular, and they suffer from periods of stiffness and limpness. Seizures may occur, and mental retardation is usually severe. Unless treatment is begun promptly, death can occur within days.

Treatment consists of a lifetime diet restricted in three amino acids (leucine, isoleucine, and valine). A variant form of the disorder can be treated with thiamine.

GLYCOGEN-STORAGE DISEASES

There are six genetic glycogen-storage diseases; two of these respond to nutritional therapy. Glycogen is the stored form of carbohydrate energy in the liver and muscles; and when energy is needed, the glycogen is converted into glucose and used as fuel. When the enzyme that assists this conversion is impaired or missing, low blood sugar can cause a life-threatening situation to develop quickly if meals are missed or even delayed. Frequent protein snacks are the most effective nutritional treatment.

The symptoms of glycogen-storage diseases vary depending on the type of disease. In Type I, called von Gierke's disease, symptoms include severe hypoglycemia (low blood sugar) in infants, anorexia, weight loss, vomiting, kidney and liver enlargement, failure to thrive, stunted growth, and gout. The symptoms of some of the other types are milder: muscle wasting and weakness, muscle cramps and weakness while exercising vigorously. Other symptoms include severe hypoglycemia, hypertriglyceridemia (excess of triglycerides in the blood), hypercholesterolemia (excess cholesterol in the blood), and increased blood urate and lactate levels. In one type, death can result from failure of the cardiorespiratory system.

Depending on the type of glycogen-storage disease present, diagnosis is made by muscle biopsy, liver biopsy, and blood test. These are used to determine enzyme activities, the response to storage of glycogen, and the presence of any other abnormalities.

VITAMIN-DEPENDENCY DISEASES

These diseases are distinct from those caused by vitamin deficiency because they occur in the presence of adequate intake of the vitamins involved. Resistant rickets is one such disease. Rickets develop in spite of adequate vitamin D intake, because the enzyme that assists in converting the vitamin is missing due to a genetic defect. Treatment consists of administering one of the substances (25-hydroxy calciferol) to which vitamin D normally would have been converted in the body.

TYROSINEMIA

A recessive gene causes the enzyme defect that blocks the conversion of the amino acid tyrosine to homogentisic acid in the body.

Blood levels of tyrosine, phenylalanine, and sometimes methionine become elevated, resulting in kidney and liver damage. The liver and spleen become enlarged, and the onset of fatal liver failure can be rapid. Diets low in the three amino acids mentioned above are the only form of nutritional therapy.

CYSTIC FIBROSIS

Although cystic fibrosis can affect many organs, its three major symptoms are pancreatic insufficiency, chronic lung disease, and abnormal electrolyte levels in perspiration. About 80 to 85 percent of the people with this hereditary disease have a malfunctioning pancreas. Mucus tends to block the pancreatic ducts and to interfere with the secretion of digestive enzymes and pancreatic juices. During periods when the disease is active, patients become malnourished. Even though they may eat heartily when they are feeling well, this often is not enough to make up for the undernourishment at other times.

Nutritional treatment stresses enzyme replacements, vitamin supplements, and frequent monitoring of the nutritional status, with dietary adjustments. Sometimes extra sodium is needed to replace the large amounts that are lost in perspiration. Selenium and other miracle cures have not proved to be effective. (Antibiotics and other therapies are used to treat the pulmonary problems.)

WILSON'S DISEASE

In Wilson's disease, also known as hepatolenticular degeneration, excess copper is accumulated in the body because of an enzyme defect due to a recessive gene. The abnormal gene seems to be found slightly more often in males than females. Characteristic symptoms include greenish-brown–pigmented rings at the outer margin of the cornea (Kayser-Fleischer rings), brain degeneration, cirrhosis of the liver, and low levels of ceruloplasmin (a blood protein into which the impaired enzyme normally would have incorporated copper). The disorder is fatal when untreated.

Nutritional therapy is combined with lifetime administration of penicillamine, a chelating agent that removes copper from the tissues and prevents its reaccumulation. Foods with a high copper content, such as shellfish, liver, mushrooms, nuts, cocoa, and chocolate, should be avoided.

ACRODERMATITIS ENTEROPATHICA

This hereditary disorder may be caused by a defect in the gastrointestinal absorption of zinc, but little more is presently known. The resulting zinc deficiency is recognized by dermatitis of the oral, anal, and genital areas, hair loss in early infancy, and severe diarrhea. Lactose intolerance, eye problems, neurological troubles, and retarded growth are frequent. Treatment consists of small daily supplements of zinc sulfate; a diet rich in zinc (especially meat and seafood) may be helpful.

REFSUM'S DISEASE

Also called phytanic-acid–storage disease, Refsum's disease is caused by an enzyme defect due to a recessive gene. Failure to convert the fatty acid phytanic acid to alpha-hydroxyphytanic acid results in an accumulation of phytanic acid in the tissues, especially those of the kidneys and liver. The chief symptoms are lack of coordination, peripheral neuropathy, skin and bone disorders, nerve deafness, and retinitis pigmentosa (a progressive hardening and coloration of the retina, ending in blindness).

Phytanic acid is not manufactured in the body and can therefore be controlled through diet. Dairy products are the chief source; fish oils and some vegetables (for example, tomatoes and squash) are minor sources. Phytol, an ingredient of chlorophyll in green plants, can be a precursor of phytanic acid but is thought not to be an important dietary source. The disease has been treated successfully by limiting the individual's intake of foods that contain phytanic acid. Reducing the phytanic acid intake to 60 milligrams per day has resulted in lower phytanic-acid levels in the blood. To normalize these levels, however, the amount consumed in the diet may need to be drastically reduced, which can involve severe restriction in the total number of calories. When this is the case, a patient's diet should be carefully supervised.

LEUCINE-INDUCED HYPOGLYCEMIA

The amino acid leucine causes major drops in the blood-glucose level of infants with this hereditary disease. Why this occurs is not known for certain, but leucine may help stimulate the production of insulin or in some way assist insulin in acting on blood glucose. The condition appears in children four months old and onward. The first symptom may be convulsions; failure to thrive and delayed mental development are typical. Acne, excessive hairiness, obesity, and osteoporosis (a bone weakness) are common.

Treatment consists of consuming a diet low in leucine. The minimum daily requirement for this amino acid is 150 to 230 milligrams per kilogram, and this amount is needed for normal development. Leucine occurs in all protein foods, and therefore all proteins must be restricted in the diet to their minimum requirements. Fruits and vegetables supplement this low-protein diet. Carbohydrates are consumed 30 to 40 minutes after each meal to counteract the effect of leucine in the proteins eaten. Once the child reaches the age of five or six, he or she can begin to consume a normal diet without adverse consequences.

HEREDITARY XANTHINURIA

An inherited enzyme deficiency, this results in reduced synthesis of uric acid in the body, with a consequent buildup of the precursors of uric acid. These precursors—hypoxanthine and xanthine—are usually harmless and do not require therapy. The one problem associated with this condition is recurrent renal calculi (kidney stones). A high-fluid, low-purine diet and maintenance of an alkaline pH in the urine are recommended.

PRENATAL GENETIC SCREENING

Couples in which both partners have genetic defects often decide not to have children rather than risk the birth of a seriously ailing child. Women pregnant late in life have similar worries. For such individuals, prenatal genetic tests have provided new possibilities. Knowing that a fetus showing signs of inherited defects can be aborted allows prospective parents to keep hoping that someday they will have a normal, healthy child. For others, however, this alternative is ethically unacceptable.

In the 1940s, physicians used Mendelian principles to calculate the risk of couples having a child with genetic defects. Since those times, many tests have been developed to detect signals of genetic disease in maternal and newborn blood and urine. In the late 1960s, amniocentesis was introduced. Women over 35 or those who already have a child with a genetic defect may take the test after the sixteenth week of pregnancy. A sample of amniotic fluid from the mother's uterus provides fetal cells for testing. Chorionic villus sampling (CVS) is a more recent test. In this procedure, placenta cells are tested after 9 to 11 weeks of pregnancy. The most recent U.S. studies have found it to be as accurate as amniocentesis, and to have comparable miscarriage rates. The advantage of CVS testing over amniocentesis is that it can be performed much earlier. The major disadvantage as of this writing is that it is only available at about 25 centers in the United States.

In conjunction with these tests, gene probes and genetic marker tests may be used to look for warning sequences of genes that may be normal themselves but are often associated with abnormal mutant genes.

19

Eating Disorders

Jerome L. Knittle, M.D.,
and David P. Katz, Ph.D.

■

INTRODUCTION

Eating disorders, especially among young people, are increasingly common medical problems afflicting large numbers of Americans. Two of the most common and complex, anorexia nervosa (self-induced starvation) and bulimia (a pattern of overeating followed by self-induced vomiting, or laxative and diuretic abuse), are becoming more prevalent. It is estimated that as many as 10 to 15 percent of adolescent girls and young women in the United States suffer from them.

Although anorexia and bulimia have been recently classified as distinctly different disorders, they share several similarities. Both are characterized by an intense preoccupation with food and body weight. Individual cases vary in severity, but in extreme cases, both bulimia and anorexia nervosa can involve life-threatening medical problems. Both disorders require special nutritional management and treatment.

ANOREXIA NERVOSA

Anorexia nervosa is an eating disorder that is characterized by a voluntary refusal of food and a subsequent severe weight loss that can jeopardize the individual's physical and psychological well-being and, in severe cases, can lead to death. Anorexia nervosa often begins during the teen years, although it has been reported in children aged 8 to 11, and can last anywhere from a few months to many years.

Recent estimates say anywhere from 1 in every 100 to 1 in every 200 girls between the ages of 12 and 18 in the United States will develop the illness. The flurry of recent publicity has created the misperception that it is a new condition, but it isn't. It was first recognized medically in England over 100 years ago by Sir William Gull, who coined its name, which means lack of appetite. This, however, is not an accurate description, since most anorexics do not lose their appetites until they are in an advanced state of starvation.

Typically, anorexics are middle- or upper-middle-class adolescent girls or young women. A minority of them, about 6 percent, are adolescent boys. Male anorexics tend to be weight-conscious athletes, such as wrestlers, gymnasts, or jockeys.

Symptoms of anorexia nervosa include fatigue, hyperactivity, and light-headedness. The anorexic has a distorted view of the world and herself, which causes her to have various psychological disturbances. She usually lacks self-esteem and believes that by losing weight and becoming thin, she will become popular and admired. Her distorted body image prevents her from seeing her body realistically. She is obsessed with her weight and, regardless of what the mirror shows or the scale registers, believes she is fat. At only 80 pounds, most anorexics will still describe themselves as too fat. Even though she is starving herself, she will stop eating after a few bites, insisting she is full.

Being intensely preoccupied with food, she may spend hours planning menus, reading cookbooks, and preparing lavish meals for others. She may develop elaborate rituals for eating, such as moving food around the plate or cutting it into tiny pieces. Despite the fatigue that can accompany her condition, the anorexic often throws herself into a rigorous exercise regimen. Other psychological symptoms include depression and social withdrawal.

Typically, anorexics come from families that are very involved with one another and place an emphasis on scholastic achievement and physical appearance. Because she tends toward perfectionism and is usually obedient and a good student, parents often describe their anorectic daughter as a model child. Some researchers theorize that some teens become anorectic to exert power over a facet of their lives that their parents cannot control—eating.

The Health Hazards of Anorexia Nervosa

Anorexia nervosa is complicated by psychological as well as endocrinological and gynecological problems. Most seriously, 10 to 15 percent will die of starvation or related problems, including hypothermia, heart or kidney failure, irreversible hypoglycemia, and pulmonary tuberculosis. Between 2 and 5 percent will commit suicide.

An anorexic will often lose more than 25 percent of her body weight; it is not unusual for her weight to slip down to as little as 60 or 70 pounds. The body responds to self-starvation as it does to that which is externally imposed. To conserve its two main organs—the brain and heart—it shuts or slows down less-than-vital bodily functions: thyroid function is reduced (which can cause dry skin, brittle and lost hair, constipation, and cold intolerance), and as a compensatory mechanism to reduce strain on the heart, blood pressure drops and heart rate is lowered (bradycardia). To compensate for the lowered body temperature that results from reduced fat, some anorexics develop lanugo, a soft body hair sometimes seen on newborns.

Amenorrhea is a major diagnostic symptom of anorexia nervosa. While a certain percentage of body fat is necessary for menses, in about 30 percent of anorexics, menstruation ceases before there has been a substantial weight loss. Researchers believe in these cases that emotional stress might be a contributory factor. Although weight gain is necessary for menstruation to return, in some, normal periods will not resume. When weight is gained, there is often a delay in the return of normal menses.

Loss of bone mass due to osteoporosis is another physical symptom. However, anorexics who are highly active are usually found to have greater bone density than those who are more sedentary, despite a low intake of calcium and estrogen deficiencies. Not all women will recover lost bone mass upon return to normal weight. Those whose bone mass does not increase with weight gain may be at greater risk for osteoporotic fractures of the wrist, hip, and vertebrae after menopause, when the rate of bone-mass loss normally accelerates.

Other symptoms anorexics can experience include mild anemia, swelling of joints, difficulty sleeping, and reduced muscle mass. With little fat for cushioning, it can be uncomfortable for the anorexic to lie in bed or in a bathtub. Anorexic boys can suffer similarly, including the interruption of normal reproductive-system development. In addition, many anorexics adopt bulimic habits, which further jeopardize their health. Most of these health problems are reversible upon return to normal weight.

BULIMIA

The word *bulimia* is derived from Greek words meaning *ox* and *hunger*, although this is a misnomer, since few bulimics experience a voracious hunger. It is an eating disorder characterized by episodic binge eating (the rapid consumption of unusual amounts of food), followed by purging (ridding the body of food by vomiting or other means). Although bulimia has long been recognized as a sister disorder to anorexia nervosa, only recently has it been documented as a separate problem.

The illness has its antecedents in ancient Rome: After gorging, banqueters tickled their throats with feathers to induce vomiting so that they could continue feasting. Whereas the Roman revelers were men, the majority of today's bulimics are women. Most bulimics, unlike those who suffer from anorexia nervosa, are of normal weight. As a result, many of them are able to hide their problem for years, even from family and close friends.

Dieting frequently precipitates the cycle of binging and purging. The dieter may cheat with an episode of binging, after which she will purge to compensate for the indiscretion. This one incident can trigger a cycle that becomes increasingly hard to break. Eventually, the individual may purge even after eating small quantities of food. At the Stanford Eating Disorders Clinic, 28 patients under treatment reported binging about 6 times a week and purging more than 14 times weekly. Some bulimics do not binge but will purge after eating certain high-calorie foods.

Binges may be planned or spontaneous. They typically last one to two hours, during which as many as 15,000 to 20,000 calories may be consumed, mostly of easily eaten, high-calorie and/or forbidden foods, such as cakes, pastries, ice cream, and bread. While binging, the bulimic feels out of control and fearful that once she starts to eat, she will be unable to stop herself. The frequency of binging and purging varies with the severity of the disorder, but it may average two or more times a week and increase during times of stress. An individual with a severe case may spend $50 per day on food. She is usually aware that her eating habits are abnormal and thus hides her behavior from family and friends.

A binge is often triggered by negative feelings—of stress, loneliness, or boredom. For the duration of the binge, these moods are suspended. However, once the episode is over, the bulimic is overcome by guilt and shame and the fear of having her behavior revealed. By ridding her body of the food, she ensures she will not gain weight and helps to minimize the tension the binging generated. However, guilt still lingers, develops into more tension, and catapults her into repeated cycles of this abnormal eating behavior.

Regurgitation is the most common method of purging. Vomiting may be self-induced by gagging brought on by sticking fingers or objects, such as toothbrushes or silverware, down the throat or by swallowing emetics, chemical substances that induce vomiting. With practice, some bulimics are able to vomit by contracting their abdominal muscles. Laxatives (between 2 and 40 tablets) and—less commonly and usually in conjunction with another method of weight loss—diuretics (drugs that increase urination) are used, in the mistaken belief that the resultant weight loss is from calories, when, in fact, only water is being lost. Fasting is yet another method the bulimic uses to counterbalance the results of binging.

The Victims of Bulimia

As with anorexics, bulimics are most often adolescent girls and young women. Because they are usually of normal weight and size, they are often able to conceal their affliction for years. Although bulimia generally begins between the ages of 17 and 25, many bulimics are not diagnosed until they are between 30 and 40.

Bulimia is believed to be more prevalent than anorexia nervosa. Although precise figures for the general population are not known, it poses a serious problem for about 5 percent of adolescent girls and young women. Some estimates place the incidence of bulimia among these women between nearly 8 and almost 20 percent.

A Gallup poll projected that approximately 2 million American women aged 19 to 39 and another 1 million teenagers are affected by one or more symptoms of bulimia, anorexia, or both. In a small survey of private schools in the Washington, D.C., area, 28 percent of female eighth graders said they considered vomiting an acceptable way to lose weight. Early in their teen years, many girls begin worrying about weight and dieting, placing themselves at greater risk for the possibility of developing an eating disorder at some time in their lives. (To determine whether someone close to you is suffering from bulimia or anorexia nervosa, see Signs of Eating Disorders on page 323.)

Men also develop eating disorders, but statistically, fewer men than women develop bulimia or anorexia. According to the *FDA Consumer*, males account for 5 to 10 percent of all cases of anorexia and bulimia. Of bulimics, the *Dairy Council Digest* reports that as many as 10 to 13 percent are male. Although people of all races can develop eating disorders, they strike a much greater percentage of whites than any other group. This may reflect certain socioeconomic rather than racial factors.

Although bulimic individuals may appear to be happy, healthy, and successful, they are depressed and have very little self-confidence. They often appear to be perfectionists. These and other symptoms of bulimia are found in 30 to 50 percent of the patients being treated for anorexia nervosa.

The Health Risks Associated with Bulimia

Binging and purging can unbalance the body's electrolytes by depleting reserves of sodium, magnesium, potassium, and calcium. The problems that result from this can include fatigue, muscle cramping, seizures, and, even in young women, osteoporosis.

If the bulimic purges by vomiting, the esophagus and stomach can be damaged. The regurgitated stomach acid can cause gums to recede and corrode tooth enamel, making the individual susceptible to caries and periodontal disease. (See Chapter 37 for more information on dental disease.) If the vomiting has been induced by syrup of ipecac, fatal poisoning is possible. When used repeatedly, ipecac accumulates in the body and can ultimately cause abnormal heart function resulting in death.

If the bulimic is involved in laxative abuse, a laxative dependency may result. The individual's intestinal system eventually cannot function without the medicine, causing chronic constipation. An addiction to laxatives can also cause severe potassium loss, dehydration, and heart-rhythm abnormalities. A bulimic who fasts between binges would be at risk for many of the related problems of malnutrition and starvation discussed previously in the section on the health hazards of anorexia.

Less severe side effects of bulimia include rashes, broken blood vessels, and swelling around ankles, eyes, and feet. In some rare instances, binging can result in pancreatic disease or possibly fatal rupture of the stomach. Some bulimics, as a result of frequent vomiting, have enlarged glands at the neck (parotid glands), which may give the appearance of mumps.

Some studies indicate bulimics have diffi-culty controlling their impulses. According to the *Journal of the American Dietetic Association,* a few investigators have noted a high rate of drug abuse and shoplifting (usually of food) among bulimics.

WHAT CAUSES THESE ILLNESSES?

While there is no single known cause for bulimia or anorexia nervosa, several theories involving psychological, environmental, and biological factors have been proposed. Whatever the cause, there are precipitating factors. Both disorders often begin with a diet.

With anorexia nervosa, a person may begin dieting reasonably but then become unable to stop. This often occurs as the individual enters puberty and begins to develop the curves of womanhood. The normal increase in body fat that accompanies sexual maturation is often viewed negatively by such a person. By becoming thin, these young anorexics may be demonstrating a desire to prevent or delay puberty by remaining childlike.

As mentioned previously, it is also true

Signs of Eating Disorders

To determine whether someone has anorexia nervosa, look for the following signs.

- Loss of 20 to 25 percent of total body weight
- Loss of menstrual period
- Compulsiveness about exercise
- Compulsive eating behavior
- Depression
- Perception of self as fat

The bulimic exhibits the following signs.

- Frequent weight fluctuations of 10 pounds in either direction
- Massive consumption of high-calorie foods
- Repeated attempts to lose weight by severely restrictive dieting or long-term fasting
- Awareness that eating pattern is abnormal
- Fear of being unable to control eating voluntarily
- Depression
- Self-deprecating behavior

that bulimia may begin when an individual is on a diet. In many cases, the individual is slightly overweight. Nobody knows what starts this process or how the desire to lose a few pounds can turn into compulsive behavior. Some psychiatrists point to the societal pressure on young women to be thin. Data collected from *Playboy* magazine and Miss America pageants over the last 20 years indicates that the fantasy woman is now thinner and more androgynous, with a smaller bust, narrower hips, and proportionately larger waist than the more Rubenesque ideal of past decades. According to U.S. census data, women now weigh, on an average, five to six pounds more than they did in 1960. This disparity between the media's ideal of feminine beauty and the average woman may explain, in part, the current national interest in weight loss and dieting and the recent rise in cases of bulimia and anorexia. Young women who are biologically prone to being overweight and/or depressed are even more vulnerable to this type of pressure. A trend away from the use of extremely thin models should be encouraged.

A dieter may be at greater risk for binging than a nondieter. Those who go off their diets and consume high-calorie foods may feel they have failed and have little incentive to continue dieting. Once this happens, overeating ensues. Studies have shown that unlike the nondieter, who is more likely to react to the consumption of a big piece of cake before dinner by eating proportionately less dessert after dinner, the dieter will more often react by overeating.

Other factors that may contribute to eating disorders include difficulty handling emotions and resolving family or other interpersonal conflicts. Personality characteristics that may place certain women at greater risk for eating disorders include poor self-image, low self-esteem, unusual dependency on others for decisions and approval, and submissiveness.

The Role of the Hypothalamus

Some researchers think that a malfunctioning of the hypothalamus, a part of the brain that controls secretion from the endocrine glands, body temperature, water balance, and sugar and fat metabolism may be responsible for eating disorders.

While abnormalities of the hypothalamus occur in anorexia nervosa and may exist prior to its onset, more research is necessary to define a connection greater than coincidence.

Depression and Bulimia

Another biological theory links a form of affective-disorder depression to bulimia. Affective-disorder depression is characterized by widely fluctuating and depressive moods and may be genetic. In one study published in the *American Journal of Psychiatry*, patients treated with antidepressant drugs were able to reduce their binge eating by 70 percent. Although there is evidence of a link between depression and bulimia, it remains unclear whether the loss of control with bulimia is the causative factor or whether depression, like anxiety, results in overeating and bulimia.

TREATMENT

Both anorexia nervosa and bulimia involve obsessive, compulsive behavior. Victims are unable to stop their destructive eating patterns without professional medical help, which must be sought. Parents are not professionals and cannot treat a child's eating disorders. They should not try to pressure an anorexic to eat by begging, scolding, or pleading. These tactics do not work and may exacerbate the behavior. Often it is this type of control over and attention from parents that the individual is seeking.

Treating these disorders, especially bulimia, can be difficult because the eating patterns often have been well established—and concealed—for years. Because of severe weight loss, anorexics are usually recognized sooner than bulimics. However, anorexics, because they do not believe they have a problem, are often defensive and resistant to treatment. Seldom will an anorexic seek treatment without prompting. Some devise ways to conceal their disease, such as placing heavy objects in their pockets before stepping on a school scale, or washing already-clean dishes so that family members will think they have eaten. Once they can cope with revealing their secret, bulimics are more likely than anorexics to seek treatment, because they realize they have an eating problem. (For a list of groups that deal with eating disorders, see Resources, below.)

Treatment for anorexia nervosa and bulimia includes psychotherapy, psychoactive medications (in cases of severe depression), and nutritional, family, and behavioral ther-apy. Because of the complexity of the disorders, no single treatment is adequate in all cases; instead, a combination of treatments, given by a collaborative team of specialists, is usually advised. For instance, a nutritionist, a psychologist, a family therapist, and a physician might work together on one case. Depending on the age of the patient and on the family situation, parents and family members may also be involved.

With bulimia, the goal is to reestablish normal eating patterns while eliminating the binge-purge cycles. Treatment for anorexics aims at getting them to eat and gain weight until they reach 95 percent of their desirable body weight. (Sometimes, the initial weight goal set for the patient will be lower than this and readjusted later.) Reestablishing normal eating patterns and regaining lost weight alone will not solve the problem. To be successful, treatment must include the resolution of psychological problems and family conflicts that may have predisposed the individual to her eating disorder. Long-term therapy may be necessary and full recovery may take three to four years, or longer.

Resources

American Anorexia Nervosa/Bulimia
  Association
133 Cedar Lane
Teaneck, New Jersey 07666
(201) 836–1800

National Anorexia Aid Society
5796 Karl Road
Columbus, Ohio 43229
(614) 436–1112

Anorexia Nervosa and Associated Disorders
P.O. Box 7
Highland Park, Illinois 60035
(315) 831–3438

Center for the Study of Anorexia and Bulimia
1 West 91st Street
New York, New York 10024
(212) 595–3449

Anorexia Nervosa and Related Eating
  Disorders
P.O. Box 5102
Eugene, Oregon 97405
(503) 344–1144

Bulimia, Anorexia Self-Help (BASH)
1027 Bellevue Avenue
St. Louis, Missouri 63117
(314) 567–4080

To tailor treatment to the individual, information should be gathered during the initial evaluation with regard to the patient's medical and psychiatric history, family life, and abnormal eating behavior. (Questions for Those Suffering from Eating Disorders, below, suggests things that usually should be asked during the initial interview.) Decisions on how to proceed with treatment and whether or not to hospitalize the patient are made at this time. The patient will usually be hospitalized if her weight loss is severe, she has life-

---

Questions for Those Suffering from Eating Disorders

The following is a list of questions a doctor might ask a patient seeking treatment for eating disorders.

Weight History
- What is the most and least you have weighed?
- What is your ideal weight?
- What is the highest stable weight you have maintained without dieting?
- How much did you weigh when your eating disorder began?
- How much do you weigh now?
- What are your weight fluctuations?
- How do you feel about your body?
- What are your preoccupations with your weight?
- What are the attitudes of other family members toward your weight; your thinness; weight in general?

Dieting Behavior
- At what age did you begin dieting?
- What were the situations or events that precipitated dieting?
- What are your patterns of eating?
- What are your feelings toward food and dieting?

Eating Patterns
- What was your eating behavior before the eating disorder?
- How much and what kinds of foods do you eat?
- How much and what kinds of foods does your family eat?

- Do you have any strong preferences or aversions to food?
- Do you have any rituals associated with eating?
- Are you taking vitamins or minerals?
- How motivated are you to change your eating patterns?

Exercise
- How much and what kind of exercise did you do before your eating disorder?
- What types of exercise do you engage in now? How much and how often do you exercise?
- What are your feelings about exercise and dieting?

For Bulimics
- How often and for how long do you binge?
- Are there certain foods, feelings, situations, or times that precipitate your binging?
- What are your feelings during, before, and after a binge?
- How have you tried to stop your binging?
- Do you vomit, or do you use laxatives or diuretics to purge?
- How often and what method do you use for purging?
- How long have you been purging?
- What events and feelings precipitate a purge?
- What is the longest time you have gone without purging?

threatening complications, she is suicidal, or if outpatient efforts have failed. An anorexic may require intravenous nutritional support if the total weight loss is life-threatening.

To regain lost weight, the anorexic does not need to consume unusual amounts of food. The quantities are small at first and are gradually increased in order for the body to acclimate to eating again and for the patient to learn to deal with her fear that food will make her obese. Rewards for eating or gaining weight may be part of a behavior-modification program. In addition, psychotherapy is often used to help the patient talk about family and social relationships and to help her gain insight into her abnormal eating behavior.

In nutritional therapy, the patient learns about good nutrition, keeps a food diary, and adheres to an individualized diet plan. With abnormal eating patterns often firmly entrenched, patients must relearn normal eating habits. Recording what is eaten reminds the patient of the quantities of foods she needs to eat. It is also useful to the dietitian in keeping track of the patient's progress and dietary trends. When eating patterns become normalized and the patient is comfortable with the new habits, the record keeping can be stopped. For bulimics especially, it is important to minimize the number of decisions about what and when to eat so that the risk of returning to the binging and purging cycle is reduced. For this reason, treatment for the bulimic involves adherence to a predetermined diet plan. The plan should exclude favorite binge foods until the bulimia is under control, at which time they can be introduced in small quantities.

The dynamics of the family is especially important because most anorexics and bulimics are young women who will continue to live at home after therapy. In family therapy, the entire family reevaluates their rela-tionships with one another, which should help to reduce family tension.

PROGNOSIS

Often, even after a return to normal weight for anorexics and to normal eating patterns for bulimics, patients suffer relapses. For this reason, follow-up therapy lasting three to five years is usually suggested. Patients who have the most difficulty recovering from eating disorders include those whose illnesses have been long untreated, those who developed them at a later age, those whose weight losses have been severe, and those suffering from a combination of anorexia nervosa and bulimia (sometimes called bulimarexia). An analysis of 12 major outcome studies of anorexics during a 15-year period revealed that about half of the patients under treatment who survived returned to their normal body weight, and more than half continued to have eating problems. Menses will return in 50 to 75 percent of cases, but menstrual irregularities may be common thereafter.

SUMMING UP

A combination of nutritional, social, psychological, and biological factors contribute to eating disorders. Although there is no single approach to treatment or prevention, professionals treating these disorders hope that with better nutritional education and an emphasis on appropriate ways to maintain desirable body weight, the incidence of eating disorders will some day decrease. Because so much is still unknown about anorexia nervosa and bulimia, however, more research is needed to assess normal and abnormal feeding behavior.

20

Medications: Food/Drug Interactions

Bernard Mehl, D.P.S.

■

INTRODUCTION

Health professionals have long known that certain drugs can interfere with nutrition—and, conversely, that certain foods can alter the effectiveness of some medications. Well-known examples include the appetite suppression caused by amphetamines, the impairing effect on absorption that milk and other high-calcium products have on some tetracycline antibiotics, and the malnutrition that accompanies chronic alcoholism. A growing body of research now indicates that interactions between diet and drugs are actually far more common than was previously thought. Given the fact that an estimated 75 million Americans regularly take prescription or over-the-counter medications, food and drug interactions pose potential problems for a great many people.

The effects of specific diet-drug interactions may vary widely among individuals, producing a dramatic change in one person and hardly affecting another. A host of variables, including drug dosage, dietary composition, and the age, sex, size, nutritional status, and general health of the individual, may influence the interaction. Whether or not the individual smokes and/or uses caffeine or alcohol also may contribute to interactions. Those most vulnerable to food and drug interactions are the elderly, the very young, the poorly nourished, and people suffering from chronic diseases.

Research indicates that people over age 65 are particularly susceptible. One reason is that as a group, older people are the largest consumers of both prescription and over-the-counter drugs. Another is that because of age-related declines in liver and kidney function, older people do not metabolize and eliminate drugs as efficiently as do younger individuals. As a result, medications may remain in their systems for a longer time and have a stronger-than-intended effect.

Until quite recently, the fact that older people frequently fail to respond to prescribed medications was usually considered to be a compliance problem; that is, a failure to follow directions. Mental confusion, forgetfulness, and stubbornness were often blamed when elderly patients didn't take their drugs as often as they should have or in the required amounts. Now, however, health professionals are recognizing that side effects from unsuspected diet-drug interactions may force older people to discontinue medications that they vitally need.

Subtle, long-term drug effects also may lead to a variety of nutritional deficiencies in the elderly. One study of 153 individuals aged

328

65 to 93 found that 23 percent had evidence of early negative balance with respect to thiamine (vitamin B_1), 19 percent to pyridoxine (vitamin B_6) and 11 percent to riboflavin (vitamin B_2). In another study of the elderly, nearly half of the examined group were found to have early negative balance for vitamin C, folic acid, and vitamin A. Although the researchers lacked clear evidence that diet-drug interactions were directly responsible for this negative-balance status, or that clinical deficiencies of these vitamins had occurred, they felt strongly that food/drug interactions did play a significant negative role.

Health professionals are becoming increasingly aware that in addition to various specific nutrient deficiencies, disorders such as chronic diarrhea, poor appetite, weight loss (or gain), and bone loss (osteoporosis) may be partly attributable to interactions between drugs and diet. It's important for you, too, to be aware that such interactions can aggravate and sometimes even create medical problems. Whenever a drug is prescribed for you, ask your doctor or pharmacist about possible interactions with diet or effects on nutrition. Likewise, if you are on a long-term course of drug therapy for a particular problem, check with your physician before making any radical changes in your accustomed diet. Many pharmacies are linked to a computer network giving immediate information on food/drug, nutrient/drug, and nutrient/nutrient interactions. Nutrients in megadoses *are* drugs.

TYPES OF INTERACTIONS

There are several classes of interactions between drugs and food. Some are based on the presence of food altering a drug's therapeutic performance. In others, the drug, although it may accomplish its medical mission, affects the body's metabolism or its ability to utilize nutrients in a way that over time can lead to nutritional deficiencies. (Table 20.1 lists common food-drug interactions.) Vitamins and minerals, in greater than RDA amounts, are drugs (even though labeled food supplements) and can have adverse drug/nutrient interactions (or nutrient/nutrient interactions).

When Food Alters a Drug's Effects

Drugs that are taken orally pass down the esophagus to the stomach, where they are wholly or partially dissolved and digested by stomach acids and other digestive enzymes. The stomach's contents are then emptied into the small intestine, in which they are further digested and absorbed and from which the major portion of most drugs is absorbed into the bloodstream. The parts that are not absorbed continue on through the large intestine and are eventually eliminated in the feces.

The drugs that are absorbed usually travel through the bloodstream to the liver, where they are further broken down and transformed (metabolized) by liver enzymes. Unmetabolized drugs and/or useful by-products of metabolism are then distributed by the bloodstream to the organs and cells where they are needed. Drugs and their by-products that are not utilized also enter the bloodstream and are passed to the kidneys for excretion mainly in the urine or to the bile for excretion in the stool.

Food components can affect this process at every step along the way. To begin, the timing and composition of meals influences the rate at which the stomach empties its contents, which, in turn, affects absorption (see Table 20.2). High-fat meals or high-viscosity liquids, such as mineral oil, will delay stomach emptying (as will protein and carbohydrate meals, albeit to a lesser extent). As a

Table 20.1. Foods and Drugs That Do Not Mix

If You Are Taking	Dietary Substance	Effects
BLOOD PRESSURE MEDICATIONS		
Thiazide diuretics (e.g., Diuril, Esidrix, Hydrodiuril)	Monosodium glutamate	↑ MSG effects (tight feeling in chest, facial flushing)
Loop diuretics (e.g., Lasix)	Diet low in potassium	↑ Risk potassium deficiency
Hydralazine	If taken with food	↑ Drug effect
	Diet low in vitamin B_6	↑ Risk vitamin B_6 deficiency
Potassium-sparing diuretics (e.g., Aldactone)	If taken with food	↑ Drug effect
	Diet very high in potassium	↑ Risk of potassium excess
Beta blockers (e.g., Inderal)	If taken with food	↑ Drug effect
HEART MEDICATIONS		
Digitalis drugs (e.g., Lanoxin, Crystodigin)	Diet low in potassium	↑ Risk of potassium deficiency
Quinine drugs (e.g., Quinaglute)	Highly alkaline diets (milk, fruit, vegetables)	↑ Risk drug toxicity
ORAL CONTRACEPTIVES		
Estrogen/Progestin combinations (e.g., Ortho-Novum, Norlestrin)	Diet low in vitamin B_6	↑ Risk vitamin B_6 deficiency
	Diet low in folic acid	↑ Risk folic acid deficiency
PAIN MEDICATIONS		
Salicylates (e.g., aspirin)	If taken on empty stomach	↑ Risk of gastrointestinal irritation
	Diet low in folic acid	↑ Risk of folic acid deficiency
	Diet low in vitamin C	↑ Risk of vitamin C deficiency
Non-steroidal antiinflammatory drugs (e.g., Indocin, Motrin)	See food interactions for aspirin	
BLOOD-THINNING DRUGS		
Oral anticoagulants (e.g., Coumadin, Dicumarol)	Cooking oils containing silicone additives, foods rich in vitamin K (leafy green vegetables, liver, etc.)	↓ Drug effects ↑ Risk of clot formation
	Foods rich in vitamin E (wheat germ, vegetable oil, nuts)	↑ Drug effects and risk of internal bleeding
ANTICONVULSANTS		
Dilantin	Diet low in folic acid and other B vitamins	↑ Risk of folic acid deficiency, anemia, and numbness and tingling of extremities
Phenobarbital	Same as above Protein-deficient diet	↑ Duration of drug's action
ANTIASTHMA MEDICATIONS		
Theophylline drugs (e.g., Theo-Dur, Elixophyllin)	Diet high in proteins, low in carbohydrate	↓ Drug effect
	Caffeine-rich beverages, chocolate	↑ Drug effect and risk of toxicity
ANTIBIOTICS		
Penicillin drugs (e.g., Ampicillin)	If taken with food	↓ Drug absorption
Erythromycins (e.g., E-Mycin, Erythrocin Stearate)	Same as above If taken on empty stomach	↑ Risk of abdominal cramping
Sulfonamides (e.g., Gantrisin, Azulfidine)	Diet low in folic acid	↑ Risk of folic acid deficiency
Neomycin (e.g., Myciguent)	Diet low in vitamin B_{12}, e.g., strict vegetarian	↑ Risk of vitamin B_{12} deficiency

Table 20.1.   Foods and Drugs That Do Not Mix *(cont.)*

If You Are Taking	Dietary Substance	Effects
ANTIBIOTICS *(cont.)*		
Quinolones	Caffeine	↑ Caffeine effects
	Iron	↓ Drug effect
	Antacids	↓ Drug effect
	Diet low in vitamin A	↑ Risk of vitamin A deficiency
	Diet low in calcium	↑ Risk of calcium deficiency
	Diet low in iron	↑ Risk of iron deficiency
Tetracyclines (e.g., Achromycin, Terramycin, Vibramycin)	If taken with milk and dairy products	↓ Drug absorption
	Diet low in vitamin C	↑ Risk of vitamin C deficiency
Zidovudine (Retrovir)	Fatty foods	↓ Drug absorption
URINARY ANTIBIOTICS		
Nitrofurantoin (e.g., Furadantin, Macrodantin)	If taken with food	↑ Drug effect
	Diet low in protein, milk and dairy products, foods which make urine alkaline	↓ Drug effect
	Strict vegetarian diets and those low in B vitamins	↑ Numbness and tingling
		↑ Risk of nerve damage
Trimethoprim (e.g., Bactrim, Septra)	Diet low in folic acid	↑ Risk of folic acid deficiency
ANTIDEPRESSANTS		
Tricyclic family (e.g., Elavil, Tofranil)	Foods that acidify urine (bread, bacon, corn, lentils, meat, fish and those high in vitamin C)	↓ Drug effect
Lithium (e.g., Eskalith, Lithobid)	If taken with food	↑ Rate of drug absorption
	Diet low in salt	↑ Risk of lithium toxicity
	Increases in dietary salt	↓ Drug effect
MAO inhibitors (e.g., Marplan, Parnate)	Foods rich in tyramine or tryptophan (fava beans, cheddar and other cheeses, certain wines, beer, yogurt, aged meats and others)	Dangerous rise in blood pressure, high fever, possible death
CORTICOSTEROIDS		
Hydrocortisone (Cortef), Prednisone (Deltasone), and many others	Diet low in calcium, vitamin K, or potassium	↑ Risk of nutrient deficiencies
	Diet low in protein	↑ Risk of protein deficiency
	Diet rich in salty foods	Sodium retention, weight gain
		↑ Risk of high blood pressure
ANTIPARKINSON MEDICATIONS		
Levodopa (e.g., Larodopa)	Diet high in vitamin B$_6$ (leafy green vegetables, whole grain cereals, meat, fish, poultry)	↓ Drug effect
THYROID MEDICATIONS		
Thyroid hormone (e.g., Synthroid, Levothroid)	Iodine-rich foods (e.g., iodized salt, seafood, soybean products, turnips, cabbage)	↓ Drug effectiveness
IRON SUPPLEMENTS		
Ferrous sulfate (e.g., Feosol)	If taken with food, milk, or wine	↓ Drug effect
	If taken with vitamin C	↑ Drug effect

result, a drug taken at mealtime will remain in the stomach and be subject to action by gastric acids for longer intervals than if it were taken between meals. Thus, such drugs as antibiotics, which are highly susceptible to stomach acids, may be too thoroughly degraded by the time they reach the absorption site in the small intestine. A drug that is chemically alkaline will dissolve rapidly, while one that is acidic will dissolve less rapidly.

Other absorption problems may be caused by food fibers that bind certain medications and delay or prevent their uptake into the blood. Carbohydrate fibers (pectin especially) appear to delay the absorption of the common analgesic acetaminophen (Tylenol, et al.). Similarly, the bran fibers in whole-grain foods may delay the heart medication digoxin's absorption from the intestine into the blood.

On the other hand, some drugs are actually better absorbed when taken with food. On a full stomach, the delivery of a drug to its absorption site is delayed, which is desirable for a slow-dissolving agent. Otherwise, portions of the drug will pass too rapidly through the intestine and may never enter the blood.

Food, in effect, meters the amount of drug that passes to the small intestine, thus preventing saturation. For example, the ulcer medication cimetidine (Tagamet) is also often recommended with meals, because the subsequent delay of absorption maintains blood levels of the drug for longer periods of time between dosages.

Absorption of other drugs may be promoted by particular food substances. The antifungal agent griseofulvin is better absorbed when fat is present in the digestive system. Propranolol (Inderal), commonly used to treat hypertension and heart conditions such as angina and cardiac arrythmias, is more efficiently absorbed with a high-protein meal.

Research carried out at the Rockefeller University in New York and at other centers indicates that specific foods or preparation methods can affect the metabolism of certain drugs in the liver. Protein foods, in general, accelerate the metabolic rate and thus hasten a drug's passage from the body. Cruciferous vegetables, such as cabbage, broccoli, brussels sprouts, and cauliflower, also tend to increase drug metabolism, as measured by blood levels

Table 20.1. Foods and Drugs That Do Not Mix *(cont.)*

If You Are Taking	Dietary Substance	Effects
CHOLESTEROL-LOWERING DRUGS		
Cholestyramine (Questran)	Diet low in folic acid, fat-soluble vitamins	↑ Risk of nutrient deficiencies
ANTACIDS		
Drugs containing aluminum hydroxide (e.g., Amphojel, Gaviscon, Maalox, Mylanta)	Diet low in phosphates	↑ Risk of phosphate deficiency
LAXATIVES		
Mineral oil, either orally or as an enema	Diet low in fat-soluble vitamins (A, D, E, and K)	↑ Risk of these vitamin deficiencies
Irritant laxatives containing cascara	Diet low in calcium	↑ Risk of calcium deficiency
	Diet low in vitamin D	↑ Risk of vitamin D deficiency
Bisacodyl (e.g., Dulcolax)	If taken within one hour of milk	Gastrointestinal irritation and cramping due to premature breakup of tablet

Adapted from *Health & Nutrition* newsletter, September 1986, Columbia University School of Public Health, with permission of the publisher.

of such agents as theophylline, phenacetin, and acetaminophen. Furthermore, substances in charcoal-broiled meat seem to speed the metabolism, and thus lower blood concentrations of drugs such as theophylline. It seems likely that these foods and food components affect the metabolism of various other medications, although specific research remains to be done.

Food and beverage composition may also alter the normal elimination of metabolized drugs by the kidneys. Drinking large quantities of citrus juices, for example, may make the urine more alkaline, which hinders the elimination of the antiarrhythmia drug quinidine (Quinidex, Quinaglute). Excess quinidine in the urine may then be reabsorbed to a greater extent by the kidneys, thus prolonging the drug's active stay in the body.

Other, sometimes severe, problems may follow from eating large quantities of certain foods while taking specific drugs. In excessive amounts, vitamin K, found in green leafy vegetables such as broccoli and spinach, can inhibit the effects of warfarin (Coumadin, Panwarfin) and other drugs given to reduce the risk of blood clots. Substances contained in natural licorice tend to cause sodium retention, which may disrupt the therapeutic action of many drugs used to treat high blood pressure. Eating large amounts of natural licorice may also produce hypokalemia (potassium depletion), which can be particularly threatening to individuals whose potassium levels are already low as a side effect of taking diuretics. The combination of hypokalemia and the heart drug digitalis (digoxin is its most

---

Table 20.2. Recommended Timing of Drug Administration in Relationship to Food

I. Drugs That Should Be Taken on an Empty Stomach: About One Hour Before Meals or Three Hours After Meals

- Antibiotics: Most penicillins, all tetracyclines (except doxycycline), erythromycins, clindamycin (Cleocin), lincomycin (Lincocin), and sulfonamides (such as Gantrisin and Gantanol)

- Appetite suppressants: phenmetrazine (Preludin)

- Cardiovascular drugs: dipyridamole (Persantine, Pentritol)

- Chelating agents: penicillamine (Cuprimine)

- Laxatives: bisacodyl (Dulcolax)

II. Drugs That Should Be Taken Half an Hour Before Meals

- Anticholinergic drugs: propantheline (Pro-Banthine), atropine, belladonna

III. Drugs That Should Be Taken with Food to Minimize Stomach Irritation

- Antibiotics: metronidazole (Flagyl), nitrofurantoin (Macrodantin, Furadantin), isoniazid (INH) and paraminosalicylic acid (PAS), sulfasalazine (Azulfidine), nalidixic acid (NegGram)

- Anticonvulsant drugs: phenytoin (Dilantin), primidone (Mysoline), phenobarbital

- Antidiabetic agents: chlorpropamide (Diabenese)

- Antigout drugs: sulfinpyrazone (Anturane), phenylbutazone (Butazolidin)

- Antiinflammatory drugs: aspirin, indomethacin (Indocin), and other nonsteroidal antiinflammatory drugs

- Antipsychotic drugs: all phenothiazines, haloperidol (Haldol)

- Diuretics: all thiazides, triamterene (Dyrenium), acetazolamide (Diamox)

- Parkinsonian drugs: procyclidine (Kemadrin), trihexyphenidyl (Artane), levodopa

- Others: all salicylate analgesics, nicotinic acid, aminophylline, potassium supplements, iron supplements, bulk-forming laxatives, reserpine compounds

IV. Drugs That Should Be Taken with Large Amounts of Water

- Antigout drugs: allopurinol (Zyloprim), sulfinpyrazone (Anturane), probenecid (Benemid), sulfonamides, zidovudine (Retrovir)

- Cholesterol lowering agents: cholestyramine (Questran)

- Laxatives: bulk-formers, psyllium preparations (Metamucil, Effer-Syllium) common form) may cause muscle spasms, weakness, fainting, and other toxic effects. For this reason, doctors often recommend potassium-rich foods, such as bananas, oranges, tomatoes, and dried fruits, or when indicated prescribe potassium supplements for people taking diuretics and/or digitalis.

Probably the most dramatic and dangerous of food-drug interactions involves a class of antidepressants known as monoamine oxidase (MAO) inhibitors, and the amino acid tyramine, found in aged cheese, Chianti wine, chicken livers, active yeast preparations, and various other pickled, fermented, and aged foods and beverages. The combination of MAO inhibitors—phenelzine (Nardil), tranylcypromine (Parnate), isocarborazide (Marplan)—and high-tyramine foods can produce a sudden rise in blood pressure, severe headaches, and even collapse and death. (Table 20.3 lists high-tyramine foods.)

Caffeine, which is present in coffee, tea, chocolate, many soft drinks, and hundreds of over-the-counter drugs, may also interact with prescribed medications. Caffeine belongs to the chemical family known as methylxanthines, of which the asthma drug theophylline (Theo-Dur, Theo-24, etc.) is a member. Theophylline has a relatively narrow therapeutic range: Too little of the drug proves ineffective; too much quickly becomes toxic. People who consume large amounts of coffee or tea along with theophylline may increase the potential for toxic side effects. Some research suggests that caffeine may impede the action of certain antipsychotic agents, such as flurphenazine (Prolixin) and haloperidol (Haldol). Caffeine can also cause cardiac arrhythmias or severe hypertension when consumed with the previously mentioned MAO inhibitors.

Effects of Nutritional Supplements

Many people self-prescribe vitamin, mineral, and other dietary supplements, usually without sound medical or nutritional reason, and usually without knowing these "harmless" supplements can interact with drugs they may be taking. For example, individuals with severe acne may be treated with isotretinoin (Accutane), which is related to retinoic acid, or vitamin A. If they are also taking vitamin A supplements, they may be risking a toxic buildup of the vitamin in the liver and elsewhere. (Excessive vitamin A from any source increases the risk of serious birth defects, hence Accutane is contraindicated during pregnancy or if there is a chance pregnancy may occur.) Excess vitamin B_6

Table 20.3. Food Sources of Tyramine

Foods Very High in Tyramine:	Foods Moderate in Tyramine:
Cheeses, aged	Broad beans (fava,
Boursalt	Chinese pea pods)
Camembert	Caffeine (in large amounts)
Cheddar	Chocolate (in large
Stilton	amounts)
Yeast Extracts	Liver, chicken, and beef
Foods High in Tyramine:	Pineapple
Bologna	Plums
Dried, salted, or pickled	Raisins
herring	Soy sauce
Dried, salted, or pickled	**Foods Low in Tyramine:**
cod	Ale
Pepperoni	Avocados
Salami	Bananas
Foods Moderately High in Tyramine:	Beer
Cheeses	Cheeses
Blue	American, processed
Brick, natural	Cottage
Gruyere	Cream
Mozzarella	Ricotta
Parmesan	Figs
Romano	Sherry
Roquefort	Sour cream
Chianti wine	White wine
Meat tenderizers	

(pyridoxine) interferes with levodopa, commonly used to treat Parkinson's disease. As noted earlier, high doses of vitamin K, whether in food or in supplement form, can interfere with warfarin. Moreover, medical literature also includes reports of vitamins C and E undermining warfarin's anticoagulant effect.

The mineral calcium, found in milk and other dairy products, canned sardines and salmon (eaten with their bones), kale, broccoli, and okra—as well as in several popular supplements and antacids—impairs the absorption of some of the drugs in the tetracycline class of antibiotics. This is reasonably well known; but the fact that magnesium, zinc, and iron may have similar effects is not. Experts recommend, therefore, that tetracycline and its cousins be taken before or several hours after meals or supplements containing these minerals. Calcium pills may interfere with iron absorption, iron pills with zinc absorption, and so on.

Finally, people taking MAO inhibitors must exercise special caution with amino-acid supplements and dietary additives containing yeast. Not only are these compounds of dubious nutritional value, they may have among their ingredients tyramine, which can interact dangerously with these antidepressant drugs.

WHEN A DRUG AFFECTS NUTRITION

Just as the presence of food or dietary supplements in the digestive tract can interfere with the absorption of a drug, the presence of a drug also may interfere with nutrient absorption. Overuse of laxatives, a practice common among elderly people, provides a classic example. Mineral-oil laxatives tend to trap fat-soluble nutrients (vitamins A, K, D, and E) and prevent their absorption. Over time and

continued laxative abuse, deficiencies in these vitamins may develop. Stimulant laxatives, such as bisacodyl (Dulcolax) and phenolphthalein (Ex-Lax) work by provoking peristaltic contractions in the digestive tract; they, too, can contribute to deficiencies by speeding nutrients through the intestine before proper absorption can take place. To ease constipation problems, a combination of eating more fruits and vegetables, increasing fluid intake, and exercising regularly is both safer and more effective in the long run than taking laxatives. When a laxative is truly required, bulk-forming products such as psyllium hydrophylic mucilloid (e.g., Metamucil) are usually the safest choice. Since Metamucil contains soluble fiber, it can moderately reduce serum-cholesterol levels.

Older people also tend to rely unduly on antacids to relieve indigestion, even though the production of stomach acids actually decreases with age. Large amounts of magnesium- and aluminum-based antacids, such as Maalox, Mylanta, and Gaviscon, can deplete the body of phosphorus, a mineral important in the formation of bones and teeth. Since older people—especially women—are already at risk of osteoporosis, antacid abuse and subsequent phosphorus deficiency can be a significant problem in this age group. Calcium-carbonate preparations (e.g., Tums) may be of little help because they can interfere with iron absorption and, in the absence of gastric acid, their calcium may be poorly absorbed.

Aspirin is yet another household drug that can produce nutrient shortages—particularly in the elderly—when large amounts are taken regularly. High doses, frequently prescribed for older people with arthritis, irritate the stomach lining and can cause microscopic bleeding (and hence, iron loss, as iron is a principal component of the hemoglobin in red blood cells). To prevent stomach irritation, it is best to use coated aspirin preparations (provided the coating is soluble in the bowel) or to take the drug with or after meals or with water as a buffer. Prolonged use of aspirin may also lead to deficiencies in folic acid and vitamin C. A diet rich in sources of iron (found in liver, meat, seafood, legumes, whole-grain and enriched breads and cereals) and vitamin C (found in citrus fruits and juices, melon, potatoes, cauliflower, and dark green leafy vegetables) is also recommended for people on long-term aspirin therapy.

Many other drugs can interfere with the absorption of specific vitamins and minerals. Fortunately, the American diet contains sufficient amounts of most nutrients to offset these subtle and often transient effects. When certain drugs are taken on a prolonged basis, however, or when an individual's nutritional status is already compromised by chronic disease, potentially serious deficiencies may result. People with inflammatory bowel disease, for example, may be deficient in folic acid. Sulfasalazine, which is frequently prescribed to treat this condition, augments this deficiency by interfering with folic-acid absorption. It is important, therefore, for individuals with this condition to include a variety of folate-rich foods in their diet, or to take supplements if their doctor specifically recommends them.

Women who take birth-control pills may also encounter nutritional effects. For example, these drugs may moderately interfere with absorption of vitamin B_6 and folic acid; if the diet is short in these nutrients, deficiencies may occur, but not if a well-balanced diet is consumed. Dietary sources high in vitamin B_6 include meat, fish, nuts, carrots, bananas, poultry, avocados, and green leafy vegetables. Foods high in folic acid include liver, wheat germ, green leafy vegetables, nuts, legumes, and many fruits.

With the recent national rise in cholesterol consciousness, cholesterol-lowering drugs such as cholestyramine (Questran) and Metamucil are being used much more widely than ever before. These drugs can interfere with the absorption of fat and several other nutrients, and there is evidence that extended use of these drugs may lead to deficiencies in fat-soluble vitamins (vitamins A, D, and E), as well as vitamin K. However, another cholesterol-lowering drug, lovastatin (Mevacor), should be taken with food to maximize absorption and thus be more effective.

Medications also may interfere with complex enzyme systems in the liver that govern much of the biochemistry of metabolism. For example, the anticonvulsive agents phenytoin (Dilantin) and phenobarbital, prescribed for people with epilepsy, can alter the liver's microsomal metabolizing system in such a way that a vitamin D shortage may result. Since vitamin D helps regulate the uptake of calcium in bone, deficiency can contribute to bone disorders such as osteomalacia and osteoporosis. There is some evidence, too, that these drugs may alter folic-acid metabolism, in part because of a structural similarity to the folic-acid molecule. Folic-acid metabolism also may be upset by methotrexate (used to treat cancer and severe rheumatoid arthritis), the antimalarial drug pyrimethamine and the diuretic triamterene (Dyrenium, and combined with another drug in Dyazide). All three of these drugs have structural similarities to folic acid and therefore can interfere with folic-acid metabolism.

Drugs and Appetite

Whereas the effects of the above interactions are subtle and sometimes slow to develop, one of the more obvious ways that medicine can interfere with nutrition is by affecting appetite and, therefore, food intake (see Table 20.4). Amphetamines, of course, have long been used deliberately to depress appetite, and they are still sometimes prescribed in weight-reduction programs, although they are good only for about two weeks and can do much harm. Such use has declined in recent years, however, due in part to the recognition of the addictive nature of these drugs and the growing understanding among clinicians that appetite is not necessarily the central problem of weight control.

Cancer-chemotherapy agents typically depress the appetite, either by causing severe nausea or by dulling or distorting taste sensations. The extreme discomfort of chemotherapy also may create negative mental associations with a particular food or foods the patient happens to eat during a treatment period. Cancer itself can adversely affect appetite.

There are, in addition, a great many other drugs—ranging from antibiotics to arthritis remedies to digitalis—that may reduce appetite by causing nausea or an unpleasant aftertaste. These side effects tend to be more pronounced in older people, who are generally more vulnerable to drug actions. Health professionals are only beginning to recognize that sudden appetite and weight loss and consequent physical failure—which often accompany chronic illness in older people—may actually be the result of the treatment rather than the disease. Digitalis, a drug used to prevent heart failure, is notorious in this regard. Nausea, vomiting, and appetite loss are common reactions to digitalis, and, particularly in older patients, even a slightly greater dose than needed can amplify these effects. To prevent appetite and weight loss, health professionals treating elderly people need to monitor carefully the amounts of digitalis and many other drugs they routinely prescribe, and to change drugs or adjust dosages whenever problems occur.

In contrast, there are a number of other drugs, including a number of psychotropic agents, that stimulate appetite as a side effect. Chorpromazine (Thorazine) and other anti-psychotic drugs used in severely disturbed individuals may even cause obesity over an extended course of therapy. Some researchers have noted, however, that these drugs may have an opposite effect in the elderly, apparently reducing interest in food. Lithium, used to treat manic-depression and other mood disorders, may also promote appetite and weight gain, as may both MAO inhibitors and tricyclic antidepressants. Cravings for sweets have been reported in people taking the tricyclic amitriptyline (Elavil).

The antihistamine cyproheptadine (Periactin) is sometimes prescribed specifically to stimulate appetite in individuals recovering from a prolonged, wasting disease. Corticosteroids, such as prednisone and triamcinolone, which are used to treat conditions such as severe allergy and asthma, also boost appetite and weight gain, although in these cases such effects are usually unwanted.

Sodium and fluid retention is another common side effect that, while not altering appetite, can result in weight gain from extra fluid. Medications that cause fluid retention include several antihypertensive agents (clonidine, guanethidine, hydralazine, and methyldopa) and antiinflammatory agents (the corticosteroids, phenylbutazone, and indomethacin, or Indocin). This problem is usually controlled by cutting down on dietary salt consumption and taking a diuretic to dispel excess fluids and sodium. Many diuretics, however, deplete the body of potassium and magnesium, along with the sodium. As noted earlier in this chapter, the combination of low potassium and digitalis (or digoxin) can increase the drug's potency to toxic strength. Since both diuretics and digitalis are commonly prescribed for heart failure, physicians should be careful to avoid this three-sided diet-drug interaction. One option is prescribing a potassium-sparing diuretic, such as spironolactone (Aldactone) or amiloride (Midamor).

Table 20.4. Examples of Drugs Affecting Food Intake

Effects	Drug Category	Examples
Reduces appetite	Allergy and cold medications containing antihistamines	azatadine (Optimine), brompheniramine (Bromphed)
	Amphetamines	methylphenidate (Ritalin)
	Anticancer drugs	cisplatin (Platinol), doxorubicin (Adriamycin), fluorouracil (Adrucil, Efudex, Fluoroplex), mercaptopurine (Purinethol)
	Anticonvulsants	phenytoin (Dilantin)
	Antidepressants	fluoxetine (Prozac)
	Heart medications	captopril (Capoten), digitoxin (Crystodigin), diltiazem (Cardizem)
	Laxatives (high-fiber types)	psyllium (Metamucil, Perdiem, etc.)
Increases appetite	Antidepressants	amitriptyline (Elavil), imipramine (Tofranil)
	Antidiabetes drugs	insulin, tolbutamide (Orinase)
	Corticosteroids	prednisone (Deltasone, Liquid Pred)
	Tranquilizers	prochloreperazine (Compazine), promazine (Sparine)
Causes stomach upset, nausea and/or vomiting	Amphetamines	aminophylline, theophylline (Slo-bid, Theo-24, Theo-Dur)
	Antiarthritic	aspirin, indomethacin (Indocin) and other nonsteroidal antiinflammatory drugs
	Antibiotics	cefazolin (Kefzol), erythromycin (E-Mycin and others), penicillins (Bicillin C-R), trimethoprim/sulfamethoxazole (Bactrim, Septra), pentamidine (Pentam 300)
	Anticancer	azathioprine (Imuran), cisplatin (Platinol), cyclophosphamide (Cytoxan, Neosar), doxorubicin (Adriamycin), diethylstilbestrol (Stilbestrol, Stilphostrol), ethinyl estradiol (Estinyl), fluorouracil (Adrucil, Efudex, Fluoroplex), mercaptopurine (Purinethol), procarbazine (Matulane)
	Anticonvulsants	phenytoin (Dilantin)
	Antihistamines	brompheniramine (Dimetane), terfenadine (Seldane)
	Antihypertensive drugs	hydralazine (Apresoline)
	Chelating agents	penicillamine (Cuprimine, Depen)
	Corticosteroids	hydrocortisone (Cortef), prednisone (Deltasone), triamcinolone (Aristocort)
	Heart medications	cholestyramine (Questran), clofibrate (Atromid-S), digitoxin (Crystodigin), digoxin (Lanoxicaps, Lanoxin), gemfibrozil (Lopid), hydralazine (Apresoline), labetalol (Normodyne, Trandate), niacin (high dose), prazosin (Minipress), probucol (Lorelco), verapamil (Calan, Isoptin)
	Painkillers	aspirin, nonsteroidal antiinflammatory drugs, propoxyphene (Darvon, Dolene)
	Potassium salts	potassium chloride (Kaon-Cl, Micro-K, Slow-K), potassium gluconate (Kaon)

Table 20.4. Examples of Drugs Affecting Food Intake *(cont.)*

Effects	Drug Category	Examples
Alters taste	Amphetamines	dextroamphelamine (Dexedrine)
	Antibiotics	pentamidine (Pentam 300)
	Anti-Parkinson's	levadopa (Dopar)
	Abuse deterrents	disulfiram (Antabuse)
	Chelating agents	penicillamine (Cuprimine, Depen)
	Tranquilizers	lithium (Lithobid)
Causes constipation	Antacids	aluminum hydroxide (Gaviscon, Gelusil, and others)
	Antidepressants	amoxapine (Asendin), doxepin (Adapin)
	Antihypertensive	clonidine (Catapres)
	Anti-ulcer	sucralfate (Carafate)
	Heart medications	cholestyramine (Questran), dilitiazem (Cardizem), verapamil (Calan, Isoptin)
	Narcotic painkillers	codeine (Empirin with codeine, Phenaphen with codeine)
Causes diarrhea	Antacids	magnesium hydroxide (Milk of Magnesia)
	Antibiotics	cefaclor (Ceclor), clindamycin (Cleocin Phosphate), amoxicillin/clavulanate (Augmentin), erythromycin (E-Mycin), lincomycin (Lincocin), tetracycline (Sumycin)
	Anticancer	fluorouracil (Adrucil, Efudex), methotrexate (Folex, Mexate)
	Antiinflammatory	diflunisal (Dolobid)
	Antimalaria	chloroquine (Aralen)
	Heart medications	guanethidine (Ismelin), gemfibrozil (Lopid), probucol (Lorelco), niacin (high dose)
	Potassium salts	potassium chloride (Slow-K), potassium gluconate (Kaon)
Causes dry mouth	Antidepressants	amoxapine (Asendin), imipramine (Sk-Pramine)
	Antihistamines	azaladine (Optimine), dimenhydrinate (Dramamine), diphenhydramine (Benadryl), meclizine (Antivert, Bonine, D-Vert), promethazine (Mepergan, Phenergan, Promex)
Increases salivation	Cholinergic	bethanecol (Urecholine)
	Antianxiety	clonazepam (Klonopin)
	Anticonvulsants	phenytoin (Dilantin)
Reduces absorption of nutrients	Antibiotics	erythromycin (E-Mycin, and others), penicillins
Interferes with the synthesis of vitamin D and the absorption of folic acid	Anticonvulsants	phenytoin (Dilantin)
Prevents absorption of vitamins A, D, E, and K	Types of mineral-oil laxatives	mineral oil
Lowers blood levels of vitamin B_6 in women	Oral contraceptives	norethindrone acetate and ethinyl estradiol (Loestrin 21, Norlestrin 21, Ortho-Novum 10/11)

ALCOHOL AND DRUGS

Alcohol is both a drug and a food and can have a profound effect when combined with some prescription medications. In fact, one treatment for alcoholism involves deliberately prescribing the drug disulfiram (Antabuse), which in combination with alcohol produces such unpleasant side effects (flushing, headache, nausea, vomiting, abdominal pain) that further drinking is strongly discouraged. Similar reactions with alcohol can be unintentionally produced by other drugs such as metronizadole (Flagyl) and furazolidone (Furoxone). Flushing and headaches may also result from mixing alcohol with the antifungal drug griseofulvin (Fulvicin, Grisactin) or with the oral antidiabetes drugs chlorpropamide (Diabinese), tolbutamide (Orinase), and tolazamide (Tolinase). Perhaps more significantly, alcohol in combination with these antidiabetic agents exaggerates the effects of lowering blood sugar, and can provoke what is known as insulin reaction: dizziness, weakness, mental confusion, and even collapse and coma.

Heavy use of alcohol depresses the appetite and food absorption and can cause malabsorption of fat, folic acid, thiamine, and vitamin B_{12}. It also directly attacks the liver, and the resulting damage from chronic alcoholism may impair the metabolism of many different nutrients. Alcoholic injury to the pancreas can hinder the production of digestive enzymes, which further contributes to absorption problems.

Alcohol also depresses the central nervous system, and thus dangerously amplifies the effects of other sedative drugs, such as tranquilizers, barbiturates, and sleeping pills. The combination of drinking and the popular tranquilizer diazepam (Valium) not only enhances the drug's sedative effects but also interferes with the drug's elimination from the body. As a result, the drug remains active for an extended period of time, heightening the risk of overdose and even death.

Finally, excessive alcohol intake can block the therapeutic action of some anticonvulsant drugs—thus causing seizures—and increase the effect of anticoagulant agents, which may lead to severe hemorrhaging. (See below for a list of drugs that may cause severe adverse reactions with alcohol.)

SUMMING UP

In this chapter, we have presented an overview of some of the myriad drug-food interactions. Whenever taking a new medication, either prescription or over-the-counter, and including over-the-counter vitamin, mineral, amino acid, or other supplements, consult your doctor or pharmacist about possible food-drug interactions, timing of drug administration and food intake, and specific substances that should be avoided.

Drugs That Should Not Be Taken with Alcohol

Antihistamines (both prescription and over-the-counter)

Narcotics: morphine, codeine, Dilaudid, Percodan, Demerol, etc.

Barbiturates: Amytal, Nembutal, Seconal, etc.

Tranquilizers: Valium, Librium, Dalmane, etc.

Antidiabetic agents: Orinase, Tolinase, Diabinese, etc.

Tricyclic antidepressants: Elavil, Tofranil, Pamelor, etc.

MAO inhibitors: Nardil, Parnate, Marplan

Anticonvulsants: Dilantin, phenobarbital

Anticoagulants: Coumadin, Panwarfin, heparin

Antidyskinetics: triheyphenidyl (Artane), benztropine mesylate (Cogentin)

21

The Nutritional Effects of Alcohol

Charles S. Lieber, M.D.

◼

INTRODUCTION

No one knows where or how mankind first discovered alcohol. Perhaps it was first encountered as honey that had fermented and become mead, or fermented grains that produced a beerlike beverage, or fruit juice that became a kind of wine. Once discovered, however, an important new industry was born—one that persists to this day. Some historians suggest, for example, that the desire to grow grains for fermentation as well as for flour may have contributed to early man's shift from hunting and gathering to the more settled life of a farmer. There is no doubt that people have been using—and abusing—alcohol since before recorded history.

Alcohol—or, to use its chemical name, ethanol—is the result of the breakdown of sugars and starches by a fungus (yeast) in a process called fermentation. Modern beer is made by fermenting barley and hops. Wine comes from the fermentation of grapes or other fruits or plants, hard liquors from the fermentation of starches derived from various grains or from potatoes. After fermentation, the resulting product is distilled to concentrate the alcohol. Our own intestinal bacteria may make some alcohol.

Over the years, alcohol has had many roles in addition to its use as a beverage. It has been used in lieu of wages, in religious ceremonies, and in the domination of one population by another. It has helped change the course of history; for example, Washington purposely crossed the Delaware on Christmas night, expecting the Hessian mercenaries fighting for England to be recovering from the excesses of their Yuletide festivities. Alcohol taxes were behind the Pennsylvania Whisky Rebellion of 1794, and drinking was the reason for one of the greatest social experiments in the United States—the attempt to prohibit the manufacture and sale of alcoholic liquors by constitutional amendment in 1920. This failed experiment revealed just how widespread alcohol use was, and how much people cherished their access to it.

Alcohol has been used as a mind-altering substance, as an anti-emetic, disinfectant, tonic, and diuretic. The Greek physician Galen referred to wine as "the nurse of old age." It has been sold as an all-purpose cure-all, disguised in some promoters' magical elixirs, and it remains a major ingredient in many cough medicines, painkillers, and tonics. Alcohol content sold the elixir Hadacol.

THE MANY FACETS OF ALCOHOL

Alcohol can be classified as a food, a drug, or a highly toxic poison. Its use and abuse are a social concern and a major health problem that span a wide cross-section of the population. About two-thirds of all Americans aged 18 years or older and three-quarters of all high school students drink alcohol. Because of the wide acceptance of social drinking—witness television and print ads linking alcohol and good times or glamour—it is unlikely that many know a great deal about its true effects.

All alcoholic beverages can be classified as foods, because they provide energy. One gram of alcohol contains seven calories, more than a gram of protein or carbohydrate, which each contain about 4 calories. Alcohol's calories are empty, however, because alcoholic beverages provide only negligible amounts of vitamins and minerals. In fact, alcohol is often called the antinutrient nutrient: Not only do its empty calories replace the nutrient-rich calories of food but it also directly interferes with the body's absorption, storage, and use of nutrients, even if they are present in adequate amounts in the diet.

As a drug, alcohol is classified as a narcotic because the body builds up an ever greater tolerance to it. For some people, it also is an addictive drug: Predisposed users can become dependent on it to the extent that strong cravings develop when it is withdrawn. Only more alcohol can *relieve* withdrawal symptoms; other drugs *suppress* them.

Alcoholism—drinking to the extent that it affects a person's health and lifestyle—is a major social problem in many countries of the world, including the United States. There is little agreement as to what exactly causes alcoholism, how to prevent it, or how to treat it, but an estimated 10 percent of those who drink are believed to do so often enough and heavily enough to experience health, social, and behavioral problems. Although long believed to be overindulgent behavior either by choice or due to personal weakness, alcoholism is now recognized as a disease, one that has a genetic predisposition.

Alcohol use has come under increasing scrutiny. In the United States, an earlier trend toward lowering the legal drinking age is now being reversed in many states and changed back to 20 or 21 years of age. This is due in large part to the alarming death rate of young people as a consequence of drinking and driving. Alcohol is thought to be a factor in half the nation's traffic fatalities—more than 20,000 deaths a year—and a large number of these accidents involve teenagers.

In addition to the role it plays in accidents—in the home and the workplace as well as on the highways—excessive alcohol use has been linked to increased risk of cancer, high blood pressure, strokes, heart disease, dementia, and other disorders. Years of excessive drinking can cause cirrhosis, a serious liver disease that is responsible for about 11,000 deaths a year in the United States. Alcohol is also implicated in innumerable cases of child abuse, rape, assault, murder, and suicide.

HOW ALCOHOL WORKS IN THE BODY

Massive amounts of alcohol, ingested over a short period of time, can be fatal. Every year, for example, there are news stories of tragic deaths as a result of excessive alcohol consumption at fraternity initiation rites or other gatherings of young people. Alcohol is also toxic in a more insidious fashion: Taken over a long period of time, it causes irreversible damage to the liver and, eventually in many cases, death.

Alcohol does not require digestion. Once ingested, alcohol quickly makes its way through the body and about 95 percent is absorbed directly and immediately into the bloodstream from the stomach and the small intestine—rather more quickly through the intestinal walls than through the thick mucous membranes of the stomach lining. The remaining 5 percent leaves the body via perspiration, respiration, and the urine. Alcohol taken on an empty stomach will be absorbed into the bloodstream within about 20 minutes.

From the bloodstream, alcohol moves into all body tissues. The effects of the same amount of alcohol, which vary depending on a person's weight, consumption, and the type of drink, will be more pronounced in a 150-pound person than in a 200-pound person, simply because the alcohol is more concentrated in the smaller body. Because fat holds less water than muscle, a flabby man weighing 200 pounds will obtain a higher blood-alcohol level than a muscular man of the same weight. Similarly, women feel the impact of a drink more quickly than men, probably because enzymes in the male stomach dispose of more alcohol than do the same enzymes in the female stomach. Thus, a woman will absorb more alcohol into her bloodstream than a man. Women also are more susceptible to the effects of a drink just before the menstrual period, when oxidization of alcohol in the liver is at its slowest.

In addition to the above differences, animal studies and those of twins indicate that genetic differences play a role in tolerance for alcohol. Most of a person's capacity to tolerate alcohol, however, has to do with drinking patterns, with increasing tolerance coming with frequent drinking.

Since about 5 percent of the alcohol ingested is eliminated from the body in perspiration, urine, and the breath, the approximate blood levels can be obtained by breathalizer and urine tests, such as those used by the police to check for drunk driving. The remainder is oxidized, or broken down, by the liver. The healthy liver oxidizes alcohol at the rate of about one-fourth to one-third ounce of pure ethanol an hour—less than one ounce of hard liquor. Meanwhile, the unmetabolized alcohol continues to circulate in the bloodstream. The alcohol in two 4-ounce glasses of wine (one-half ounce of ethanol per drink) circulates for three to five hours before being completely broken down. The more alcohol that is consumed, the more time that is required to metabolize it.

Contrary to popular belief, the rate at which the body (liver) processes alcohol cannot be speeded up by a cold shower, a brisk walk around the block, a cup of strong coffee, or other strategies. Instead, they may produce a wide-awake drunk and are dangerous in that they may mislead the drinker into thinking that he or she is sober enough to drive or perform other tasks. Only the passage of time will clear the alcohol from the bloodstream.

THE PROCESS OF INTOXICATION

Within minutes of being ingested, alcohol reaches the brain. In the brain, alcohol acts as a depressant and a sedative, producing a sense of calm; as an anesthetic, producing numbness; and finally as a hypnotic, producing sleep. Paradoxically, however, its initial effect is a stimulating one, producing a feeling of well-being, even of euphoria. (See pages 344–45 for information on the effects of different types of drinks and the factors influencing alcohol absorption.)

The first brain functions to be depressed are those in the frontal lobe, which controls judgment and behavior. The drinker will usually be more talkative and outgoing, perhaps more aggressive. There will often be a release of sexual inhibitions; unexpected mood swings may be exhibited.

With higher levels of alcohol in the blood, the parts of the brain that control speech, vision, and the voluntary muscles will be affected. Reaction time, depth perception, night vision, and muscle coordination will all be impaired. In most states, a drinker at this stage is legally intoxicated, with a blood concentration of 0.1 percent—one part pure alcohol per thousand parts of blood. (It should be noted that responses to a given blood-alcohol concentration vary from individual to individual, and even in the same person at different times.)

If drinking continues to a blood-alcohol concentration of 0.4 percent, brain function will be depressed to the state of unconsciousness. At a blood-alcohol concentration of about 0.5 percent, complete paralysis of the breathing functions can occur, resulting in death. This seldom occurs, however; either the alcohol is vomited out of the stomach or the drinker passes out before a fatal dose can be taken. Occasionally, rapid, marathon drinking leads to death because enough alcohol is consumed before the drinker loses consciousness so that the blood-alcohol concen-

Effects of Different Types of Drink

The alcohol content of a drink varies according to how a beverage was made: The distilling process used to make whiskey and other hard liquors, as well as brandy, cognac, and cordials, produces a more concentrated beverage, at 40 to 50 percent. Table wines have a 10 to 14 percent alcohol content, most American beers about 4 percent, and light beers about 3 percent (see The Meanings of *Light* on page 351).

The term *proof* refers to the concentrations of alcohol. Standards vary from one country to another, but in the United States proof is two times the alcohol content: 80-proof whiskey contains 40 percent alcohol. There is an equivalent amount of alcohol (½ ounce) in 1½ ounces of 80-proof liquor, 4 or 5 ounces of wine, and 12 ounces of beer. It is therefore not true, as some believe, that drinking wine or beer is not drinking.

The body's initial reaction to alcohol depends to a large extent on the type of drink. In studies done in the 1960s, subjects were given gin or vodka, whiskey, wine, or beer amounting to 0.6 grams of alcohol per kilogram of body weight. Those who received gin or vodka had a blood-alcohol concentration of 0.1 percent within about 15 minutes. Whiskey produced a slightly lower blood-alcohol concentration (0.09 percent) in the same time period. However, table wine and beer produced significantly lower maximum levels: 0.06 percent after about 30 minutes for wine and 0.045 percent in 90 minutes for beer. After about two hours, the blood-alcohol concentration of all the subjects was essentially the same: about 0.04 percent. The level fell to zero in about seven hours, whatever the drink.

When all three types of beverages—distilled spirits, wine, beer—are consumed with food, the peak levels of blood-alcohol concentration are lower (in one study, 0.04 for spirits, 0.03 for beer). The most important factors affecting peak blood-alcohol concentration, in addition to the type of drink, appear to be body weight and the rate at which the stomach empties.

These studies illustrate what many drinkers have long known: Hard liquor produces a stronger initial kick, but over time, alcohol is alcohol. Of course, although it is quite possible to become drunk on wine or beer, these beverages do not provoke the surge in blood-alcohol concentration, with the attendant relaxation of inhibitions and rapid intoxication, that hard liquor does. However, in terms of the long-term effects of alcohol, it is the total amount consumed that is important.

tration continues to rise thereafter to the fatal level. However, people who drink and are taking medications that also depress the central nervous system, such as tranquilizers or barbiturates, may suffer respiratory failure at lower levels of alcohol.

THE HANGOVER

The hangover has plagued mankind since alcohol was discovered. Symptoms vary from person to person, but they generally include a throbbing headache, thirst, nausea, upset stomach, diarrhea, and irritability. The headache is the result of dilation of the blood vessels in the brain. The thirst and dehydration are due to alcohol's diuretic action (alcohol inhibits release of the antidiuretic hormone vasopressin from the pituitary). The gastrointestinal symptoms are caused by increased secretion of hydrochloric acid in the stomach.

The severity of a hangover may be related, in part, to substances in alcoholic beverages called congeners, present as by-products of fermentation. Congeners are responsible for a beverage's taste, color, and aroma. The more congeners in a beverage, the worse the hangover can be. Vodka has the least congeners and reportedly produces the

Factors Influencing Alcohol Absorption

Absorption will be somewhat slowed if the stomach has food in it, particularly fatty or protein foods that tend to delay the emptying of the stomach. Watery drinks such as beer or a wine spritzer are absorbed more slowly than drinks with a higher alcohol content. Carbonated beverages speed up passage of the stomach's contents into the small intestine, where absorption is quicker.

mildest hangover, followed in ascending order by gin, white wine, whiskey, rum, red wine, and brandy.

Over the centuries, there have been numerous cures for the hangover, as well as some remedies to be taken before or during a drinking bout. The cures range from the owlets' eyes of the Romans to today's chili peppers, Worcestershire sauce, oysters, inhalations of oxygen, and vigorous exercise. A hair of the dog—more alcohol—has long been popular; the Bloody Mary, among other mixtures, was originally a hangover cure. As noted earlier, none of these remedies really helps. A hangover is essentially a withdrawal state; treating it with more alcohol simply postpones recovery. Time and medications to relieve the symptoms (an analgesic for the headache and an antacid for the upset stomach) are the best remedies.

A panel convened by the Food and Drug Administration to review over-the-counter remedies found than no product or single ingredient was "unique in relieving the symptoms of a hangover." The panel also reviewed several products that claimed to prevent inebriation if taken before or during drinking, and found them all to be ineffective. The effectiveness of fructose, claimed to prevent or reduce drunkenness (supposedly by lowering blood-alcohol concentrations), awaits further studies; thus far, toxic effects on the liver (hepatotoxicity) had been reported. Currently, any product that claims to produce sobriety is considered a drug and must be approved for both safety and effectiveness by the FDA prior to going on the market.

EFFECTS OF ALCOHOL ON BODY ORGANS

The chronic use of alcohol has damaging effects on virtually every organ system in the body, including the liver, the pancreas, the gastrointestinal tract, the brain, the heart, the muscles, and the gonads.

The Liver

Unlike most sources of energy, alcohol is not broken down significantly anywhere in the body except the liver. In the liver, disposing of the alcohol takes precedence over other functions. Alcohol breaks down in the liver via different enzyme systems to form acetaldehyde, which is toxic to both heart and brain. This, in turn, is broken down into carbon dioxide and water. One of the systems also breaks down virtually all toxic substances including drugs, becoming more active in the presence of alcohol. The liver of a habitual drinker thus develops a tolerance for alcohol, breaking it down faster than that of a nondrinker. It also degrades drugs much more rapidly (see Alcohol and Drug Interactions on page 348). As a result, dietary protein and fat are not metabolized as readily and, instead, are stored in the liver. The stored protein can absorb ten times its volume as water and thus causes the liver to swell. Unmetabolized fat deposited in the liver produces a fatty liver, which further impairs the organ's function. The inability of the liver to metabolize fat adequately also results in high levels of lipids in the blood.

The liver rapidly accumulates fat: After only a weekend of heavy drinking, fatty deposits will be evident. A fatty liver is the first step in the organ's deterioration and is characteristic of heavy drinkers. With continued alcohol abuse, many heavy drinkers go on to develop alcoholic hepatitis (not related to infectious or serum hepatitis), in which the liver becomes inflamed and hardened. If the person stops at this point and follows a nutritious diet, the changes may be reversed and the liver will return to normal. When drinking is heavy and continues over years, however, fibrous scar tissue replaces normal liver cells and the organ will be unable to perform its numerous functions. An estimated 10 to 20 percent of alcoholics progress to this final stage of liver disease, cirrhosis, which is not reversible by good nutrition and can lead to liver failure and death. (See Chapter 31.)

With the decline in function, the liver cannot make glucose from the stored glycogen. Abnormalities in the metabolism of vitamins and increases in the lipoproteins and accumulation of toxic substances in the body are among the consequences of liver dysfunction.

The Brain

Excessive long-term use of alcohol destroys the neurons, producing a decline of intellectual function, memory loss, and inability to concentrate. The brain of a heavy drinker ages prematurely. Sometimes, however, a period of abstinence brings improvement in brain function. Alcohol also affects the brain's normal production or use of the neurotransmitter serotonin and endorphins, the body's natural opiates.

Chronic alcohol use can reduce blood flow—and oxygen—to the brain and may result in blacking out. During a blackout, the drinker functions as usual and seems to be aware of his or her surroundings but later cannot remember anything that happened. Not all heavy drinkers have blackouts and whether or when they occur is unpredictable.

A type of alcoholic dementia also may occur among heavy drinkers. This is sometimes difficult to differentiate from Alzheimer's and other forms of dementia, but X rays of the head often will show a characteristic shrinking of the brain.

Recently, a large study reported an increased risk of stroke even in those characterized as light drinkers. Dementia related to recurrent ministrokes, or transient ischemic attacks, is also thought to be more common among heavy drinkers.

The Cardiovascular System

Alcohol can affect the heart and blood vessels in many ways, ranging from dilation of peripheral blood vessels, producing flushing and warmth, to damage of the heart muscle, which can result in sudden death. Even a single episode of heavy drinking may produce arrhythmia (irregular heartbeat), and those who abuse alcohol have an increased risk of hypertension and heart-muscle disease, or cardiomyopathy.

In alcoholic cardiomyopathy, the heart becomes enlarged and cannot pump effectively, resulting in a backup of blood into tissues and organs. The disorder usually is confined to men who are chronic abusers and is often reversible with bed rest and abstinence.

Some studies have shown that moderate alcohol consumption (5 to 10 grams daily) is positively correlated with higher levels of high-density lipoproteins (and lower cholesterol). Other researchers note that the type of HDL cholesterol that increases with drinking has no protective effect against heart attacks. (See also Chapter 6.)

The Gastrointestinal Tract

Alcohol is an irritant to the entire digestive tract, damaging the mucosal linings of the mouth, esophagus, and stomach. Especially in heavy smokers, there is strong evidence of a link between alcohol and cancers of the gastrointestinal tract, the mouth, the pharynx, the larynx, and the stomach.

In the stomach, alcohol increases the output of hydrochloric acid, irritating the lining and producing heartburn, nausea, and ulcers in both the stomach and duodenum. Peptic ulcers are more common among heavy drinkers. Chronic alcohol use also impairs the stomach's ability to move food into the intestine. In the small intestine, it damages the absorption and movement of nutrients including lactose (milk sugar)—resulting in lactose intolerance—folic acid, vitamin B_{12} and thiamine. Added to the poor diet of many heavy drinkers, this often results in severe malnutrition.

Alcohol also causes inflammation of the pancreas and impaired production of pancreatic enzymes needed for the digestion of proteins and fat. The inflammatory effects continue through the large intestine and to the rectum.

ALCOHOL AND SEXUAL FUNCTION

In small doses, alcohol releases inhibitions and increases self-confidence, which is responsible for its reputation as a sex stimulant. In larger doses, however, sexual performance suffers and interest in sex declines. Alcoholic men frequently become impotent.

A moderate amount of alcohol can interfere with erection and ejaculation; heavier use results in reduced sex drive and in impotence in the majority of alcoholic men. Reduced levels of testosterone and increased ones of estrogen may result in growth of breast tissue and soft, atrophied testicles. In women, heavy drinking may lead to ovarian malfunctions and the cessation of menstruation.

ALCOHOL AND PREGNANCY

Heavy drinking during pregnancy—especially during the first trimester—can have devastating effects on the fetus. The baby may be born suffering from a condition known as fetal alcohol syndrome. These babies are below normal in weight, height, and head circumference. They have characteristic face malformations and frequently suffer from poor motor development and mental retardation. The abnormalities are irreversible.

Scientific investigation has not yet determined what level of alcohol consumption is safe during pregnancy, or whether there is a safe level at all. There is some evidence that women who drink as little as one ounce of alcohol a week have an increased rate of spontaneous abortion, and that one ounce a day can lead to a low-birth-weight baby. This was borne out in a study of over 30,000 pregnant women in which researchers at the National Institute of Child Health and Human Development found that consumption of one or two drinks a day was associated with a "substantial risk" of producing a lower-birth-weight infant, and that those who had three to five drinks a day gave birth to infants who weighed about six ounces less than babies of nondrinkers. An editorial that accompanied the study when it was published in 1984 stated that "women who are pregnant and wish to have healthy babies should not drink alcohol at all." The issue remains unresolved, but many doctors advise their pregnant patients to avoid all alcohol, including the alcohol in drugs such as cough syrups, and so on. (See also Chapter 12.)

ALCOHOL AND DRUG INTERACTIONS

The presence of alcohol in the blood alters the way in which the body handles other drugs. One group of enzymes in the liver that is responsible for metabolizing alcohol is also responsible for breaking down drugs. Since these enzymes become more active when chronically exposed to alcohol, drugs will be removed more rapidly from the system in drinkers than in nondrinkers. Thus, generally, a drug will have less of an effect, and wear off more quickly than intended. However, if the person is drinking heavily at the time the drug is taken, the alcohol will compete successfully with the drug, which will remain in the body relatively unchanged and, if the drug dose is repeated, high and potentially dangerous levels will build up. (See Chapter 20.)

Alcohol need not be taken at the same time as a drug for there to be an effect. The determining factor is how much of each substance is in the blood. Substantial amounts of alcohol may still be present the morning after a night of heavy drinking and will react with a drug when it is taken.

Of the 50 most frequently prescribed drugs, more than half contain ingredients that react adversely with alcohol. The effects of depressants of the central nervous system—including narcotics, barbiturates, sedatives, some sleeping pills, and codeine-containing pain medications—are potentiated when alcohol is also present. Alcohol interferes with the action of anticonvulsants and anticoagulants. Beer and wine taken along with MAO inhibitors (a group of antidepressants) produce headache, extreme rises in blood pressure, rapid heartbeat, nausea, and vomiting. Heavy use of aspirin (for example, in the treatment of arthritis) combined with chronic alcohol use can lead to bleeding in the stomach. In a heavy drinker, acetaminophen, present in many over-the-counter analgesics and often taken to alleviate symptoms of hangovers (such as headaches), may become toxic to the liver in amounts usually considered safe. (For a list of other drugs that interact with alcohol, see Table 21.1).

Whether alcohol use is heavy or light,

care must be exercised when taking other drugs. The patient should inform the doctor about the level of alcohol consumption so that any needed adjustments in drug dosages can be made. Any change in drinking habits should be reported to the doctor for the same reason. For instance, some gastric acid inhibitors (H_2-blockers) may increase blood-alcohol levels. Read the labels on over-the-counter medications carefully for information about interactions with alcohol.

At least 500 drugs, some prescription and some sold over the counter, contain alcohol. The majority are vitamin preparations, decongestants, and cough medicines. (See Table 21.2.) Some cold remedies contain as much as 25 percent alcohol. As with other alcoholic consumption, medications containing 10 per-

Table 21.1. Drugs That Interact with Alcohol

Drug Category	Examples	Effects When Taken with Alcohol
Antianxiety and sleeping drugs	alprazolam (Xanax) lorazepam (Ativan) diazepam (Valium) flurazepam (Dalmane)	Can cause excessive sedation and increased effects on the central nervous system.
Antipsychotics	thioridazine (Mellaril) chlorpromazine (Thorazine) fluphenazine (Permitil)	Increases sedation, thereby leading to a severely impaired ability to drive or operate machinery. Judgment, alertness, and coordination will be diminished. When taken in excess amounts with alcohol can depress breathing, leading to death.
Antihistamines	dimenhydrinate (Dramamine) meclizine (Antivert)	Alcohol enhances the sedative effects of antihistamines, even in small doses. Be especially careful to avoid driving a car or operating machinery.
Anti-ulcer drugs (H_2-blockers)	cimetidine ranitidine nizatidine	These drugs increase blood alcohol levels.
Analgesics	aspirin (Bayer) indomethacin (Indocin) ibuprofen (Motrin and Advil)	Use of alcohol with analgesics can aggravate an already-existing condition of intestinal bleeding.
Narcotic analgesics	codeine meperidine (Demerol)	Adding alcohol can lead to serious depression of the central nervous system, respiratory arrest, and death.
Antidiabetic drugs	chlorpropamide (Diabinese) glyburide (DiaBeta) insulin	The combination of alcohol with these drugs can cause excessive hypoglycemia, a dangerous lowering of the glucose (sugar) level in the blood, which can lead to coma.
MAO inhibitors	isocarboxazid (Marplan) Phenelzine (Nardil) tranylcypromine (Parnate)	Using alcohol-based products with MAO inhibitors can result in increased blood pressure, headache, and fever.
Cephalosporin antibiotic	cefadroxil (Duricef) cefaclor (Ceclor) cefamandole (Mandol) cefazolin (Ancef) cefonicid (Monocid) cefonarine (Precef) cefotaxime (Claforan)	Drinking alcoholic beverages while receiving these medicines and for several days after stopping them may cause increased side effects such as abdominal or stomach cramps, nausea, vomiting, headache, fainting, fast or irregular heartbeat, difficult breathing, sweating, or redness of the face or skin.

cent or more alcohol can stimulate gastric secretion and provoke erosions of the gastrointestinal lining.

People who take vitamin supplements or other medications in elixir (liquid) form must be careful that any alcohol present is not reacting adversely with a regimen of prescription drugs. For example, an elderly person who is taking the oral medication Diabinese for diabetes may have a reaction to alcohol-containing medications similar to the reaction experienced by an alcoholic receiving disufiram (Antabuse), in which the face and neck flush, a headache develops, the body sweats, and the heart rate increases. (See also Chapter 20.)

ALCOHOL AND WEIGHT CONTROL

Anyone watching calorie intake in order to attain or maintain ideal body weight must count the calories in alcohol and in the mixers with which alcohol is often served. Not only are these calories displacing needed nutrients found in foods—if not monitored, they can quickly mount up as a significant part of the daily intake. Based on national consumption data, the estimated contribution of alcohol to the average American diet is 4.5 percent of total calories.

A single five-ounce glass of table wine has 110 calories. A 12-ounce regular beer has approximately 150 calories; a light beer has approximately 95. (See The Meanings of

Table 21.2. Alcohol in Pharmaceuticals

Drug	Percent Alcohol	Drug	Percent Alcohol
Diphenhydramine HC1 elixir	12–15	Pertussin 8-Hour Cough Formula	9.5
Dramamine liquid	5	Pertussin Night-Time Cold Medicine	25
Dristan Cough Formula Syrup	12	Phenobarbital elixir	12–15
Eldertonic	15	Potassium Gluconate elixir	5
Feosol elixir	5	Prolixin elixir	14
Genvitol	5	Quibron elixir	15
Geralix liquid	12	Reserpoid elixir	14
Geriatric elixir	12	Robitussin	3.5
Geri-Pen elixir	5	Romilar CF	10
Geritol	12	Secobarbital elixir	10–14
Gerix elixir	20	Seconal elixir	12
Kaochlor 10% liquid	5	Stannitol elixir	23
Lomotil liquid	15	Symptom, 1,2,3 and Multi	5
Lufyllin-GG elixir	17	Tedral elixir	15
Mellaril solution	4.2	Theolixir	20
Nembutal elixir	18	Triaminic Expectorant	5
Neo-Synephrine	8	Tylenol liquid	7
Novahistine DMX	10	Valerian	68
NyQuil	25	Vicks Day-Care	7.5
Oxtriphylline elixir	18–22	Vicks Formula 44	10
Periactin syrup	5	Viro-med	16.63
Peri-Colace syrup	10		

Adapted with permission from: Dukes, G. E., Kuhn, J. G., and Evens, R. P., "Alcohol in Pharmaceutical Products," *American Family Physician,* 16:97, September 1977.

Light, below.) A typical one-and-one-half-ounce serving of 80-proof liquor has 100 calories; when a mixer—for example, cola, quinine water, Tom Collins mix—is added, the calorie count may double. A wine cooler, favored by many because of its seeming lightness, has between 200 and 300 calories per 12-ounce can. Very high-calorie drinks include Brandy Alexanders and White Russians (made with cream); pina coladas, daiquiris, and whiskey sours (with added sugar); and heavily sweetened after-dinner cordials such as apricot brandy and coffee liqueur.

Two glasses of wine with dinner represents 10 percent of the total daily-calorie budget for someone aiming for 2,000 calories of food intake. Alcohol is a luxury item as far as controlled calorie intake is concerned; it pro-

vides only insubstantial nourishment and makes dieting difficult. Only when very large amounts of alcohol are taken do these calories not "fully count."

ALCOHOL ABUSE

Definitions of alcoholism vary widely from one expert to another, just as there is disagreement among health professionals about what causes the disease. One commonly accepted definition is regular drinking to the extent that it affects a person's health or home and work life. (See quiz on page 352.)

By any definition, alcoholism is a major social problem, touching people without re-

The Meanings of *Light*

To satisfy what one brewer identifies as "current lifestyle interests in physical fitness, health, diet, and moderation," the liquor industry has launched on the market a variety of light beers and dealcoholized wines. This has produced considerable confusion as to what these terms mean. A glossary follows.

- Alcohol-free beers contain no alcohol (but have a beer taste).

- Non-alcoholic malt beverages contain no more than 0.5 percent alcohol.

- Light beers have nearly as much alcohol (3 percent) as regular beers (4 percent), but often fewer calories (about 100 per 12 ounces, as opposed to 150 for regular beers). However, calorie counts are not uniform and may range from as few as 70 per 12 ounces to as many as 134 per 12 ounces.

- Dealcoholized wines usually have no more than 0.5 percent alcohol, but no FDA guidelines are in force.

- Wine coolers (reconstituted fruit juice, carbonated water, white wine, sugar) are low in alcohol (3.5 to 6 percent) compared to regular wine (11 to 12 percent) but high in calories (about 220 calories per 12-ounce can).

- Light wines have more alcohol (6 to 10 percent) than regular coolers but fewer calories than either the coolers or regular wine (65 versus 110 per 5 ounces).

Light, as applied to a beverage, traditionally meant a lighter color or taste. Today, it is often taken to mean lower in calories, but the older meaning may still apply. In an attempt to correct misperceptions, the Bureau of Alcohol, Tobacco and Firearms has proposed that the caloric content of beverages designated as *light* or *lite* must be given on their labels. This would help consumers compare light products with one another but would be no guide in comparing light with regular.

gard to age, race, sex, or socioeconomic status. It is the most common form of substance abuse in both the United States and Russia and costs tens of billions of dollars each year in medical costs and lost work. In the United States, an estimated 10 million adults and 3.3 million adolescents are thought to have drinking problems.

Long-term alcohol abuse has serious health consequences. Alcoholics have overall mortality and suicide rates two and a half times greater than average and an accident rate seven times greater. Moreover, an alcoholic abusing only alcohol is very rare. Heavy drinkers tend also to smoke heavily and to misuse other drugs ranging from tranquilizers to cocaine.

There may be as many causes of alcoholism as there are alcoholics. No common cause has been found despite extensive re-

What Are the Signs of Alcoholism?

Here is a test to help you review the role alcohol is playing in your life. These questions incorporate many of the common symptoms of alcoholism. This test is intended to help you determine whether you or someone you know needs to find out more about alcoholism.

Yes No

☐ ☐ 1. Do you occasionally drink heavily after a disappointment, a quarrel, or when the boss gives you a hard time?

☐ ☐ 2. When you have trouble or feel under pressure, do you always drink more heavily than usual?

☐ ☐ 3. Have you noticed that you are able to handle more liquor than you did when you were first drinking?

☐ ☐ 4. Did you ever wake up on the "morning after" and discover that you could not remember part of the evening before, even though your friends tell you that you did not "pass out"?

☐ ☐ 5. When drinking with other people, do you try to have a few extra drinks when others will not know it?

☐ ☐ 6. Are there certain occasions when you feel uncomfortable if alcohol is not available?

☐ ☐ 7. Have you recently noticed that when you begin drinking you are in more of a hurry to get the first drink than you used to be?

☐ ☐ 8. Do you sometimes feel a little guilty about your drinking?

☐ ☐ 9. Are you secretly irritated when your family or friends discuss your drinking?

☐ ☐ 10. Have you recently noticed an increase in the frequency of your memory "blackouts"?

☐ ☐ 11. Do you often find that you wish to continue drinking after your friends say they have had enough?

☐ ☐ 12. Do you usually have a reason for the occasions when you drink heavily?

☐ ☐ 13. When you are sober, do you often regret things you have done or said while drinking?

☐ ☐ 14. Have you tried switching brands or following different plans for controlling your drinking?

search. Genetic susceptibility, home environment, childhood experiences, learned behavior, and various other possibilities have all been investigated; each may play a role.

The alcoholic can be easy to identify—the stereotypical skid row bum—or indistinguishable from the nonabusing population; for example, the housewife who drinks secretly or the businessman who functions successfully despite several drinks at lunch, drinks after work on the way home, and more drinking at home before dinner. Alcoholism may start gradually, or some people may drink to intoxication from their first drink. More commonly, alcoholism is a progressive disease that starts with ordinary social drinking but over time—often many years—progresses to the point at which alcohol must be consumed every day or periodically—for example, on the weekends. Eventually, with an increased tolerance

What Are the Signs of Alcoholism? (cont.)

Yes No

☐ ☐ 15. Have you often failed to keep the promises you have made to yourself about controlling or cutting down on your drinking?

☐ ☐ 16. Have you ever tried to control your drinking by making a change in jobs, or moving to a new location?

☐ ☐ 17. Do you try to avoid family or close friends while you are drinking?

☐ ☐ 18. Are you having an increasing number of financial and work problems?

☐ ☐ 19. Do more people seem to be treating you unfairly without good reason?

☐ ☐ 20. Do you eat very little or irregularly when you are drinking?

Yes No

☐ ☐ 21. Do you sometimes have the "shakes" in the morning and find that it helps to have a little drink?

☐ ☐ 22. Have you recently noticed that you cannot drink as much as you once did?

☐ ☐ 23. Do you sometimes stay drunk for several days at a time?

☐ ☐ 24. Do you sometimes feel very depressed and wonder whether life is worth living?

☐ ☐ 25. Sometimes after periods of drinking, do you see or hear things that aren't there?

☐ ☐ 26. Do you get terribly frightened after you have been drinking heavily?

Any yes answer indicates a probable symptom of alcoholism.

Yes answers to several of the questions indicate the following stages of alcoholism:

Questions 1–8: early stage
Questions 9–21: middle stage
Questions 22–26: the beginning of final stage.

To find out more, contact the National Council on Alcoholism in your area.

This test is reproduced with the permission of the National Council on Alcoholism, Inc.

for alcohol, accompanied by decreased control, drunkenness becomes habitual.

Only in recent decades has alcohol been recognized as an addictive drug and alcoholism as a disease. The alcoholic is no longer viewed as someone lacking in morals or willpower, but as someone who needs help. This has cleared the way for effective treatment of alcoholism. However, like other chronic diseases, such as diabetes or arthritis, there is no cure, only treatment to keep the disease at bay. For the alcoholic, the only treatment is lifelong abstinence. It is for this reason that the drinker's desire to stop drinking is a critical factor and membership in a support group such as Alcoholics Anonymous is so important.

The health effects of alcoholism run from poor nutritional status to permanent brain damage, from hepatitis to cirrhosis to death.

WITHDRAWAL

Because alcohol is an addictive drug, stopping drinking produces withdrawal symptoms. Mild withdrawal symptoms begin within 12 to 48 hours after cessation of drinking and include nausea, vomiting, irritability, weakness, and sweating. Severe withdrawal symptoms include delirium tremens (the DTs), which usually develops two to four days after drinking ends. Symptoms of the DTs include increased low-grade fever, delirium, and auditory and visual hallucinations. DTs are treated with tranquilizers such as Librium and Valium, fluids in cases of dehydration, the B vitamins, and, most of all, reassurance. The mortality rate from the DTs used to be as high as 15 percent.

ALCOHOLISM AND NUTRITION

Several decades ago, the popular notion was that alcoholism was caused by malnutrition, a conclusion reached because so many alcoholics were found to be malnourished. Repeated studies have shown this not to be the case at all. Rather, the reverse is true: Heavy drinking has a variety of effects on the body's digestive and metabolic systems, which, cumulatively, lead to malnourishment. Alcoholism is one of the major causes of true nutritional deficiency in this society. One estimate is that 20,000 alcoholics in the United States suffer from serious illnesses due to malnutrition.

At the peak of their disease, alcoholics typically ingest half their calories in the form of alcoholic beverages.

Some are overweight, even obese, as the result of this caloric intake. Others are underweight, both because of neglect in eating regular meals and the appetite-suppressing effect of large amounts of alcohol. Because of the effects of alcohol on absorption and the use of nutrients, even the alcoholic who does eat protein, carbohydrates, and so on, will frequently be malnourished. When the caloric intake from alcohol exceeds 30 percent of the total intake, significant decreases in protein and fat consumption occur and the intake of virtually all vitamins and minerals may fall far below the recommended dietary allowances. An exception is iron, particularly if wines that contain iron are regularly consumed or the alcoholic takes an iron-rich tonic. In contrast to its effects on other nutrients, alcohol in excess increases iron absorption, making an iron overload likely.

Not only is intake affected by excessive alcohol consumption, the nutrients that are present are ineffectively utilized. Chronic alcohol consumption damages the linings of the stomach and the small intestine. It alters gastric-acid secretion, first increasing and then decreasing it, the emptying of the stomach, and the wavelike contractions of the intestine (peristalsis) that move nutrients along. Profound deficiencies of thiamine and low levels of folic acid, pyridoxine, and riboflavin are common among alcoholics. The body's vitamin A balance is also disturbed. Recent research has found that the presence of alcohol increases the amount of vitamin A in some tissues, depletes it in others (such as the liver), and speeds up or alters the process by which the vitamin is converted into metabolic byproducts. One consequence is the loss of night vision observed in alcoholics. There is also ample evidence that alcoholics have problems related to a deficiency of vitamin D: decreased bone density and mass and increased susceptibility to fractures. The deficiency is believed to be caused by lessened dietary intake, poor absorption, and lack of sunlight due to the alcoholic's lifestyle.

The absorption of proteins, fats, and carbohydrates also is impaired by alcoholism. The liver secretes diminished amounts of bile, needed for the digestion of fats. Impairment of pancreatic function leads to further problems with fat absorption. Malabsorption of fats can lead to steatorrhea, a condition in which undigested fats appear in the feces. Further, alcohol promotes extra insulin release from the pancreas in response to glucose, causing hypoglycemia. At the same time, alcohol depletes the liver's glycogen stores and impairs its capacity for formation of new glucose.

Among the specific medical conditions associated with nutritional deficiencies due to alcoholism is the Wernicke-Korsakoff syndrome, caused by excessive alcohol intake and a severe deficiency of the B vitamins, particularly thiamine. The syndrome has two components: Wernicke's encephelopathy, characterized by uncoordinated movement (ataxia), and Korsakoff's psychosis, the inability to re-member recent events. In the latter, the patient makes up details—often sounding believable to strangers—in order to fill the memory gaps, a phenomenon known as confabulation. To prevent the brain damage from becoming permanent, large doses of B vitamins must be given promptly.

Thiamine deficiency also affects the outer or peripheral nerves, causing leg cramps, numbness, partial paralysis of the toes, and a burning sensation in the feet, which is worse at night. With an adequate diet, abstinence, and vitamin supplementation, it can be reversed.

NUTRITIONAL THERAPY FOR ALCOHOLISM

The first step in nutritional therapy for the alcoholic is the cessation of drinking. Without this, little can be done to move the nutritional status toward normal.

With cessation of drinking, an alcoholic will usually respond quickly to a balanced, appetizing diet. Complications such as cirrhosis, B-deficiency anemias, or secondary illnesses caused by vitamin deficiencies or other malnourishment should be treated. To compensate for the poor diet of many alcoholics, this improved diet should contain about 3,000 calories a day and consist of complete protein along with fats and carbohydrates. An alcoholic who is overweight may be placed on a more restricted diet aimed at reducing weight while reversing the ravages of alcohol.

If there are complications, nutritional therapy often will be a balancing act that involves moving as quickly as possible toward recovery without triggering further problems. For example, a liver damaged by alcohol abuse is particularly sensitive to the amount of protein in the diet. Too much protein may precipitate hepatic coma, which can be fatal; too little delays recovery. (See Chapter 31.)

Thiamine is usually prescribed for all alcoholics, since most have a deficiency and there is no problem toxicity from overconsumption. Folic-acid deficiency is most easily dealt with by adding folate-rich foods to the diet, but sometimes a supplement is given. (There has been a proposal that folic acid be added to alcoholic beverages, since many alcoholics display the deficiency and it would do no harm to other drinkers.) Pyridoxine and riboflavin deficiencies are usually treated with a daily multivitamin preparation. Vitamin A therapy is more complicated, since the vitamin when given as a supplement can become toxic. Most doctors prescribe minimal amounts of vitamin A in outpatient situations.

In contrast to vitamin supplements given under medical supervision to correct deficiencies, many heavy drinkers believe that vitamin supplements can prevent liver damage and take them far in excess of the RDA. In other cases, alcoholics who may have been advised

Drinking in Social Situations

The cocktail party has often been described as the worst possible setting in which to drink moderately. Tension levels are high—many of the guests are meeting each other for the first time—and the room is likely to be hot, noisy, and full of smoke. All these factors encourage people to gulp down their drinks. Circulating waiters, or bars scattered around the room, make it all too easy to get the next drink.

With a smaller, more relaxed group of friends, such problems need not occur. An open bar in the same room as a gathering should be avoided. When mixing drinks, the host or hostess should use a jigger or similar measure rather than eyeballing the alcohol in the glass. The host need not rush to refill a guest's glass. Frequently, a guest whose glass is empty is not eager for an immediate refill but out of politeness will not refuse one. More and more, people now prefer wine at social functions; the potent hard liquor can remain in the cabinet.

When attending a party, large or small, the host/guest who wants to hold down alcohol and calorie consumption can use several simple tactics:

- Be aware of the pressures of a party and carefully pace the drinking.

- The host/hostess should premeasure the drinks; one drink being 5 ounces of wine, 12 ounces of beer, or 1½ ounces of spirits.

Guests can then approximate a safe amount to drink by figuring weight, body type, sex, and so forth. For example, a 160-pound man can safely have one drink in an hour.

- If thirsty while drinking, remember that alcohol has a dehydrating effect. Have water or soda, not another drink.

- Return to the bar midway through a drink and ask for more ice or club soda to further dilute the drink. Drink wine diluted with club soda or seltzer (a spritzer). Switch to soda with a slice of lime after one or two drinks.

- Put the glass down and circulate through the party with empty hands.

Salty foods, such as pretzels, peanuts, potato chips, and saltine crackers should be avoided because they increase thirst. Fatty foods coat the lining of the stomach and delay stomach emptying. It is often helpful to eat a small meal before a party. Failing this, a few hors d'oeuvres should precede the first drink.

Keep in mind how much energy you need to burn to work off the calories of the drink. To work off the calories from 12 ounces of beer requires a brisk half-hour walk; those from 1½ ounces of 80-proof gin or vodka, 20 minutes of rowing.

by a physician to take supplements as prophylaxis against deficiencies take megadoses—on the theory that if a little is good, more is better. Self-treatment with megadoses can lead to toxic buildups.

Should alcoholics drink low-alcohol beverages? Some experts on alcoholism express concern that the so-called nonalcoholic beers and dealcoholized wines (which contain 0.5 percent alcohol) might trigger a relapse rather than being safe for recovering alcoholics as substitutes for their former drink. There is less danger from the tiny amount of alcohol present—even drinking up to 8 nonalcoholic beers in an hour would not appear as an elevated concentration of alcohol in the blood or make a person feel drunk—than from the familiar taste and smell of these beverages, and the atmosphere surrounding their consumption. These associations might prove to be more powerful than any physiological effects from the small amounts of alcohol.

SAFE AND MODERATE DRINKING

There is no doubt that people who drink socially will continue to do so. And unless they are taking drugs that interact adversely, they will do themselves no harm by taking an occasional drink. Prudence and nutritional awareness require that the drinking be moderate and controlled. The key is to avoid entering or creating situations where excessive drinking is easy. There is ample evidence that emotions, habits, environment, and cultural background play a role in the level of alcohol consumption. These factors should be considered when drinking or serving alcohol to guests. (See Drinking in Social Situations on page 356.)

Causes of Nutrient Deficiency in Alcoholics*

There are six ways to get a nutrient deficiency—three inadequacies and three excesses. The three inadequacies are:

1. Inadequate ingestion (i.e., not eating enough of a nutrient).
2. Inadequate absorption (i.e., some damage to the ability of the nutrient to be absorbed from the intestine into the bloodstream).
3. Inadequate utilization (i.e., damage to the metabolic machinery of the body's cells).

The three excesses are:

4. Increased requirement.
5. Increased destruction.
6. Increased excretion.

The reason that more than 80 percent of people with alcoholism have deficiency of the vitamin folic acid is that alcohol produces all six problems with respect to folic acid, as studies in our and other laboratories have shown.

*This section written by Victor Herbert, M.D., F.A.C.P.

22

Nutrition and the Use of Tobacco, Caffeine, and Other Mood-Altering Substances

Leonard Handelsman, M.D.

■

INTRODUCTION

Throughout history, man has smoked or ingested any number of plant-derived substances such as opium from the poppy, marijuana from the cannabis plant, peyote from a cactus, and nicotine from tobacco. Modern man has not only these plant-derivative drugs to alter his moods or modify his behavior but also the drugs that he has synthesized—barbiturates, amphetamines, LSD, and tranquilizers such as Valium and Librium. The synthesized drugs produce similar or even more pronounced results. These substances and many others, including some that are not usually thought of as drugs, alter the basic chemistry of the brain in ways that are as yet not fully understood. Some alterations are temporary, with brain chemistry returning to normal in a few hours, or a day or two at most. Others are profound, with the body's chemistry so affected that it is difficult for the brain to recover.

ABUSE VERSUS DEPENDENCE

There has been considerable debate over the definitions of *abuse* and *dependence*. To be di-

agnosed as abusing a drug, a user will display one or both of the following behaviors: He or she may repeatedly jeopardize personal safety and perhaps that of others with its use—for example, driving while under the influence of a drug; and he or she will continue drug use even though aware of the physical, social, psychological, or work-related problems that its use causes or worsens. To be considered abusive of drugs, the individual will continue this pattern of behavior for at least one month. For example, someone who abuses drugs could have a duodenal ulcer but continue drinking even though a physician had cautioned against it, or could take cocaine every few weeks and then miss several days of work or school as a consequence. Other symptoms need not be present.

Those who are said to be dependent on a drug exhibit some but not necessarily all of the following symptoms: Larger amounts of the drug are taken for a longer period of time than desired; there is the desire or attempt to curtail its use; excessive time is spent attempting to procure, take, or recover from a drug; other activities are renounced or limited; an increased amount is needed to induce desired feelings; there are symptoms of withdrawal; the drug may be taken to prevent or relieve withdrawal symptoms; intoxication or withdrawal makes it impossible for the person to function when personal or professional responsibilities require it; and, as with abuse, an individual continues to use the drug even though he or she recognizes that it causes psychological, physical, or social problems and thus interferes with other aspects of life. The extent of dependence ranges from mild to severe, depending on the number and severity of the symptoms present.

The physiological nature of drug addiction, both generally and, in the case of individual drugs, specifically has been the subject of substantial medical research. In general, addictive drugs are believed to affect neurotransmitters in the brain, biochemicals that carry messages. Neurotransmitters are produced by the basic cells of the brain, the neurons, and are the substances that carry the electrical impulses across the synapse. These impulses are the basis of all brain and nerve activity, and their transmission is a complex process that varies depending upon the specific nature of the neuron, the body function in which it is involved, and the particular neurotransmitter.

While abusable substances affect many classes of neurotransmitters, they all share the ability to stimulate dopamine neurotransmission in the so-called brain reward circuitry. Enkephalins and endorphins, for example, are two naturally occurring opiates that are involved in the perception of pain and the integration of emotional experiences. Drugs such as heroin and Demerol—a synthetic drug obtainable only by prescription—apparently interact with natural brain receptors for enkephalins and endorphins and produce characteristic sensations and the resulting addiction, which can develop rapidly.

It is believed that chronic users of marijuana develop a need for the drug to get them through the day. Cessation of its use, however, usually does not produce withdrawal symptoms. Although marijuana's active ingredient obviously alters brain chemistry when it is circulating in the blood and passing across the blood-brain barrier, we do not know whether it alters neurochemistry on a long-term basis. Many scientists hope that an increased understanding of the subtleties of drug abuse and associated brain-chemistry changes will lead to new treatments for drug addiction that are more effective than the current approaches, which have a high failure rate.

EFFECTS ON NUTRITIONAL STATUS

Users of addictive drugs pay a nutritional price for their habit. Some drugs suppress the appetite. Others produce a marked increase in motor activity and mood elevation; as a result, an individual may be unaware of the need for food for long periods of time. Illegal drugs or alcohol may be so expensive that there is little money left for food. Eating is often focused on low-nutrition foods—jelly doughnuts, cream-filled cakes, chips, pretzels, and soft drinks. Vegetables, fruits, and dairy products are often forgotten. Malnourishment is common among drug addicts, as are vitamin and mineral deficiencies.

Some drugs have effects that compromise nutrition beyond this level. In one study, it was shown that the potentially dangerous eating disorder bulimia occurred in a higher percentage of cocaine users than in those who did not use the drug. Marijuana causes "the munchies," a craving for sweets and an increased appetite. There is some evidence that cigarette smoking lowers the blood levels of HDL cholesterol—the so-called good cholesterol that is believed to protect against heart disease. New experiments suggest that heroin addicts may prefer sweets because high blood-sugar levels can suppress signs of physical withdrawal from heroin.

Addictive behaviors and their physical and nutritional consequences can be controlled. An estimated 37 million Americans have stopped smoking. In recent years, society has mobilized to reduce the incidence of cocaine addiction, although the success of these efforts remains to be seen. Still, the evidence is clear that in many cases addiction can be controlled and the body returned to near normal, including a sound nutritional status.

NICOTINE ADDICTION AND CIGARETTE SMOKING

The scientific evidence that smoking cigarettes is a serious health hazard and that addiction to nicotine is the primary cause of cigarette smoking has become overwhelming. Evidence also is accumulating that cigarette smoking has significant nutritional effects.

Public-health experts report that tobacco use is the number-one preventable cause of illness and death in the United States. The U.S. Surgeon General's first report on smoking and health was issued in 1964, but cigarette smoking continued to increase each year until 1975, after which point the number of adults who smoked began to decline. In 1975, 32 percent of adults smoked, compared to 42 percent a decade earlier. However, since 1975 smoking has increased among teenagers, particularly among adolescent girls. The latest statistics reveal that 53 million Americans smoke, consuming 570 billion cigarettes a year.

The medical bill for smoking-related illnesses was put at $60 million a day in a 1985 study by the Congressional Office of Technology Assessment. The Surgeon General estimates that tobacco use, primarily cigarettes, accounts for 350,000 excess deaths each year. Nearly 40 percent of these deaths are believed to result from heart disease and 20 percent from lung cancer.

The Surgeon General has stated that "cigarette smoking is clearly identified as the chief preventable cause of death in our society." Smokers are three times more likely to die of cancer than nonsmokers. Smoking is the chief cause of lung cancer; a major cause of cancers of the mouth and throat; a contributing cause of cancer of the kidney, bladder, and pancreas; and a major cause of pulmonary diseases. Heavy smokers' risk of death from coronary heart disease is up to ten times that of nonsmokers.

The addictive factor in cigarettes is nicotine, an alkaloid found in the leaf of the tobacco plant. Once nicotine binds to its receptor in the brain, it can influence chains of neurons. In this way, nicotine specifically affects a class of neurotransmitters known as catecholamines (including dopamine), which play a wide variety of roles in brain function.

Research has shown that nicotine is a highly addictive drug. Its use leads to increasing tolerance and craving. If it is no longer present in the blood and the brain, distinct withdrawal symptoms result. In one study, people addicted to opiates reported that it was easier for them to go without these drugs than to be deprived of cigarettes.

Nicotine in cigarette smoke is absorbed rapidly through the mucous membranes of the mouth and throat. Inhaled into the lungs, it passes across the membrane that separates the air sacs of the lung from the bloodstream and is quickly distributed through the body. About 15 percent goes directly to the brain, where it is immediately taken up. The time lapse from the passage of nicotine into the blood at the lungs until it affects the brain's catecholamines is only seven seconds. The resultant secretion of adrenaline causes the heart rate and blood pressure to rise immediately, in turn raising the body's overall metabolic rate. Every puff on a cigarette introduces another hit of nicotine into the blood and the brain, maintaining the physiological changes. So closely connected is the act of puffing on a cigarette to the resulting changes that smokers quickly learn to maintain a level of nicotine in the blood and brain that satisfies their craving without producing dizziness or other side effects. Falling levels of nicotine in the blood and brain lead to classic withdrawal symptoms, one of the major barriers to stopping smoking. Headache, nausea, diarrhea or constipation, a slower heart rate, falling blood pressure, fatigue, and insomnia are common, as are irritability, anxiety, inability to concentrate, and depression. Although not necessarily associated with withdrawal symptoms, a deep craving for a cigarette is common. These symptoms generally become less troublesome in seven days, but they may take weeks or months to disappear completely.

Nutritional Effects

Metabolic Rate. Recent research has produced some intriguing findings about nicotine's effect on the body's metabolic rate and expenditure of energy. In one study, it was found that the volunteer subjects' bodies consumed 10 percent more energy when they were smoking than when they were not. The research suggested that someone who stops smoking needs 200 fewer calories per day due to the lowered metabolic rate that results from quitting. If dietary intake remains constant, weight gain is inevitable. The need to have something in their mouths that many smokers feel, or their deliberate use of snack food to replace cigarettes, combined with the lower

metabolic rate, with its reduced need for calories, undoubtedly act to produce the added pounds associated with quitting smoking. New studies suggest that the use of nicotine gum prescribed by a physician may reduce weight gain after the cessation of smoking cigarettes.

Nutrients. Numerous studies have found that smokers have lower levels of vitamin C in their blood than nonsmokers. One study found 25 percent less vitamin C among those who smoked fewer than 20 cigarettes a day and 40 percent less among those who smoked more than 40 cigarettes a day. However, this lower blood level of vitamin C is still well within normal limits. The suggestion that smokers should take vitamin C supplements is counterproductive because there is evidence that large amounts of vitamin C drive nicotine out in the urine and thereby prompt smokers to reach for the next cigarette that much faster. The treatment for the lowered (albeit normal) levels of vitamin C in smokers is to stop smoking, not to take supplements.

Lower blood levels of carotene (a precursor of vitamin A) have also been found in studies of smokers, as have lower levels of folic acid. The nutritional consequences of these findings, if any, remain obscure. Smoking also can cause an optic neuropathy, a condition in which functional disturbances affect the optic nerve. One study of patients suffering from this condition found low levels of vitamin B_{12}. Of the 77 patients studied, 17 had vitamin B_{12} levels chronically so low that they suffered from pernicious anemia.

Numerous studies of the body's calcium metabolism have found that smoking also reduces the levels of calcium in the blood, although the mechanism is not understood. There is also a substantial body of research showing that women who smoke pass through menopause earlier. A study of more than 15,000 women in Australia found that those who smoked 10 or more cigarettes a day reached menopause 1.3 years earlier than non-smokers. Some researchers think that this may account in part for the fact that women who smoke have an increased risk of osteoporosis, the "brittle bone" disease to which postmenopausal women are especially prone. (For more information, see Chapter 34.) However, doctors disagree about whether reduced calcium levels in the blood are directly related to increased osteoporosis among smokers or whether the known relationship of smoking and earlier menopause is responsible.

Smoking and Heart Disease

Evidence continues to accumulate that tobacco use is a significant risk factor for heart disease, stroke, arrythmia, and angina. Angina, the chest pains that result when the coronary arteries are narrowed (usually by fatty plaque) is more prevalent in smokers, and they experience it following less exertion than is the case with nonsmokers. There are several possible mechanisms for this. There is considerable evidence that smoking increases atherosclerosis, the buildup of fatty deposits in the blood vessels. Nicotine also increases the risk of cardiac arrythmias and spasms of the coronary arteries, both of which can cheat the heart muscle of its necessary blood flow and produce chest pains.

Smokers who give up cigarettes—even after years of smoking—can diminish their risk of heart disease. For example, studies of former smokers under age 65 have shown a marked reduction in the risk of heart attack compared to people still smoking. People who have suffered a heart attack and then stop smoking are half as likely to die of a subsequent heart attack as are those who continue to smoke.

Traditionally, the risk of heart disease in women who have not reached menopause has been significantly lower than for men. Specialists warn, however, that the growing prevalence of smoking among young women could increase the incidence of coronary artery disease among them, especially those who compound their risks by both smoking and using oral contraceptives. In one study of women under age 50 who had had a heart attack, the incidence of subsequent heart attack among those who smoked 35 or more cigarettes a day was 20 times greater than among nonsmokers.

The role of cholesterol and the lipoproteins in the development of heart disease is becoming better understood. Studies show that an increased blood level of high-density lipoproteins (HDLs), the "good" lipoproteins, is related to a lower incidence of heart disease. Researchers have found that smoking decreases HDL levels but that these lowered levels can return to normal within a year after stopping smoking. There is clear evidence that even people who consume fewer saturated fats and increase their HDL levels as a result can undo the benefits by continuing to smoke cigarettes.

It remains unclear how smoking causes HDL levels to decrease. Studies with animals have suggested that it may be due in part to the carbon monoxide in cigarette smoke. Carbon monoxide has a far greater affinity than does oxygen for the hemoglobin in blood. Carbon monoxide binds to the hemoglobin, reduces available oxygen, and makes the heart work harder to deliver this essential substance to the body's cells. Studies with rabbits found that when they are exposed to carbon monoxide for several months, they begin to show changes on the walls of their arteries that could lead to atherosclerosis (narrowing of the arteries) in time. When cholesterol was added to the rabbits' diet, the levels of cholesterol in the blood of the animals exposed to carbon monoxide was significantly higher than in the blood of those who breathed normal air. Similar studies in primates have produced corroborating results. Some researchers believe that carbon monoxide and nicotine work synergistically, increasing the fatty deposits on artery walls. Smoking low-tar, low-nicotine cigarettes does reduce the amount of nicotine in the body and some of the risk of heart disease. However, the carbon monoxide content is unaffected, and the risk of heart disease is still significant.

Smoking and Pregnancy

Smoking cigarettes during pregnancy has been clearly shown to have an adverse effect on the pregnancy and the fetus, and its effects follow the baby into its early years of life. In a 1979 report, the U.S. Surgeon General said that smoking remains one of the most controllable risk factors in pregnancy.

Adequate nutrition during pregnancy—to produce a weight gain of about 26 pounds or more—reduces the risk of delivering a low-birth-weight baby, but smoking can counteract the effects of sound nutrition. Women who smoke are nearly twice as likely to deliver low-birth-weight babies—infants who weigh less than five and a half pounds and are more likely to have health and developmental problems after birth. The decrease in birth weight is dose-related; babies born to heavy smokers are more affected than babies born to light smokers. Smoking throughout the pregnancy is more harmful than smoking during only part of the pregnancy. Studies also have shown that mothers who smoke have an increased risk for spontaneous abortion, premature birth, stillbirth, and complications involving the placenta. The risk of delivering a baby who dies soon after birth is also higher.

Of the many potentially toxic chemicals in cigarette smoke, carbon monoxide is believed to be the major cause of fetal problems. The carbon monoxide binds to the hemoglobin in the blood, depriving the placenta and the fetus of oxygen. In the mother, the carbon monoxide and the associated oxygen starvation (hypoxia) can cause the heart to work harder, lead to the development of a larger placenta, and result in the redistribution of blood flow. Some researchers have suggested that smoking leads to lower caloric intake by the mother and that her resultant smaller weight gain accounts for the lower birth weight of the baby.

Nicotine easily crosses the placenta and enters the fetus's blood. Its presence in laboratory animals has been shown to cause a rise in blood pressure, tachycardia (rapid heartbeat), and hypoxia. There also is evidence that it impedes the transport of amino acids across the placenta, which may contribute to growth retardation in the fetus.

Research groups have attempted to determine whether children born to mothers who smoke suffer long-term consequences. The results have been conflicting. In some studies, no difference was found one year after birth between the children of women who smoked during pregnancy and those whose mothers did not smoke. Other studies found some differences at various ages. For example, one British study found that at age seven, the children of smokers were shorter in stature and had learned to read later. However, other lifestyle variables might possibly explain the differences. (For more information, see Chapter 12.)

"Smokeless" Tobacco

Health warnings over a quarter century have convinced many people to stop smoking.

Others have switched from cigarettes to the so-called smokeless tobaccos—snuff and chewing tobacco. An estimated 22 million people now use these products, which also carry health and nutritional risks. Chief among these are serious gum and tooth problems and an increased incidence of oral cancer in long-term users, particularly those who use snuff and place a pinch of it between lip and gum. Some researchers have also warned about the possible harmful effects of the sugar and salt that manufacturers add to the smokeless tobaccos to make them more flavorful. One researcher, who analyzed 10 brands of loose-leaf and plug tobacco, found from 500 to 1,050 milligrams of sodium per container. Four out of six brands of snuff had more than 1,000 milligrams of sodium per container. It is not known how much of this sodium might be absorbed into the body, but since some people use as many as 12 pouches of loose-leaf tobacco per day, the amount may be considerable.

Benefits of Quitting

Each year, millions of people attempt to stop using cigarettes; a significant number succeed. The health benefits of quitting are great. Ten to fifteen years after quitting, an ex-smoker's risk of shorter life expectancy, and of cancer of the lungs, mouth, and larynx, is close to that of someone who has never smoked. The risk of coronary heart disease drops one year after quitting and after 10 years is the same as a nonsmoker's. The ability to breathe improves immediately.

There is no single way to stop smoking. Some people stop cold turkey; others gradually taper off cigarette consumption. Although about 95 percent of those who stop do it on their own, many find it helpful to join a stop-smoking clinic (such as those offered by the American Lung Association, the American Heart Association, local hospitals, and others) or a commercial group such as Smokenders. Hypnosis, counseling, and behavior modification are other methods. Nicotine chewing gum, available by prescription, sometimes eases withdrawal.

One of the consequences of stopping—and one of the excuses some people use to avoid stopping—is the weight gain that often follows. Some studies have shown that about 60 percent of men and 50 percent of women gain some weight when they stop smoking. For most, the gains are modest, about five to nine pounds. Some of the initial gain is due to the retention of water associated with withdrawal from nicotine, but this effect soon subsides. The real culprits are the absence of the higher metabolic rate that went with smoking (this alone can account for a weight gain of two pounds a month) and the substitution of food for cigarettes in an attempt to satisfy the oral cravings associated with cigarettes. As mentioned, the use of nicotine gum may be a way to minimize the weight gain associated with stopping smoking.

Someone who has stopped smoking may be able, for the first time in years, even decades, to taste and smell food once again. People may begin eating more just because of these rediscovered sensations. For many smokers, moreover, part of smoking is the ritual of handling a cigarette and match or lighter or the feeling of the cigarette in the mouth; others use cigarettes as a psychological crutch in times of stress, or in business and social situations. With the cigarette gone, they turn to candy, gum, snack foods, or soft drinks. Caloric intake from such replacements can mount up quickly.

Most smoking-cessation experts advise not worrying about weight gain at first. A small weight gain can be dealt with several weeks or months after the ordeal of stopping smoking is past. Helping to put the matter of weight gain in perspective, one American Cancer Society assessment stated that "to present the same health hazard as smoking a pack of cigarettes a day, one must be 125 pounds overweight." Nevertheless, someone who is about to stop smoking can take specific steps to keep weight gain to a minimum. Some of these steps are outlined below.

CAFFEINE

If Americans can be said to have a national dietary addiction, it is their taste for caffeine, the bitter alkaloid present in coffee, tea, cola and many other soft drinks, cocoa, a variety of other foods and beverages, and hundreds of over-the-counter medications. It is estimated that on a per capita basis Americans consume between 150 and 200 grams of caffeine annually. Most adults and large numbers of children consume one or more pharmacologically active doses of caffeine—about 100 milligrams—at least once a day. A person who drinks four or five cups of coffee a day consumes about 400 milligrams daily.

There is no question that caffeine is a drug, but whether it is a truly addictive one is not certain. However, caffeine use is not equated with the ruined lives that the truly addictive drugs are noted for. Nevertheless, millions of Americans will attest to how much they depend upon caffeine, particularly in their morning cup of coffee, to provide a lift.

It is this lift that scholars believe early man discovered in the leaves, roots, and berries of various plants, including coffee beans, the cola nut, tea leaves, and the cocoa plant. Tea is known to have been cultivated as early as 4700 B.C., and caffeine was recognized historically as a stimulant and antisoporific. Caffeine can lift a person out of boredom or fatigue, making it possible to focus on the task at hand. Its general systemic effects include increased mobilization of free fatty acids, which are used for prolonged exertion—for example, marathons. It does not, however, significantly alter mood.

Caffeine is one of the methylated xanthines. The two other principal members of this chemical class are theophylline and theobromine. All three are quickly absorbed

Tips to Avoid Weight Gain After Stopping Smoking

Begin an exercise program to coincide with stopping smoking. As the days without cigarettes lengthen into weeks, the ability to jog, play tennis, swim, or do aerobic exercises will increase and the shortness of breath common to smokers will decrease. Soon, exercise will be a pleasure. In addition, it burns up extra calories.

Examine daily diet. Since stopping smoking can lead to a rediscovery of food, there is a temptation to overeat. Avoid high-calorie foods and keep a supply of low-calorie snacks on hand. These might include carrot and green pepper sticks, unsalted and unbuttered popcorn, high-fiber crackers, and other low-calorie foods. Determine how many calories per day are needed based on age, height, and ideal weight and try not to eat more than this target.

Pick a convenient date for quitting. Avoid setting a target date for quitting smoking that coincides with a major holiday when rounds of parties and family get-togethers will increase the temptation to eat and drink too much.

Curtail the consumption of alcoholic beverages. The calories in such beverages are empty.

Consider the pros and cons of using nicotine gum during the first three months of abstinence.

into the body. They stimulate the central nervous system and the heart, have a diuretic action, and cause some of the body's smooth muscles, such as those in the bronchial tubes, to relax. They provoke increased synthesis of glucose and increase the basal metabolic rate slightly. Of the three, caffeine is the strongest central-nervous stimulant and in large doses increases the capacity for muscular work. It also causes increased secretion of gastric juices in the stomach and small intestine.

Studies of the effects of caffeine on the human body have been conducted for decades. A common difficulty with such studies is the fact that over time the body develops at least a partial tolerance to caffeine. Thus, someone who is what medical investigators call caffeine-naïve will have a more marked response than someone who regularly ingests caffeine. In one now-classic investigation, a randomized crossover study in which neither the investigators nor the research subjects knew who was receiving caffeine and who was not, a group of caffeine-naïve young men was given oral doses of caffeine. It was found that an oral dose of caffeine equivalent to two or three cups of coffee produced significant physiological effects. The activity of renin, the enzyme associated with control of blood pressure, increased dramatically, as did blood pressure itself, gradually subsiding over a three-hour period. Bradycardia, a slowing of the heartbeat, was noted 45 minutes after caffeine ingestion and lasted for an hour. Bradycardia may decrease cardiac output, leading to feelings of fatigue and a decrease in the ability to exercise. Other studies, some of which used people accustomed to regular caffeine consumption, also have noted temporary alterations in the heart's rhythm. In a significant number of people, high doses of caffeine cause rapid heartbeat and twitching.

Caffeine and Heart Disease

Despite more than three decades of research, the overall picture regarding the effects of caffeine on cardiac function remains unclear. Some studies have found a connection between caffeine and coronary heart disease and other heart problems, while others have found no link. A fundamental problem that has plagued such studies has been the difficulty of controlling the amount of caffeine ingested and relating it to a host of other lifestyle factors that can vary widely from person to person, such as tobacco and alcohol use, diet, occupation, and level of exercise. There even has been a wide discrepancy over the years about levels of caffeine used in the studies, marked by wide variations in the size of a cup of coffee, the method by which the coffee was prepared, and the number of cups consumed each day. Some studies have been flawed because they were based on a research subject's recall of coffee consumption rather than on actual measured consumption.

When research volunteers were asked to recall their coffee consumption, an association with heart attacks was frequently found: People who had heart attacks recalled drinking more coffee than matched subjects who had not had heart attacks. Other retrospective studies could not find an association, however. The wives of 649 men who had died of coronary heart disease were interviewed about their husbands' lifestyles and the data was then subjected to extensive analysis. The risk of dying of heart disease because of coffee drinking was found to be very small. This study was marred, however, by the fact that the diagnosis of coronary heart disease was made from death certificates rather than from prior clinical observations or autopsy.

Prospective studies are those in which a group of subjects is selected and then followed over time. One of the best-known of these is the Framingham study, in which more than 5,000 people in a Massachusetts community outside Boston have been followed since 1948. In this group, a statistically significant risk is associated with increased coffee drinking only in the category of "death from all causes." However, coffee drinking was linked with cigarette smoking in this analysis. Similar studies have found that the combination of coffee drinking and smoking can increase the risk of death from heart disease. When the effect of cigarettes is removed in the statistical analysis, coffee plays no role in the development of coronary artery disease.

In another prospective study, the coffee-consumption habits of more than 1,000 male graduates of Johns Hopkins Medical School were followed for 25 years. The more coffee the men drank, the higher the incidence of heart disease. The investigators had accounted for smoking, high blood pressure, and variations in cholesterol levels, but they did not account for exercise, stress levels, and diet, all of which are also important in the development of heart disease.

Doctors also have investigated whether coffee consumption has an effect on the levels of fats in the blood, which could lead to increased heart disease by promoting buildup of blockages within the arteries. Again, the results have been mixed. Some studies find little or no effect, while others indicate a possible risk. For example, a study of more than 5,000 men of Japanese ancestry being followed in the Honolulu Heart Program found that increased consumption of coffee—but not of tea or cola—was associated with increased levels of cholesterol in the blood, suggesting a deleterious effect from caffeine. It is not possible to say whether these men will experience more heart disease as a result.

Such research results point up the difficulty of reaching a definitive answer about coffee and heart disease. Nevertheless, many doctors advise patients who are concerned about heart disease to limit coffee consumption to one or two cups a day and to select caffeine-free soft drinks. Patients who have heart conditions that involve either disturbed rhythms or problems with the function of the heart's valves are usually advised to avoid coffee and other sources of caffeine—or to curtail their consumption sharply—because of the effect that caffeine can have on heartbeat.

Coffee and Smoking

The relationship between coffee and smoking has been the subject of increasing research in recent years. Investigators have sought to discover whether caffeine ingestion affects smoking behavior and whether the nicotine, carbon monoxide, and other chemicals in tobacco somehow interact with caffeine. Results have suggested that cigarettes have a stronger effect if the smoker also drinks coffee. For example, a 1987 study of men at the Veterans Affairs Medical Center in Los Angeles found that smokers drinking regular coffee seemed to inhale more smoke from their cigarettes than those who consumed decaffeinated coffee. A study by a research group in Oregon found that smokers and ex-smokers tended to drink more coffee (and alcohol) than non-smokers.

Decaffeinated Coffee

Concern about coffee's possible harmful effects has led many people to switch to decaffeinated coffee, in which caffeine is removed from the coffee bean by using a chemical treatment. The traditional chemical, methylene chloride, has come under attack because it has been shown to cause cancers when inhaled in large amounts by laboratory animals.

The federal Food and Drug Administration banned it from use in hair sprays because of the danger that it would be breathed in when aerosol cans were used to apply the spray. However, the FDA ruled that methylene chloride could continue to be used to remove caffeine from the coffee bean because so little of the chemical remains at the end of the decaffeination process. The FDA reported that even if someone drank five cups of decaffeinated coffee a day, there was only a one-in-a-million chance of developing cancer.

Public interest and consumer groups challenged the decision and the resulting publicity raised questions about decaffeinated coffee in the minds of many. Some coffee manufacturers responded by altering the decaffeination process, using the chemical ethyl acetate to dissolve the caffeine out of the coffee beans. (Ethyl acetate occurs naturally in some fruits and vegetables and has not been shown to cause cancer in laboratory animals.) Manufacturers who prepare their coffee this way advertise that their decaffeinated coffee is natural. Caffeine also can be removed using treatments based on carbon dioxide and water or coffee oils and water. The handful of research studies seeking to determine whether decaffeinated coffee prepared with methylene chloride caused any ill effects has found none.

Other Concerns

In recent years, there also have been warnings about consumption during pregnancy of too much coffee and caffeine from other sources. For example, in 1980, the Food and Drug Administration formally warned pregnant women to be cautious about their caffeine consumption. There is some evidence suggesting that *heavy* coffee drinking may be associated with an increased incidence of miscarriage and retarded fetal growth. This has prompted many obstetricians to advise pregnant patients to use caffeine in moderation— for example, not more than two cups of brewed coffee (or not more than a total of 200 milligrams of caffeine) spread over an entire day. Caffeine is secreted in breast milk; thus accumulated caffeine might affect very young infants, who eliminate it slowly from their bodies. (For more information, see Chapter 12.)

Often, individuals experience a special sensitivity to caffeine. Sometimes this develops early in life; in other cases, it appears in adulthood. Such people must avoid caffeine in coffee and elsewhere in the diet, and they may also need to avoid the methylxanthines found in chocolate and cocoa. No clinical test for such susceptibility exists. Rather, the individual, by dietary trial and error, identifies caffeine as the culprit. (For more information on caffeine, see Chapter 10.)

ILLICIT AND MOOD-ALTERING DRUGS

Drugs such as heroin, cocaine, and marijuana, which are illegal today, have been used since ancient times to treat a variety of illnesses and for their mood-altering properties. Other synthetic drugs such as amphetamines and anti-anxiety drugs have been developed in recent decades. These have legitimate uses in medicine, but their ability to alter mood makes them candidates for abuse.

By most measures, use of illicit drugs by Americans has been rising in recent years, and increasing federal, state, and local government resources are being spent to combat their production, sale, and use. Treatment centers for chronic drug abusers can now be found in many communities, and civic and medical groups are giving increased attention to educating both young and old about drug abuse, its dangers and treatments. While there are indications that the use of marijuana and cocaine by some groups may be slackening, use of these two drugs remains considerably elevated compared to use 20 years ago. The number of people addicted to heroin is not increasing alarmingly, but neither is there evidence that it is decreasing. Few experts see any signs that drug abuse is lessening, or will end in the near future.

Drug abuse takes an enormous toll in terms of work lost, money spent on buying illegal drugs, and lives ruined, including the lives of those close to a person who abuses. A drug habit can cost hundreds of dollars a week, and the need for money can eventually lead to selling the drug itself to earn enough to buy personal supplies. Sometimes other criminal activities follow.

Drug abuse also has nutritional consequences. The effects on the body vary from drug to drug. Chronic abuse of addictive drugs frequently results in generally poor nutritional status, either because the addict has no money left for food after purchasing drugs or because appetite is diminished. Some drug addicts believe that snack foods, particularly cakes, cookies, soft drinks, candy, and potato chips, will enhance the effects of a drug. In general, milk, fruits, and vegetables are lacking in the diets of such drug users. Family members and others who are close to a drug addict and seeking to intervene need to be conscious of the poor overall nutritional status of such people. Adequate attention must be given to nutrition while at the same time dealing with the addiction itself.

Drug abuse also often goes along with alcohol abuse, leading to the nutrient deficiencies common to alcoholism, such as deficiencies of folic acid, thiamine, niacin, riboflavin, and vitamin A and C deficiencies. Deficiencies of the minerals magnesium, potassium, and zinc are sometimes seen. (For more information, see Chapter 21.)

Adolescents are particularly vulnerable to the nutritional problems that accompany drug abuse. When drug use begins in prepuberty and continues into adolescence, the nutritional requirements to support growth and physical maturation may not be met, leading to serious developmental problems. Even if drug abuse begins after the adolescent growth phase, a teenager can develop nutritional problems because there are no nutritional reserves on which the body can draw. Teens and young adults also normally have limited financial resources, and diet may suffer simply because all their money is used to buy drugs.

Marijuana

Marijuana users are predominantly younger persons—teens, young adults, and people in their thirties. Marijuana use rose in the 1970s, from about 500,000 people in 1971 to over 3 million at the end of the decade. Since then, there has been evidence that its use has declined slightly, although gathering reliable statistics is difficult because marijuana use is illegal and severely prosecuted in some states.

From a psychotropic standpoint, it is not known whether long-term use of marijuana has serious harmful effects, or whether its occasional use is no more harmful than an occasional drink of alcohol. Tetrahydracannabinol, the primary active chemical in marijuana, is soluble in fat and is absorbed in the lungs from smoke. It is believed to be taken up by the lipoproteins and is transported throughout the body. Traces of marijuana tend to remain in the body for a week or more after smoking a single cigarette. Marijuana alters perceptions of time and space, produces a mild euphoria, and reduces the ability to think logically and communicate clearly. In some users, it may produce distortions of sense perception akin to hallucinations, feelings of panic, or paranoia. Other effects are faster heartbeat, dry mouth and throat, poor short-term memory, and impaired motor skills, decreased reaction time, and altered depth perception. These latter effects make operating automobiles or machines particularly dangerous. In adolescents, marijuana use sometimes can result in a loss of motivation and disinterest in school and in social relationships.

Marijuana's most serious long-term consequence for the heavy user—someone who smokes five or six cigarettes a day over a long period—is the danger of lung cancer. Marijuana smokers typically inhale more deeply and hold the smoke in the lungs longer to increase the amount of tetrahydracannibol reaching the blood, and smoke a cigarette down to the butt. Together with the high level of tars in the smoke, all this suggests that marijuana smoking may be more likely to lead to lung cancer than cigarette smoking. It is known that long-term marijuana use causes metaplasia, a precancerous condition of lung tissue.

A pronounced nutritional consequence of marijuana use is an increased appetite and craving for sweets. One study of college students aged 17 to 21 found that 69 percent using marijuana reported increased appetite. Other studies have found that the types of foods preferred when high on marijuana (in descending order of preference) were sweet foods, soft drinks, meat, fruits, vegetables, salty snacks, bread, and crackers.

Cocaine

The use of cocaine has grown rapidly in recent years, particularly among young adults in poor areas, although it is also used by young adults from the middle and upper-middle classes, young professionals, and white-collar workers. In the early 1980s, cocaine was associated with popular figures in the entertainment field. For many others, it is the euphoriant drug of choice. It is estimated that between 5 and 10 million Americans use cocaine with some frequency. In the last decade, the number of deaths related to the use of cocaine tripled.

Contrary to previous beliefs, cocaine is an addictive drug. In recent years, numerous experts have warned that those who become addicted to it experience real withdrawal symptoms when they stop using it. Laboratory monkeys given a choice of intravenous cocaine or food will choose cocaine almost every time. Edward B. Mohns, M.D., head of the division of psychiatry and behavioral medicine at the Scripps Clinic in La Jolla, California, notes that laboratory animals who are given an unlimited supply of cocaine will not sleep or eat because they are so occupied with using cocaine. Such behavior quickly kills them. He warns that humans may be equally vulnerable.

The addictive nature of cocaine appears to be related to the form in which it is taken. In recent years, crack—a highly addictive form of cocaine that is smoked—has become increasing popular, especially among disadvantaged urban youths.

Cocaine, or coke as it is commonly known, is derived from the leaves of the coca plant, grown in the mountainous regions of central South America. Although it is illegal to produce, distribute, or use cocaine today, it has a long history as a local anesthetic and, until 1906, it was a primary ingredient of Coca-Cola. It was replaced by caffeine.

Cocaine is a powerful stimulant of the central nervous system. It causes restlessness, excitement, and a feeling of well-being accompanied by a sense of extraordinary mental prowess and a lessening of fatigue. High doses can lead to impaired motor activity, tremors, and convulsive movements. Respiration rate, heart rate, and body temperature become elevated, as does blood pressure.

Chronic cocaine users suffer loss of appetite, with resulting weight loss and malnutrition. Some therapists report even more severe nutritional problems. At the Fair Oaks Hospital in Summit, New Jersey, which runs the national cocaine hot line, researchers found that more than 30 percent of the cocaine abusers who called in suffered from bulimia or anorexia nervosa or both. (Bulimia is the gorge-and-purge eating disorder; anorexia nervosa involves slow self-starvation.) The researchers hypothesized that the cocaine abuse itself did not cause the eating disorders but that the individuals with the eating disorders were prone to addictive or compulsive behavior that would lead to abuse of either drugs or food. They warned that physicians should be alert for excessive cocaine use in patients who have eating disorders and suggested that cocaine users who seek treatment should also be examined for the presence of eating disorders. (For more information, see Chapter 19.)

Heroin

Compiling reliable statistics is particularly difficult in the case of heroin, but estimates are that between 500,000 and 750,000 people in the United States are addicted to the drug. Although the overall number of heroin addicts is believed to be relatively steady, heroin is regarded as one of the country's longest term, most destructive drug-addiction problems.

Heroin is made from the opium poppy and is a chemical derivative of morphine, but it is three or four times more potent. It is quickly absorbed through the mucous membranes and can be snorted like cocaine. It can also be taken orally. Many heroin users inject it into a vein to obtain a faster response. There is no disagreement that heroin is highly addictive, producing tolerance to higher and higher doses, dependence on its presence in the body, and distinctly unpleasant withdrawal symptoms. Some experts believe that many heroin addicts use the drug as much to stave off painful withdrawal symptoms as they do for the euphoric effect it produces. Death from heroin overdose is an always-present danger for addicts. An overdose rapidly depresses the central nervous system, slowing or stopping breathing and the heart.

Apart from overdose, the complications arising from heroin use are related to the adulterants with which it is cut, and to unsterile injection practices, rather than to the narcotic properties of the drug itself. The adulterants include maltose, lactose, and quinine, all of which are readily soluble in the blood. Talc is also sometimes mixed with heroin. Some addicts add other drugs, hoping for a heightened effect. Unsanitary methods of preparing and injecting heroin are further sources of serious side effects. Addicts often experience liver problems, pneumonia, and lung abscesses. Skin ulcers, phlebitis, bacterial endocarditis, and scarring of the arms and other areas where injections are given come from the use of dirty needles. In recent years, the incidence of Acquired Immune Deficiency Syndrome (AIDS) has increased dramatically among drug addicts, passed from one to another through sharing needles contaminated with virus-infected blood.

Heroin addicts are frequently so consumed by their habit that all available funds go to buy the drug. They are often malnourished and display deficiencies of vitamins and minerals, including vitamins A, C, B_6, B_{12} and the minerals magnesium, potassium, and zinc. A study of a group of heroin addicts found that 30 percent had abnormal liver function and about one-fourth showed vitamin deficiencies, particularly of folic acid and vitamin B_6. Lowered thiamine levels were also found. Like marijuana users, when heroin addicts do eat, many tend to consume sweet foods, resulting in a lack of fruits, vegetables, and dairy products in their diets.

Addicts are unlikely to do anything about their nutritional status while they are actively using heroin. In a treatment setting, whether the synthetic opiate methadone is substituted for heroin or the program is drug-free, part of the approach is to return the addict to a sound nutritional basis. Malnourishment often must be treated, along with vitamin and mineral deficiencies.

Amphetamines and Other Drugs

A variety of other drugs have become popular, including amphetamines, LSD, and prescription drugs such as barbiturates and benzodiazepines (tranquilizers). They carry risks that range from psychological and/or physical dependence to the danger of death from overdosing or mixing different types of drugs. Users often suffer from a compromised nutritional status and pay little attention to diet. Malnourishment sometimes is seen, and vitamin and mineral deficiencies similar to those of other drug abusers are not uncommon.

Amphetamines were first synthesized in the late 1920s and initially appeared as anticongestant inhalants. They were widely used later to combat fatigue and subsequently saw prescription use as antidepressants and appetite-suppressant diet pills. Their medical uses are sharply curtailed today, but illegally prescribed or manufactured amphetamines are sold on the street to abusers known as speed freaks. Amphetamines are called speed,

bennies, pep pills, diet pills, and uppers. Amphetamines are usually taken orally, but some hard-core abusers inject them.

Amphetamines cause release of adrenaline, which stimulates the central nervous system. Their euphoric effects and their ability to allow the user to overcome fatigue account for their popularity with truck drivers, musicians, students, and others. The drug causes decreased appetite, a dry mouth, enlarged nasal and bronchial passages, increased heart rate and blood pressure, and increased respiratory rate. Large doses produce dizziness, a racing heart, and aggressive behavior. The appetite-suppressant side effect can lead to malnutrition and vitamin and mineral deficiencies in the chronic abuser. Amphetamines, like cocaine, are addictive and produce both physical and psychological dependence. Some abusers take amphetamines for days on end and then crash, experiencing extreme fatigue, depression, anxiety, and hunger.

Barbiturates are sedative-hypnotic drugs, usually prescribed as sleeping pills and tranquilizers. They lessen anxiety and promote calmness and sleep. Some well-known brand names are Seconal, Nembutal, and Tuinal. Abusers often obtain prescriptions by duping doctors or finding a cooperative doctor. Another class of sedative-hypnotics subject to abuse are the benzodiazepines, the minor tranquilizers, best known by the brand names Valium, Librium, and Xanax. They, too, are prescribed to combat anxiety, produce a feeling of calmness, and promote sleep. Both types of drugs when taken in small doses produce relaxation and mild euphoria. In larger doses, they result in unsteady gait, slurred speech, and drowsiness. Too large a dose can cause unconsciousness and, rarely, death through the suppression of breathing and heartbeat.

These drugs can produce dependence. Therefore, those patients who require these medications for treatment of serious anxiety disorders, such as panic attacks or agoraphobia, should discuss the benefits as well as the risks of using benzodiazepines. Sedative-hypnotic addicts behave like alcoholics, often neglecting work, family, and diet in favor of their drug habit. As a consequence, the chronic abuser can become malnourished and develop some of the same nutritional deficiencies seen in alcoholics. Severe withdrawal symptoms are associated with cessation of use in heavy abusers of both classes of the sedative-hypnotics. Withdrawal can be difficult and should be carried out under a doctor's supervision. As the withdrawal phase ends, increasing attention must be paid to nutritional status and the introduction of a balanced diet to maintain health and address any deficiencies.

Alcohol and the sedative-hypnotics both depress the central nervous system and should therefore never be taken together, even in small doses. The result can be a fatal overdose, particularly when someone who has been drinking heavily takes a larger than normal dose of barbiturates to combat insomnia brought on by the alcohol.

Lysergic acid (LSD), a popular drug in the 1960s, is a synthetic hallucinogen known commonly as acid. Along with peyote and mescaline, which are derived from cactus, and psilocybin, which comes from mushrooms, it is one of the so-called psychedelic or mind-expanding drugs. They are not addictive in either a psychological or physical sense, but they cause highly unpredictable reactions, including distorted sense perceptions, a sense that time is standing still, difficulty in speaking and communicating, sharply lowered appetite and sexual desire. Some people have experienced panic or paranoia after taking psychedelics, and in some cases their use has triggered a psychosis lasting long after the drug wore off and requiring hospitalization.

SEEKING HELP

Many services are available for substance abusers seeking help to overcome their addictions. Each state has a toll-free drug-abuse information line so that callers can obtain confidential referrals for treatment and find out what resources are available within their community. The number should be listed in the government listings in the blue pages at the back of the telephone book. In most states, the number also is broadcast on public-service announcements, and printed in various ads. Private and religious-sponsored treatment centers are listed in the Yellow Pages under Rehabilitation.

There are basically three types of drug-free treatment programs offered for drug addiction. They vary in the intensity of the therapy.

Outpatient programs are the least intensive of the three and are generally for those who might already have been through a residential treatment or may not need 24-hour care. Patients in these programs usually have some means of support—whether it be from family members or employers—that provides an incentive for breaking a drug habit.

In most states, outpatient programs are funded by state and federal monies, supplemented by some local funding. The state administers the funding and monitors the services, which are operated by a nonprofit organization, some with religious affiliation, or by a local or county government agency. Patients usually visit the program two or three times during a week.

The most intensive drug-free addiction therapy is offered by residential programs that provide 24-hour care. These are generally for the serious abuser and those with prominent socioeconomic problems, many of whom have lost their jobs or are homeless. These are primarily state-operated and are supported by federal and sometimes local funding. There are also private residential treatment centers, such as the Betty Ford Clinic in California, and Smithers Center in New York City.

Day-service programs are the second most intensive of the drug-free rehabilitation programs. Care is administered five days a week, usually during regular business hours.

Methadone-maintenance programs are drug-based treatments provided for those with opiate addictions, including heroin. Whereas the drug-free programs provide care on a short-term basis, methadone-maintenance programs usually provide care for several years.

In addition to programs that receive government funding—whether it be from federal, state, or local sources—there is a wide range of private programs. These are primarily funded through the fees paid by patients or by their employers or health insurance. Many of the private residential facilities offer 28-day programs, because this is the period of time typically reimbursed by health-insurance providers. Private drug therapies offer outpatient, residential, and methadone services. Those who avail themselves of private facilities generally have a higher average income than those in government-sponsored programs.

Within each of these types of treatment programs there are therapies geared specifically for different subgroups, such as women and children of substance abusers, or the young, the homeless, or the employed substance abuser.

Unfortunately, the demand for treatment for drug addiction far outstrips the supply of services. New York State has the most extensive drug-treatment system of any state, but it also claims one of the worst problems. As of this writing, the waiting list for treatment in a residential-care facility in New York State was over 2,000, with some people waiting up to six months to be admitted.

23

Nutrition for Hospitalized Patients

David Gentili, M.D., Peggy O'Sullivan, R.D., M.S.,
and Thomas J. Iberti, M.D.

■

INTRODUCTION

The need for good nutrition takes on added importance in a hospital setting because illness can be a double-edged sword in its effects on nutritional well-being. On the one hand, symptoms common to a number of illnesses, as well as prolonged hospitalization, increase the risk of nutrient depletion in a number of ways.

1. Fever increases the body's metabolic rate and can deplete its nutrient stores.

2. Anorexia is a common manifestation of many diseases and impairs the body's ability to maintain adequate nutrition.

3. Severe diarrhea can cause dehydration and loss of vital elements.

On the other hand, the treatment of disease can create nutrition problems. For example, the use of certain drugs, as in cancer chemotherapy, can inhibit a patient's appetite and the stress of surgery can increase the need for protein and other nutrients.

Just as disease can foster poor nutrition, a sound eating regimen is essential to the heal-ing process. A nutritious diet that compensates for previous deficiencies or illness-related losses can help in the recovery of cancer victims, surgical patients, burn victims, and alcoholics, among many others.

The fact that proper nutrition can promote health has caused a virtual revolution in hospital care. As recently as 15 years ago, medical schools all but ignored nutrition as a specialty except as a postgraduate elective course. As scientific knowledge and public awareness have grown, nutritional support has become increasingly sophisticated. Nutritional assessment and intervention is part of each patient's care.

The enhanced status of nutrition in the medical arena gives the patient an additional role, as well as a responsibility, in his or her relationship with the physician.

GOALS OF NUTRITION SUPPORT

A prescribed hospital diet usually complements medical and surgical care, but often the diet itself is the specific treatment for a disease.

Nutrition support differs from hospital to hospital but includes one or more of the following goals.

- Maintenance of normal nutrition during hospitalization.

- Correction of a nutritional deficiency.

- Countering impaired ability of the body to process various nutrients.

- Providing relief to a specific organ by supplying nutrients in a different form or changing the timing of meals.

Diet Therapy

In most hospitals, the physician (in consultation with the nutritionist) will order a patient's diet regimen, in the same way medication and other therapy is prescribed.

After the patient's medical status is established, nutritional assessment by a staff dietitian can begin. The patient will be asked about weight changes, past medical problems, and eating problems. In addition to the standard laboratory tests given upon hospital admission, further procedures may be ordered if nutrient deficiencies are suspected. If the patient has a satisfactory appetite and no special nutritional needs, an appropriate eating regimen is prescribed from the hospital's diet manual (see pages 378-81).

The nutritionist will make recommendations to the physician regarding the feeding regimen, as well as formulating specialized care plans for patients requiring additional nutrition support.

The Standard Hospital Diet

Also called a regular diet, this regimen falls under the broader classification of an *oral*

diet. It provides the standard recommended daily dietary allowances of proteins, vitamins, minerals, as well as carbohydrates, fat, and trace elements.

Patients on a standard diet who find it difficult to tolerate hospital food can get food from outside, if it is allowed by the physician and nutritionist.

Modified Diets

A modified diet is essentially a standard diet that has been adjusted to meet special nutritional needs. Such diets might be modified for the following reasons.

- To regulate or eliminate certain foods (e.g., a lactose-restricted or gluten-free diet).

- To adjust the level of nutrients (high- or low-protein, high- or low-carbohydrate, high- or low-fat, low-sodium, or low-potassium diets).

- To provide a particular consistency of food (liquid, soft, or low-residue diets).

In addition, a diet might be modified to conform to a patient's personal or religious preferences, as in the case of a kosher or vegetarian diet.

How to Eat Well in the Hospital

Nutrition is one of the most important aspects of hospital care in which a patient can participate. Indeed, depending on the level of nutrition services in a particular institution, you may need to be your own consumer advocate. This is especially true for the patient who will be hospitalized a long time, regardless of his or her nutrition status upon admission.

Studies have shown that not only can patients enter the hospital with some degree of malnutrition, they also can develop further nutritional problems. Prolonged hospitalization can lead to poor nutritional status and delayed recovery if proper steps are not taken to correct these problems.

The following tips explain how to safeguard nutritional health and speed recovery.

1. Be honest with the staff in the assessment process. Unless a patient has obvious signs of malnutrition, the physician and dietitian will learn much about nutritional status based on what you tell them when they take the admission history. The physician will most likely write the diet order, but the dietitian will supervise its implementation and suggest modifications as the need arises.

   Be specific in describing your eating and drinking habits, including recent weight changes, dietary restrictions, and known food allergies or intolerances. Mention any prescription or over-the-counter drugs—including any and all vitamin and other supplements—you are taking, as these may interact with nutrients or new drugs prescribed. Volunteer this information.

2. Know the risks. From a nutritional standpoint, a patient admitted to a hospital is considered at high risk for any of the following reasons:

   - obesity (generally defined as more than 20 percent above desirable weight)

   - underweight (weighing less than 80 percent of desirable weight)

   - any recent unintentional loss of 10 percent or more of normal body weight

   - alcoholism.

   In addition, the following factors pertaining to already-hospitalized patients can contribute to malnutrition:

   - a lack of adequate dietary intake for five to seven days; for example, a patient on intravenous fluids without nutrient supplementation

   - extensive loss of nutrients due to dialysis, draining abscesses and wounds, and various intestinal disorders

   - increased metabolic needs arising from severe burns, infection, fever

   - the use of drugs and therapies that inhibit normal nutrient metabolism. These include steroids, chemotherapy, and radiation.

   Patients and family members should discuss any of these factors, if relevant, with the physician and nutritionist so that proper nutritional support can be implemented.

3. Know the options. If meal choices are unsatisfactory, ask the nutritionist what alternates are available. Food may be brought in from outside the hospital, provided that it falls within the particular diet regimen.

4. Be assertive but cooperative. Those who are too ill to feed themselves have the right to assistance and sufficient time for feeding. Problems with meals should be made known to the nurse or nutritionist.

5. Ask questions. Use the nutritionist as a resource person for questions: the reason behind a special diet, food and medication interactions, how to maintain the diet upon discharge, and so forth.

Diet Manual

The diet manual is a comprehensive guide to all the diets a hospital provides. It gives information on when to use a specific diet, what foods are allowed and not allowed, sample menus, and summaries of the diet's nutritional composition.

These are some sample pages from Mount Sinai Hospital's diet manual:

I. Regular Diets:

(a) The regular diet is indicated for patients who do not require specific dietary modifications.

(b) The vegetarian diet is a regular diet that is characterized by the omission of animal products. (There are different diets to which the vegetarian name has been added and that may represent nutritionally inadequate or dangerous nutritional fads, but these should not be mistaken for the balanced vegetarian diet.) Milk products are not omitted.

(c) The diet for the elderly is a regular diet that will be individually altered to satisfy nutrient needs that are a part of the aging process.

(d) These include diets for pregnancy and lactation.

II. Diets Modified in Consistency:

(a) The soft diet contains a minimum of fiber and connective tissues but does contain a moderate amount of residue.

(b) The semisoft diet contains foods modified in texture for use as a transition from full fluids to soft diet.

(c) The mechanical soft diet contains foods that are easily chewed.

(d) The clear fluid diet includes only those foods that are translucent, low-residue, and are liquid at room temperature.

(e) The full fluid diet adds milk and egg-based products as well as strained cereals to the clear fluid diet.

(f) The pureed diet is a modification of the mechanical soft diet, and offers foods that have been blenderized and therefore require no chewing.

(g) These include diets modified in type and amount of fiber.

(h) Bland diets continue to be used in patients with a variety of gastrointestinal disorders. The manual discusses the rationale and propriety of these regimens.

(i) The postgastrectomy diet is designed to minimize the symptoms and severity of the "dumping syndrome."

(j) The low-residue diet is designed to reduce the amount of residue remaining in the lower bowel after digestion.

III. Diets Modified in Energy Value:

(a) The calculated calorie, carbohydrate, protein, and fat diet is a variation of the regular diet and is designed to meet individual nutritional needs, to achieve normal metabolic functioning; for example, as in diabetes.

(b) These include the diet for the pregnant diabetic.

IV. Diets Modified in Sodium:

(a) The sodium-restricted diets are prescribed for the specific treatment of disease. They are ordered by the amounts of sodium desired rather than by sodium chloride.

1. 3500 mg. sodium: regular diet without salt shaker and omitting obviously salty foods.

2. 1000 mg. sodium: Unsalted foods only are used.

3. 500 mg. sodium: No salt is allowed.

4. 250 mg. sodium: Dialyzed milk is used in place of fresh cow's milk.

5. 1000 mg. sodium: All unsalted foods are used, with the exception of regular bread, butter/margarine, and regular desserts.

NOTE: Unnecessary sodium restriction may result in relatively less palatable food, which may pre-

OPTIONS FOR NUTRITIONAL SUPPORT

Oral Supplemental Foods (Nourishments)

Disease, injury, and illness can diminish the appetite, leaving a patient unable to eat adequately to meet his or her nutritional needs. When this occurs, a physician may call for oral supplemental foods to be added to the prescribed diet. Such nourishing supplements are easier to ingest than solid food and can increase caloric and protein intake.

Among the more common such supple-

Diet Manual (cont.)

dispose to decreased intake with other nutrient deficiencies!

V.   Low-Fat Diets:
   (a)   These include diets for the reduction of high blood cholesterol levels.
   (b)   A low-cholesterol, low-saturated-fat diet for weight maintenance in patients with elevated blood cholesterol.
   (c)   A low-fat diet may be useful in the management of disorders of the pancreas and biliary tract. Nutritional adequacy may be difficult to achieve.

VI.   Diets Modified in Protein:
   (a)   The objective of the modified Giovannetti diet is to provide essential amino acids while minimizing nonessential amino acids.
   (b)   The 40-gram protein diet provides protein of a high biological value along with appropriate calories. It may be useful to patients with severely impaired renal or liver function.
   (c)   The controlled protein, sodium, and potassium diet is designed for the dialysis patient.
   (d)   Diets individually modified for the patient on Continuous Ambulatory Peritoneal Dialysis (CAPD) are individualized and include modifications of protein intake.

VII.   Miscellaneous Diets:
   (a)   These include the lactose-restricted diet.
   (b)   The low-tyramine diet may be used in patients taking monoamine oxidase inhibitors.
   (c)   Low-purine diets are used for patients with hyperuricemia.

   (d)   These include the low-calcium diet.
   (e)   These include the low-phosphorus diet.

VIII.   Pediatric Diets:
   (a)   Appropriate age-related diets are discussed in the diet manual.
   (b)   The ketogenic diet is a high-fat, low-carbohydrate diet designed as a potential therapy for children with intractable seizures.
   (c)   The nutritional management of the patient with cystic fibrosis is a highly individualized matter for which guidelines are provided in the manual.

IX.   Supplementary Feedings and/or Tube Feedings:
   (a)   A wide variety of supplementary feedings and nutritional modules are available. They have specific formulations and specialized applications. Their use should be planned to overcome specific metabolic, physical, or constitutional deficiencies.

NOTE: In pediatrics, the use of these special products is limited to the Pediatric Nutritional Support Service.

X.   Dietary Tests and Procedures:
   Special procedures relating to impending tests (usually of gastrointestinal function) must be specifically ordered by the physician, although the manual provides some widely used guidelines.

XI.   Appendix:
   The appendix contains tables and charts that may be of considerable use to the individual seeking more information relating to nutritional intake.

ments are items such as milk shakes, pudding, and instant breakfast preparations. These supplements are fortified with protein, calories, vitamins, and minerals to boost their nutritional value. Other options include commercially prepared liquid oral supplement formulas such as Ensure, Sustacal, or Meritene.

Liquid supplements are just what the name implies—supplements to solid food. Often they provide only some of the vital nutrients needed for a balanced diet. Sometimes they contain all necessary nutrients and are thus called nutritionally complete formulas. When liquid oral supplements are the sole source of nutrition, they should always be a complete formula.

Enteral Feeding

Enteral means through the gastrointestinal tract. Technically, all oral nutrition is enteral, but in a hospital setting, the term is most often synonymous with tube feeding. The basic principal of enteral nutrition is to supply food directly to the intestine via a tube.

A patient is considered a candidate for enteral feeding if he or she has normal digestive and absorptive function but cannot take enough nutrients by mouth. In general, this problem occurs within the following categories:

- disease or injury that makes it difficult to chew or swallow, as in complications arising from oral surgery, cancer of the mouth or esophagus, head and neck injuries, or coma

- disease or injury that greatly increases the body's metabolic needs, as can happen from severe burns, systemic infection, and trauma

- severe malnutrition related to illness that has led to inadequate oral nutrition.

Regular Diet

Description
The regular diet is indicated for patients who do not require specific dietary modifications. There is no restriction on the type of food served or the method of preparation.

Adequacy
The regular diet is planned to meet or exceed the recommended daily allowance (1) for essential nutrients in accordance with the requirements of a moderately active, normal adult male or female age 25 to 50 years.

Approximate Nutrient Value*

NUTRIENT	RANGE
Calories	2000–2700
Protein	80–90 gm.
Fat	90–100 gm.
Calcium	800–1,000 mg.
Phosphorus	1,200–1,400 mg.
Iron	10–18 mg.
Sodium	4,000–6,000 mg.**
Potassium	3,000–4,000 mg.
Vitamin A	7,000–10,000 IU
Thiamine	1.0–1.4 mg.
Riboflavin	1.7–1.9 mg.
Niacin	11–20 mg.
Ascorbic acid	90–100 mg.

*Figures represent average based on sample daily menu that follows.
**Figures do not represent sodium added to food in cooking or salt added to food at the table.

Enteral nutrition has been greatly improved in recent years. Feeding tubes are now made from pliable polyethylene, come in smaller diameters and cause far less discom-

Regular Diet *(cont.)*

Sample Daily Menu

Milk		1 pint
Eggs		1
Meat, fish, poultry, cheese		6 oz.
Bread or substitute		3 servings or more
Cereal		1 serving (½ cup cooked, ¾ cup dry)
Vegetables		3 servings (½ cup)
Fruit		3 servings (½ cup)
Butter or margarine		1½ T (5 t)
Other fats		2 or more servings
Sugar		3 packets or more
Jelly		1 packet
Vegetable	Buttered asparagus	1 serving (½ cup)
Bread or roll		1 serving (1 slice or 1 roll)
Butter or margarine		3 servings (3 t)
Fruit or dessert	Chocolate brownie	1 serving (1 square)
Milk		1 serving (1 cup)
Coffee or tea		
Sugar		1 serving (1 packet)

Sample Meal Plan

BREAKFAST		
Fruit	Orange Juice	1 serving (½ cup)
Cereal	Cream of rice	1 serving (½ cup cooked, ¾ cup dry)
Milk		1 serving (1 cup)
Egg	Scrambled egg	1
Bread	Toast	1 serving (1 slice)
Butter or margarine		2 servings (2 T)
Coffee or tea		
Sugar		1–2 servings (1–2 packets)
Jelly		1 serving (1 T)
LUNCH		
Egg, cheese, poultry, meat, fish	Leg of lamb	1 serving (3 oz. cooked)
Bread substitute	Buttered linguine	1 serving (½ cup)
DINNER		
Meat, fish, poultry	Roast beef au jus	1 serving (3 oz.)
Bread substitute	Rice	1 serving (½ cup)
Gravy		1 serving
Vegetable	Green beans	1 or more servings (½ cup each)
Salad with dressing	Relish plate	1 serving (½ cup)
Bread or roll		1 serving (1 slice or 1 roll)
Butter or margarine		2 servings (2 t)
Fruit or dessert	Chilled apricot halves	1 serving (½ cup)
Coffee or tea		
Sugar		1 serving (1 packet)
Nourishments (1 or more)		
Juice	Orange juice	½ cup per serving

fort than the stiff "garden hoses" of the past. Once inserted, position of the tube must be checked to ensure proper placement. If a patient cannot tolerate a tube inserted through the nose, or when the esophagus is blocked, the tube may be placed directly into the stomach; this is called gastrostomy. (Patients who cannot be fed through the stomach may have a tube inserted into the small intestine.) While such a procedure requires surgery, it may prove more convenient to the long-term enteral patient. Placement of a tube directly into the stomach

may also be done for disoriented patients who might try to pull a nasogastric tube out. (Recent developments enable the tube to be inserted endoscopically through the mouth or nose rather than surgically through an incision.)

The psychological impact of tube feeding can be a difficult situation with which to deal. (See Avoiding Complications of Tube Feeding on page 383.) The loss of the sensory and cultural pleasures of eating and self-consciousness due to the presence of feeding equipment can trigger feelings of isolation and

Figure 23.1. Types of Nutritional Support

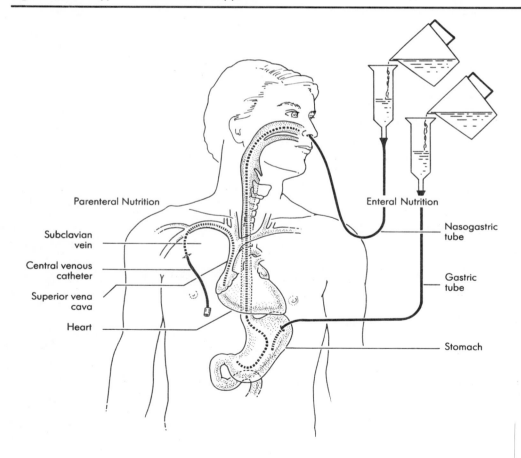

depression. Patients who will need tube feeding on a long-term basis may want to seek counseling to help them through the initial adaptation period. Focusing on the benefit to health rather than the equipment is important. If the nursing staff's schedule and feeding pattern permit, the procedure may be done in the evening or during the night to allow freedom of movement during the day. Some patients may be able to take nutrients orally along with the tube feeding.

Many patients requiring long-term enteral nutrition must learn to manage feedings in the home once they have been discharged from the hospital. (See Tips for Tube Feeding at Home on page 388.)

Parenteral Nutrition

Parenteral nutrition refers to the intravenous administration of fluid, amino acids, carbohydrates, fats, vitamins, and minerals. Nutrients are delivered by a catheter directly into the bloodstream. When this type of feeding is a patient's sole source of nutrients, it is called total parenteral nutrition (TPN).

TPN is called for when enteral feeding cannot meet the patient's nutritional needs. It is often used in response to a malfunction of the intestine (obstruction, severe absorption problems). Other indications are to rest the gastrointestinal tract following surgery, or more permanently if large sections of the intestine have been removed.

As with tube feeding, long-term parenteral patients must adjust to the loss of the sensory pleasures associated with eating, a change in body image caused by the presence of the catheter, and, at times, depression. However, this is often more than compensated for by restored health after surgery to remove diseased intestine, the comfort of returning home following a long hospitaliza-

Avoiding Complications of Tube Feeding

Careful monitoring by members of the nutrition support team can avert the potential complications listed below. It is also the responsibility of the patient and family to help out by reporting early signs of difficulty to staff members, as well as by familiarizing themselves with the procedure if tube feeding is to be continued at home after discharge.

Diarrhea. Bacterial contamination of the formula solution that is either too concentrated or being infused too rapidly can cause diarrhea, which, if severe enough, can lead to dehydration. Opened cans of formula should be refrigerated and marked as to date opened.

Dry Mouth. Patients with nasogastric tubes usually find it easier to breathe through the mouth and may experience dryness as a result. Ask the nurse for lemon/glycerine swabs to moisten lips and mucous membranes and ice chips to suck on if allowed by the physician.

Aspiration. Improper positioning of a nasogastric tube or lying down too soon after the feeding can result in the liquid being regurgitated and inhaled into the lungs. The patient should remain in a sitting position for at least a half hour after a feeding. If unable to sit without assistance, the head of the bed should be raised for the same length of time.

Infection. The incision site for a tube inserted into the stomach or intestine may be exposed to small amounts of stomach acid, which can irritate the skin, leading to infection. The area should be cleansed daily and the patient should report any redness, tenderness, warmth, or swelling to the nurse or physician.

tion, and the freedom to resume normal activities.

Once they are medically stable, candidates for parenteral nutrition to be continued at home, known as HPN, are evaluated by the nutrition support team for their ability to follow the instructions for catheter care, use of the pump, and infusion procedure. Medicare and some insurance companies may cover the cost if TPN is medically indicated.

It should be stressed that patients can and do successfully adapt to long-term TPN. Often, feeding schedules are arranged to coincide with patients' lifestyles; many patients can eat in addition to TPN. The use of TPN facilitates recovery from surgery in patients who would otherwise suffer from the severe consequences of malnutrition.

NUTRITION AND SURGERY

Patients with surgical problems are particularly at risk for developing nutritional problems. Statistics show that well-nourished patients sustain lower mortality rates and fewer postoperative complications than do malnourished patients. Ideally, nutritional defects should be corrected before any operations. However, this option may not be available in acute surgical conditions. Patients' responses to surgery are affected by their preoperative status, the extent of surgical injury, and their ability to maintain their metabolic demands after the operation.

Preoperative Nutrition

For those who are well nourished prior to surgery, there is little need for preoperative support. These patients usually continue with the same type of diet that followed before entering the hospital, whether on a regular or a modified diet. Many surgical patients, however, are poorly nourished. Chronic disease, pain, loss of appetite, nausea, and vomiting may have contributed to reduced nutrient intake or increased losses.

When surgery is on a scheduled (elective) rather than emergency basis, a supplemented diet helps to correct deficiencies and bring the patient to surgery in an improved state. The diet should provide a balance of all essential nutrients, with special emphasis on protein, calories, vitamins, and minerals.

Being overweight does not necessarily imply adequate nutrient stores. Amount of body fat has no relation to available reserves of protein and other vital nutrients. Obese but malnourished patients should not be put on weight-reduction diets immediately before or after surgery.

Immediate Preoperative Period

Patients are not given any solid foods or liquids for at least eight hours prior to surgery in order to prevent vomiting or aspiration during anesthesia or in the immediate postoperative period. Although this requirement is usually designated by a sign, NPO (Latin for *nothing by mouth*), by the bed, this may be omitted inadvertently. Therefore, patients who will be having surgery within hours and are presented with a breakfast tray should check with the physician or nurse before eating or drinking.

Postoperative Nutrition

The goal of postoperative nutrition is twofold: first, and most immediate, to maintain the body's balance of fluids and electrolytes or restore those lost during surgery;

second, to help the patient resume consumption of solid foods.

Well-nourished patients who undergo a relatively minor surgical procedure usually require only routine intravenous fluids (mainly water with electrolytes and dextrose, or sugar, rather than the complete TPN solutions) for hydration in the immediate postoperative period. A return to normal feeding is begun as soon as gastrointestinal function returns. The function of the small intestine returns rapidly, whereas it may take 24 hours or longer for the stomach to regain its normal muscular function (motility). The colon may require three or four days to regain its motility. Resumption of oral intake depends on the extent and type of surgery, as well as the individual patient's progress. After minor surgery, the patient can usually tolerate liquids within a few hours. However, oral feeding may be delayed for two to three days with more major surgery.

When to reintroduce solid food depends on the body's response to surgery and the patient's overall nutritional health. Generally, a physician will look for two signs of readiness for solid food: (1) gastrointestinal secretions are being produced, and (2) normal bowel activity has resumed. To check for these, a stethoscope is placed on the patient's abdomen to detect the gurgling sounds that signal the resumption of intestinal muscular movements known as peristalsis.

Typically, clear liquids are initiated as soon as normal bowel activity has returned. (To avoid swallowing excess air, which can cause gas pains, drinking through a straw and drinking carbonated beverages should be avoided. Eating slowly and in small amounts can also reduce the amount of air that the patient swallows.) The patient is then progressed to full liquids according to his or her tolerance, then to a soft diet, and then to his or her normal diet prescription. Although the sched-

ule varies with the individual, it is not unusual to be back on a regular diet by the second or third postoperative day.

Special care is taken to see that adequate amounts of important vitamins are supplied. For example, B-complex vitamins aid in the metabolism of protein, carbohydrate, and fat; vitamin C helps promote the healing of wounds; and vitamin K fosters proper blood clotting. A regular diet provides these.

Special Nutrition Considerations for Surgical Procedures

Head and Neck Surgery

Surgery for cancer of the oral cavity or to repair a broken jaw or major dental work can make chewing or swallowing difficult to manage. The patient may be unable to eat solid foods for a period of weeks and the diet followed during hospitalization will have to be maintained when the patient returns home.

The patient and/or caregiver will be given guidelines by the physician or nutritionist as to the foods allowed and in what consistency they should be served (i.e., finely chopped or completely blenderized). Nevertheless, many find they go through a trial-and-error process at home in the course of adjusting to new ways of preparing food.

Whether the patient is being fed through a tube or can take small amounts of food by mouth, he or she should be generally served the same foods as the rest of the family. A person recuperating from oral surgery is likely to have an impaired appetite to begin with, and serving special foods or relying solely on liquid supplements only reinforces the feeling of being sick and can diminish appetite. (For more information on maintaining a soft diet after hospitalization, see Tips on Preparing Soft or Blenderized Meals at Home, page 389.)

Gastrectomy

In this procedure, part or all of the stomach is surgically removed as a treatment for gastric cancer, following trauma to the organ or complications of severe peptic ulcers, or perforation, among other reasons. A number of nutritional problems may develop following gastric surgery, such as severe weight loss and nutrient deficiencies, especially anemia.

Of particular concern after a gastrectomy is the dumping syndrome, in which the patient becomes pale and weak following a meal, particularly one high in simple carbohydrates. Perspiration, rapid heartbeat or palpitations, and diarrhea may also occur. This problem occurs because removal of all or part of the stomach leaves the body unable to process food at a controlled rate. The high particle concentration of the food dumped directly into the intestine without stomach processing attracts fluid, distends the intestine, and causes diarrhea.

Although the dumping syndrome can subside, persistent symptoms require a modified diet high in protein and fat—which are broken down less rapidly in the intestine— and low in simple carbohydrates (sugar, candy) and hard-to-digest fiber. The patient should eat only a small volume of food for several days in order to assess tolerance. Meals should be divided into five or six small feedings (low in carbohydrates, high in proteins and fats). Many patients progress more rapidly if they do not take liquids with meals. The diet should be modified according to individual tolerance. For example, a modified diet may not be required by patients who have had a proximal gastric vagotomy, a surgical procedure in which the vagus nerve, which serves the stomach and other abdominal organs, is severed to reduce production of digestive acids, thus increasing the amount of time food that remains in the stomach.

Intestinal Surgery/Ileostomy

This surgery is used to treat ulcerative colitis, Crohn's disease, or other conditions affecting the intestinal tract that do not respond to medication. (See also Chapter 30.) An opening, which may be permanent or temporary, is made in the abdominal wall for the removal of waste. Newer surgical alternatives include ileo-anal pull-throughs and Koch pouches. Not every patient is a candidate for these alternative procedures, so this should be discussed with your surgeon.

The postoperative diet generally proceeds from clear liquids to low-fiber solids, to prevent irritation and promote healing of the stoma. Most ileostomy patients resume a normal eating regimen within two to three weeks, but in the interim there is usually a period of adjusting the diet to counteract various complications, including the following.

Diarrhea. Excessively watery stools often occur because the colon is not present to reabsorb liquids. Foods to avoid include prune juice, alcohol, baked beans, broccoli and leafy vegetables, highly spiced foods, and raw fruit. However, a food that causes diarrhea in one patient may not in another, and trial and error is often required to determine individual responses.

Gas. Avoiding foods commonly associated with gas reduces odor and gas pain. Offending substances include dried beans and peas, cabbage, and beer and carbonated beverages. (See list on page 532 in Chapter 30.) Individuals should also chew meals slowly.

Fluid/sodium and potassium loss. Patients should increase their intake of fluid and sodium (the capacity to reabsorb both is lost with removal of the colon) to avoid dehydration. Vitamin B_{12} absorption may be diminished and the patient should check with the physician and nutritionist about vitamin supplements.

Colostomy

Less extensive than an ileostomy, here only the rectum, anus, and part of the colon are removed, and a pathway for wastes is made from the remaining part of the colon. The consistency of fecal material depends on what portion of the colon is removed; as food residue passes toward the rectum, water is increasingly absorbed, producing a more solid stool. While a colostomy usually allows a patient to resume normal eating sooner than an ileostomy, some of the same problems with gas and odor can occur. In addition, patients can suffer from constipation, which can be alleviated by increasing intake of fluids, as well as a moderate amount of fiber in cooked fruits and vegetables, seeds, and cereals.

In general, surgery of the small or large intestine results in an impairment of nutrient absorption that lasts until the remaining portion of the gastrointestinal tract adapts. Once this occurs, a patient can usually progress to a nutritionally adequate diet of solid foods.

Colorectal surgery inevitably requires coping with a changed body image, becoming involved in the normally taken-for-granted function of excretion, and adjusting to other reactions to the surgery. Many hospitals now have ostomy nurses who assist with both physical and psychological rehabilitation, and most ostomy patients can resume fairly normal lives with a minimum of restrictions; achieving a proper, well-balanced diet is an important first step.

There are several support groups patients can contact if additional help is needed after hospital discharge. The National Foundation for Ileitis & Colitis, 444 Park Avenue South, New York, NY 10016, 212–685–3440, supports research on inflammatory bowel disease and publishes educational pamphlets. The United Ostomy Association (phone: 213–413–5510) publishes *The Ostomy Quarterly* ($25 per year), which provides practical advice on living with an ileostomy or colostomy, including a regular column called "Foods for Fitness."

SUMMING UP

The impact of nutritional status on a patient's response to medical and surgical therapies is a burgeoning field of knowledge that has already resulted in improved hospital care. Even as physicians and nutritionists learn more and more about new ways to apply the benefits of nutrition to hospitalized patients, so must the patients endeavor to play a more active role in their own nutritional support, both in the hospital and at home.

THE SPECIAL CONCERNS OF HOSPITALIZED CHILDREN*

All of the risks that hospitalized adults face due to malnutrition are greatly magnified in children. Infants and children must take in sufficient nutrients to meet growth needs even when ill. Simply being stable, while acceptable for adults, is never acceptable for the pediatric patient. Depending upon their ages, varying growth rates are essential. Moreover, most children by nature have little concern for or knowledge of proper nutrition. When sick

*This section written by Neal S. LeLeiko, M.D., Ph.D.

and hospitalized, they are even less likely to show much interest in food. For these reasons, physicians, dietitians, and parents must pay special attention to a hospitalized child's nutritional needs.

Risk Factors

Even a well-nourished child who requires hospitalization is at risk for becoming malnourished. Severe complications of malnutrition such as the failure of the immune system to function properly and the inability to heal occur only in extreme cases. Among the factors that contribute to malnutrition problems are the priorities of hospital care: During mealtimes, patients are often absent from the ward for diagnostic or therapeutic procedures; they may be unable to take food by mouth; the medications they have to take may dull the appetite.

Proper nutritional care is especially important for premature babies and for children with any of the following conditions:

- chronic kidney or liver disease
- gastrointestinal disease
- growth failure associated with chronic heart or lung disease
- major trauma, such as severe burns
- cancer, which can be especially critical because malnutrition can often be induced by the treatment (chemotherapy, radiation) as well as by the disease.

In addition, as with adults, children who undergo major surgery have greatly increased nutritional needs that must be addressed in the effort to promote recovery.

Early Intervention

Any child facing long-term hospitalization should receive nutritional consideration soon after admission. Early on, the physician and nutritional support staff should develop a

---

Tips for Tube Feeding at Home

Patients who are otherwise medically stable but require long-term tube feeding may be sent home with complete instructions for self-care. Returning to familiar surroundings and being able to independently care for oneself can provide a psychological lift. In addition to information given by the physician or other members of the nutrition support team, the following tips will prove helpful in dealing with some common complaints of tube feeding.

- Chew sugarless gum or rinse the mouth frequently to prevent excessive thirst.
- To relieve throat irritation from a nasogastric tube, try gargling with a mixture of warm water and mouthwash. If runny nose is a problem, gently blow the nose. Keep the tube clean by frequent rinsing with water and lubricate it with a water-soluble or other physician-approved lubricant.
- Sit down both during and after a feeding to help ease feelings of fullness.

- Gastrostomy patients may experience irritation around the incision site. The physician or nurse may be able to recommend a skincare product to relieve this.
- Contact the Oley Foundation, a research and education group dealing with home parenteral and enteral nutrition. Write or call them at 214 Hun Memorial, Albany Medical Center, Albany, NY 12208 (518–445–5079).

strategy that anticipates the drawbacks of a long hospital stay as well as the effects of the disease itself.

Prior planning can help prevent the need for some of the more drastic forms of nutritional care, including special enteral-tube and parenteral feeding. Moreover, the continuing participation of a dietitian or physician nutritionist in a child's care throughout his or her hospital stay will assure that nutrition therapy properly responds to the ongoing impact of the disease, tests, and treatments.

Assessment of the Growing Child

Aside from routine questions regarding general medical history taken on admission to the hospital, the assessment of children differs in significant ways from that of adults, just as their needs differ.

The following discussion addresses some of the specific differences.

Nutritional history. Parents or, if old enough, children themselves will be asked to provide details about dietary habits to help the physician determine possible problem areas. For infants, the following information will be solicited: type of feeding, quantity of formula/breast milk per day, vitamin/mineral supplementation, intake of solids, food allergies, unusual feeding behavior, foods avoided or not tolerated.

For older children, along with the relevant items mentioned above, the physician

---

Tips for Preparing Soft or Blenderized Meals at Home

Food processors, blenders, and meat grinders simplify the preparation of soft and liquid meals and help provide the patient with a balanced diet.

- Remove gristle and tough skins from meat and vegetables before blending or grinding. Blend meat first, then add liquids, gravies, sauces, or creams for texture.

- Choose softer baked or boiled meats and fish rather than fried. Likewise, opt for rare rather than medium or well-done meats in order to preserve softness and moisture.

- For breakfasts, pour hot milk or fruit juice over dry cereal and let soak for an hour or two.

- Create blenderized casseroles by combining boneless meat, fish, vegetables, and/or pasta. Add sour cream or mayonnaise for a more liquid texture.

- Note that large volumes of blenderized food may prove unappetizing. Serve smaller portions at more frequent intervals. Keep the components of a meal separate from each other, either in different bowls or dishes that contain separate compartments for each food.

- Promptly refrigerate leftovers; do not reuse uneaten food that has been left uncovered in a warm room.

- To boost the caloric or nutrient values of the foods, add one to three tablespoons of any of the following: grated or creamed cheese, yogurt, pureed meat, fish, vegetables or fruit, powdered milk, margarine, butter, fruit juices, or softened bread.

- Provide sufficient liquids to help a patient chew and swallow. These can include water, coffee, fruit juice, or milk.

- Garnish individual portions with paprika, mint, or parsley for color.

- Supply plenty of napkins, paper towels, or facial tissues to help the patient stay clean.

- Be sure the patient has plenty of time to eat. People with impaired oral function take longer to get through a meal.

may want to know about any special diets, the number of meals and snacks per day, the frequency of intake of foods found in the four main food groups, as well as sweets and other snack foods, and any behavioral problems experienced at mealtimes.

At Mount Sinai Hospital, a detailed seven-day record of food consumption, compiled prior to the child's admission to the hos-

pital, has been found to be especially useful in determining the actual quantity and quality of the child's intake. This dietary analysis enables the physician to compare actual intake of carbohydrates, proteins, fats, calories, fluids, and vitamins/minerals with accepted nutritional standards, and thus to determine possible excesses and deficiencies.

Figure 23.2. Girls: 2 to 18 Years Physical Growth NCHS Percentiles*

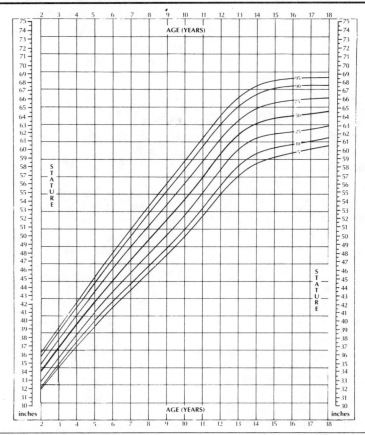

*Adapted from: Hamill, P. V. V., Drizd, T. A., Johnson, C. L., Reed, R. B., Roche, A. F., Moore, W. M.: Physical growth: National Center for Health Statistics percentiles, *American Journal of Clinical Nutrition* 32:607-629, 1979. Data from the Fels Research Institute, Wright State University School of Medicine, Yellow Springs, Ohio. Used with permission of Ross Laboratories, Columbus, OH 43216, © 1982 Ross Laboratories.

Physical examination. In addition to assessment of organ systems, measurement of growth (anthropometry) provides a physician with vital information that is used to determine the nutritional status of the patient.

A physician will routinely measure a child's weight, height, and head circumference. Additional evaluations may be made of fat reserves by measuring skin-fold thickness of the triceps, and of muscle mass by measuring the circumference of the mid-upper arm. This data is then plotted on standardized graphs in order to compare the child's actual state of growth with established norms. (See figures 23.2 and 23.3.) If a child's actual measurements deviate substantially from the established norm for his or her weight for height, that child may be suffering from a serious medical problem. For example, if a child whose height and weight has been consistently in the 75th percentile drops to the 25th percentile, it may indicate a medical problem.

The single best indicator of a child's long-term nutrition status is rate of growth. This rate, especially during expected periods of development in adolescence, is particularly sensitive to the quality of nutrition intake. A child's growth should be checked at six-month to 12-month intervals.

It should be noted that a normal growth

Figure 23.2.   Girls: 2 to 18 Years Physical Growth NCHS Percentiles* *(cont.)*

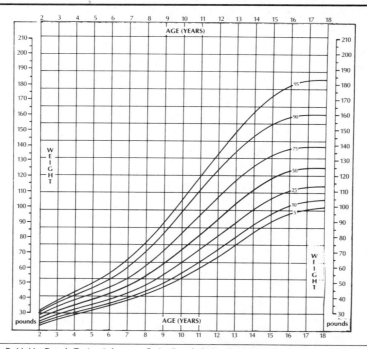

*Adapted from: Hamill, P. V. V., Drizd, T. A., Johnson, C. L., Reed, R. B., Roche, A. F., Moore, W. M.: Physical growth: National Center for Health Statistics percentiles, *American Journal of Clinical Nutrition* 32:607-629, 1979. Data from the Fels Research Institute, Wright State University School of Medicine, Yellow Springs, Ohio. Used with permission of Ross Laboratories, Columbus, OH 43216, © 1982 Ross Laboratories.

rate is not necessarily synonymous with good health or proper nutrition; however, a deviation from normal is more likely than not to reflect poor nutrition or disease.

Biochemical evaluation. Measurements of total body water, nitrogen, fat, glycogen, and the various minerals help determine whether the body's metabolism has been disturbed by nutritional depletion. Such tests, performed by chemical analyses of body fluids, are called for at the physician's discretion. Total body water may be determined in any of several ways, as discussed in Chapter 17.

Nutritional Support of the Child

If a child is well nourished at the outset of his or her hospital stay, the goal of nutri-

Figure 23.3.   Boys: 2 to 18 Years Physical Growth NCHS Percentiles*

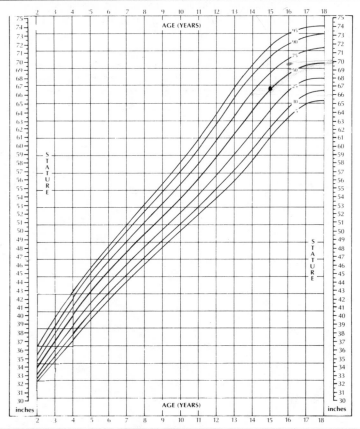

*Adapted from: Hamill, P. V. V., Drizd, T. A., Johnson, C. L., Reed, R. B., Roche, A. F., Moore, W. M.: Physical growth: National Center for Health Statistics percentiles, *American Journal of Clinical Nutrition* 32:607-629, 1979. Data from the National Center for Health Statistics (NCHS), Hyattsville, Maryland. Used with permission of Ross Laboratories, Columbus, OH 43216, © 1982 Ross Laboratories.

tion support is to m   panionship and helping a
nutrient stores are   y with being in the hospi-
pleted, the patient's st   must act as a go-between
parenteral feeding fo   ncooperative child follows
particularly when chro   tions, or to speak up if the
present.   'hat the dietitian ordered.

Inadequate intake   ting well, parents may be
a common problem fou   the child's favorite foods
children. Proper nutriti   so-called junk foods,
clude monitoring of a   rcumstances should be
The nursing staff shoul   important calories in a
meals served during a ch   to the patient. When a
ward are not returned to   lequate, the physician
should play a watchdog   supplements to the diet.

In any case, parents   Many liquid defined-formula diets, which can
partners in nutrition support, as well as offer- be taken by mouth or tube, are available ei-

Figure 23.3.   Boys: 2 to 18 Years Physical Growth NCHS Percentiles* *(cont.)*

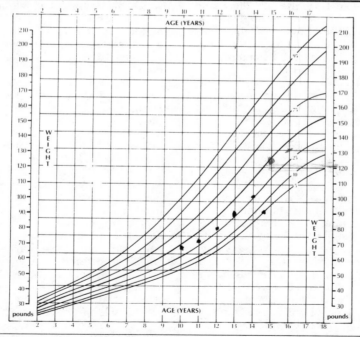

*Adapted from: Hamill, P. V. V., Drizd, T. A., Johnson, C. L., Reed, R. B., Roche, A. F., Moore, W. M.: Physical growth: National Center for Health Statistics percentiles, *American Journal of Clinical Nutrition* 32:607-629, 1979. Data from the National Center for Health Statistics (NCHS), Hyattsville, Maryland. Used with permission of Ross Laboratories, Columbus, OH 43216, © 1982 Ross Laboratories.

ther to complement solid food or to serve as the total diet.

Defined-formula supplements come in a wide variety and can be tailored to meet nearly all requirements. Nevertheless, a physician will want to monitor closely the child placed on a special diet regimen so that he or she can check for possible complications, including overhydration, hyperglycemia (excess blood sugar), and diarrhea.

Whenever possible, a child's nutritional needs should be met by oral intake. The child should be fed by tube directly into the gastrointestinal tract only if he or she is unable to take adequate nourishment by mouth, and parenteral feeding should be used only when the child's gastrointestinal tract cannot process food. In addition to its high cost, parenteral feeding carries an increased risk of complications. Moreover, feeding by mouth or enteral tube permits easier delivery of a more nutritionally complete diet.

Special Needs of AIDS Patients*

AIDS, or autoimmune deficiency syndrome, is a disease characterized by severe weight loss and wasting. In fact, AIDS patients die from starvation more often than from the HIV virus (the organism that causes the disease) itself. This is partly because the AIDS virus attacks the stomach and damages its ability to release enzymes and acids needed to digest food. Even more important, the immune-system deficiency that is a hallmark of AIDS enables a variety of tiny parasitic organisms to grow in the small intestine, producing gradually progressive diarrhea and the inability to absorb the nutrients in food. This results in starvation, even though the AIDS patient may be eating an adequate diet.

The best advice for anyone who is diagnosed as infected with the HIV virus is to consume a nutritious diet as high in calories as possible, even if symptoms of AIDS have not yet developed. A patient facing AIDS should not be concerned about getting fat; as the disease progresses, the extra pounds will be needed.

In recent years, many AIDS patients have fallen victim to nutrition quackery. Aside from consuming a high-calorie diet, there is no dietary treatment for this dread disease. Indeed, some of high-dose vitamin supplements actually hasten the progression of AIDS. For example, some nutrition charlatans advocate high doses of vitamin C for AIDS patients, claiming that this will bolster their faltering immune systems.

In reality, the high-dose vitamin C actually accelerates the progress of AIDS because it promotes diarrhea. There have been instances in which high-dose vitamin C has led to severe, life-threatening diarrhea and electrolyte imbalances among AIDS patients. Similarly, the semistarvation regimens advocated for AIDS patients by some nutrition quacks hasten rather than forestall death.

Feeding via hyperalimentation, either intravenously or via a gastric feeding tube, should begin as soon as there is any evidence of diarrhea or weight loss. Studies in New York and San Francisco indicate that hyperalimentation may be beneficial even earlier, since even before there is obvious weight loss or diarrhea, there is reduced absorption of nutrients, as demonstrated by lower blood levels of carotene, a negative vitamin B_{12} balance, and other abnormalities.

The importance of maintaining body weight and good nutritional status in the treatment of AIDS has been demonstrated in studies by Dr. Donald Kotler and his associates at New York's St. Luke's–Roosevelt Hospital Medical Center. These researchers have found that death occurs when an AIDS patient falls to about 56 percent of desirable body weight. This is the same as was observed two decades ago in starvation in Africa—namely, that people die when they fall to about 56 percent of desirable weight.

*This section written by Victor Herbert, M.D., F.A.C.P.

A major factor in the success of tube feeding is the manner in which children's resistance to it is handled. The natural reaction is to resist having the tube inserted, and once it is in, to try to remove it. For a physician or parent, gaining the child's confidence and explaining why a tube is necessary can go a long way toward acceptance. Using the tube as a threat or punishment frequently leads to even more resistance.

For the child who repeatedly pulls the tube out, prompt reinsertion in a matter-of-fact manner generally stops the practice. Most children soon realize that removal of the tube means they must undergo reinsertion.

In general, the complexity of nutritional therapy increases with the complexity of the illness. The ultimate watchword is *prevention*. It is much easier to prevent malnutrition than to correct it.

24

The Nutritional Needs of Athletes

David T. Lowenthal, M.D., Ph.D., and Yair Karni, B.Sc.

■

INTRODUCTION

Many athletes firmly "believe" in special diets, or megadoses of vitamins or minerals, or ergogenic (work-enhancing) dietary additives. Since people who take part in sports put greater demands on their bodies than sedentary people do, they assume that they need something extra to boost performance. If additives can be put in gasoline to improve efficiency, they ask, why not in food? In fact, however, once the basic nutrient needs have been met by a well-balanced diet, the only special requirement for most athletes is a greater intake of calories to meet the body's increased energy needs.

Although it is not possible to change average athletes into Olympic champions simply by changing their diet, the importance of nutrition should not be underestimated. Poor eating habits erode one's endurance, reduce energy levels, and result in a subpar performance. Special diets are usually rip-offs.

FOODS FOR ENERGY: CARBOHYDRATES AND FATS

The body is an engine, in that it converts food to fuel in the form of chemical energy that, in turn, can be converted into the mechanical energy of muscular movement. However, the body differs from a combustion engine in at least one important way: It does not derive instant energy directly from the fuel it consumes. Instead, it uses energy already stored in its tissues. An athlete cannot hope to convert a particular food into instant energy. It must be broken down and processed first.

The approximately 600 groups of muscles in the human body make up about 40 percent of its weight. Every muscle is composed of hundreds of thousands of tiny fibers, each of which is able to shorten or lengthen, causing the muscle to contract or relax.

The energy required for this muscular action comes primarily from the burning of fatty acids (the product of fat breakdown) and glucose, a simple sugar which is the end product of digestion of all carbohydrates (sugars and starches). Fatty acids are found in small quantities in the muscles and are stored in much larger quantities in the body's fat cells. Glucose is stored in liver and muscle cells as glycogen (a series of glucose molecules linked end to end). Liver glycogen stores are reconverted to glucose as needed to keep blood-sugar levels normal, while muscle glycogen serves as a reserve source of energy for the specific muscles in which it is stored.

Whether fatty acids, glucose, or a mixture of the two will be used as fuel for muscular activity depends on the individual athlete's capacity for taking in and using oxygen, on the individual's previous diet, and on the duration and intensity of the exercise. Glucose can be burned as fuel with oxygen (aerobically) or without oxygen (anaerobically); fatty acids, however, always need oxygen. Thus, in short (two to three minutes), all-out exercise such as sprinting, where muscles work faster than the heart and lungs can supply them with oxygen, stored muscle glycogen and blood-borne glucose are the prime contributors of energy.

Anaerobic exercise can continue for only short periods of time, as this method of energy production results in the formation of a by-product, lactic acid. As exercise continues, this lactic acid accumulates, changing the acid balance in the muscle and interfering with normal muscle contraction. When strenuous activity stops, the body is able to provide adequate oxygen to the tissues to break down the accumulated lactic acid and then muscle function returns to normal.

During less intense but sustained exercise such as long-distance running, the circulatory system is better able to keep pace with oxygen demands and both glycogen stores and fat stores help fuel the body. Initially, glycogen provides about 40 to 50 percent of the energy requirement, but even trained athletes store only enough glycogen for about two hours of nonstop exercise. So as exercise continues, an increasingly greater percentage of energy is supplied by the body's abundant fat stores, sparing the limited glycogen reserves. Fatty acids may provide as much as 80 percent of the energy needs of endurance athletes.

The potential energy from stored fat is almost unlimited (one pound of fat has enough energy to fuel 30 to 40 miles of running), but muscles can't function effectively on fat alone; they need a simultaneous supply of glucose. As glycogen stores become depleted, glucose levels in blood and muscle fall, efficiency and performance deteriorate quickly, and exhaustion occurs. Marathon runners commonly refer to this sensation of fatigue as "hitting the wall."

THE ATHLETE'S DIET

Both training and proper diet are important to optimize athletic performance. A well-balanced diet stocks the body with the needed fuel sources, ensuring plentiful glycogen stores and adequate calories, as well as supplies the vitamins and minerals that play indirect, supporting roles in the use of energy. Training, on the other hand, helps improve the body's utilization of that fuel. A more fit individual has an increased ability to store glycogen, and can use fat as a fuel source during exercise.

A well-balanced diet for the athlete is based on the same principles of variety, moderation, and balance that ensure adequate nutrition for less active individuals. No one food or beverage contains all the nutrients in the amounts necessary to promote health. The diet should be based on the Basic Four food groups and should contain a minimum of two servings from the meat group, two servings from the dairy group (four servings for adolescents), and four servings each from the fruit/vegetable group and from the bread/cereals group. Such a plan can serve as the basic diet regardless of whether the goal is weight loss, weight gain, or weight maintenance. Since this basic diet provides only about 1,200 calories, extra servings can be chosen from the Basic Four and selections can be made from the calorie-dense "others" category (sweets, fats, and moderate amounts of alcohol) based on individual food preferences and caloric needs. (For more information on the basic diet, see Chapter 1.)

Carbohydrates

Carbohydrates are the body's most important source of fuel. An athlete's initial levels of carbohydrate stores (muscle and liver glycogen) are directly related to his or her ability to sustain prolonged vigorous exercise. The average person stores 1,500 to 2,000 calories of energy as blood glucose and glycogen, but this level can be modified considerably through the diet. For example, fasting for as few as 24 hours or eating a low-carbohydrate diet results in a large reduction in glycogen reserves. On the other hand, maintaining a carbohydrate-rich diet for several days enhances the body's carbohydrate stores to a level almost twice that obtained with a normal, well-balanced diet.

The average American diet contains about 46 percent of total calories as carbohydrates. Athletes and other active people need more to ensure ample glycogen reserves, however. Most experts recommend that 55 to 60 percent of the daily caloric intake should be in the form of carbohydrates. Athletes training exhaustively on a daily basis or competing on successive days should try for an even higher percentage: 65 to 70.

There are two types of carbohydrates, simple and complex. Simple carbohydrates are sugars, such as glucose, fructose (fruit sugar), lactose (milk sugar), and sucrose (table sugar). Foods such as fruits, honey, and juices are composed largely of naturally occurring sugars. Foods such as syrup, jams, and candies contain mostly refined sugars. Complex carbohydrates, also called starches, contain long chains of many glucose units linked together. Examples of complex carbohydrates include vegetables, cereals, breads, grains, beans, potatoes, and pasta. The bulk of an athlete's carbohydrate allowance—80 to 85 percent—should come from starches, and the balance from sugars.

Fats

Fat is the body's most concentrated source of energy, providing nine calories per gram, compared with four per gram for carbohydrates and protein. Pound for pound, body fat contains more than twice as much stored energy as muscle glycogen. This fat provides most of the energy required for bodily functions at rest as well as during prolonged moderate exercise. However, while some fat is essential, both in the diet and as an energy source, there is no rationale for a high-fat diet. Even a very lean (8 percent body fat) 150-pound athlete stores approximately 42,000 calories in his body fat deposits—enough to power a run from San Francisco to Los Angeles. Any surplus carbohydrates and proteins in the diet are readily converted into body fat, so fat stores are easily maintained without relying on a high fat intake.

Fat also takes longer to digest and to metabolize than carbohydrates, making fat a less efficient source of quick energy, particularly for the casual athlete. Endurance training increases the muscle's ability to use fat as a fuel.

If a high-fat diet is not optimal, however, how much fat is? There is still no clear-cut answer to this question. In the typical American diet, fat provides approximately 37 percent of the calories. A diet containing this much fat is almost always too low in carbohydrates to ensure optimal glycogen stores, however. Diets high in fats, particularly saturated fats, are also associated with an increased intake of cholesterol and a risk of coronary heart disease. As a general recommendation, a fat intake of about 20 to 25 percent of total calories would be prudent and would allow for adequate intakes of protein and carbohydrate.

Protein

The most important role of protein is to build, maintain, and repair tissue, and to produce hormones and enzymes. Muscles also can utilize protein for energy. Like carbohydrate, protein yields four calories per gram; however, the body must make a greater effort to transform protein into a fuel, making it a less efficient energy source. Proteins are made up of chains of subunits called amino acids. The breakdown of amino acids usually contributes between 5 and 15 percent of the body's total energy requirement. During sustained exercise, protein has the potential to provide the working muscle with even more energy, especially when glycogen stores are depleted or very low. The use of protein for energy produces a by-product (urea) that must be eliminated from the body through the urine. This requires water, and when an athlete is metabolizing excessive amounts of protein, it can increase the risk of dehydration.

The RDA for protein is .36 grams per pound of body weight for all adults. That's about 50 grams for an average woman, and 63 grams for an average man. Yet athletes and individuals involved in training programs often eat four to five times the amount they need in the hope that extra protein will enhance their athletic abilities or build bigger muscles. It will not.

Accumulating evidence suggests that some individuals—endurance athletes such as long-distance runners and strength/power athletes such as weight lifters—may need more protein than more sedentary individuals. They often obtain this increase through a general rise in total caloric intake. Estimates of protein requirements for athletes range from .45 grams to .73 grams per pound of body weight. This additional protein does not mean that athletes should eat high-protein diets or take protein supplements, however. Government surveys indicate that most Americans already eat one and a half times the RDA for protein. Active individuals, because of their higher energy needs, generally consume even more, meeting their higher protein needs automatically.

Intakes above requirement cannot be stored for future use. Excess protein is broken down by the liver and is either burned for energy or stored as body fat, not muscle. High-protein diets are usually also high in fat and, thus, often deprive the athlete of the most efficient fuel, carbohydrates.

However, while excessive protein intakes can hinder performance, neither should the protein content of the diet be neglected, as it is by some overly carbohydrate-conscious athletes. Individuals who are keeping caloric intakes low in order to lose weight or maintain a low body weight sometimes load up on carbohydrates while eliminating high-protein foods because they also contain calorie-dense fat. A diet providing 12 to 15 percent of calories from protein is generally adequate for all active individuals when a minimum of 1,200 calories is consumed by women and 1,500 calories by men.

Vitamins

Vitamins, themselves, do not provide energy; however, they are essential for the various energy transformations that occur in the body. Without an adequate supply of vitamins, many of the body's vital chemical processes slow down or even stop. It is well known that a deficiency of key vitamins can impair physical performance, but in America today, an athlete is much more likely to suffer from an excess of vitamins than from a lack of them.

Over the past 45 years, many studies have investigated the effect of supplemental vitamins on physical performance, particularly vitamins C, E, and those in the B-complex group. The general findings are that vitamin supplementation is not necessary or advantageous in well-nourished athletes. Athletes who feel they must take a vitamin pill for insurance against unlikely dietary deficiencies should choose a daily multivitamin pill containing no more than 100 percent of the RDA. Megadoses of any vitamin—including the water-soluble ones—carry a risk of toxicity.

The B Vitamins

Because the B vitamins are essential cofactors in the breakdown of carbohydrates, proteins, and fats to energy, supplements of one or more of this group are frequently taken by athletes in the hope that an intake of these vitamins above and beyond the normal RDA will produce extra energy. The need for thiamine (B_1) is dependent upon energy expenditure; thus, athletes have higher requirements than sedentary individuals. However, the increased needs for thiamine can be met easily by the larger quantities of foods consumed by the active person, provided a well-balanced diet is chosen.

Likewise, several studies carried out at Cornell University in Ithaca, New York, suggest that women who exercise regularly may have a higher requirement for riboflavin (B_2). This does not seem to apply to other B vitamins, however; the same studies failed to show any beneficial effects of niacin (B_3) supplements on performance. Any increased need can be met easily through diet. Active women on low-calorie weight-loss regimens should

be sure to include riboflavin-rich foods such as milk, cheese, and yogurt in their daily diets.

Recommended Dietary Allowances for niacin are also commonly related to energy expenditure, but there is little evidence that niacin requirements actually parallel energy expenditure. Moreover, some studies suggest that niacin in large doses may hinder endurance performance.

Pyridoxine (B_6) acts as a catalyst in the conversion of stored glycogen back to glucose. Studies also have shown that blood levels of vitamin B_6 increase with endurance exercise and with B_6 supplementation. Because of these facts, it has been theorized that this vitamin could be helpful in endurance-type activities. However, when this theory was tested, B_6 supplementation had no significant effect on the endurance of the athletes studied. High-dose supplements of vitamin B_6 can cause severe nerve damage and should be avoided.

Taking supplements of vitamin B_{12} in pill form, by injection, or as a nasal gel is a common practice throughout the athletic world. Advertisements in fitness magazines commonly promote this vitamin as giving an instant energy high. However, several studies investigated vitamin B_{12} supplementation and physical performance and found no beneficial effects whatsoever. Vitamin B_{12} is found in all animal foods. The only athletes who are at risk for vitamin B_{12} deficiency are strict vegetarians who eat only plant foods.

Vitamin C

Vitamin C is one of the most popular supplements used by active individuals, although its deficiency is very rare in them. Various claims have been made for vitamin C, including the assertion that it has a beneficial effect on the cardiovascular system during workouts. However, no well-designed study has shown that vitamin C supplements have any significant effect on endurance performance. Megadoses are harmful.

Vitamin E

Vitamin E is touted as increasing energy as well as improving stamina and circulation, but several recent studies have shown that supplemental vitamin E has no effect on the physical performance capacity. Vitamin E deficiency is extremely rare, occurring only in premature infants and in individuals who cannot absorb fat normally. Wheat germ's reputation for being a so-called ergogenic food is due to its high vitamin E content. It is not ergogenic, nor is vitamin E.

Minerals

Minerals are also important regulators of the physiological processes involved in physical performance, and mineral supplements receive much popular attention from athletes. As with vitamins, however, the high caloric intake of most athletes helps to ensure that all mineral needs are met. The minerals that are most likely to be low in the diets of athletes are the same ones that all Americans tend to get in short supply—iron and calcium. The electrolytes—sodium, potassium, magnesium, and chloride—are the other category of minerals that are of particular interest to athletes.

Iron

Although iron is needed in only small amounts, it is of particular importance because it is a key component of hemoglobin, the protein in blood that transports oxygen to the working muscle. Iron-deficiency anemia is well known to affect athletic performance adversely. Mild iron deficiency without detectable anemia is even more common and can also affect an individual's ability to perform physically.

Since women lose iron during menstruation, they are much more likely to be iron-deficient. Women at highest risk are vegetarian women and those who eat little meat, poultry, or fish—all rich sources of highly absorbable iron.

Most men obtain sufficient iron in their diets, and iron deficiency among male athletes is usually limited to rapidly growing adolescents whose diets do not meet the additional iron needs imposed by their growth. However, both male and female long-distance runners sometimes develop iron deficiency despite well-balanced diets. Athletes with this problem have usually been running more than 50 to 60 miles per week for long periods of time. Causes of this iron deficiency are uncertain, but contributing factors may include decreased iron absorption and increased iron losses in perspiration, urine, and the stools.

Men and women who fall into these high-risk groups and others who suspect that they may be iron-deficient should have their iron status checked by measuring the level in their blood, and then have any deficiency treated under medical supervision.

Men, in particular, should not take supplements as insurance against iron deficiency. One male in 250 has a genetic abnormality which causes him to absorb at least twice the normal amount of iron from food. If such a man takes supplemental iron, it can damage his pancreas, liver, heart, and joints. Women can also have iron-overload disease, although iron buildup and subsequent damage is slower in premenopausal women. Fatigue can be a symptom of iron deficiency *or iron overload*. (For more information about iron deficiency or iron overload, see Chapter 29.)

Sports Anemia

A pseudoanemia called sports anemia is also seen in male and female athletes, especially in the early stages of training. Most doctors agree that this condition is not caused by a deficiency of dietary iron but is probably a normal, beneficial adaptation to exercise. Unlike the anemia of iron deficiency, the number of red blood cells is normal in sports anemia. Because there is an increase in blood volume, however, the concentration of red blood cells is diluted, making hemoglobin concentration appear to be too low. Blood tests then make it seem as if the athletes are slightly anemic, but they are not. They just have thinner blood than their sedentary counterparts. No treatment is required for this "hemodilution."

Calcium

Adequate calcium intake is essential for all individuals—whether they are active or sedentary—throughout life. Approximately 99 percent of the calcium in the body is found in the skeleton. The other 1 percent is found in the blood, where it is essential to regulate muscular contraction, blood clotting, and nerve transmission. When calcium intake is low, the body draws calcium from the bone to ensure adequate blood levels. If dietary calcium is not sufficient to replace calcium lost from the bones, bone density is reduced, increasing the risk of fracture or shin splints.

Calcium deficiencies are primarily a concern for women, because they tend to have lower calcium intakes than men and because they have less dense bone structures. After menopause, all women begin to lose bone unless they take estrogen, regardless of their calcium intake. Research has shown, however, that exercise stimulates the formation of new bone and can slow the rate of bone loss in this age group. For younger women, adequate dietary calcium intake, plus exercise, is the prime defense against thinning bones.

Other Minerals

The effects of exercise on the requirements of some trace minerals such as zinc, copper, and chromium are also under study. Some research suggests that heavy sweating or strenuous exercise may place a drain on the body's stores of these essential minerals. However, at this time there is no agreement as to how or to what degree body levels of these minerals affect exercise performance, and supplements are not recommended. Not only are all minerals toxic in large quantities but dosing oneself with single mineral supplements can cause an imbalance that will alter needs for other nutrients, as well.

Electrolytes

The elements sodium, potassium, magnesium, and chloride are collectively termed *electrolytes* because when dissolved in body fluids, they separate into electrically charged particles called ions. Electrolytes play indispensable roles in transmitting nerve impulses, contracting muscles, keeping a proper level of fluids in the body, and maintaining the proper acid-base balance of these fluids.

Potassium. Potassium (along with magnesium) is found primarily in the fluid within body cells. A deficit of potassium is associated with muscular weakness and fatigue, but potassium depletion is rarely a concern for the athlete. Potassium losses in perspiration are negligible, except under the most extreme conditions of heat in a person unadapted to the environment. Even in these cases, potassium loss is easily replaced by consuming a high-potassium food. For example, a glass of orange juice or tomato juice will replace the amount of potassium excreted in two to three quarts of perspiration.

Sodium. Sodium (along with chloride) is found primarily in the fluids that surround the cells. It is the chief ion in perspiration and a significant amount may be lost in profuse and protracted sweating. However, only under extreme circumstances is salt deficiency a problem. The American diet has an overabundance of sodium. Salt is lavished on commercially prepared food. Canned peas, for example, contain 90 times as much salt as fresh peas, and one TV dinner can provide all the salt an average adult needs for several days. Even individuals who consciously avoid salty food and ignore the salt shaker consume more than an adequate supply. A balanced diet will supply all the salt an athlete needs, with the possible exception of an endurance athlete competing in hot weather to which he or she is not accustomed. The consumption of salt tablets is unwise and may be harmful. The tablets frequently cause nausea, vomiting, and gastric distress. Excessive salt increases the load on the kidneys and can aggravate dehydration unless an adequate amount of fluid is taken, as well.

Fluids

Water accounts for approximately 60 percent of the body weight of the average person. Water serves many vital functions, but the one of particular importance to the athlete is that water cools the body. During exercise, heat is generated within the body by the working muscles. If this heat builds up, the body temperature rises, performance suffers, and the risk of heat injury increases. The body's main mechanism for getting rid of this heat is through evaporation of perspiration from the skin. Heavy sweating, however, results in large losses of body water. Unless a substantial portion of this sweat loss is replaced, the body quickly becomes dehydrated and its cooling mechanism cannot function effectively.

Unfortunately, it is widely believed that drinking water before or during exercise will weigh down an athlete or upset the stomach, interfering with performance. Other individuals are under the misguided notion that fluid deprivation during training and competition will help the body adapt to dehydration, making athletes less dependent on fluids during athletic events. No evidence exists to support either of these beliefs, and, in fact, the need for fluid before and during exercise—as well as afterward—cannot be overemphasized.

Dehydration is one of the major factors that limits the body's capacity for strenuous exercise. As water is lost through perspiration, the blood volume decreases, reducing circulation to the skin—preventing heat dissipation—and to muscles, where nutrients and oxygen are needed. A loss of as little as 2 percent of body weight as perspiration (3 pounds for a 150-pound person) can bring the first signs of dehydration: generalized discomfort, fatigue, headache, and apathy. A 5-percent loss leads to heat cramps and then heat exhaustion, characterized by a weak, rapid pulse rate and fever; at 7 percent, an athlete may suffer hallucinations; at 10 percent, heatstroke and circulatory collapse are likely.

Exercise during hot, humid weather can lead to heat injury more quickly than exercise during cool, dry—or even hot, dry—weather. When the humidity is high, sweat does not evaporate readily, so heat builds up in the body faster. Working out in heavy sports gear, heavy clothing, or in plastic or rubber exercise suits also can interfere with the evaporation of perspiration, causing a dangerous buildup of body heat.

Athletes cannot depend on thirst to alert them to the need for fluid. The thirst response is controlled by brain cells that react to salt concentration in the blood rather than to sudden fluid loss. Although perspiration contains salt, the blood's salt concentration is lowered more slowly than the body's water content. Adaptation to heat results in a lower salt concentration in perspiration. The brain, therefore, does not initiate a thirst response until well after water loss has occurred. For this reason, athletes should force themselves to drink even when they are not thirsty, both before and during competition.

A good rule is to consume about 20 ounces (30cc = 1 ounce) of water an hour or two before exercise; have another 10 to 15 ounces 15 minutes before the activity begins; and then drink 3 to 6 ounces at 10 to 20 minutes intervals during events that last more than a half hour. (See Guide to Water Replacement, below.) Cold water is absorbed most rapidly and can help to reduce body temperature.

However, even following these recommendations may not be sufficient to replace all fluid losses. Endurance athletes competing in warm climates may lose as much as two to four quarts of perspiration (about four to eight pounds body weight) in an hour in spite of their efforts to keep up their fluid intake.

The most effective way for athletes to monitor their fluid needs is to weigh themselves both before and after an event. For each pound of weight lost, an athlete needs 16 ounces of water. Thus, a weight loss of five pounds means a deficit of 80 ounces (two and a half quarts) of water. Obviously, replacing such large amounts of water will take time. When weight loss is 4 to 7 percent of body weight, up to 36 hours may be needed for complete rehydration.

Sports Beverages

Commercial sports beverages are intended to deliver a combination of fluid, carbohydrate, and electroytes to boost performance. Whether or not they achieve their goal is a topic of considerable debate.

Past research has suggested that bev-erages used for fluid replacement should not contain more than 2.5 percent sugar. (Most sports beverages contain 4 to 10 percent sugar.) This recommendation was based on the observation that as the sugar concentration of a beverage increases, the rate of gastric emptying (the time it takes for the beverage to leave the stomach) decreases.

However, more recent research, which has also looked at other physiological parameters of importance to fluid absorption during exercise, suggests that beverages containing up to 10 percent sugar (glucose or sucrose) actually enter the blood at rates similar to water. Furthermore, the higher-sugar solutions have been shown to improve endurance in long-distance events, over two to three hours, by providing carbohydrates to the exercising muscles and by staving off depletion of glycogen stores. On the other hand, some hypertonic solutions that contain more than about 10 percent sugar may cause nausea, bloating, cramps, and diarrhea.

Some of the newer sports beverages contain glucose polymers (glucose molecules linked in a short chain) instead of loose sugar molecules. Manufacturers claim that these beverages can provide a higher concentration of carbohydrate calories and deliver them faster than other sports beverages, but research to determine whether polymers are superior to simple sugars is inconclusive. Glucose-polymer solutions probably do have

Guide to Water Replacement

Weight Lost During Exercise	Amount of Water Needed
1 pound	Two 8-oz. glasses
3 pounds	Six 8-oz. glasses
5 pounds	Ten 8-oz. glasses
8 pounds	Sixteen 8-oz. glasses

an absorption advantage over glucose solutions when the concentration of sugar in the drink is greater than 5 percent, due to the lower osmolality (the concentration of particles in a solution) of the polymer drinks. Also, sports beverages containing glucose polymers do not have an unpalatable sweet taste or produce upset stomach the way concentrated sugar solutions do.

Athletes in such events as marathons or fifty-mile bicycle races may find carbohydrate-containing beverages valuable, particularly if their muscle-glycogen stores are less than optimal. Competitors in relatively short events are better served by water.

Most commercial sports beverages also contain electrolytes, but electrolyte intake during exercise is generally unnecessary. Perspiration contains a far greater amount of water than minerals, so the concentration of extracellular electrolytes (sodium, chloride) in the body fluids actually increase during periods of heavy sweating. Intracellular electrolytes (potassium, magnesium) are lost from the cell and can increase in body fluids that are extracellular. They are lost possibly through perspiration. The body's main need is for water to bring the concentration of the electrolytes in the body back into balance. Meals eaten after exercise readily compensate for any electrolytes lost in perspiration.

It is only when sweat losses are excessive (i.e., over three to four quarts) that electrolyte replacement may be necessary. Since athletes who are acclimated to hot weather excrete fewer electrolytes in their sweat, endurance athletes participating in intense heat conditions to which they are not accustomed are most likely to experience problems.

A few cases of hyponatremia (low levels of sodium in the blood) have also been reported in athletes who consumed large amounts of plain water during endurance events such as triathlons or ultramarathons. Symptoms of hyponatremia include headache, nausea, fatigue, drowsiness, muscle weakness, muscle twitching or cramping, mental confusion, seizure, and coma.

Sports beverages spiked with vitamins are definitely better left on the supermarket shelf. No significant amount of vitamins are lost during exercise and taking extra vitamins will not improve performance. Drinking large amounts of such beverages also could lead to dangerous vitamin overdoses.

ENERGY COSTS

The energy cost of exercise varies with the intensity, frequency, and duration of the exercise, and with the individual's age, sex, weight, and height. For example, the energy cost of a marathon is greater than that of a short-distance event; a lighter person uses less energy than a heavier one for any given activity.

Among some male athletes in training, the energy needs range from 3,500 to 5,500 calories per day or more. In contrast, some female dancers, gymnasts, and figure skaters maintain their competitive weight by consuming only 1,400 to 2,000 calories a day. Under normal conditions, caloric intake is automatically adjusted—by appetite and the sense of satiety—to meet increased energy requirements. However, these sensitive regulators are not always reliable under stressful conditions—such as training and competition—and an athlete may eat too much or, more commonly, too little.

Knowing a sport's energy requirement (see Table 24.1) can help an athlete determine approximately how many extra calories are needed to fuel a chosen physical activity. However, maintenance of desirable body weight is the best criterion of long-term adequacy or inadequacy of energy intake. Selecting additional foods from all four food groups with emphasis on complex carbohydrates such as dried peas and beans, whole-grain and enriched grain products, and fruits and vegetables is the best way to satisfy caloric needs, meet vitamin and mineral requirements, and ensure adequate glycogen stores. If energy needs are high, frequent snacking may be necessary in order to attain adequate calories.

EFFICIENT BODY WEIGHT

Height-weight charts have been developed for both men and women and are commonly used to determine whether a person is overweight or underweight. However, these tables are of limited usefulness to many athletes because they do not distinguish between a heavy body weight due to well-developed muscles and a heavy body weight caused by excess fat. For example, a six-foot-tall body builder with a medium frame may weigh 200 pounds with little excess fat, but according to some charts, he would be from 30 to 45 pounds overweight. The real issue in many sports is not body weight but body fat.

Some body fat is essential to protect organs from injury, insulate against cold, and store extra energy. The complete absence of body fat is neither possible nor desirable. Excess body fat decreases muscular efficiency, however: More energy and more oxygen are required to produce a given amount of muscular work.

There is no one ideal body-fat level for athletes; body composition varies between the sexes and from sport to sport. In general, body-fat levels in male athletes range from 4 to 12 percent of body fat; in female athletes, 10 to 20 percent. (In nonathletes, values up to 15 percent for men and 20 percent for women are acceptable.)

However, while too much body fat can hamper performance, leaner is not necessarily better. In one survey of the nation's top women runners, no correlation was found between the thinnest runner and the fastest time. When athletes become too thin, they also lose muscle and strength.

WEIGHT CONTROL

To compete effectively, athletes must be at their ideal weight, have an appropriate body composition, and, at the same time, be well nourished and well hydrated. Any desired gain or loss should be accomplished gradually, one to two pounds a week, starting well before any competitive event. Diet modifications for both gaining and losing weight should be based on the four food groups to assure an optimal intake of all essential nutrients. (See Chapter 17 for more information on weight control.)

Unfortunately, drastic and sudden measures are often used by athletes—both those who need to lose weight and those who need to gain it.

Athletes, such as wrestlers and boxers, who have to "make weight" (be under a certain weight at the time of an event) frequently use weight-reduction methods dangerous to their health. Among these are fasting, crash diets, liquid-restricted diets, diuretics (water pills), laxatives, induced vomiting, and excessive sweating in a plastic sweat suit or sauna. All of these methods can impair performance. Starvation and near starvation cause mainly a loss of muscle and water—not fat—and such regimens also decrease aerobic power, speed,

Table 24.1. Approximate Energy Expenditure During Performance of Various Physical Activities*

Activity	120 lbs. 54.5 kg.		150 lbs. 68 kg.		200 lbs. 90.9 kg.	
	10 min.	60 min.	10 min.	60 min.	10 min.	60 min.
Aerobic dancing	92	553	115	691	153	922
Badminton (singles)	53	318	66	396	88	529
Basketball	75	452	94	564	126	753
Bicycling						
6 mph.	35	210	44	262	58	349
12 mph.	92	553	115	691	154	922
Bowling	25	150	30	180	35	210
Calisthenics	36	216	45	270	60	360
Canoeing (leisure)	24	144	30	180	40	240
Dancing						
Slow	28	167	35	209	46	278
Fast	92	550	115	687	153	916
Football	72	432	90	540	120	720
Golf (walking and carrying bag)	46	278	58	348	77	450
Hockey	60	360	70	420	75	450
Jumping rope	60	360	70	420	75	450
Lacrosse	55	330	68	410	85	512
Rugby	60	360	75	450	94	564
Running or jogging						
5 mph.	74	442	92	552	122	736
7.5 mph.	105	630	132	792	175	1,050
10 mph.	137	824	171	1,030	229	1,375
Sailing	30	180	36	216	44	254
Skating (ice or roller)	41	245	51	307	68	409
Skiing						
Downhill	50	280	63	360	78	450
Cross-country	65	390	81	487	108	649
Soccer	55	330	68	410	85	512
Squash	60	357	74	446	99	595
Swimming (fast freestyle)	70	420	87	522	116	698
Tennis						
Singles	60	357	74	446	99	595
Doubles	35	210	44	262	58	350
Volleyball	27	164	34	205	46	273
Walking						
3 mph.	34	206	43	258	57	344
4 mph.	51	308	64	385	86	513
Upstairs	79	471	98	589	131	786
Weight training	60	340	74	420	90	520
Wrestling (practice)	110	600	140	800	180	1,020

Caloric Expenditure (kcal) by Weight and Time

*Energy expenditure depends not only on the activity but the intensity with which the activity is carried out. Thus, individual variation in energy expenditure for a given physical activity can be quite large. In addition, the duration of the activity can be quite variable.

This table was originally published in *Nutrition Today*, March/April 1986. It was compiled by the staff at the Nutrition Clinic at Penn State under the supervision of Marian I. Hammond, M.S., R.D., with assistance from E. R. Buskirk, Ph.D., from numerous sources. Used with permission.

coordination, and judgment. Likewise, studies show that water restriction combined with other dehydration techniques lower glycogen levels, decrease endurance, and impair the sweating-cooling mechanism. Young athletes who repeatedly participate in crash weight-loss programs risk permanently compromising their growth.

Those participating in strength-dependent sports—for example, football and weight lifting—often aim for a quick gain in weight. Bulking up, as this is sometimes called, does not always enhance performance, however. Only weight gain that is due to an increase in muscle can improve one's potential as an athlete. Increasing body fat will only reduce speed and endurance.

The addition of muscle mass can be accomplished only through regular muscle work (weight training or similar conditioning) coupled with a caloric increase. A little extra protein is also required to supply the amino-acid building blocks for new lean tissue, but if additional calories come from a variety of foods, abundant protein also will be present. A high-protein diet or protein supplements offer no advantages and are not recommended. Any extra protein that is eaten is simply broken down and burned as energy or stored as body fat. Tryptophan supplement promotes diet harm.

Muscle building also takes time. A muscle must be exercised at 60 to 80 percent of its capacity several times a week to increase in size and strength. Furthermore, a gain of one pound of muscle requires about 2,500 extra calories, in addition to the calories needed for the training. Ideally, an addition of 700 to 1,000 calories to the daily diet should support a gain of one to two pounds of lean muscle each week, as well as the energy needs for the additional exercise. Realistically, however, individual differences and the type, intensity, and frequency of training factors also affect weight gain.

FOOD AND DRINK BEFORE COMPETITION

There is no magic meal that will guarantee an athlete the competitive edge. Performance during an event is more dependent on food consumed in the days prior to the event than on immediate pregame eating. However, there are some general guidelines that may help the athlete maximize the benefits of the pre-event meal. They are based on common sense.

High-protein, high-fat foods such as the traditional pregame steak are seldom recommended today. Both protein and fat delay the emptying of the stomach, and neither contributes to the glycogen stores needed during exercise. Instead, foods that are high in carbohydrates, low in fat, and low to moderate in protein are the best choice. Some pregame suggestions are: hot or cold cereal with low-fat milk and fruit; pasta with a low-fat sauce; lean meat sandwich without mayonnaise. In terms of timing, the meal should be eaten at least three hours before the event so that the stomach and upper bowel are empty at the time of the event. Exercising immediately after a heavy meal causes oxygen-rich blood to be diverted from the digestive system to the working muscles, which may cause stomach cramps or a painful side stitch. The size of the meal will vary among athletes but should be sufficient to prevent hunger during competition. Fluids such as water, juice, and skim milk should be included as desired.

In general, only fluids—preferable plain water or perhaps a low-sugar sports beverage—should be consumed after the pre-event meal. Eating honey, chocolate or other candy, sweetened beverages or other sources of concentrated sugar in hopes of boosting energy is particularly not recommended. Some research has suggested that eating or drinking sweets within an hour of exercise may actually decrease endurance. As sugar is released into the bloodstream, blood-glucose levels jump, causing the pancreas to release a surge of insulin. If exercise commences when insulin is elevated, the uptake by muscle of glucose from the blood will be enhanced, producing a decline in blood sugar that can sometimes cause transient hypoglycemia, making the athlete feel weak and shaky. At the same time, insulin interferes with the body's ability to burn fat for energy, so the body is forced to turn to its glycogen stores, causing premature exhaustion of their energy supplies and hastening the onset of fatigue.

All athletes attempting to increase their glycogen stores should be aware that 2.7 grams of water are stored in the body for every gram of glycogen. This extra water increases body weight and causes some athletes to feel heavy or stiff. On the positive side, however, as glycogen stores are burned off in competition, this water is released as perspiration, cooling the body.

Although a high-carbohydrate diet is beneficial for all athletes, carbohydrate loading (consuming a high-carbohydrate diet for several days before an event) is effective only for athletes whose event requires nonstop activity for at least 90 minutes, or for those who may be in daylong, multi-event competition such as swimming or track meets, wrestling tournaments, and so forth. It is of no value in short events or in such intermittently strenuous ones as football. (See Table 24.3 for a sample carbohydrate-loading meal plan.)

A high-carbohydrate diet (70 percent carbohydrate) also may be beneficial during strenuous activity at high altitudes (above 8,000 feet), where oxygen is less available and greater demands are placed on the anaerobic metabolism of carbohydrate.

Athletes attempting to plan diets high in carbohydrates should consult food-composition tables. (Table 24.2 lists foods high in carbohydrates.) Foods high in calories are not automatically high in carbohydrates. Many high-calorie sweets, for example, are also very high in fats.

THE ELEMENTARY SCHOOL ATHLETE

The best overall advice for all children, regardless of physical activity, is simply to follow a balanced diet based on the four basic food groups. This is not the age to get into such practices as carbohydrate loading or low-calorie dieting, nor the time for particular emphasis on any special food or food group. Special dietary supplements, drugs, and steroids are particularly dangerous in this age group. More exercise brings a better appetite, which, in turn, almost assures adequate nutrition as long as the rules of variety, balance, and moderation are followed.

The one nutritional problem that is of special concern in this age group is fluid replacement. Children have a lower sweating capacity than adolescents or adults, which means that a child is less efficient in regulating his/her body temperature. Young athletes are also slower to adjust to exercise in warm weather.

Exercise and training in the heat must be carefully supervised to make sure children wear lightweight clothing and drink enough to replace their fluid losses.

THE ADOLESCENT ATHLETE

Teenage athletes are often surprised and disappointed when they learn that the proper training diet differs little from the well-balanced diet needed by all teenagers. Energy requirements are generally higher for the adolescent athlete than they are for his or her more sedentary peers, but the additional 500 to 1,500 calories needed for training and competition are usually automatically supplied because of an increase in appetite. Snacking frequently becomes important in helping to provide these calories, especially when practice interferes with scheduled meals. Failure to consume adequate calories can jeopardize both growth and physical performance.

The overwhelming wish of adolescent male athletes is to increase their body size and strength in order to enhance their playing potential in a particular sport. To this end, they will sometimes pursue ineffective, counterproductive, or potentially dangerous nutrition-related practices. Coaches, trainers, and parents must be constantly on the lookout for athletes who "believe" that the key to big muscles lies in unbalanced diets, nutritional supplements, and drugs and the like rather than in weight training in conjunction with a proper diet.

Both coaches and adolescent athletes also must be aware that there is a normal maturation sequence experienced by young men as they acquire adult body size, weight, and strength. They first experience a rapid gain in height. Toward the end of this linear growth spurt, they will begin to gain weight through an increase in muscle size, which is naturally accompanied by an increase in strength. These normal stages of growth are regulated and controlled by the normal hormonal changes

Table 24.2. Selected Foods High in Carbohydrates

	Grams of Carbohydrate		Grams of Carbohydrate
MILK GROUP		**FRUIT-VEGETABLE GROUP** (cont.)	
Milk shake, chocolate, 10.6 oz.	63	Potato, sweet, ½ medium	18
Yogurt, strawberry, 1 cup	42	Beans, lima, ½ cup	17
Pudding, chocolate, ½ cup	30	Corn, ½ cup	16
Milk, chocolate, 1 cup	26	Orange, medium	16
Cocoa, ¾ cup	19	Squash, winter, ½ cup	14
Ice cream, vanilla, ½ cup	16	Potatoes, mashed, ½ cup	13
Milk, low-fat and skim, 1 cup	12	Grapefruit, pink, ½ medium	13
Milk, whole, 1 cup	11	Orange juice, ½ cup	13
		Watermelon, 1 cup	13
MEAT GROUP			
Refried beans, ½ cup	26	**GRAIN GROUP**	
Black-eyed peas, mature, ½ cup	17	Corn bread, 2½ by 3 inches	30
		Roll, hard	30
FRUIT-VEGETABLE GROUP		Bagel	28
Raisins, 4 T	33	Rice, ½ cup	25
Potatoes, French-fried, 20 pieces	31	Roll, hamburger or frankfurter	21
Potato, baked, large	30	Noodles, egg, ½ cup	19
Applesauce, sweetened, ½ cup	30	Waffles	17
Banana, medium	26	Cornflakes, ¾ cup	16
Peaches, canned in syrup, ½ cup	26	Hominy grits, ½ cup	14
Pear, medium	25	Tortilla, corn, 6-inch diameter	14
Fruit salad, ½ cup	25	Biscuit, baking powder	13
Pineapple, large slice	24	Bread, white, 1 slice	12
Grape juice, ½ cup	21	Oatmeal, ½ cup	12
Apple, medium	20	Bread, whole-wheat, 1 slice	11
Potatoes, boiled, 2 small	18		

that occur during adolescence and are related directly to sexual maturation rather than to chronological age. Until young men arrive at the appropriate level of maturity, weight training will not result in significant major gains in muscle mass and body weight.

Adolescents who mature late should not be pushed beyond their physical capabilities by parents and coaches. Instead, the young athlete should be encouraged to work on his skills and to participate in sports that are not dependent on strength and size until his muscle development and coordination catch up with his height. Only then can his muscles respond to the demands of a supervised weight-training program that will result in the desired increases in size and strength. Some adolescent athletes are more concerned with the need to minimize body fatness and reduce body weight. This can be a particular problem among female athletes involved in sports such as gymnastics, figure skating, and ballet, which have relatively high energy requirements but also demand slimness. It may also occur among young men participating in wrestling and boxing (see section on weight control on page 406). Fasting, crash diets, overuse of laxatives or diuretics, vomiting, using diet pills, and other extreme weight-loss measures all have performance-robbing consequences and can create a variety of medical problems, including damaging the adolescent's growth and maturation, sometimes permanently.

THE VEGETARIAN ATHLETE

There's no question that an athlete can enjoy good health and perform well on a meatless diet, although the vegetarian athlete must pay a little more attention to planning balanced eating. All animal protein (except gelatin) contains adequate amounts of all nine essential amino acids, while almost all vegetable protein sources are low in one or more. If properly selected, however, a vegetarian diet can provide the same high-quality protein as animal food.

Those vegetarians who do not eat any animal products must use foods fortified with vitamin B_{12} or take a B_{12} supplement. Lack of this vitamin can result in anemia and irreversible nerve damage. Calcium, iron, zinc, and vitamin D are other nutrients that may be lacking in a strict vegetarian diet. Extreme types of vegetarianism, such as macrobiotic diets or fruitarian diets, are not balanced and can lead only to poor performance as well as poor health. Luckily, the vast majority of American vegetarians do eat milk products, which contain animal protein, and also vitamin B_{12}. Of Seventh-Day Adventist vegetarians, 69 percent eat some meat. (For more information on vegetarianism, see Chapter 25.)

Table 24.3.   Carbohydrate-Loading Meal Plan

Sample Menu: approximately 3,200 calories

BREAKFAST:	8 oz. orange juice
	1 cup Grape-Nuts
	1 medium banana
	8 oz. low-fat milk
	1 whole-wheat English muffin
	1 t margarine
LUNCH:	2 oz. turkey
	2 slices bran bread
	lettuce/tomato slices
	8 oz. apple juice
	1 cup lemon sherbet
SNACK:	⅔ cup frozen yogurt
DINNER:	2 cups spaghetti (6 oz. uncooked)
	⅔ cup tomato sauce with mushrooms
	2 T Parmesan cheese
	4 slices French bread
	1 cup apple sauce with 2 T raisins
	12 oz. cranberry juice
	½ cup ice cream
SNACK:	6 cups popcorn, hot air
	3 gingersnaps
	8 oz. seltzer water with lemon

THE DIABETIC ATHLETE

Exercise offers the same benefits to diabetics as it does to individuals without medical problems. However, because exercise affects blood-sugar levels and insulin requirements, it is essential that insulin-dependent diabetics monitor their blood-glucose levels before, during, and after exercise and adjust insulin dosages and food intake accordingly.

If the diabetic athlete fails to make an appropriate reduction in insulin dosage or fails to eat adequate amounts or types of food when participating in prolonged or vigorous exercise, blood sugar may fall to low levels and produce symptoms of hypoglycemia. Diabetics should carry some source of simple sugar such as sugar cubes or hard candies with them at all times and should inform their coaches, teammates, and partners of their diabetes and how to react if help is needed.

Diabetics who control their diabetes with oral drugs instead of insulin also can develop exercise-induced hypoglycemia, although these individuals usually have more stable blood-glucose levels than insulin-dependent diabetics. (For more information about diabetes, see Chapter 28.)

GINSENG, BEE POLLEN, AND OTHER FADS

Advertisements abound for "scientifically balanced energy foods" that are supposed to provide a competitive advantage in sports. The pills and powders are often labeled all-natural, raw, pure, ergogenic, mega, or sustained-release. There is no sound data demonstrating that any of these preparations can improve performance, however.

Some of these supplements such as octacosanol (a substance found in raw wheat germ and in many plant oils) or para-amino-benzoic acid (PABA—a vitamin for bacteria but not for humans) are not needed in our diets and offer no known dietary benefits.

Glandular extracts, which consist of tiny amounts of dried animal organs such as the pituitary gland, thyroid gland, adrenal gland, hypothalamus, and testicles, are alleged to strengthen corresponding organs in the human body. This idea is nonsense, however. When these substances are taken orally, they are broken down by digestion and do not reach the body's cells intact.

Food concentrates such as dessicated liver pills, brewer's yeast, wheat germ, royal jelly, protein powder, and spirulina (a blue-green algae) are all unnecessary expenditures, and none is a unique supplier of any essential or therapeutic ingredient. Buying these substances is just an overpriced way to get the same nutrients that can be obtained easily from a variety of foods purchased in any supermarket. Some can be harmful.

Other "wonder" foods can be harmful. Bee pollen can produce life-threatening allergic reactions in pollen-sensitive individuals, and ginseng contains estrogens and potentially toxic chemicals. Pangamic acid, also called "Vitamin B_{15}," is not a vitamin. According to the Food and Drug Administration, it is "not an identifiable substance," since the chemical composition of the compound seems to vary with the manufacturer. The chemicals present in some pangamic-acid supplements may have dangerous drug effects. Taking single amino-acid supplements can interfere with the absorption of other amino acids, upsetting the body's natural balance of these protein building blocks. Furthermore, animal studies have shown that consumption of excessive amounts of some amino acids can have serious side effects.

DRUGS

Caffeine

Caffeine may enhance endurance under some conditions. According to studies by David Costill of the Ball State Human Performance Laboratory in Indiana, 250 milligrams of caffeine (about two cups of brewed coffee) taken one hour before exercise can delay fatigue and prolong performance in sports lasting one hour or longer. It seems that caffeine facilitates the body's use of free fatty acids for fuel, conserving the body's limited glycogen stores.

However, in other investigations, caffeine has failed to produce a carbohydrate-sparing effect or has improved performance only under certain conditions. For example, in one recent study, researchers found that a high-carbohydrate diet seemed to negate the metabolic effects of caffeine during exercise. Furthermore, individuals with a low tolerance to caffeine may find that it hinders performance by causing increased anxiety, nervousness, or diarrhea.

Athletes should also be aware that caffeine has a diuretic effect and may promote dehydration by increasing urination. Coffee, tea, cocoa, chocolate, many soft drinks, and some drugs, such as pain relievers and decongestants, contain varying amounts of caffeine.

Alcohol

Even small amounts of alcohol taken before a workout or event can reduce alertness, interfere with judgment, slow reaction time, and alter coordination, balance, and visual perception. Prolonged heavy drinking may also lead to many undesirable changes in the cardiovascular system and the nervous system. Alcohol is also a diuretic and can increase urine production and fluid loss.

Amphetamines

Amphetamines (also called pep pills or uppers) stimulate the brain and cardiovascular system, increasing metabolism and blood glucose, elevating blood pressure and heart rate, and accelerating breathing. Athletes sometimes use these potentially dangerous drugs in an effort to increase self-confidence or to suppress feelings of fatigue. However, any "benefits" of these dangerous drugs are of short duration and are more than offset by their potential negative side effects, which include impaired judgment, depressed appetite, headaches, dizziness, and insomnia. Long-term use can lead to either physiological or psychological dependence.

Steroids

Anabolic (tissue-building) steroids are synthetic derivatives of testosterone, the male sex hormone that helps the body build muscle and synthesize proteins. Many athletes, particularly body builders, weight lifters, wrestlers, football players, and discus throwers, believe these drugs will build bigger muscles and enable them to improve their performance. Despite their popularity, however, the ability of these drugs actually to increase muscle mass or improve performance is a very mixed blessing. Many studies of steroids show either modest strength gains or no significant performance gains. However, while the capability of these drugs to enhance strength is uncertain, the numerous adverse side effects of steroids are unquestioned. Men may develop acne, a decreased sperm count, atrophied testes, enlargement of the breasts, and serious liver disorders. In women, steroids' masculinizing effect often causes deepening of the voice, growth of facial and body hair, male-pattern baldness, and aggressiveness, as well as shrinking of the breasts and irregular or absent menstrual periods. Many of the changes in women tend to be irreversible. The drugs can stunt growth permanently in children and adolescents.

DISORDERS

Menstrual Disorders

Menstrual disorders are common among adolescents and women participating in rigorous training programs. Some young athletes experience a delayed onset of menstruation as compared to their peers who do not exercise vigorously. Other female athletes may have irregular menstrual cycles (oligomenorrhea) or a complete cessation of menstrual periods (amenorrhea). These irregularities are particularly common in ballet dancers and competitive or long-distance runners, but they are also seen in women participating in cycling, rowing, gymnastics, and other sports. In general, as training increases, so does the prevalence of amenorrhea.

The exact cause of athletic amenorrhea is unknown. One theory is that it may be related to reduction of body fat below a certain critical level. However, while the lean-to-fat ratio of the body may be one factor, it is clearly not the complete answer. One recent study on women runners found no difference between normal and amenorrheic runners in either body composition, weight, or running mileage, but it did find that those with abnormal menstrual cycles consumed fewer calories. Support cells in body fat make hormones.

Fortunately, athletic amenorrhea is rever-sible. Once rigorous training stops, menstruation begins again and future fertility does not seem to be compromised. Nevertheless, this condition should not be dismissed as a harmless side effect of physical training. Amenorrheic women have low levels of the female sex hormone estrogen, and a loss of estrogen results in accelerated bone loss, similar to that seen in postmenopausal osteoporosis. Studies also have confirmed that, on average, amenorrheic athletes have bones that are less dense and a higher incidence of bone fractures than those of athletes with regular cycles.

Athletes who are amenorrheic should see a doctor for a careful evaluation to rule out medical reasons for the problem. If the amenorrhea is exercise-related, it is seldom necessary or recommended to give up exercising completely, since exercise stimulates bone formation and may partially compensate for the bone loss that is associated with estrogen deficiency. Eating a well-balanced diet containing an adequate number of calories and at least the recommended dietary allowance of calcium is also important. (For more information about osteoporosis, see Chapter 34.)

Eating Disorders

Whether certain sports cause eating disorders or attract people who already have these disorders is open to debate. However, the emphasis on the advantages of minimum body fat for some sports causes weight loss to becomes an obsession among some athletes, leading to serious disorders such as anorexia nervosa (deliberate self-starvation) or bulimia (binge eating followed by self-induced purging). Both of these self-punishing and dangerous disorders have serious consequences. Athletes engaged in such practices need medical, psychological, and nutritional counseling. (See Chapter 19 for more information.)

25

"Vegetarianism"

Victor Herbert, M.D., J.D.

■

INTRODUCTION

For many people, the interest in food extends far beyond the boundaries of mere sustenance. Diets are selected for numerous other reasons, including promotion of weight loss, prevention of disease, and support of philosophical or religious perceptions.

Vegetarianism, a popular nutritional practice in many parts of the world, has been extolled by its proponents throughout history. Advocates have included followers of many Eastern religions, Trappist monks of the Roman Catholic Church, and people such as Albert Schweitzer, Leonardo da Vinci, Benjamin Franklin, and George Bernard Shaw. Many follow a vegetarian diet because they believe it to be healthier than one with red meat. Others cite social and economic reasons for minimizing meat from the diet; for example, they point out that nine pounds of grain (which can be used to meet human needs) are required for an animal to produce one pound of meat for the table. In economically depressed areas, meat is simply too expensive or unavailable. Others believe that the killing of animals is fundamentally wrong, and they therefore refuse meat and sometimes avoid animal products such as fur and leather, as well. Overzealous "vegetarian" practices are discussed in James Worthon's book *Crusaders for Fitness: A History of American Health Reformers* (Princeton University Press/Consumers Union, 1982). Worton includes the story of Horace Fletcher, a famed faddist who eventually "fletcherized" himself to death from anorexia nervosa. In this chapter we will review the nutritional and health implications of the various "vegetarian" diets.

TYPES OF VEGETARIANISM

Are vegetarian diets healthful? In the past, some nutritionists have questioned whether people can be adequately nourished without animal protein. Studies of the diets and nutritional status of people from poor countries who have a limited food supply are now helping to provide some answers about vegetarian diets. One of the difficulties in clarifying this issue is the diversity among various groups and individuals in their *definitions of what constitutes a vegetarian diet*. Practices range all the way from those who eliminate only red meat to those who limit their diets to a single food. Some objective definitions help to clarify various vegetarian practices:

Vegans, or strict vegetarians. These people consume no animal products, including no eggs or dairy products, but eat only food from plant sources: grains, legumes, fruits, vegetables, nuts, and seeds. They are only about 2 percent of American "vegetarians."

Ovolactovegetarians. They avoid all meat but include in their diet eggs and dairy products, along with all foods from plant sources. Groups that advocate avoidance of animal slaughter generally subscribe to this practice.

Lactovegetarians. This group eliminates only meat and eggs, not dairy products. This form of vegetarianism is practiced by groups such as Hare Krishnas, some Yoga groups, and Trappist monks.

Semi- or partial vegetarians. Such people usually refuse red meat but may include chicken and/or fish along with ovolacto-vegetarian fare, and small amounts of meat.

Classifying the degree of vegetarianism solely on the consumption or exclusion of animal food does not take into account the additional diet modifications practiced by many vegetarian adults. For example, some vegans eat only raw plant food. One group, fruitarians, limits diet to fruits, nuts, seeds, olive oil, honey, and, in some cases, whole grains. Some individuals often devise their own eclectic variations. Other variables frequently associated with vegetarianism include the use of "organically grown" (i.e., without artificial fertilizers or pesticides) or natural foods, avoidances of refined sugar and processed foods, use of megadoses of vitamin supplements, and inclusion of certain foods in the misguided belief that they have special health-promoting or disease-preventing properties.

Because of the many variations on the theme of vegetarianism, generalizations about the adequacy of vegetarian diets are difficult. Some vegetarian diets are well-balanced and healthful; others are too restrictive; and still others are borderline. Thus, each must be evaluated on its own merits.

Many individuals and groups have practiced their types of vegetarianism on a long-term basis and demonstrate excellent health. As with other nutritionally sound diets, those traditional vegetarian diets that are characterized by variety, balance, and moderation pose fewer risks than do those that involve extensive food avoidance or excesses. Dietary restrictions are most hazardous to those whose well-being is already stressed, such as those who are ill or recovering from disease, women who are pregnant or lactating, and infants and growing children.

POSSIBLE HEALTH BENEFITS OF A "VEGETARIAN" DIET

A well-planned vegetarian diet can provide all the food elements necessary for good health, but whether such a diet is actually more healthful or leads to greater longevity than a diet that includes meat has not been established. Conflicting evidence from scientific studies attests to the difficulty in proving that a given finding is attributable to diet alone. It is important to note that many vegetarians alter their lifestyle in addition to diet. For example, Seventh-Day Adventists advocate a vegetarian diet; they also eschew the use of tobacco and alcohol. It may well be a combination of these practices that accounts for the reduced incidence of heart disease among Seventh-Day Adventists, but which practice is most important is difficult to determine. Although the lower incidence of health problems among this group is often attributed to their vegetarianism, it should be noted that they follow a wide range of dietary practices. The Adventist Health Study at Loma Linda University, California, reported that among

Seventh-Day Adventists, 2 percent are vegans, 29 percent are ovolactovegetarians, 25 percent eat meat once a week, 29 percent eat meat one to four times a week, and 15 percent eat meat five or more times a week. In recent years, millions of Americans have similarly changed their eating habits to decrease consumption of red meat and increase consumption of poultry, fish, and complex carbohydrates, and some experts think that this, or its accompanying reduction in saturated fat intake, may be a factor in the marked decrease in heart attacks in recent years.

Studies of members of the Church of Jesus Christ of Latter-Day Saints (Mormons) have found that they enjoy a similarly greater longevity and less chronic disease than the general American population, although their church does not recommend vegetarianism. What Seventh-Day Adventists and Mormons share is abstinence from smoking and alcohol consumption, a strong emphasis on education and family life, and deep commitment to their religion and its teachings. These lifestyle factors may also play a role in their generally favorable health statistics. An interesting sidelight is that sugar consumption in the Mormon capital, Salt Lake City, is one of the highest in the United States.

Perhaps the best-documented benefits of a diet that includes no meat are the following:

Decreased obesity. Vegans are rarely overweight and, on average, even ovolactovegetarians are leaner than meat eaters. The reduced incidence of obesity among vegetarians is probably because vegetables, fruits, and whole grains tend to be high in fiber, making them bulky and more filling than less fibrous foods. Furthermore, since plant foods generally contain little fat—which, gram for gram, contains over twice the number of calories as carbohydrates or proteins—they are less calorie-dense (have fewer calories relative to bulk). Overconsumption of calories produces obesity, which brings out a number of health problems.

It should be noted, however, that vegetarianism does not guarantee slimness. Ovolactovegetarians, who shun meat in favor of rich, high-fat entrées such as quiche, pasta with cream sauces, cheese-laden casseroles, and other dishes loaded with cream, cheese, and butter, can easily consume as many calories, or more, than meat eaters.

Less risk of coronary heart disease. All vegetarians tend to have lower blood-cholesterol levels than meat eaters, and vegans typically have levels that are very low. This is not surprising, since a diet made up solely of plant foods is not only completely devoid of dietary cholesterol but, more importantly, usually very low in saturated fat, as well. Studies have shown most saturated fats, which are predominant in animal foods such as red meat, dairy products, butter and eggs, and the fats from tropical oils (palm and coconut), increase blood-cholesterol levels, while some unsaturated fats, which are predominant in most vegetables, grains, and nuts, help keep blood-cholesterol levels low. High levels of cholesterol in the blood have been correlated with an increased incidence of cardiovascular disease, the number-one cause of death in the United States. Thus, for many people at high risk for atherosclerosis, a diet low in cholesterol-raising fatty acids offers clear benefits.

Less hypertension. Vegetarians have lower blood-pressure levels and are less likely than nonvegetarians to develop hypertension, but why this is true is unknown. The differences cannot be explained solely by lower body weight, although this is probably an important factor, nor by differences in dietary sodium. Possibly, the increased content of potassium, magnesium, polyunsaturated fat, vegetable protein, or fiber in vegetarian diets is related to lower blood pressure. However, the lifestyle often associated with a vegetarian diet may also be a consideration.

Fewer intestinal disorders. Population studies have shown that vegetarians have less constipation and a lower incidence of diverticulosis (a common condition in which small sacs, or diverticula, bulge outward from the lining of the intestine). Vegetables, fruits, and whole grains provide dietary fiber, which tends to produce stools that are bulkier, softer, and pass more quickly through the intestines. An increase in fiber intake relieves constipation and seems to reduce the incidence of and symptoms from diverticular disease in omnivores, as well. An important caution is that too much fiber, eaten all at once, such as two heaping bowls of high-bran cereal for breakfast, can produce intestinal obstruction requiring surgery. There is nothing wrong with one bowl, but two is ridiculous, and grossly violates the rule of moderation, as does pouring high-fiber bran on high-fiber vegetables, which some advertisements suggest.

Vegetarianism has also been credited with a lowered risk of other disorders such as osteoporosis, kidney stones, gallstones, and adult-onset diabetes. Again, appropriate-calorie diet along with many other factors, such as genetic predisposition, hormonal factors, exercise level, smoking, alcohol consumption, and environment, all impact on the occurrence and severity of these problems. Vegetarian diets must also follow the rules of moderation, variety, and balance. For example, high oxalate–high vitamin C vegetarian diets may promote oxalate kidney stones.

CONCERNS REGARDING VEGETARIAN DIETS

For most healthy adults, vegetarian diets planned with care for nutritional adequacy present no known health hazards. Cause for concern increases, however, if the diet becomes restrictive and as individual nutritional requirements increase. Risks of dietary deficiency of important nutrients are highest for growing children and pregnant or lactating women.

Semivegetarians, who eliminate red meat but include fish, fowl, or both in their diets, are at no greater risk than omnivores for malnutrition. Red meat is higher in saturated fats than many other foods, so eating excessive amounts is not prudent. Red meat is nutrient-dense, so modest amounts are a dietary plus.

Similarly, lactovegetarians and ovolactovegetarians have adequate sources of essential nutrients in their diets, since both eggs and milk provide generous amounts of high-quality protein. Care must be taken, however, to assure enough absorbable iron in the diet, since dairy products are poor sources of it and the iron in plant foods is on average only one-fifth as absorbable as the iron in meat, fish, and poultry.

A greater challenge awaits those who eliminate all animal products from their diets. Careful planning must be practiced to ensure that the vegan diet provides a good balance of essential amino acids, sufficient calories, and adequate sources of vitamins D, B_{12}, and B_2 (riboflavin), calcium, iron, and zinc. A closer look at each of these nutrients will help to explain why they are potential problem nutrients for strict vegetarians, and later in this chapter we will discuss ways to assure adequate intake.

Protein and amino acids. Most American adults average about one and a half times the RDA for protein, and protein-deficiency diseases are rare in the United States, except among alcoholics and the very poor. Analyses of the diets of ovolactovegetarians and total vegetarians have consistently shown that while they tend to eat less protein than meat eaters, vegetarians still eat enough.

However, the requirement for protein is not for protein per se, but, rather, a requirement for the 20 amino acids that are the building blocks of human protein. Eleven of the amino acids required by the body for growth and maintenance of body tissues are considered nonessential, because they can be synthesized in the body. However, the other nine amino acids cannot be manufactured in the body and it is essential that the diet supply them. If even one of these essential amino acids is not available in adequate amounts, the body's protein needs will not be met.

To determine whether the protein consumed supplies these essential amino acids, first consider its source. Animal foods such as milk, cheese, meat, and fish contain all the essential amino acids in proportions optimal for human use. Thus, animal proteins are often referred to as complete or high-quality protein. Plant proteins, with the exception of soybeans, are incomplete, meaning that they are deficient in one or more of the amino acids from the essential category. (Soy protein is closer to animal protein than plant protein in its pattern of amino acids.) Fortunately, however, the limitations of other plant proteins can be overcome easily by pairing plant foods that provide complementary proteins. This means that the essential amino acid deficient in one food will be provided by its complementary food. For example, cereal grains, such as wheat, which are poor in the essential amino acid lysine but rich in methionine, can be effectively combined with legumes—dried peas and beans—which provide abundant lysine but little methionine. (See Table 25.1 for a chart of complementary protein sources.)

Choosing food combinations that provide complementary protein may seem complicated in theory, but, in actuality, it's difficult for an adult not to eat complementary proteins if meals follow the guidelines of balance, moderation, and variety. And, while it was once believed that complementary proteins had to be eaten at the same meal to achieve a balanced amino-acid intake, data now suggest that eating different plant proteins in separate meals during the course of a day is adequate for adults, although possibly not for children.

The addition of even a modest amount of any animal protein (except gelatin) will compensate for any essential amino acid underrepresented in any plant food. Thus, partial vegetarians or ovolactovegetarians needn't worry about getting enough high-quality protein.

How much protein is enough? The RDA for protein for an adult is .36 grams per pound of body weight. For most Americans, this figure not only meets requirements but also contains a margin of safety. However, the RDA is based on a diet that includes both animal and vegetable protein. Since plant proteins are somewhat less digestible than animal proteins, the RDA for a strict vegetarian should be about 25 percent higher. For example, a 150-pound omnivore or ovolactovegetarian would need to eat 54 grams of protein to meet his or her RDA, while a 150-pound vegan would need about 68 grams. However, this slightly increased need should not be cause for concern. Any adult vegetarian who consumes adequate calories from a wide variety of nutritious foods is almost certain to meet protein needs also.

Pregnant and lactating women and children require more protein per pound of body weight and RDAs have been set for each of these groups. (See Chapter 4.)

Calories. While vegetarians as a group are leaner than omnivores, obtaining enough calories for energy needs is rarely a problem among adult vegetarians. Very active vegans with a high caloric requirement can maintain their weight by consuming generous amounts of legumes, nuts, nut butters, dried fruits, seeds, and breads. The moderate use of sweets, sweeteners, and added fats (margarine and oils) can also provide extra calories. Meeting caloric needs when only plant foods are consumed is much more difficult for small children.

Vitamin D. Vitamin D is manufactured in the body when the skin is exposed to sunlight and is also plentiful in fortified milk, egg yolks, and fish oils, so deficiency is rare. However, vitamin D-deficiency rickets, a disorder in which the bones are weak and malformed, has been reported in breastfed infants of vegan mothers and in vegan children who have little exposure to sunlight.

Vitamin B$_{12}$. Adequate intake of this vitamin poses a particular problem for vegans because, while vitamin B$_{12}$ is widely available in foods of animal origin, it is not found in plants except when they are contaminated by B$_{12}$-synthesizing microorganisms.

Vegetarians who avoid all animal foods should use fortified soy milk, fortified cereals, fortified meat analogues, or vitamin supplements. Foods such as fermented soy, spirulina, and similar products are often touted to be rich in B$_{12}$, but they are not reliable sources of this vitamin. Studies have shown that a substantial amount of the alleged B$_{12}$ content in these nonanimal foods are actually analogues (warped molecules) of B$_{12}$, which are active only for bacteria, not for humans. Label "B$_{12}$" content is for bacteria.

The requirement for vitamin B$_{12}$ is very small, and it can take years for deficiency to develop. The earliest warning sign of impending B$_{12}$-deficiency anemia may be modest nerve damage, which is curable. A severe de-

Table 25.1. Complementary Vegetable Proteins

The following are examples of complementary vegetable proteins that can be combined to obtain complete proteins.

Combine	With
Legumes: beans, chick-peas, lentils, peas, peanuts, soybeans	Grains: barley, buckwheat, cornmeal, oats, rice, rye, wheat

EXAMPLES OF MEALS: rice-bean casserole, peanut butter sandwich, bean soup with roll, corn tortillas with beans, corn bread and baked beans

Combine	With
Legumes: beans, chick-peas, lentils, peas, peanuts, soybeans	Nuts and seeds: pumpkin, sesame, sunflower

EXAMPLES OF MEALS: dip made with chick-peas, sesame seeds, garlic, lemon and oil, handful of sunflower seeds, and soybeans; lentil salad with sprinkling of sesame seeds; "trail mix" of peanuts, soy nuts, and sunflower seeds; pea soup with pumpkin-seed topping.

Grains: barley, buckwheat, cornmeal, oats, rice, rye, wheat	Milk products: cheese, milk, yogurt

EXAMPLES OF MEALS: macaroni and cheese, cheese sandwich, bread and milk, rice pudding, cereal and milk, corn bread and buttermilk, rice-cheese casserole

The number of vegetable proteins that complement each other in the following combinations are limited to a few foods in each group.

Combine	With
Nuts and seeds: pumpkin, sesame, sunflower	Milk products: cheese, milk, yogurt

EXAMPLES: cheese balls rolled in sesame seeds, milk with sunflower or pumpkin seeds

Nuts and seeds: pumpkin, sesame, sunflower	Grains: barley, buckwheat, cornmeal, oats, rice, rye, wheat

EXAMPLES: breadsticks rolled in sesame seeds, bread with sunflower or sesame seeds, rice with sesame seeds

Legumes: beans, chick-peas, lentils, peas, peanuts, soybeans	Milk products: cheese, milk, yogurt

EXAMPLES: green-pea soup with cheese topping, peanut butter sandwich and milk, pole or butter beans and milk, cooked dried beans with cheese sauce

ficiency, however, can result in severe anemia and irreversible neurological damage. Infants whose only source of food was the milk from their vegan mothers have developed vitamin B_{12} deficiency.

Riboflavin (vitamin B_2). Vegetarian diets that do not contain milk products tend to be marginal in riboflavin, but intakes are still usually adequate. Riboflavin is essential to the function of enzymes that promote the release of energy from food. Dark green leafy vegetables, legumes, whole-grain and enriched-grain products, and brewer's yeast are also good sources of this nutrient and should be stressed in the vegan diet.

Calcium. The strict vegetarian may have difficulty obtaining adequate calcium without dairy products. Typically, dairy products provide about three-fourths of the calcium in American diets, while fruits and vegetables, including potatoes, legumes, nuts, and soy products, provide only one-tenth the total calcium intake. Furthermore, the high-fiber content of calcium-containing vegetables such as broccoli, collard, kale, mustard, and turnip greens may impede the absorption of calcium from these foods. Other high-calcium plant foods—spinach, Swiss chard, beet greens, rhubarb, and sesame seeds—also contain high levels of oxalic acid, a compound that combines with calcium during digestion and prevents its absorption.

Calcium is essential throughout life in order to have strong bones. It also plays important roles in the function of nerves and muscles, enzymes, and in blood coagulation, so it is important that both children and adults have adequate intakes. Dairy products are the best source. However, vegan children and adults can ensure adequate calcium intakes by the regular use of sufficient amounts of fortified soybean milk and tofu (soybean curd) that has been processed with calcium sulfate.

Iron. Iron is essential for the formation of oxygen-carrying blood cells, and an inadequate intake of this mineral causes iron-deficiency anemia. About 40 percent of the iron in animal foods is heme iron, which is absorbed in a particularly efficient way. The other 60 percent of animal iron and all plant iron is nonheme iron, which is absorbed on average only one-fifth as well as heme iron. Thus, vegetarians, especially growing children and women of childbearing age, who have increased iron needs, are at an increased risk for becoming iron-deficient. This is also true of ovolactovegetarians, since neither eggs nor milk are good sources of absorbable iron. Legumes, enriched breads and grains, blackstrap molasses, prune juice, raisins, and some other dried fruits provide moderately absorbable iron for the individual who does not eat meat, poultry, or seafood. Cooking food in iron cookware can increase the iron content of the food significantly, especially acid foods that are simmered for a period of time, such as vegetarian chili and tomato-based soups and sauces.

Dietary factors affect the availability of nonheme iron after it is eaten. For example, a substance called phytic acid, which is found in cereals and whole grains, reacts with plant iron to form insoluble compounds in the intestines. Coffee, tea, and fiber also interfere with nonheme iron absorption. Conversely, vitamin C (ascorbic acid) and other organic acids (malic, tartaric, etc.) enhance the absorption of nonheme iron. Vegetarians should include a dietary source of vitamin C at each meal. Meats contain an "animal protein factor" that enhances the absorption of plant iron, so small amounts of meat in a vegetarian diet go a long way toward preventing iron deficiency.

Zinc. Zinc, which is found in highest concentrations in seafoods (especially oysters), meats, and eggs, has been reported to be below the recommended allowance in the diets of some lacto-, ovolacto-, and total vegetarians. The RDA for zinc was too high, and was reduced in 1989, along with reductions in the RDAs for vitamin B_{12} and folic acid. Although zinc is present in whole grains, this source has several limitations. The amount of zinc in plant foods is affected by the zinc content of the soil in which they are grown. Even when the soil is rich in zinc, grains contain much less zinc than animal and seafood sources. To further complicate matters, the intestinal absorption of zinc from vegetable sources is impaired by dietary fiber, phytate, and possibly other substances that tend to bind the mineral. Thus, vegetarians who limit their diets to foods of vegetable origin may need higher intakes of zinc to assure adequate supplies are absorbed. Hard cheeses, tofu, miso, nuts, wheat germ, and legumes also contain zinc.

See Table 25.2 for a summary chart of problem nutrients for vegetarians.

Table 25.2. Problem Nutrients for Vegetarians

Nutrient	Function	Usual Sources	Vegan Source	Ovolacto	Comments
Vitamin D	Helps body absorb and use calcium. Promotes normal development of bones and teeth.	Sunshine, egg yolks, fish oils (such as cod-liver oil), liver, fortified milk	Sunshine, fortified foods, supplements	Sunshine, fortified milk, egg yolks	
Vitamin B_2	Is essential to the function of enzymes that promote the release of energy from carbohydrates, fats, and proteins.	Milk and milk products, liver, pork, meat	Dark green leafy vegetables, wheat germ, brewer's yeast, enriched and whole-grain breads and cereals, legumes, nuts	Milk, eggs	
Vitamin B_{12}	Is essential for formation of red blood cells and proper functioning of nervous system.	Meat, poultry, seafood, eggs, milk and milk products	Fortified foods, supplements	Eggs, milk and milk products	
Calcium	Is the major building material for bones and teeth; essential for blood clotting, nerve transmission, and muscle contraction.	Milk and milk products, canned sardines and salmon eaten with small bones	Fortified soy milk, tofu (especially when processed with calcium sulfate), calcium, dark green leafy vegetables, blackstrap molasses, fortified foods, supplements	Milk and milk products	Some plant foods contain oxalic acid, which binds with calcium, preventing its absorption. Fiber also interferes with calcium absorption.

A SPECIAL WORD OF CAUTION

A particularly dangerous form of vegetarianism is seen in conjunction with various groups who eat a very restrictive vegetarian diet. One such group subscribe to the Zen macrobiotic diet, which consists of 10 dietary stages. Followers of such macrobiotic diets believe that sequentially eliminating more and more specified foods from the diet as one progresses through the 10 stages will result in a happy, harmonious life. As the individual progresses through the stages, desserts, fruits and salads, animal foods, soup, and vegetables are eliminated one by one and replaced by increased amounts of cereal grains. All dietary stages also encourage fluid restriction. This continues until, at the highest level, only brown rice and small amounts of water or herbal tea are consumed. When a young woman eating such a diet died of undernutrition in New Jersey, a grand jury indictment was brought against her guru.

The lower-level diets can meet nutritional needs, but strict adherence to the higher-level diets has resulted in serious malnutrition and even death. Such restricted diets are especially hazardous to growing children.

Young infants of parents who use the Zen macrobiotic diet are typically fed a food mixture called kokoh, which is made up of ground seeds, brown rice, beans, wheat, oats, and water. Kokoh has been found to be deficient in several vitamins and minerals, includ-

Table 25.2.   Problem Nutrients for Vegetarians *(cont.)*

Iron	Is an integral part of hemoglobin, which carries oxygen in the red blood cells; component of enzymes involved in energy metabolism.	Liver, red meat, poultry, seafood	Enriched and whole-grain breads and cereals, wheat germ, seeds, nuts, blackstrap molasses, raisins, prune juice, potato skins, green leafy vegetables, tofu, miso, brewer's yeast, foods cooked in cast-iron cookware	Same as for vegan	The nonheme iron in plants is much less well absorbed than the heme iron in meat. The fiber in plants also interferes with plant iron absorption, as do coffee, tea, and calcium supplements when taken with or shortly before or after a meal.
Zinc	Is essential to the composition or function of over 70 enzymes in the body; necessary for protein synthesis in body cells; role in reproduction, taste acuity, and function of immune system.	Shellfish (esp. oysters), liver, red meat, dark-meat poultry, egg yolks	Nuts, legumes, miso, pumpkin and sunflower seeds, wheat germ, whole-grain yeast breads, whole-grain cereals	Milk and milk products, egg yolks (+ vegan sources)	The phytate in whole grains and the fiber in many plant foods bind zinc, interfering with its absorption. Calcium and iron supplements can also interfere with zinc absorption.

ing calcium, iron, and vitamin B_{12}. Since Zen followers frequently refuse nutrient supplementation, extreme growth retardation and death have been reported in infants on this diet.

SPECIAL CONSIDERATIONS

Pregnant and Lactating Women

The development and growth of the fetus is affected by the mother's nutritional state. Malnutrition during the critical period of development can result in a variety of negative manifestations, ranging from suboptimal growth to poor dental health to mental retardation. The pregnant woman has an increased need for many nutrients, including calories, protein, B vitamins, vitamin C, calcium, phosphorus, iron, magnesium, iodine, and zinc. Although some of these are plentiful in the strict vegetarian diet, the requirements for others can be met only by careful planning or supplementation. The vegan diets of pregnant and lactating women who do not take vitamin supplements have frequently been found to be deficient in iron, calcium, zinc, and vitamins B_{12} and D.

The Food and Nutrition Board of the National Academy of Sciences recommends that pregnant women eat an average of 300 extra calories per day during their pregnancy. Breastfeeding women require an extra 500 calories per day. Adequate caloric intake is important not only to assure that sufficient energy is available for the growth of the fetus but also to assure that protein will be used for its intended purpose of building new tissue, and not broken down for energy. The pregnant vegetarian woman, like the pregnant meat-eating woman, should gain 25 to 30

pounds during the course of her pregnancy. Expectant mothers whose caloric intake is inadequate for the recommended gain are likely to give birth to a baby of low birth weight and subsequently to produce inadequate milk.

Pregnant women also require about 10 grams of extra protein each day, while lactating women require an additional 15 grams. Ovolactovegetarians should have no problem meeting this increased requirement, but vegans should plan their diets carefully. Soy products (soy milk, soybeans, tofu, meat analogues, etc.) are highly recommended, since soy protein is the only complete protein of vegetable origin.

Iron is needed to support the increased maternal blood volume and to provide iron stores for the fetus. Since iron found in sources other than meat is less well absorbed, it is especially difficult to avoid depletion of maternal iron stores and subsequent anemia in this group. At birth, an infant should have enough stored iron obtained from the mother's iron reserves to supply needs for the first few months of life. Iron requirements of the pregnant vegetarian woman are best met by appropriate supplementation. Large amounts of iron block zinc absorption, so iron supplements should be modest in pregnant vegetarian women, to avoid zinc deficiency in the newborn.

Similarly, the mother supplies the calcium needed for the mineralization of fetal bones and later for milk production. When calcium levels in the mother's blood are not adequate for her needs and those of the fetus, calcium deposited in her bones is withdrawn for other essential functions. Pregnant or breastfeeding ovolactovegetarians easily can meet their increased calcium needs by consuming four portions of milk, cheese, and yogurt daily. If the vegan uses fortified soy milk to replace dairy products, her calcium needs also can be met easily. However, the vegan who does not use soy milk will have considerable difficulty consuming adequate calcium during pregnancy and lactation. Almost seven cups of chopped broccoli or three and a quarter cups of almonds are required to provide the daily requirement of 1,200 milligrams of calcium, and the absorbability of the calcium from these sources is questionable. Calcium supplements are another alternative, but the form of the calcium salt in some calcium pills makes the calcium very poorly absorbed. Studies indicate that calcium citrate is well absorbed, as is calcium carbonate unless there is reduced gastric acid, a frequent problem in the elderly.

Breastfeeding, especially during the first six months of life, is a generally encouraged practice because of the many nutritional and other health benefits provided by human milk. The nursing mother also requires more of many nutrients than the nonpregnant woman. Both the quantity and the nutritional quality of maternal milk is important in order to sustain good growth in the infant for the first six months of life. The composition of nutrients in human milk is remarkably constant and a nutrient shortage in the mother's diet is more likely to reduce the quantity than the quality of the mother's milk.

One nutrient that is present only in low concentration in human milk regardless of the mother's diet is vitamin D. Vitamin D is important in the absorption of calcium from the intestine. Vitamin D-fortified milk or a supplement is usually recommended for pregnant and lactating vegetarian women. Breastfed infants should also receive vitamin D supplements.

Similarly, vitamin B_{12} supplements or foods fortified with vitamin B_{12} are recommended for pregnant and lactating vegan women as well as for their breastfed infants because this vitamin is found in significant amounts only in foods of animal origin. In omnivores, vitamin B_{12} stores in the newborn are adequate for the first year of life. However, the vegan mother's diet may not provide adequate amounts for these reserves. The problem is compounded by the fact that inadequate B_{12} in the infant's diet may result in anemia and neurologic abnormalities.

Children and Teens

The rapid growth and relatively high nutrient needs of infants and children and teens create special nutritional risks for those whose diets do not include animal products. Although some of the concerns are the same as for adults, the consequences of inadequate nutrition for the young are potentially more harmful.

The most apparent problem is that growing children on vegetarian diets may be unable to meet their needs for energy. Simply stated, kids with their relatively small stomach volumes just can't eat enough vegetables, fruits, and grains to supply their caloric needs. Most of these foods are high in fiber, making them bulky and quite filling, but they are not very high in calories. For example, a cup of beans would be a very large portion for a five-year-old, yet this amount provides only 240 calories, which is just 14 percent of the energy requirements at this age. In comparison, a young child would have no problem drinking a cup of milk (about 150 calories) along with a full meal or as part of a snack.

What happens when energy needs are not met? Protein, the source of vital amino acids, is broken down to provide fuel for the body and is not available for its intended purpose of growth and repair.

A balanced ovolactovegetarian diet easily can meet the nutritional needs of children and teens. Clear evidence of this is seen in Seventh-Day Adventist cultures in which this type of vegetarianism has been practiced by several generations without adverse health effects.

More strict vegetarian diets may not meet the nutritional needs of the young and can lead to health problems. Several studies have found that vegan children are of shorter stature and lower weight than those who consume animal products. The Committee on Nutrition of the American Academy of Pediatrics, the Food and Nutrition Board of the National Research Council–National Academy of Sciences, and the American Dietetic Association have all expressed concern about the hazards of very restricted vegetarian diets for young children.

Parents who insist on a vegan diet for their child should consult a registered dietitian who works with a pediatrician for help in meal planning. Children on such diets should also be routinely monitored by a pediatrician who will work with the dietitian to assure normal growth and development.

Table 25.3. Sample Menus for Various Types of Vegetarians

The following menus are designed to provide a balance of essential nutrients without including meat.

Ovolacto Vegetarianism

BREAKFAST	Orange juice	DINNER	Vegetable lasagna
	Whole-grain cereal		Marinated white beans
	Low-fat milk		Spinach salad
	Cranberry nut muffin		Angel food cake with frozen yogurt (or
LUNCH	Zucchini and cheese omelette		fresh fruit)
	Carrot raisin slaw		Beverage
	Corn bread	SNACK (optional)	Yogurt with freesh berries
	Fresh fruit		Cheese with whole-grain wheat or
	Beverage		graham crackers

Ovolacto-Fish/Seafood

BREAKFAST	Stewed prunes	DINNER	Baked salmon with lemon
	French toast with wheat germ and honey		Steamed broccoli
	Low-fat milk		Wild rice
LUNCH	Lentil soup		Mixed green salad with vinaigrette
	Macaroni salad with tuna		dressing
	Fresh apple		Vanilla ice milk
	Beverage		Beverage
		SNACK (optional)	Graham crackers
			Low-fat milk

Vegan

BREAKFAST	Pineapple juice	DINNER	Bean and tomato soup
	Oatmeal with raisins		Tofu† and vegetable stir-fry
	Date nut bread		Whole-wheat pasta
	Soy milk*		Mixed salad
LUNCH	Soybean burger on whole-wheat bun		Sesame breadsticks
	Leaf lettuce and tomato		Rice pudding*
	Sliced peaches		Beverage
	Peanut butter and raisin cookie	SNACK	Oatmeal muffin
	Beverage		Soy milk*

*B$_{12}$- and calcium-fortified soy milk
†calcium-precipitated tofu

PLANNING THE NUTRITIOUS VEGETARIAN DIET

Many of the concerns that motivate new eating patterns are valid, but it isn't necessary to eliminate all animal products from the diet to achieve the health benefits associated with vegetarianism, which are primarily those of not overeating. Less radical measures can also offer the same advantages. Vegetarians correctly claim that it's not necessary to eat meat at every meal, or even every day. At some meals, one can replace it with dishes that include milk, cheese, eggs, or legumes as the primary source of protein. When meat is included in a meal, one can keep servings small and emphasize a variety of vegetables, fruits, and grains. These practices add fiber to the diet and reduce fat and caloric intake. Furthermore, the selection of a wide variety of foods is the best way to assure a nutritious diet. Small amounts of animal, fish, and poultry meats help.

Two of the best sources of information on nutritious vegetarian diets are the Proceedings of the First International Congress on Vegetarian Nutrition, published as a 222-page supplement to the looseleaf *Diet Manual Including a Vegetarian Meal Plan,* published by The Seventh-Day Adventists Dietetic Association of Loma Linda, California (P.O. Box 75, 92354). The Second International Congress on Vegetarian Nutrition is planned for spring of 1992 in Washington, D.C., by the Loma Linda University Department of Nutrition.

Part V

The Role of Nutrition in Common Diseases

26

Nutrition and Heart Disease

W. Virgil Brown, M.D.

■

INTRODUCTION

Cardiovascular disease remains our leading cause of death despite a significant decline in fatal heart attacks in recent years. According to the American Heart Association, more than 60 million Americans have some form of heart or blood-vessel disease, and nearly a million die of these disorders annually. Heart attacks claim the most lives—about 540,000 a year. In addition, about 150,000 die each year from strokes, and 30,000 more die from other effects of high blood pressure.

Both heart attacks and strokes can strike people in the prime of life. Nearly half of the 1.5 million people who suffer a heart attack in the course of a year are under the age of 65. In a large percentage of heart attacks, the victims have had no obvious symptoms to suggest that they were walking about with a potentially fatal disease. Despite modern medical techniques that now save thousands of lives that would have been lost in earlier years, first heart attacks still kill about a third of their victims.

The toll of heart disease, both financial and human, is tremendous. The American Heart Association estimates that cardiovascular disease adds a whopping $85.2 bil-lion to the nation's medical bill each year. The numbers of people involved are staggering. According to American Heart Association estimates, 59 million Americans have high blood pressure and more than 5 million are affected to varying degrees by angina or other manifestations of coronary disease. Their lost productivity adds to the total cost of heart disease. Of course, the economic losses do not take into account the human suffering to both the victims and their loved ones. In this chapter, we will concentrate on the associations between nutrition and our most common forms of cardiovascular disease—namely, coronary heart disease and high blood pressure.

ATHEROSCLEROSIS AND CORONARY HEART DISEASE

The cause of coronary heart disease is almost always atherosclerosis, a form of arteriosclerosis (hardening of the arteries) in which fatty deposits build up on the inner arterial walls and interfere with blood flow to the heart muscle. Although all of the body's blood passes through the heart every few minutes, the heart itself does not derive its oxygen and nutrients from the blood it pumps through its chambers and into the general circulation. Instead, a small fraction of that blood flow enters the coronary arteries, which encircle the heart like a crown (thus the word *coronary*), and is responsible for nourishing the heart muscle. If one or more of these coronary arteries becomes blocked or very narrowed, the heart muscle in that area is deprived of adequate oxygen, a condition referred to as myocardial (heart muscle) ischemia (lack of oxygen). This can cause the chest pains called angina (meaning pain) pectoris (of the chest), but very often the ischemia is "silent," or symptomless. If a vessel becomes completely blocked—usually by formation of a blood clot (coronary thrombosis) in the narrowed artery—a heart attack occurs. This is referred to as a myocardial infarction, which literally means heart-muscle death.

Figure 26.1.

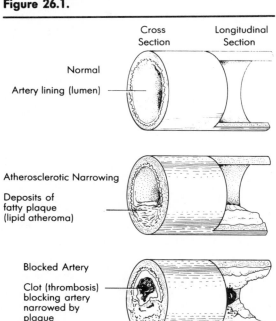

Cross Section | Longitudinal Section

Normal
Artery lining (lumen)

Atherosclerotic Narrowing
Deposits of fatty plaque (lipid atheroma)

Blocked Artery
Clot (thrombosis) blocking artery narrowed by plaque

If the degree of heart-muscle destruction is not too severe, the heart may continue to beat and pump enough blood to sustain life and even reasonably normal function. In many instances, however, the infarction causes the heart to lose its synchronous beat—a condition known as ventricular fibrillation. Instead of pumping blood with each beat, the heart muscle quivers in an uncontrolled fashion and is unable to continue vital circulation. Unless quickly reversed, ventricular fibrillation results in death. Death also may occur if so much heart muscle is destroyed that the heart cannot pump enough blood to support life.

Atherosclerosis is a slowly progressive disease. Although it is thought to begin quite early in life, it rarely becomes sufficiently advanced to produce symptoms or cause a heart attack until middle age. The precise causes of atherosclerosis are unknown, but people with high levels of blood cholesterol and a clotting protein called blood fibrinogen are known to have a greater incidence of the disorder. Recent studies have demonstrated that lowering an elevated amount of cholesterol circulating in the bloodstream can actually cause a reduction in the fatty deposits. Atherosclerosis and the consequent coronary heart disease are often described as the epidemic diseases of today's industrialized, economically advanced societies. Epidemic diseases seldom have a single cause; a number of factors must be present for them to become rampant in a society. Tuberculosis, for example, was a major epidemic disease until the early part of this century. Although the causative tuberculosis bacterium was necessary to spread the disease, this alone did not account for the massive epidemics that made TB the leading cause of death in many countries. The other prerequisites were a result of the Industrial Revolution: crowded slums, malnutrition, poor sanitation, child labor, unhealthy work places, and inadequate public health and medical care. When these contributing conditions were eased, tuberculosis began to decline, even before the discovery of curative antibiotics.

Similarly, most experts today stress that our modern epidemic of cardiovascular disease has multiple causes, many of which can be traced to an accumulation of social, economic, and cultural factors. Although we think that diet is a major contributing factor, it is by no means the only one; a number of other factors that increase the risk of a heart attack have been identified. Whereas it is impossible to predict whether any particular individual will have a heart attack, we know that the chances are increased in the presence of specific risk factors. Some of these are beyond our control, but many can be modified or reduced. The major cardiovascular risk factors are the following.

Gender. Men of all ages have more heart attacks than women, although the incidence among women rises after menopause, and as women age, they almost catch up with men. Why men should be more vulnerable is not fully understood, although it is thought that women derive some protection from estrogen, the major female sex hormone. Studies have found that postmenopausal women who do not take replacement estrogen have a rise in LDL cholesterol, which is thought to increase atherosclerosis, and a decrease in the protective HDL cholesterol. In contrast, men tend to have higher levels of LDL and lower levels of HDL throughout adulthood. This may be due to testosterone, the male sex hormone, which is known to raise both total cholesterol and lower protective HDL cholesterol. (See also Chapter 6.)

Age. The chance of having a heart attack increases with age. About 55 percent of all heart-attack victims are over the age of 65. Of those who die, almost four out of five are 65 or older.

Heredity. Heart attacks and atherosclerosis tend to run in families. The risk is highest in people who have a first-degree relative (parent or sibling) who suffered a fatal heart attack before the age of 50.

Race. Among Americans, black men have a higher incidence of heart disease than men of other races. This is in large part due to the fact that blacks have a 33 percent greater chance of having high blood pressure, but other factors, such as diet and stress, also may play a role.

The above risk factors are beyond individual control, although people who fall into these groups can take extra precautions to minimize controllable risk factors—specifically, those that can be avoided or altered. They include the following factors.

Cigarette smoking. Smokers have almost a threefold increase in heart attacks compared to nonsmokers. Cigarette smoking is also considered the major risk factor for sudden cardiac death. A heart attack in a smoker is more likely to be fatal than in a nonsmoker. In addition, smoking is the leading risk factor in peripheral vascular disease, the narrowing of vessels that carry blood to the arms and legs. The benefits of stopping cigarette use have been demonstrated. Studies have found that regardless of how long a person has smoked, the risk of a heart attack declines after stopping. Within 10 years of stopping, the risk of a heart attack for ex-smokers is about the same as for people who have never smoked.

Smoking is known to affect the heart in a number of ways. Nicotine causes an almost immediate rise in blood pressure and heart rate. In a person susceptible to disturbances in the heart's rhythmic beat, repeated exposure to nicotine can increase the risk of serious arrhythmias. Smoking raises levels of fibrinogen, which increases the blood's tendency to clot, which, in turn, may increase the likelihood of a coronary thrombosis. Smoking tends to lower HDL cholesterol, and some researchers also think that tobacco use may be instrumental in initiating atherosclerosis.

High blood pressure. People with undetected or inadequately treated high blood pressure—defined as 140/90 or higher—have an increased risk of heart attacks, congestive heart failure, and strokes. The risk is even greater when combined with other risk factors, particularly cigarette smoking. (See the section on high blood pressure on page 456 for a more detailed discussion.)

High blood cholesterol. People under the age of 50 who have cholesterol levels of more than 240 milligrams per deciliter (mg./dl.) of blood plasma are considered at risk for a heart attack, and the higher the cholesterol, the greater the risk. Anyone whose cholesterol level is more than 240 milligrams per deciliter should be tested further to determine levels of LDL and HDL cholesterol. LDL cholesterol over 160 is too high in any adult; if there are other risk factors, such as high blood pressure or cigarette smoking, an LDL of 130 or greater should cause concern about the risk of a heart attack.

Diabetes mellitus. People with diabetes have an increased incidence of heart attacks and other cardiovascular diseases. Most people who develop adult-onset diabetes, which usually occurs during middle age, also are overweight, a contributing factor for cardiovascular disorders. Diabetics also have a higher prevalence of high blood pressure and elevated blood cholesterol.

Obesity. The Framingham Heart Study, insurance statistics, and other large-scale studies show that people who are markedly overweight are prone to a number of illnesses, including cardiovascular disease. Obesity also increases the risk of high blood pressure, diabetes, and high blood cholesterol.

Stress. Although most people believe that psychosocial stress is important in causing heart attacks, the scientific evidence for this is extremely weak. There is considerable evidence that sudden, unusually heavy exercise can trigger a heart attack in a susceptible individual, and this has led some people to attribute such an event to stress in a broader, more prolonged context. Animal studies indicate that monkeys that develop increased blood pressure and higher pulse rates when under stress are more likely to develop atherosclerosis when fed a high-cholesterol diet than their counterparts who do not show these physical responses. In some way, this may be linked to the personality characteristics discussed subsequently, but this has not been proved.

Personality characteristics. Some studies have found that people who have Type A personalities, as defined by particular psychological tests, have an increased risk of heart attacks. Not all experts agree as to what the Type A personality designation means, but, in general, its traits include aggressiveness and increased time awareness, anger, hostility, and a drive to succeed. Recent studies at Duke University indicate that of these traits, anger and hostility may be the ones that increase heart-attack risk. The Duke researchers found that patients who score high in hostility have more atherosclerosis and coronary disease than other Type A's who were not so angry or hostile. More research is needed, however, to determine whether anger and hostility are, indeed, cardiovascular risk factors.

Sedentary lifestyle. Although a lack of exercise has not been clearly established as increasing the risk of a heart attack, it can contribute to other risk factors, such as obesity. Studies also have shown that people who exercise regularly have a lower incidence of heart attacks. This may be due to a number of factors, including reduced weight, lowered blood cholesterol, or the development of collateral circulation to increase the heart muscle's blood supply.

THE RELATIONSHIP BETWEEN DIET AND HEART DISEASE

For more than forty years, the effect of the American diet on the heart has been a subject of investigation. A large number of epidemiological studies have compared dietary factors with heart-disease statistics. Although data from these studies point to diet as a major factor in cardiovascular health, there still are many unanswered questions. Over the last few decades, for example, almost every component of the diet has been linked in some way with heart disease, and consumers have been bombarded by often-conflicting advice. Fat, cholesterol, sugar, salt, caffeine, alcohol, protein, excessive calories, and even the mineral content of drinking water are but a few of the dietary factors that have been purported—in some cases on very shaky grounds—to increase risk of heart disease. In contrast, protective effects have been attributed—again, often without scientific proof—to a variety of substances, including unsaturated fats, fish oil, various vitamins and minerals, and fiber, among others.

In many instances, the evidence linking a specific dietary factor to cardiovascular health is too skimpy and insufficient to warrant recommending changes in eating habits. Frequently, further study reverses earlier conclusions. A case in point involves sugar. Some

years ago, a group of researchers postulated that the high sugar consumption in industrialized countries contributed to the coincidental increased incidence of heart attacks, compared to population groups that ate little or no refined sugar. Although the data did not separate cause and effect from coincidence, a number of popular nutrition writers such as the late Adelle Davis and J. I. Rodale took the message that sugar causes heart attacks to the general public. Current scientific evidence indicates that sugar per se has little if any relationship with heart disease. Still, this notion persists among many, especially purveyors of natural foods, as well as people who are genuinely concerned about eating a heart-healthy diet. They often pay inflated prices for sugar-free health foods that may be loaded with ingredients such as saturated fats and oils, which in fact do have an established link with heart disease.

More recently, there has been a mushrooming interest in fish oils, fiber, and various vitamin regimens as preventives for heart attack. Again, claims are based on emerging or incomplete data. At this point, there is no scientific basis to recommend fish-oil supplements (even though this is the message in many advertisements for these products) or the consumption of megadoses of vitamins and minerals in the hopes of reducing deaths from heart attack. Indeed, these measures may create a whole new set of health problems.

Given our current knowledge, moderation and prudence should be the basis for any nutritional guidelines to improve cardiovascular health. Although there are some experts (both recognized and self-styled) who advise massive overhauling of the American diet from cradle to grave, the consensus—as reflected in recommendations from the American Heart Association, National Cholesterol Education Program and other such organizations—calls for moderate changes in very specific areas. More rigid changes, such as a strict low-fat diet, are recommended only after careful evaluation by health professionals.

We believe there is enough good evidence to advise people on a few very important issues—namely, cholesterol, fat and sodium intake, weight control, and tobacco and alcohol use. Some of the most frequently asked questions regarding cholesterol are listed on page 437. The following sections review some of the major studies linking coronary disease and diet and outline specific dietary guidelines. (Please refer to Chapter 6 for further background information and guidelines regarding these two components, and to Chapter 17 for other material relevant to heart disease and diet.)

THE CHOLESTEROL FACTOR

Without a doubt, cholesterol is the most familiar nutritional factor affecting cardiovascular health; it is also one of the most misunderstood. As stressed in Chapter 6, misconceptions abound regarding the role of dietary cholesterol as a risk factor for heart attack. Many people fail to distinguish between dietary cholesterol—what you eat—and serum cholesterol—what circulates in your bloodstream. Elevated levels of the latter are strongly associated with an increased risk of heart attack. While a diet high in cholesterol-rich foods—eggs, whole milk, cheese, meat, and other animal products—will raise blood cholesterol, there are other major factors involved. Some people consume large amounts of cholesterol yet have low serum-cholesterol levels, while others may eat a low-cholesterol diet and still have high serum-cholesterol levels. The controlling factors appear to be the amount of saturated fat and calories in the diet, as well as hereditary controls of cholesterol metabolism and transport in the blood. *Type* of saturated fat also counts.

The Evidence to Date

The relationship between cholesterol, atherosclerosis, and heart attacks is probably the most-studied aspect of coronary disease. Even in the 1930s, some farsighted researchers were reviewing studies by a Russian scientist named Anitshkov, who noted that rabbits fed a high-cholesterol diet developed atherosclerosis. They began trying to determine whether the same was true of human beings. However, it was not until after World War II that large numbers of studies were undertaken, often comparing a number of different population groups in an attempt to pinpoint why some had high cardiovascular death rates and others were relatively unaffected.

One of the most extensive early projects—the International Cooperative Study on the Epidemiology of Cardiovascular Disease (commonly referred to as the Seven-Country Study)—screened 12,000 men from 18 different population groups in seven countries. During the 10-year study, marked differences in the prevalence of heart disease among the men, who were 40 to 59 years old when they entered the project, were noted. Men from eastern Finland had the highest prevalence of heart disease, with groups from western Finland, the Netherlands, and the United States not far behind. Japan, Greece, and Yugoslavia displayed the lowest rates.

In analyzing the diets of these men, the researchers noted differences in fat and cholesterol intake. The Japanese ate very little fat of any sort. In other countries, *total* fat seemed less important. Almost 40 percent of total calories came from fat in the diets of inhabitants of Crete, Zutphen in the Netherlands, the

Some of the Most Frequently Asked Questions and Answers About Cholesterol

Q. How often should a person have his or her blood-cholesterol level checked?

A. Doctors are increasingly making such a blood cholesterol test part of the routine physical examination, and patients should request it if it is not suggested. For a low-risk adult whose reading was below 200 on at least two occasions, measurement every five years should be sufficient. Children who are at high risk for developing atherosclerosis (i.e., with close family members who had a heart attack or heart disease before the age of 50) should be tested by the time they are six or seven. All people should have a baseline test when they are about 20, regardless of risk factors.

Q. At what blood-cholesterol level should a person become seriously concerned about the possibility of a heart attack?

A. One should be concerned when the level is above 240. Remember, however, that having a cholesterol level of 180 is better than one of 200, and that coronary heart disease accelerates above the 220 level. An increase in blood cholesterol to 265 represents a 200 percent increase in risk over that at 200.

Q. How much can a person realistically expect to lower his or her elevated blood cholesterol by going on a low-cholesterol diet?

A. Reduction varies with the individual. Usually a 10 to 15 percent lowering in LDL can be expected. Blood cholesterol can be reduced by as much as 30 percent in three to four weeks by some people on a very strict diet. However, most diets do not produce fast results, and as a consequence, they are often abandoned before they have a chance to become effective. It may take six months to establish new dietary habits necessary to a meaningful reduction in the blood level. The important issue is how long cholesterol stays down, not how quickly it comes down.

Q. Concerning saturated fats, what are the most deceptive products in the supermarket?

A. Probably bakery goods and cream substitutes, which may have highly saturated palm and coconut oil as ingredients. In general, products that do not specify the type of vegetable oil may contain either of these.

Q. Are there any dangers in a low-cholesterol diet?

A. None, so long as a balanced diet is followed and the alterations are reasonable, such as those recommended by the American Heart Association for adults and the American Academy of Pediatrics for children.

Q. Why not take cholesterol-lowering drugs instead of going on a diet?

A. Drugs are not a substitute for diet. Drug therapy is used in combination with diet therapy only when diet alone is not successful in lowering cholesterol. A diet high in saturated fats can negate some of the medication's effects. Drugs do not cure high cholesterol, must be taken indefinitely, and many have unpleasant or even potentially dangerous side effects.

Q. How is it that some people can eat saturated fats and cholesterol and yet have a normal blood-cholesterol level?

A. Genetically, people have different capacities to process fats and other lipids in the body. Some can eat what they want and develop no problems. If HDL is normal or high, and the LDL is under 100 milligrams per deciliter, heart disease is rare. On the other hand, dietary cholesterol may add to the risk even in persons with average or below-average blood-cholesterol levels. There are factors about diet and heart disease that are not fully explained by the blood-cholesterol or even the blood-lipoprotein levels. For example, eating fish may lower the risk by reducing the ability of blood to clot and yet this may not change blood-cholesterol levels, and dietary cholesterol may increase the risk without raising blood cholesterol.

United States, and eastern Finland. However, the men from Crete enjoyed a much lower incidence of heart disease than those from Finland, the United States, and the Netherlands. Further analysis showed that most of the fat in the Cretan diet came from olive oil, which is high in monounsaturated fatty acids, with only a small portion (8 percent of total calories) from saturated fats. In contrast, the fats consumed in Finland, the United States, and the Netherlands contained many more saturated animal fats (18 to 22 percent of calories). Men from these countries also were found to have blood-cholesterol levels that were significantly higher than those of the Cretan men. The consistent message is that consumption of large amounts of saturated fats leads to high blood cholesterol and high rates of heart disease within a population.

Since this landmark project, which was carried out in the 1960s, scores of other studies have concentrated on further defining the link between diet and heart disease, with the emphasis on saturated fats and cholesterol. For example, the Framingham Heart Study, a 40-year-long research project involving several thousand people in this Boston suburb, found that men with an average cholesterol level of 260 milligrams per deciliter of blood plasma suffered heart attacks three to five times as often as men with levels below 195. Even more modest blood-cholesterol levels of 220 to 240—the average for middle-aged American men and a range that had long been considered normal by most American physicians—correlate with an increased risk, especially if the ratio of LDL to HDL cholesterol is high. More recent Framingham reports suggest that these conclusions are much stronger for people 60 or younger; after 60, cholesterol levels are less predictive of a heart heart attack. (It should be noted, however, that HDL and LDL levels are still useful predictors, even in this older age group, par-

ticularly for risk related to low HDL values.)

On a nationwide level, the most extensive study has been the Multiple Risk Factor Intervention Trial, or MR FIT, as it is popularly known. From 1973 to 1985, researchers at 22 MR FIT clinics in 18 cities followed a total of 356,222 men between the ages of 35 and 57. In a 1986 report by Dr. Jeremiah Stamler of Chicago and his colleagues at the MR FIT Coordinating Center at the University of Minnesota, the researchers stressed that cardiovascular risk was not confined to the highest cholesterol levels. Instead, they found a continuously rising risk of heart attack beginning with blood-cholesterol levels of 180 milligrams per deciliter. This level was lower than had been expected, leading the researchers to warn that even slightly elevated blood cholesterol "powerfully affects risk for the great majority of middle-aged men."

Analysis of MR FIT data showed that, when compared to those with cholesterol levels of less than 182 over a six-year period, the heart-attack death rate was increased by 29 percent for men with blood-cholesterol levels of 182 to 202; by 73 percent for those with levels of 203 to 220; by 121 percent for those with levels of 221 to 244; and by 242 percent for those with levels above 245. The study emphasized that the danger of high blood cholesterol was amplified by the coexistence of high blood pressure, cigarette smoking, obesity, diabetes, and so forth.

On the other hand, lower blood cholesterol means less heart disease in all groups with comparable risk factors. This is most clearly manifested in societies such as Japan where a low rate of heart disease accompanies low cholesterol even when high blood pressure, smoking, and other risk factors abound.

In the face of these and other scientific studies, there seems little doubt that elevated blood cholesterol increases the risk of a heart attack. Will lowering blood cholesterol actually decrease the risk, however? The MR FIT study did not provide an answer. Experts have debated this crucial question for decades, but recent research suggests the answer is yes.

A study of people with high serum cholesterol, conducted by Dr. David Blankenhorn and his colleagues at the University of Southern California, found that a strict low-fat, low-cholesterol diet combined with cholesterol-lowering drugs (colestipol and niacin) resulted in slowing the coronary disease in most men and, for about one out of six participants, an actual shrinking of the fatty deposits in the coronary arteries. The two-year study involved 162 men who did not smoke and who had undergone earlier coronary-bypass surgery. The men were divided into two groups: One followed a diet that allowed no more than 125 milligrams of cholesterol a day and no more than 22 percent of calories consumed from fats. These men also took the cholesterol-lowering drugs. The other group ate a less restrictive diet and took placebos instead of the actual drugs.

At the end of two years, the researchers reported an average 43-percent drop in LDL cholesterol and a 37-percent rise in protective HDL cholesterol. In contrast, the control group showed an average improvement of no more than 5 percent. Additional fatty deposits had formed in 61 percent of the placebo group, compared to 39 percent of the men in the treatment group. More encouraging was the fact that 16 percent of the men in the diet-drug group showed less blockage of their arteries than when they had entered the study. Only 2 percent of the placebo group showed improvement.

In describing the significance of these findings, Dr. Blankenhorn said the study demonstrated "that the basic process that causes coronary artery disease can be reversed at the level of the artery wall." Dr. Claude Lenfant, director of the National Heart, Lung and Blood Institute, added that, in his opinion, the California study also supported the belief that a low-fat, low-cholesterol diet alone can be beneficial. "Only if diet fails should one go to drugs," he stated.

Of course, it should be noted that the California study was small and involved a special subset of patients. Still, it did show that a marked reduction in blood cholesterol by drugs plus diet may reverse earlier damage to the coronary arteries.

Dietary Guidelines

As noted in Chapter 6, it is generally agreed that the average American, as well as people in other industrialized countries, consumes a diet too high in saturated fat and cholesterol. Diets in Western developed countries also tend to be relatively high in refined carbohydrates (i.e., sugar) and animal protein and low in dietary fiber. In contrast, diets in Oriental and undeveloped countries tend to be comparatively low in fats, particularly animal fats, and high in complex carbohydrates. Exercise as physical labor also produces a better caloric balance in these countries, and there is less obesity. (It is not the excess calories as much as the lack of burning those calories that leads to obesity in Western society. We eat about the same but do less.) Sorting out which dietary differences are significant can be difficult and misleading, as witness the earlier example of sugar. However, when the epidemiologic data are combined with direct experimental studies, more accurate theories can be developed.

The Seven-Country Study, for example, showed that total fat appears to be a less important factor than the nature of the fat. The olive oil used to prepare much Mediterranean food gives it a high fat content, about equal to that of the American diet. However, olive oil is very low in saturated fats (high in monoun-saturated fats), whereas the American diet is rich in animal fats (highly saturated), which raises blood cholesterol.

Heart Association Guidelines

In an attempt to unify previous, some-times conflicting dietary advice and to focus on the total nutritional picture, the American Heart Association issued new guidelines in 1986. These guidelines emphasize "a gradual but steady modification in the diets of healthy adults." (Some of the recommendations have since been refined in the 1987 guidelines by the National Cholesterol Education Program, which is discussed on page 446.) Since a per-son's nutrient needs vary according to size, activity, and special situations, such as preg-nancy, the guidelines are based on percent-ages of calories consumed. Specifically, the dietary goals instructed the following.

1. *Saturated fat intake should be less than 10 percent of calories.* Presently, about 12 to 18 percent of the calories in the typical American diet come from saturated fat, mostly from ani-mal products and the coconut and palm oil and cocoa butter in commercial baked goods. A reduction in these foods is usually sufficient to bring saturated fat intake to the 10-percent goal (see Chapter 6, Tips on Low-Fat Cooking and Shopping on page 71).

2. *Total fat intake should be less than 30 per-cent of calories.* This compares with the pres-ent average intake of 35 to 40 percent of calories. Again, the Heart Association stresses that the reduction should be from saturated fats. In fact, polyunsaturated and monoun-saturated fats could be consumed in the amounts currently eaten by Americans with-out effect on blood cholesterol. The cho-lesterol-lowering effect is derived primarily from reducing saturated fat. The monounsatu-rates, which also come primarily from meats, will fall naturally when there is a reduction in the intake of this primary source of saturated fat—unless purposefully added back as in olive, peanut or canola oils. Polyunsaturates have no specific benefit, but it appears safe to consume up to 10 percent of calories from this source, based on observations in other coun-tries.

3. *Cholesterol intake should not exceed 300 milligrams per day.* (Originally, the guidelines urged no more than 100 milligrams of dietary cholesterol per 1,000 calories consumed [the average man consumes about 2,400 calories per day], but this has since been modified to bring the Heart Association guidelines in line with those of the National Cholesterol Educa-tion Program.) Cholesterol is essential to sus-tain life, but the body is capable of making all that it needs. Even strict vegetarians, who shun all animal products and thereby con-sume less saturated fat and no cholesterol, will not develop a shortage of cholesterol. In-deed, vegetarians tend to have low blood-cho-lesterol levels and a low incidence of heart attacks. Dietary cholesterol appears to have the most impact on blood cholesterol when consumed along with saturated fat. (See Chapter 6 for specific suggestions on reducing cholesterol intake.)

4. *Protein intake should be approximately 15 percent of calories.* Protein is essential to build and repair body tissue and to manufacture vi-tal enzymes, but it does not take much to meet our daily needs. The average American diet provides more than enough protein. Even athletes or people who participate in heavy physical labor need less than one gram of pro-tein per pound of body weight. There are many good sources of protein other than meat, fish, and poultry (see Chapter 4). The Heart Association cautions that excessive meat consumption is likely to result in a high intake

of saturated fat, which, in turn, raises blood cholesterol, and it recommends that several meals each week be built around vegetable protein—things such as grains combined with dried beans, peas, or other legumes.

5. *Carbohydrate intake should make up 50 to 55 percent of calories, with emphasis on increasing sources of complex carbohydrates.* Population groups who enjoy a very low prevalence of coronary disease typically consume large amounts—60 to 75 percent of their total calories—of vegetables, grains, and other complex carbohydrates. In contrast, the typical American diet derives only 40 to 50 percent of its calories from carbohydrates, and a third to half of these come from refined sugars. The recommended goal can best be met by increasing consumption of pasta, whole-grain cereals and breads, legumes and other vegetables, and fruits, while at the same time reducing sugar intake. Foods high in complex carbohydrates, or starches, have a number of advantages: They are usually low in calories, they contain a variety of important vitamins and minerals, and they are our main sources of dietary fiber. The latter may be of value in improving cardiovascular health in light of recent studies indicating that certain soluble fibers, such as pectin, guar, and the fiber found in beans, peas, fruits and certain vegetables (broccoli), and grain (oats), help lower blood cholesterol. (See Chapter 9 for a more detailed discussion.)

6. *Sodium intake should be reduced to approximately one gram per 1,000 calories, not to exceed three grams per day.* The human body can get by on a very small amount of sodium, about a quarter of one gram per day. The typical American diet, however, provides many times this: four to five grams per day, or the amount in two to four teaspoons of salt. Much of this salt comes from processed foods, often in things such as cereal, bread, canned or frozen foods, and other items that may not even taste salty. The question of whether sodium causes high blood pressure is still unresolved, but it is known that people who eat diets naturally lower in sodium have a lower incidence of high blood pressure than Americans and others who consume a high-salt diet. About 20 percent of the people with established high blood pressure will show a sizable reduction when they limit their sodium intake.

7. *If alcoholic beverages are consumed, the limit should be 15 percent of total calories, not to exceed 50 milliliters (one and two-thirds ounces, or the amount in about two mixed drinks, two 4-ounce glasses of wine, or two 12-ounce beers) of alcohol per day.* Over the last three decades, alcohol consumption by Americans has increased markedly. Recent studies have found that up to 5 percent of all calories consumed in this country come from alcohol, and among people who drink, 10 percent of their calories come from alcohol. Even moderate alcohol consumption is associated with an increased risk of stroke, and many people think that the Heart Association's limitations are too generous. (See Chapter 21.)

8. *Total calories should be sufficient to maintain the individual's best body weight.* To arrive at one's best body weight, the Heart Association recommends using the 1959 Metropolitan Height and Weight Tables rather than the updated version that allows for a wider range in the upper limits of what is considered normal (see Table 26.1). The Framingham Heart Study has found that even a moderate increase in weight—10 to 30 percent over the ideal—is linked to an increased risk of heart disease. (See Chapter 17.)

9. *A wide variety of foods should be consumed.* This point has been stressed repeatedly throughout this book, and it bears repeating.

A varied diet will provide adequate amounts of the vitamins, minerals, and other nutrients essential for good health. It is also more palatable; after all, eating should be a pleasure and not a chore.

Cholesterol and Atherosclerosis

It is well established that excess blood cholesterol eventually leads to atherosclerosis, the buildup of fatty plaque in the arterial walls. Atherosclerosis has been compared to the accumulation over the years of rust inside metal water pipes. With age, a certain amount of wear and tear is unavoidable, but it is possible to minimize the damage. The average age at which arterial obstruction from the gradual accumulation of plaque may potentially occur varies with the blood-cholesterol level, as shown below.

Blood Cholesterol Level: mg./dl.	Critical Age
200	70
250	60
300	50

If other risk factors are present, as they often are, that person's likelihood of a heart attack at a younger age is further increased. For example, if a person with a cholesterol level of 200 also smokes, the critical age drops from 70 to 60; if high blood pressure is also present, the critical age may be lowered to 50.

Ideal Cholesterol Levels

For years, physicians in this country regarded blood-cholesterol levels of 250 or even higher in the normal range, and generally they did not recommended treatment until the level approached 300 or more milligrams per deciliter. This has changed dramatically in recent years. Experts are beginning to agree as to what constitutes an ideal blood-cholesterol level and at which point treatment should be initiated. In an attempt to provide uniform guidelines for the diagnosis and treatment of elevated cholesterol, the National Cholesterol Education Program issued new guidelines late in 1987, and it is now encouraging doctors to follow this approach, which is outlined on page 446.

In general, an adult blood-cholesterol level of 200 milligrams per deciliter or less is desirable, and people who fall into this range need only to be retested every five years. (Obviously, they should not throw all caution to the wind and should continue to follow a moderate, varied diet.) Readings of 200 to 239 milligrams per deciliter fall into the borderline-to-high-cholesterol category. Such people should be rechecked annually and should also receive dietary information on how to reduce blood cholesterol. The exceptions are people who already have coronary disease, or who have two other risk factors (see the list of other risk factors on page 444); they fall into the high-risk category, and should undergo the same approach to treatment as people whose cholesterol levels are over 240.

In recent years, a cholesterol reading of 200 milligrams has been the level usually cited as a reasonable goal to minimize the risk of atherosclerosis. Studies show, however, that even 200 can represent an increased risk, especially if LDL levels are above 130 milligrams per deciliter. Analysis of MR FIT data indicates that the ideal cholesterol levels for adults range from 130 to 190 milligrams per deciliter, with LDL levels below 120, and the lower the better. If the entire American population was to achieve this goal, it is conceivable that the rate of coronary heart disease could be reduced by more than 50 percent, according to extrapolation of MR FIT data. Even more modest reductions may result in considerable lowering of cardiovascular deaths. According to Dr. Claude Lenfant, ''We could reduce the nation's toll from heart attacks by 100,000 lives a year if we could lower average cholesterol by 10 percent.''

Is such an ideal achievable? Many experts think it is, but it would require considerable public education, resulting in changes in eating habits and other lifestyle factors. Many experts think that a more realistic goal for adults with no other cardiovascular risk factors would be cholesterol levels ranging from 200 to 225 milligrams per deciliter. Dr. Scott Grundy of the Center for Human Nutrition at the University of Texas in Dallas, in a review (*Journal of the American Medical Association,* Nov. 28, 1986) of recent cholesterol studies, wrote that this range should prevent premature coronary disease (defined as under the age of 65) in most healthy adults. He stressed, however, that the 130 to 190 range throughout adulthood would be preferable in preventing coronary disease when people are over 65. ''A shift in peak incidence of coronary heart disease,'' he wrote, ''from late middle age to old age, because of a decline in other risk factors, should focus attention on the problem of mildly elevated plasma cholesterol levels as the major causative factor of coronary disease in older people.''

Role of Diet in Lowering Cholesterol

As explained in Chapter 6, the human liver manufactures about 1,000 milligrams of cholesterol per day, making it the major source of the serum cholesterol that circulates in the bloodstream. When the levels are too high, atherosclerosis results. A number of factors prompt the liver to increase cholesterol production. For years, consumers have been cautioned against eating eggs, organ meats,

Table 26.1. 1959 Metropolitan Height and Weight Tables

	Men					Women		
	SMALL FRAME	MEDIUM FRAME	LARGE FRAME			SMALL FRAME	MEDIUM FRAME	LARGE FRAME
Height (without shoes)	Weight in Pounds (without clothing)				Height (without shoes)	Weight in Pounds (without clothing)		
Feet Inches					Feet Inches			
5　1	105–113	111–222	119–134		4　9	90–97	94–106	102–118
5　2	108–116	114–126	122–137		4　10	92–100	97–109	105–121
5　3	111–119	117–129	125–141		4　11	95–103	100–112	108–124
5　4	114–122	120–132	128–145		5　0	98–106	103–115	111–127
5　5	117–126	123–136	131–149		5　1	101–109	106–118	114–130
5　6	121–130	127–140	135–154		5　2	104–112	109–122	117–134
5　7	125–134	131–145	140–159		5　3	107–115	112–126	121–138
5　8	129–138	135–149	144–163		5　4	110–119	116–131	125–142
5　9	133–143	139–153	148–167		5　5	114–123	120–135	129–146
5　10	137–147	143–158	152–172		5　6	118–127	124–139	133–150
5　11	141–151	147–163	157–177		5　7	122–131	128–143	137–154
6　0	145–155	151–173	166–187		5　8	126–136	132–147	141–159
6　1	149–160	155–173	166–187		5　9	130–140	136–151	145–164
6　2	153–164	160–178	171–192		5　10	133–144	140–155	149–169
6　3	157–168	165–183	175–197					

Prepared by Metropolitan Life Insurance Company. Source of basic data: *Build and Blood Pressure Study,* 1959, Society of Actuaries and Association of Life Insurance Medical Directors of America. Used with permission.

and other high sources of dietary cholesterol. Consumption of such foods should be restricted even though the normal liver reduces its cholesterol synthesis in response to absorbed dietary cholesterol. Dietary cholesterol in excess changes blood cholesterol. In addition, dietary cholesterol can be related to the risk of heart disease directly. Most Americans consume more cholesterol than some experts consider desirable: The average intake for men is about 500 milligrams a day; women consume about 320 milligrams. This is less than the average of nearly 800 milligrams 30 years ago but it's still considerably more than the 200 to 300 milligrams a day that is recommended under the National Cholesterol Education Program's dietary therapy. (See page 446.) Although there is still disagreement as to what the cholesterol intake for a person with normal blood cholesterol should be, we recommend 300 milligrams as an average

Other Risk Factors to Be Considered in Treating High Blood Cholesterol

- Male gender
- Family history of early coronary disease (i.e., a heart attack or sudden death before the age of 55 in a parent or sibling)
- Cigarette smoking (more than 10 cigarettes a day)
- Hypertension
- Low HLD cholesterol (less than 35 mg./dl. confirmed by repeat measurements)
- Diabetes mellitus
- History of cerebrovascular (i.e., stroke or transient ischemic attacks) or occlusive peripheral vascular disease
- Severe obesity (30 percent or more overweight)

limit for daily consumption. This is a prudent and reasonable amount, and it makes possible a very palatable diet.

Although cholesterol consumed in foods increases serum cholesterol, experts now agree that other factors, such as a diet high in saturated fats or individual physiologic characteristics, are probably more important. Carefully controlled studies have shown that consuming 250 milligrams of dietary cholesterol per day increases blood-cholesterol level by an average of 17 milligrams per deciliter, although there is much individual variation. Under normal circumstances, the liver cuts back on cholesterol production and the body steps up its cholesterol excretion to compensate for what is eaten and absorbed into the bloodstream. For all too many people, however, this change is inadequate to maintain a low blood cholesterol. The key element seems to be the rate at which LDL cholesterol is removed from the bloodstream, which is regulated by the cholesterol content of the liver and by the individual's genetically determined capacity to handle LDL. Also, the normal cholesterol feedback mechanisms may grow more sluggish as we age, resulting in high blood cholesterol and an increased risk of developing atherosclerosis and eventual coronary disease.

In view of the widespread prevalence of atherosclerosis and coronary disease related to high blood cholesterol, the American Heart Association, the National Institutes of Health, and other authorities have recommended that the entire population follow a diet aimed at reducing cholesterol levels. There are a number of dissenters who argue that urging everyone to adopt dietary restrictions that are based on studies involving patient populations who already have coronary disease is not justified. The problem with this argument is we do not know the optimal cholesterol level. Clearly, a middle-aged adult whose lifelong serum cholesterol has hovered around 130 milligrams per deciliter is not likely to have fatty streaks in his or her arteries and has little risk of developing coronary disease.

Cholesterol levels in this low range are common in some parts of the world, mostly in noindustrialized societies that have a very low incidence of heart disease. This is not the case in the United States and most other Western nations: Less than 5 percent of our population has what may be considered average cholesterol levels (i.e., less than 165 milli-

Standard Guidelines for Diagnosing Elevated Cholesterol

CHOLESTEROL LEVEL	CATEGORY
Under 200 mg./dl.	Desirable level
200–239 mg./dl.	Borderline, high cholesterol
Over 240 mg./dl.	High blood cholesterol

Recommended Follow-up for Each Group

CHOLESTEROL LEVEL	ACTION
Under 200 mg./dl.	Repeat test in 5 years; provide general dietary and risk-factor education.
200–239 mg./dl.	Repeat test to confirm results.
If 2nd test is still over 200–239 mg./dl.:	
For persons *without* coronary disease or 2 other risk factors:	Go on a cholesterol-lowering diet; have cholesterol tested annually.
For persons with coronary disease or 2 other risk factors:	Retest for LDL/HDL levels and treat according to LDL level.
Over 240 mg./dl.:	Retest for LDL/HDL levels and treat according to LDL level.

Classification of Risk Based on LDL Levels

LEVEL OF LDL CHOLESTEROL	CATEGORY
Under 130 mg./dl.	Desirable LDL level
130–159 mg./dl.	Borderline/high-risk LDL level
Over 160 mg./dl.	High-risk

Treatment Recommendations Based on LDL Levels

START DIETARY TREATMENT IF:	MINIMUM GOAL
LDL cholesterol is at or above 160 mg./dl. *and* person has no coronary disease or 2 other risk factors	<160 mg./dl.*
LDL cholesterol is at or above 130 mg./dl. *and* person has coronary disease or 2 other risk factors	<130 mg./dl.†

START DRUG TREATMENT IF:	MINIMUM GOAL
LDL cholesterol is at or above 190 mg./dl. *and* person has no coronary disease or 2 other risk factors	<160 mg./dl.
LDL cholesterol is at or above 160 mg./dl. *and* person has coronary disease or 2 other risk factors	<130 mg./dl.

*Roughly equivalent to total cholesterol <240 mg./dl.
†Roughly equivalent to total cholesterol <200 mg./dl.

Reprinted with permission from the National Heart, Lung and Blood Institute.

grams per deciliter) in nonindustrialized countries. Indeed, the 195 to 205 milligram cholesterol levels that are the mean for 40-year-old Americans would be considered abnormally high in countries that have low cardiac mortality. Proponents of widespread dietary change argue that, for adults at least, no one will be harmed by following a cholesterol-lowering diet and the large majority will likely benefit. (This may not apply to young children, as explained subsequently.) Obviously, a person whose blood cholesterol falls in the 5th percentile and who is normal weight does not need to be as diligent about following a low-fat, low-cholesterol diet as someone in the 75th percentile or higher. (See Table 26.2.) Also, people with a favorable HDL/LDL cholesterol ratio may not have as high a risk of coronary disease as someone with high LDLs and low HDLs. (See Chapter 6.) For large numbers of Americans, if not most, however, the recommendations from the National Cholesterol Education Program make sense. Specifically, these recommendations call for:

1. Intensive dietary therapy (as outlined in the Step One and Step Two diets) for all persons whose blood-cholesterol levels fall into a high-risk category (see Recommended Diet Modifications on page oo).

2. Dietary changes also are recommended for persons with blood-cholesterol levels between 200 and 240 and LDL above 130 if they have other cardiovascular risk factors.

3. Cholesterol-lowering drugs may be added to dietary therapy for those who do not achieve adequate cholesterol lowering in six to eight months.

4. Ideal weight should be achieved and maintained by a combination of reduced food intake and regular exercise.

Table 26.2. Blood-Cholesterol Levels by Age and Percentile

Age (year)	Percentiles				
	5	50	75	90	95
MALE CHOLESTEROL LEVELS (MG./DL.)					
5–19	115	155	170	185	200
20–24	125	165	185	205	220
25–29	135	180	200	225	245
30–34	140	190	215	240	255
35–39	145	200	225	250	270
40–44	150	205	230	250	270
45–69	160	215	235	260	275
69 +	150	205	230	250	270
FEMALE CHOLESTEROL LEVELS (MG./DL.)					
5–19	120	160	175	190	200
20–24	125	170	190	215	230
25–34	130	175	195	220	235
35–39	140	185	205	230	245
40–44	145	195	215	235	255
45–49	150	205	225	250	270
50–54	165	220	240	265	285
54 +	170	230	250	275	295

Reprinted with permission from The National Heart, Lung and Blood Institute.

Although these guidelines are important in establishing basic parameters for preventive treatment, a number of questions remain. These include the following.

Do women need to be as concerned as men about lowering their cholesterol levels? Most of the cholesterol studies have involved high-risk middle-aged men. Not as much is known about the benefits of a cholesterol-lowering diet for women with normal lipid levels. Women of all ages have a lower risk of heart attack than men, even though they tend to have comparable total blood-cholesterol levels. Women enjoy a more favorable HDL level all of their lives, but their LDL levels rise, often to levels even higher than in men, after the age of 55 or so. While women may well benefit from reducing total calories and fat consumption, there are trade-offs. For example, dairy products and meat—two of the most common food categories slated for cutbacks—are major sources of calcium and iron, two nutrients that are inadequate in many women's diets. Still, a large number of women have blood-cholesterol levels that are too high, and for these women, a prudent approach that lowers cholesterol without compromising other nutritional needs can be recommended. For example, skim milk and products made from it contain very little cholesterol and no saturated fat but still provide calcium. There also are good sources of iron, such as lean meat and poultry, that are low in saturated fats.

How far should we go in restricting the diets of young children? This is another recommendation that is hotly debated. There is general agreement that a cholesterol-lowering diet is advisable for children with an inherited predisposition to elevated cholesterol (familial hypercholesterolemia). However, the American Academy of Pediatrics disputes the contention that all children over two should be placed on a cholesterol-lowering diet. Dr. Alvin Mauer, chairman of the Academy's Committee on Nutrition, has stressed that "there is no evidence that diet in childhood influences the development of atherosclerosis in adult men." He further emphasizes that undue restriction of calories, dairy products, meat, and other such foods may unnecessarily hinder growth and development, both in young children and during the adolescent growth spurt. Again, common sense and moderation should dictate the approach to a child's diet. Studies have repeatedly shown that elevated cholesterol and atherosclerosis begin early in life, and a strong case can be made for beginning a preventive diet early before poor eating habits become deeply ingrained. This does not mean adopting an extreme low-fat, low-calorie diet that compromises normal growth. For example, there can be more than adequate calories and protein in the prudent diet recommended by the American Heart Association.

What is the best way to lower serum cholesterol? The dietary guidelines from the National Cholesterol Education Program, combined with the cholesterol- and fat-lowering tips in Chapter 6, are good starting points. The prudent diet recommended by the American Heart Association and others is low in saturated fat and cholesterol and high in complex carbohydrates. Vegetarian diets are high in complex carbohydrates, fiber, and polyunsaturates; Mediterranean diets are high in olive oil, a mostly monounsaturated fat, and complex carbohydrates. Thus, a wide variety of foods can be eaten while lowering saturated fat and cholesterol intake. To us, a prudent, varied diet that follows the general caloric recommendations of the American Heart Association seems preferable to one that emphasizes large amounts of one or two items, such as fish oil or olive oil. Regular vigorous exercise and weight control lower LDL cholesterol. These changes plus stopping smoking may also help raise HDL. For people with very high cholesterol, especially those with established atherosclerosis, cholesterol-lowering drugs in addition to dietary changes may be recommended. (See discussion on drug treatments on pages 452–53.)

Will following these measures prevent having a heart attack? Of course, this is the biggest question, and unfortunately, there is no pat answer. When we refer to increasing or lowering risk, we are talking about population groups and not individuals. It is impossible to predict with certainty who will or will not have a heart attack. There are people whose blood cholesterol is normal and who follow all the rules and still wind up with a heart attack. There are others whose lives are a study of excesses who live to an old age without a sign of heart disease. We have numerous instances of people who eat virtually identical diets but have different blood-cholesterol levels. Some people who go on a rigid cholesterol-lowering diet achieve little change and others on the same diet will note dramatic improvement.

Some experts argue that it's all a matter of genes, and what you eat and how you live makes little difference. There is strong contrary evidence. Japanese who moved to Honolulu or San Francisco and who adopted the American diet developed blood-cholesterol levels and heart-disease rates very similar to their American neighbors of European ancestry. Clearly, genetics is important, but diet

Recommended Diet Modifications to Lower Blood Cholesterol

	Choose	Decrease
Meat, poultry, and fish	Fish, poultry without skin, lean cuts of beef, lamb, pork, or veal, shellfish. Reduce portion sizes to 4 ounces or less.	Fatty cuts of beef, lamb, pork, spare ribs, organ meats, regular cold cuts, sausage, hot dogs, bacon, sardines, roe
Dairy products	Skim or 1%-fat milk (liquid), powdered, evaporated, buttermilk	Whole milk (4%-fat): regular, evaporated, condensed; cream, half and half, 2%-fat milk, imitation milk products, most nondairy creamers, whipped toppings
	Nonfat (0%-fat) or low-fat yogurt	Whole-milk yogurt
	Low-fat cottage cheeses, farmer or pot cheeses (all of these should be labeled no more than 2.6 gm. fat/ounce)	All natural cheeses (e.g., blue, Roquefort, Camembert, cheddar, Swiss)
		Low-fat or light cream cheese, low-fat or light sour cream
		Cream cheeses, sour cream
	Sherbet, sorbet	Ice cream
Eggs	Egg whites (2 whites = 1 whole egg in recipes), cholesterol-free egg substitutes	Egg yolks
Fruits and vegetables	Fresh, frozen, canned, or dried fruits and vegetables	Vegetables prepared in butter, cream, or other sauces

and other lifestyle factors alter your risk. The dramatic reduction in cardiovascular deaths in the last two decades seems to support this thesis, because there is little doubt that Americans are changing the personal factors—cigarette smoking, diet, blood-pressure control, among others—that increase the risk of heart attack.

Other Dietary Factors Affecting Cholesterol

Although saturated fats and dietary cholesterol may have the most significant impact on blood cholesterol, there are a number of other foods that raise or lower lipid levels or alter the LDL/HDL ratio. These include the following.

Alcohol. Although alcohol contains no fats or cholesterol, its heavy consumption may provide a significant percentage of total calories. By stimulating liver synthesis of triglycerides, alcohol increases the manufacture of VLDL, for very low density lipoprotein, the molecule that transports mostly triglycerides. When consumed in moderate amounts (one or two drinks a day), alcohol seems to have little direct effect on LDL, but in many people, it elevates the protective HDLs. When this effect was first announced a few years ago, a

Recommended Diet Modifications to Lower Blood Cholesterol *(cont.)*

	Choose	Decrease
Breads and cereals	Homemade baked goods using unsaturated oils sparingly, angel food cake, low-fat crackers, cookies	Commercial baked goods, pies, cakes, doughnuts, croissants, pastries, muffins, biscuits, high-fat crackers, high-fat cookies
	Rice, pasta	Egg noodles
	Whole-grain breads and cereals (oatmeal, whole-wheat, rye, bran, multigrain, etc.)	Bread in which eggs are major ingredient
Fats and oils	Baking cocoa	Chocolate
	Unsaturated vegetable oils: corn, olive, rapeseed (canola oil), safflower, sesame, soybean, sunflower	Butter, coconut oil, palm oil, palm kernel oil, lard, bacon fat
	Margarine or shortening made from one of the unsaturated oils listed above	
	Diet margarine	
	Mayonnaise, salad dressings made with unsaturated oils listed above	Dressings made with egg yolks
	Low-fat dressings	
	Seeds and nuts	Coconut

Reprinted with permission from the National Cholesterol Education Program.

number of articles appeared in the popular media indicating that a drink or two a day may actually reduce the risk of a heart attack. There is little justification for these claims, and more recent studies have found that even a moderate alcohol intake markedly increases the risk of a stroke. Regular consumption of three or more drinks per day has been linked to increased blood pressure in some people. Excessive alcohol consumption also can damage heart muscle, leading to a potentially fatal condition called alcoholic myocardiopathy. (See Chapter 21.)

Fiber. Dietary fiber—the nondigestible portions of fruits, vegetables, grains, and other plant foods—is widely promoted as having a cholesterol-lowering effect. This varies considerably depending upon the type of fiber consumed, however. For example, bran fiber, generally from the outer layer of the whole-wheat kernel, does not lower blood cholesterol or increase the body's excretion of cholesterol products. Still, many people are consuming large amounts of bran cereals or fiber supplements in the mistaken notion that bran reduces the risk of heart attack. In contrast, the soluble fibers—pectin and guar, which are used as food thickeners; oat bran; and the fiber in beans, peas, and other legumes—can lower blood cholesterol. We do not understand how this effect is achieved. One hypothesis is that these fibers may interfere with intestinal reabsorption of bile acids, which are replaced by converting cholesterol to bile acids. This results in a reduction of the liver cholesterol content. A study at Northwestern University, in which two ounces of oat products (the amount in one cup of cooked oatmeal and an oat-bran muffin) were added daily to a cholesterol-lowering diet, produced an additional drop of almost 3 percent in blood cholesterol in six weeks. Thus, the effect may be small, but on a population

basis, a 3-percent reduction in cholesterol could produce a 6-percent reduction in heart disease. That translates to 20,000 American lives per year. (See Chapter 9 for a more detailed discussion.)

Coffee. What role, if any, that coffee may play in heart disease has not been established. The Framingham Heart Study has failed to find any correlation between coffee consumption and heart attacks. In contrast, a 25-year study of male graduates of Johns Hopkins Medical School found that the incidence of heart attacks among men who drank five or more cups of coffee a day was two and a half times greater than those who drank none. However, researchers conducting the study caution that this statistic alone is not enough to conclude that heavy coffee consumption increases the risk of a heart attack; a number of other factors, such as whether the coffee drinkers also smoked, had high blood pressure or were overweight, may account for the apparent differences between coffee drinkers and abstainers.

The relationship between coffee consumption and increased blood-cholesterol levels is better established: Heavy coffee consumption may raise blood cholesterol significantly. A study involving 5,858 middle-aged Japanese men living in Hawaii found that those who drank more than two or three cups of coffee a day had higher mean cholesterol levels than those who drank no coffee. The researchers did not find any cholesterol increase from drinking tea, cola, or other sources of caffeine, leading them to conclude that some other ingredient in coffee may be responsible. On the other hand, a study in the California community of Rancho Bernardo found that blood cholesterol was related to the amount of caffeine consumed. Researchers at Stanford University also found that drinking more than two cups of coffee a day raised blood cholesterol, especially LDL levels. In Scandinavia, only heavy coffee drinkers (more than five cups per day) and only those drinking coffee prepared by boiling the grounds had increased cholesterol.

Caffeine has been linked to other cardiovascular effects that may pose a risk to some people. Large amounts of caffeine, especially when taken along with phenylpropanolamine, a common ingredient in diet pills, can upset the heart's normal rhythm. This can be especially dangerous in people with diseased heart valves or with other conditions that predispose them to cardiac arrhythmias. Even moderate amounts of caffeine can raise blood pressure and force the heart to work harder by increasing vascular resistance.

In summary, it seems that healthy individuals have nothing to worry about from moderate coffee consumption. But people with heart disease or high blood pressure may be wise to limit their intake of coffee to one or two cups a day.

Shellfish. For years, people concerned about reducing cholesterol intake have been cautioned to avoid shellfish. This stand has been softened considerably due to the revised lower estimates of the cholesterol content of shellfish. Since shellfish are very low in fat, particularly saturated fat, they are no more likely to raise blood cholesterol than lean meat or skinless poultry. Table 26.3 shows the cholesterol, fat, and calorie contents of popular shellfish; it should be noted, however, that the cholesterol and fat content may vary by 20 percent above or below the stated values, depending upon the season and the location where the fish are caught.

Fish oils. Taking fish-oil supplements derived from cold-water fish, such as cod or salmon, has become the latest cholesterol-lowering fad. These fish oils are high in omega-3 fatty acids, a polyunsaturated fat that can lower blood triglycerides if taken in large quantities. They also reduce the tendency for the blood to clot. However, contrary to popular belief, they do not lower LDL cholesterol.

The current fad is based on observations that Greenland Eskimos and others who consume very large amounts of fatty fish have very low heart-attack rates, even though their diet is very high in fat and cholesterol. Other studies in industrialized communities in Holland and the United States have found a reduction in heart-attack rates among people who eat fish regularly. However, we do not know whether fish oil or some other factor is responsible. It is important to note that these studies are with whole fish, which contain many substances in addition to oil and fatty acids. In 1990, the Food and Drug Administration ordered fish oil supplement sellers to stop claiming that their pills reduce heart disease risk, because the evidence is too shaky. We endorse the American Heart Association's recommendation against taking fish-oil supplements except under medical supervision. It appears that two or three servings of fish a week can provide the desired benefits without

Table 26.3. Cholesterol and Fat Content of Selected Shellfish

Amount: 4 ounces, raw	Cholesterol (mg.)	Calories from Fat	Total Calories
Clams	39	10	85
Crab, Alaska king	48	6	96
Crab, Dungeness	67	10	98
Crayfish	159	11	102
Lobster, northern	109	9	103
Lobster, spiny	80	16	128
Mussels, blue	32	23	98
Oyster, eastern	63	26	79
Scallops	38	8	101
Shrimp	174	17	121
Squid	266	15	105

Source: United States Department of Agriculture.

running the risk of excessive blood thinning and other consequences of taking the concentrated amounts of omega-3 fatty acids found in many supplements. (See Chapter 6 for more complete discussion on fish oils and other cholesterol-lowering strategies.)

Cholesterol-Lowering Drugs

The recent introduction of new kinds of cholesterol-lowering drugs has been hailed as a major advance in treating coronary disease. Even so, drug therapy should be reserved for patients with dangerously high cholesterol and should be used only after documenting that adequate lowering has not been achieved through diet, exercise, and other lifestyle changes. In the past, cholesterol-lowering drugs have been less than satisfactory because of side effects or, for some types, their gritty, unpleasant taste. Also, some produced only minor reductions in cholesterol. However, if the drugs are selected carefully for the individual, effective, long-term reductions have been possible, and recent studies have documented a subsequent reduction in heart attacks. Some newer drugs can reduce blood cholesterol by more than 40 percent, but we still do not know whether they cause potentially harmful long-term effects. Thus, the National Cholesterol Education Program recommends that the physician first try the drugs whose long-term safety has been established.

In any event, drugs should not be considered a substitute for diet and other nondrug treatments. All work best to prevent heart disease when a person consumes a prudent low-fat, low-cholesterol diet, does not smoke, exercises regularly, and so forth. Classes of cholesterol-lowering drugs include the following.

Bile-acid sequestrants. These are among the older cholesterol-lowering drugs and include cholestyramine (Questran) and colestipol (Co-

estid). They take the form of powders that are suspended in a liquid, such as fruit juice, and work by binding to bile acids in the intestine. This forces the liver to use more cholesterol to manufacture bile acids, and forces the body's cells to draw LDL from the bloodstream to supply the extra cholesterol. LDLs are thus reduced, often by 25 or 30 percent. There is also a small increase in HDLs. The major problem with these drugs is their inconvenience and their sandy texture. They also can produce constipation and, in some people, intestinal gas and bloating. Manufacturers have reduced the texture problem by producing finer granules and by concealing it in a chewable candy bar.

Although the side effects can be annoying, most people take these drugs without undue problems. Beginning with a low dose and increasing it after a few weeks to the full dose needed often prevents the constipation. Increasing fiber intake or taking a mild high-fiber laxative can also overcome constipation problems. Mixing the powder in applesauce, oatmeal, or other such food helps conceal the texture. On the plus side, the safety record of these drugs is unsurpassed, in great part because they work in the intestine without actually being absorbed into the body. Most importantly, a study lasting over seven years clearly demonstrated that heart disease is reduced with one of these agents.

Nicotinic acid (niacin). This drug is actually the vitamin niacin, which is used in very large quantities. (When taken in doses of more than 20 milligrams a day, niacin should be considered a drug.) It is is the oldest of the cholesterol-lowering agents, as well as one of the most effective. It decreases the liver's output of VLDL, thus lowering triglycerides and LDLs. Unfortunately, at the high doses required to lower cholesterol, large numbers of people experience unpleasant side effects—

hot flushes, itching of the skin, and intestinal upsets. More serious side effects such as liver dysfunction, cardiac arrhythmias, and a buildup of uric acid in the blood may occur. Large doses should never be taken unless under the direction of a physician.

Recent studies have found that some people derive benefits at dosages of 1,000 to 3,000 milligrams a day, but others may need the higher doses of 5,000 to 8,000 milligrams, as previously recommended. More people can tolerate niacin at the lower dosages, especially if the medication is started at very low doses of 50 to 100 milligrams after meals and is increased slowly over a period of several weeks. An added word of caution: Some people try to avoid the side effects of nicotinic acid by taking nicotinamide instead. This should be avoided because this derivative is not effective in lowering cholesterol.

Fibric acids. Drugs in this category include gemfibrizol (Lopid) and clofibrate (Atromid S), with others in the testing stage. They speed up the body's breaking down of VLDL, thus lowering triglycerides. They also increase the removal of LDL and raise HDL levels. Some drugs in this category cause transient liver and muscle disorders, which disappear when the drugs are stopped. Clofibrate caused a higher number of gallbladder problems, but gemfibrizol and some of the newer agents are said to be free of this side effect. However, more research is needed to be certain.

Probucol. This drug, sold under the trade name of Lorelco, is believed to change the structure of LDL cholesterol, prompting a faster turnover. Unfortunately, some studies have indicated that the drug has the possible disadvantage of also reducing HDL levels. In addition, its benefit has not been demonstrated in long-term studies.

Enzyme inhibitors. This is the newest category of anticholesterol drugs, and the first to be marketed is Lovastatin (Mevacor), which gained FDA approval in the fall of 1987. Others are being tested and are expected to be approved soon. These drugs work by blocking an enzyme that the liver needs to make cholesterol. As a result, cells needing cholesterol draw more from the bloodstream by specifically taking up LDL and breaking it down to take its cholesterol component. With this drug, blood levels fall by as much as 45 percent. Even larger reductions may be achieved if the person follows a cholesterol-lowering diet and increases exercise. This agent can cause muscle and liver dysfunction. Treatment with the first of these enzyme inhibitors is expensive—$700 to $2,500 a year—but this cost is expected to go down as more drugs of this type are approved for prescription use.

Effectiveness of Drug Therapy

Several recent studies have found that long-term use of certain cholesterol-lowering drugs, specifically the bile-acid sequestrants, gemfibrizol, and nicotinic acid, reduce the incidence of heart attacks. Most of the studies involved middle-aged men with high levels of cholesterol. Whether the same preventive effects will hold for people who do not fall into these categories, or apply to other drugs, is not yet known.

Dubious Remedies

Chelation therapy. There has been no reliable scientific demonstration that chelation therapy widens narrowed coronary arteries, and practitioners have been sued for allegedly producing osteoporosis by removing calcium from the bone. Still, the "treatments" are widely available, notably in popular retirement communities of the Southwest. Chelation therapy entails administering EDTA (ethylendiamine tetraacetic acid), an artificial amino acid that is used to treat heavy-metal poisoning from lead, mercury, or other such substances. The EDTA chelates (binds on to) heavy metals, enabling the body to excrete them in the urine.

The notion that EDTA might work in atherosclerosis is based on the fact that the substance chelates with calcium. As fatty plaque builds up in the arteries, some calcium also accumulates. Promoters of chelation therapy often describe the EDTA as a magnet that draws the calcium from the plaque, thereby causing the fatty deposits to disintegrate. To a lay person, this may sound perfectly reasonable, but there is no scientific evidence that chelation therapy lessens atherosclerosis.

In one study of chelation therapy, the project was abandoned after two of the thirty patients in the group died and the rest showed no improvement. Possible side effects of the treatments include osteoporosis, kidney failure, bone-marrow depression, shock, low blood pressure, convulsions, irregular heartbeat, and respiratory arrest.

Despite the lack of efficacy and safety, and repeated warnings against chelation therapy from the Food and Drug Administration and numerous medical and consumer groups, thousands of Americans each year undergo the full course of 20 to 50 treatments, which can cost $5,000 to $15,000. The treatments usually are administered at special clinics or "alternative-medicine" centers. Chelation therapy is among the "top ten health frauds" listed by the Food and Drug Administration, hence these doctors risk hefty damage suits, and, indeed, a number have been sued. Frequently, the treatments are combined with a diet and exercise program, and the benefits that many patients attribute to the chelation therapy are more likely due to these additional components or to the placebo effect; very often, if a person believes in a treatment, he or she will feel better, even when there is no benefit from the therapy itself.

Megadoses of vitamin E. For more than 40 years, large doses of vitamin E have been promoted—without any proof of effectiveness—for the treatment or prevention of many diseases, most notably high blood pressure, angina, and coronary disease. Many of the claims can be traced to the late Dr. Evan Shute, a Canadian obstetrician/gynecologist, whose book *The Heart and Vitamin E and Related Matters* was published in 1948. With his brother, Dr. Wilfred Shute, he established the Shute Institute and Shute Foundation for Medical Research. Over the years, these organizations have kept the vitamin E myths alive through a publication entitled *The Summary*, which was established, as Evan Shute once reported, because of "the inability of the Shute Foundation to gets its presentations published in North American medical journals." To a knowledgeable observer, such an admission is a tip-off that the reports have not met the scientific standards required by reputable journals. Even so, many people are convinced that vitamin E somehow protects against heart disease—something that researchers have been unable to show in scientific studies.

Lecithin. Lecithin is a phospholipid, a naturally occurring emulsifier that can react with both water and fats. It is added to many foods to prevent the fats and water from separating. In the body, lecithin stabilizes cholesterol in bile and prevents gallstones from forming. The body makes all that it needs, and there is no evidence that lecithin supplements lower cholesterol or perform any of the other benefits claimed by their purveyors. (See Chapter 6 for a more detailed discussion.)

Fad diets. Each year, dozens of diet books are published, and many of these are directed to heart patients or people concerned about heart disease. Some are based on solid, authoritative information; many of these carry the imprimatur of world-renowned institutions or organizations and others are by reputable authorities. A distressing number, however, are by self-styled nutritionists whose diets are based more on imagination and commercial appeal than facts. Sorting the legitimate diets from the fad ones, many of which can be dangerous, is often difficult for a lay person, especially when the author has an M.D. or impressive-sounding credentials. In general, any diet that promises a quick, easy cure, especially for a serious disorder such as heart disease, which has no proven cure, should be suspect, regardless of who the author is. A recent example is the *Eight-Week Cholesterol Cure* by Robert E. Kowalski. The diet, low in calories, saturated fat, and cholesterol, will indeed lower blood cholesterol, but there is no "cure" for high cholesterol. The problem can be controlled by a lifelong change in diet and other lifestyle habits that contribute to the elevated cholesterol. Even so, a large number of people will not gain the desired cholesterol reductions through diet alone, and will require drug therapy, often for life. The author promises his cure is without drugs, and then recommends high doses of niacin, presumably assuming that since this is a vitamin, it is not a drug. This is not true: When taken in large doses, any vitamin or mineral takes on pharmacologic properties and becomes by definition a drug. High-dose niacin, like any drug, carries a risk of dangerous side effects and should be used only under a doctor's supervision. (See Chapter 3 for a more detailed discussion of food fads and health fraud.)

OTHER BLOOD LIPIDS

Although cholesterol is the most studied and publicized of the blood lipids, it is not the only one that has been linked to an increased risk of heart disease. Triglycerides—the most abundant of all the lipids—also may play a role, but not as much is known about the effects of elevated blood triglycerides (hypertriglyceridemia). Since their role in heart disease has not been established, there has been a tendency to ignore elevated triglyceride levels and, instead, to concentrate on cholesterol. In general, people with elevated triglycerides have an increased risk of heart disease. People whose levels are in the 250-to-500-milligram range have an increased heart-attack rate, but it is not known whether the high triglyceride levels or other related factors are responsible. For example, elevated triglycerides often indicate other lipid abnormalities, such as low HDL and high LDL cholesterol, or disorders clearly linked to atherosclerosis. People with a disorder known as familial combined hyperlipidemia have an overproduction of VLDL, causing high levels of VLDL triglycerides and, because of their conversion to LDL, elevated blood levels of this component. These individuals appear to have a higher risk of a heart attack, probably because they also have high cholesterol levels. Thus, this relationship between high triglycerides and other lipoprotein abnormalities appears to explain their link to cardiovascular diseases.

These genetic lipid disorders are relatively common but often exist in very mild forms that are markedly exaggerated by excessive alcohol consumption or by obesity. A number of drugs, including thiazide diuretics, oral contraceptives, estrogen supplements, and some of the beta-blocking drugs, can increase triglyceride levels. Kidney and liver disease, diabetes and certain other metabolic or hormonal disorders, heart attacks, serious infection, and even stress are other potential causes of high triglyceride levels.

A 1983 National Institutes of Health consensus panel of experts in lipid disorders recommended that patients whose blood triglyceride levels are in the 250-to-500-milligram range be examined for possible causes. It is important to measure the LDL and HDL levels in order to assess the risk of cardiovascular disease. Treating the underlying causes usually will lower the triglyceride levels. Even if no causes for the elevated lipids can be found, a diet similar to the one used to reduce high cholesterol usually will lower triglycerides, too. Losing excess weight and cutting back on alcohol consumption, if this is a factor, will also lower triglycerides. In patients with triglyceride levels over 500 milligrams per deciliter, it is particularly important to find effective treatment in order to avoid consequences such as pancreatitis (inflammation of the pancreas). If dietary changes, exercise, and other lifestyle changes fail to bring the triglyceride levels below 500, drug therapy may be recommended.

HIGH BLOOD PRESSURE

As noted earlier, high blood pressure, or hypertension, is the most common circulatory disorder in human beings. With a few exceptions (for example, in remote parts of the South Pacific, South America, and Africa), it occurs worldwide, most often in middle-aged or elderly men and women. It is estimated that as many as 60 million adults and 2.7 million children aged 6 through 17 in the United States have high blood pressure and nearly half of all Americans have it by the time they reach the age of 74.

Although people can live for many years with high blood pressure, it does have serious health consequences. It is the leading cause of stroke; it is also a major risk factor for heart attack and kidney failure. In recent decades, great advances have been made in the diagnosis and treatment of high blood pressure. There are now numerous effective drugs to lower blood pressure. Increased emphasis on early diagnosis and treatment have contributed to the more than 50-percent decline in the stroke death rate over the last 20 years. More effective control of high blood pressure is also believed to be a major factor in the marked reduction in fatal heart attacks in recent decades.

Blood pressure is the force (tension) that blood exerts against artery walls. It can vary considerably during the course of a day. Blood pressure is generally lowest during sleep, and tends to be higher in the daytime. Exercise, anger, and other conditions can produce temporary rises in blood pressure. It is the average blood pressure that seems best related to the future disease.

Blood pressure is stated in two numbers, such as 120/80. The larger number reflects the maximum force and is called the systolic pressure. The minimum force, exerted as the blood leaves the arteries between heartbeats and enters the capillaries, is called the diastolic pressure.

Normal resting blood pressure for people between the ages of 18 and 50 varies, but is usually less than 140/90 (systolic/diastolic). Both readings are important, but studies show that an average diastolic reading of greater than 85 and an average systolic pressure greater than 130 are the levels above which risk of complications increases. (Table 26.4 lists classifications of blood pressure.)

Causes of High Blood Pressure

High blood pressure is a complicated set of disorders caused by the interaction of a number of regulatory systems. In rare situations is it due to an abnormality in just one system or organ, such as the kidney.

Nutrition for the Heart-Attack Patient

Whenever a person is hospitalized, he or she can expect that their usual meal routines will be upset. When and how food and liquids are administered, especially in the first few hours and days after a heart attack, can be very important to the outcome. The idea is to provide adequate liquids and nutrition without increasing the heart's work load.

During and immediately after a heart attack, many patients feel nauseated, and while this persists, nothing should be consumed by mouth, so that any vomiting and retching will be minimized. At first, most heart-attack victims do well after the pain ends and need only careful observation to be certain that recovery occurs without irregular heart rhythms. Some patients also may develop poor heart function and go into "shock." To minimize circulation needs, body fluids temporarily leave the vascular system and move into the interstitial spaces. This shift in body fluids will make a person feel very thirsty, as if dehydrated. Although a heart-attack patient will complain of extreme thirst, no fluids should be taken in by mouth while the person is in shock. The fact that not as much fluid is circulating in the bloodstream will stimulate the body's thirst responses, even though the body does not need, and may even be harmed by, extra oral fluids at this time. Fluids given by vein can help fight certain types of shock, but heart attack–related shock causes excess pooling of fluid in the lungs. To relieve the feelings of thirst, the patient can be given ice chips—which will not add much water to the system—to suck on. This also helps relieve nausea.

Small amounts of water can be given as the shock diminishes. If the nausea persists, intravenous fluids will be started to provide a route for medications and to maintain the right amount of fluids in the body.

For the first few days, small and frequent feedings are advised. Taking in too much food at a time should be avoided, because this can cause stomach and diaphragmatic discomfort, which may be confused with further heart pain. Foods should be bland and room temperature; consuming foods with strong odors or that are very hot or cold can stimulate the vagus nerve—the large nerve that serves the neck, chest, and abdomen, with branches to the heart and lung. Vagus-nerve stimulation can slow the heart rate and should be avoided in this phase of recovery. Stimulants such as caffeine-containing drinks are avoided.

Initially, the patient's diet should be limited to 1,000 to 1,200 calories a day; again, to minimize the extra demands on the heart posed by the digestive process. Most hospitals restrict caffeine during the first few days but will permit decaffeinated coffee and tea. Sodium should be restricted, and alcohol should not be consumed at least for the first few weeks.

After 5 to 10 days of following this regimen, the patient's meals can be increased gradually until he or she is again on a normal schedule. Throughout the recovery period, the person should eat slowly and avoid activity before and after meals.

Many cardiologists find that the final days of the hospital stay are an ideal time to begin nutrition counseling. Understandably, a heart attack is a life-changing event. Before, the person may have been the hale and hearty type who joked about exercise and dieting. This is likely to change dramatically after a heart attack; a person who has faced death suddenly gains new perspectives and values life in a new way. At this time, the typical patient avidly seeks advice and wants to know what he or she can do to prevent a recurrence. Sadly, it often takes something as serious as a heart attack to motivate a person to lose excess weight, cut down on fat consumption, and make other dietary changes. Ideally, cardiac rehabilitation should include intensive dietary counseling, along with a progressive exercise program, and other lifestyle changes, such as smoking cessation and behavior modification to learn how better to cope with stress and modify Type A personality characteristics.

All disorders related to high blood pressure involve the arterioles, millions of tiny arteries that conduct blood from large arteries to capillaries. Arterioles are vital to the regulation of blood pressure because they are composed of a layer of muscle cells that enables them to widen (dilate) or narrow (constrict) as needed. If, for example, more blood is needed for digestion, the arterioles in the intestine open up and those farther away—in the arms and legs, for instance—constrict. During aerobic exercise, the opposite may occur. Such operations are controlled by chemicals from the nervous and endocrine systems.

The body's protective reflexes maintain blood pressure in such a manner as to ensure that all tissues and organs receive an adequate supply of blood. For example, when you suddenly stand up, the body responds almost instantaneously by increasing blood pressure enough to ensure that adequate blood will reach the brain. This is accomplished by chemical messengers that signal the tiny muscles controlling the sides of the arterioles to constrict. Imbalances or high levels of some of these chemical messengers can result in high blood pressure. For reasons that are not completely understood, in some people the arterioles' muscle cells tend to constrict more than normal, and this results in chronic high blood pressure.

In about 5 to 10 percent of hypertensive patients, high blood pressure can be traced to an identifiable cause, such as kidney disease, a narrowing of the arteries leading to the kidneys (renovascular hypertension), or to a tumor or overactivity in the adrenal glands. Some of those problems—and the resulting high blood pressure—may be corrected by treating the underlying cause. For example, expanding a narrowed renal artery often will resolve the problem of renovascular hypertension. (This can be accomplished in a relatively new procedure using a catheter and a balloon.) In 90 to 95 percent of cases, however, no specific cause can be found for the high blood pressure. This is referred to as primary or essential hypertension.

Treatment of High Blood Pressure

High blood pressure usually does not produce symptoms until it reaches an advanced stage; thus, large numbers of hypertensive people are unaware that they have a potentially life-threatening disease. Many of the symptoms often attributed to high blood pressure—headaches, dizziness, light-headedness, feelings of fullness in the head and tightness in the scalp, numbness and tingling in the arms and fingers—may, in reality, turn out to have other causes. Thus, routine health checkups, including blood-pressure measurement, are important, especially for anyone who is in a high-risk group. (Since about one

Table 26.4.	Classification of Blood Pressure in Persons 18 or Older*

Range (mmHg)	
DIASTOLIC	
Below 85	Normal
85–89	High normal
90–104	Mild hypertension
Above 105	Moderate to severe hypertension
SYSTOLIC	
Below 140	Normal
140–159	Mild elevation
Above 160	Moderate to severe elevation

Examples:	
145/95 ———	mild hypertension
160/105———	moderate hypertension
175/115———	severe hypertension

*Based on an average of 2 or more readings on 2 or more occasions.

Adapted with permission from the 1988 Report of the Joint National Committee on Detection, Evaluation and Treatment of High Blood Pressure, National High Blood Pressure Education Program, May 1988.

out of every five or six adults has high blood pressure, it can be argued that all of us are at risk, but as noted in the previous listing of risk factors, some people are more likely to develop the disease than others.)

A diagnosis of high blood pressure often means lifelong treatment, but the approaches to therapy vary according to the severity of the disease. Modern antihypertensive therapy began in the 1950s, and over the last 30 years, dozens of highly effective medications to lower blood pressure have been developed. Today, the large majority of people with high blood pressure can achieve normal or near-normal blood-pressure readings with minimal side effects. Because there are so many dif-

ferent drugs, it may take several months to find the one (or the combination) that works best for the individual patient. In most cases of mild to moderate high blood pressure with no evidence of organ damage (for example, no sign of an enlarged heart or impaired kidney function), a trial of nondrug therapy may be recommended. This would include reducing salt intake, losing excess weight, and increasing exercise. Other nondrug strategies may include reducing or eliminating caffeine and alcohol from the diet, increasing intake of dietary fiber, calcium, potassium, and magnesium, and behavior modification (for example, meditation or relaxation exercises). Always remember that successful treatment

Risk Factors for High Blood Pressure

Factors associated with an increased risk of high blood pressure include:

Heredity: A family history of hypertension is a strong predisposing factor.

Age: The chances of developing high blood pressure increase with age. Men tend to develop it earlier, but by age 45 or 50 (or after menopause), women become as susceptible as men.

Race: Blacks of all ages and either sex are at a higher than average risk of developing high blood pressure. The disease also occurs at a higher rate among some Oriental populations, notably the Japanese.

Obesity: Overweight people are also more susceptible to develop both high blood pressure and coronary heart disease. Diabetes, which increases the risk of high blood pressure, is also more common among the obese.

Salt: Sodium chloride (table salt) increases high blood pressure in those with a genetic predisposition to the disease. Several factors may be involved, including the brain's response to sodium stimuli, a possible deficiency of potassium, a response to chloride, or other factors.

Others: A number of other factors, such as excessive alcohol use, cigarette use, and stress have been linked to increased blood pressure or cardiovascular risk. Scientific evidence supporting these factors is not as conclusive as for the risk factors listed above, but it makes sense to moderate or avoid as many of these as possible. This is particularly true for cigarette smoking, which is clearly related to an increased risk of heart attack.

requires monitoring by your physician. You may feel better but your blood pressure may still be high.

Weight Loss and Weight Control

Numerous studies have documented a positive relationship between obesity and hypertension. For example, surveys of hypertensive patients have found that up to 60 percent are obese (defined as being at least 20 percent above normal weight). In addition, the prevalence of hypertension among people aged 20 to 39 is two to three times higher for those who are overweight.

There are a number of ways in which obesity can raise blood pressure. For instance, the extra weight requires that the heart work harder to supply blood to excess tissue. As noted earlier, obesity increases the risk of Type II, or adult-onset, diabetes, which, in turn, increases the likelihood of high blood pressure.

This does not mean that all obese people develop high blood pressure, or that all people with high blood pressure are obese or even overweight. Because the relationship between hypertension and obesity is so widely accepted, however, most doctors encourage hypertensive patients who are overweight to lose weight. In fact, weight reduction is often the initial treatment for obese patients with hypertension.

In one study where obese hypertensives were placed on a low-calorie diet, a significant decrease in both systolic and diastolic blood pressure was noted after the loss of approximately 20 pounds. This occurred despite the fact that in this particular study, no attempt was made to reduce sodium intake. The results do not mean that salt reduction is not important in the total eating plan for a person with high blood pressure; it does, however, show that weight reduction even without a change in sodium intake can lower blood pressure.

Unfortunately, losing excess pounds and maintaining that weight loss are easier said than done. The National Center for Health Statistics reports that despite the national preoccupation with dieting and weight, Americans weigh more now than ever before. Interestingly, the average American actually eats less than his or her counterpart at the turn of the century. Instead, the difference is at least partly attributed to the reduced amount of physical activity characteristic of today's lifestyle compared to earlier times. (A number of other factors, including increased fat consumption and genetics, also contribute to excess weight; for a more detailed discussion, see Chapter 17.)

Obese hypertensive patients are advised to follow a commonsense program that entails reduced consumption of total calories, moderate salt restriction, and increased physical activity. The source of calories also is important: The bulk (about 60 percent) should come from carbohydrates, about 12 percent from protein, and less than 30 percent from fats, with emphasis on monounsaturated and polyunsaturated fats. Such a program not only helps reduce excess weight, it also may lower blood-cholesterol levels and improve glucose metabolism, thereby lowering other important cardiovascular risk factors. (See also chapters 6 and 17.)

Salt Reduction

Salt restriction has long been considered an important nondrug treatment of hypertension. Before the development of modern antihypertensive medications, strict salt restriction was the major treatment for high blood pressure. Dr. Walter Kempner of Duke University demonstrated the effectiveness of this approach with his rice and fruit diet—a boring but effective regimen that did lower blood pressure in many patients. Today, salt restriction is no longer the mainstay treatment for high blood pressure, but it is still considered important, both in its prevention and treatment.

It's a well-established fact that Americans consume large amounts of salt: on the average, 6 to 20 grams a day. This is probably not dangerous to those who are not sodium-sensitive (salt is made up of sodium and chloride), but for those who are, this amount can be a major factor in raising blood pressure.

People who are sodium-sensitive tend to retain fluid with excessive salt intake; for reasons that are not fully understood, their kidneys may be more efficient at conserving sodium. To compensate for the extra sodium, the body increases its fluid (blood) volume and the circulation of excess blood makes the blood vessels overly sensitive to nerve stimulation, which causes them to constrict, thereby raising blood pressure. The heart also must work harder to circulate the extra blood and to maintain the increased blood pressure. For these salt-sensitive individuals, reducing sodium intake will lower blood pressure and ease the work load of the kidneys, heart, and blood vessels.

Although salt reduction is recommended for hypertensive patients, not all will achieve the desired blood-pressure lowering. For one thing, only about 20 to 30 percent of them may be sensitive to sodium. Blacks tend to be more sodium-sensitive than whites, and this is thought to be a factor in the higher incidence of hypertension among blacks.

Ongoing research is attempting to identify people who are sodium-sensitive. For example, one line of research is studying the relationship between the kidney's production of renin—a hormone that regulates the body's sodium balance—and high blood pressure. Salt-sensitive people who retain sodium will suppress their renin output. Therefore, low renin is a result of salt retention. People who have a primary defect in renin secretion (i.e., overproduce renin) will not be salt-sensitive. However, they will retain sodium because of the high renin-to-angiotensin-to-aldosterone linkage.

In contrast, people whose kidneys retain sodium for other reasons are low renin secretors. Other people who are high renin secretors tend not to be sodium-sensitive. Many black people are low renin secretors because of a problem in sodium retention. While this theory seems promising, it is probably not the whole answer to identifying salt-sensitive individuals; some people secrete normal amounts of renin and are still salt-sensitive and hypertensive. Continued research is necessary to determine other factors that identify salt-sensitive individuals.

Even though we may not be able to identify people who are most likely to benefit from sodium restriction, enough is known to advise a prudent approach to salt intake. For example, many hypertension specialists recommend that children of hypertensive parents avoid excessive salt consumption from an early age. Animal studies have found that even rats who have a genetic predispostion to develop high blood pressure when given a high-salt diet do not do so if they are fed a low-salt diet. Whether the same holds for humans is not known, but specialists point out that cutting down on salt cannot hurt, and it may be helpful in preventing a potentially lethal disease. Population groups around the world have been studied. Those with habitually low salt intakes have a low incidence of high blood pressure, and those with high intakes have much higher blood pressure. (The low-salt menu in Table 26.5 and the information in Table 26.6 show how salt can be reduced in the diet; for additional general information on salt and guidelines on reducing salt in the diet, see Chapter 8.)

Exercise

Some studies have found that physical exercise may produce a modest lowering in blood pressure among some individuals, especially if it is part of an overall program to reduce excess weight and other lifestyle factors related to an increased risk of cardiovascular disease. Even though exercise alone is not enough to lower blood pressure in the large majority of hypertensive patients, it is an important factor in healthy lifestyle.

When embarking on an exercise program, the degree and intensity of activity depend upon many factors, including the work capability of the heart, age, weight, circulation in the lower legs and feet, and the condition of muscles and joints. Aerobic exercise is the best type for those with hypertension; weight lifting and other static exercises should be avoided because they can increase blood pressure to dangerous levels. Blood pressure also rises during aerobic exercise, but the increases are more moderate and the activities themselves contribute to overall improved cardiovascular function. Examples of aerobic exercise include walking, jogging, swimming, and bicycling. The term *aerobic exercise* refers to the fact that the muscles being exercised require extra oxygen. To deliver the required oxygen, the heart must pump more blood to the muscles. Normally, the heart pumps about six quarts of blood a minute in an adult non-exercising man who weighs about 150 pounds. During peak exercise, this increases to about 25 quarts a minute. To deliver this much blood, the heart has to pump harder and faster; the blood vessels will become more dilated (or wider and opened), allowing blood to flow through more easily.

As might be expected, systolic blood pressure rises during vigorous exercise, but it re-

Table 26.5.   Cutting Down on Sodium

Giving up salt in one's diet does not mean giving up eating pleasure. Here is a sample menu that shows how easy it is to reduce sodium content in a single day's meals. The following menu provides less than 2,000 milligrams of sodium. It is also low in total calories and fat.

Breakfast

Low-salt cereal (e.g., oatmeal or shredded wheat) with low-fat or skim milk
Toast with jelly and unsalted margarine
Orange juice
Beverage (coffee, tea, Postum, etc.) with low-fat milk and sugar (optional)

Lunch

Tuna-salad sandwich (made with water-packed, low-salt tuna)
Fruit salad
Vanilla yogurt
Beverage

Dinner

Unsalted cream of celery soup
Pasta with chunky tomato-vegetable (low-salt) sauce
Green salad with vinegar/oil dressing
Bread with unsalted margarine
Poached pears
Low-fat milk
Beverage

Snacks

Fresh fruits or vegetables, low-salt crackers, yogurt, and other low-salt foods in moderation

Table 26.6.   Switching to Low-Salt Foods

Many major food manufacturers offer low-salt alternatives to foods that are traditionally high in sodium. Substituting some of these items can make a big difference in overall sodium consumption. The following are examples of low-sodium foods compared to regular ones.

Low Sodium	Food	Serving Size	Regular
18 mg.	Canned tomato juice	6 oz.	658 mg.
32 mg.	Canned green-pea soup	1 cup	987 mg.
34 mg.	Canned white tuna in water	3 oz.	309 mg.
1 mg.	Canned green beans, drained	½ cup	170 mg.
6 mg.	Peanut butter	2 T	150 mg.
14 mg.	Cottage cheese	½ cup	455 mg.

Look also for labels that indicate no added salt on items such as processed vegetables, cereals, and other processed foods.

turns to its usual level after exercise. Diastolic pressure rises less and may actually fall during exercise. Studies in Australia, at Duke Medical Center and elsewhere, have shown a lowering of blood pressure in some patients with mild hypertension, especially when the exercise was combined with weight reduction and decreased sodium intake. However, this does not happen in all hypertensive patients. Among those who do achieve a lowering, it often is not sufficient or tends to be temporary. Still, exercise conditioning is considered an important part of the overall treatment of high blood pressure; it is also a wise preventive measure for people whose blood pressures are in the high to normal range.

Regular exercise may also influence other cardiovascular risk factors. The effect on weight was mentioned earlier; studies also have found that people who exercise regularly are less likely to smoke than those who are sedentary. Exercise can increase the protective HDL component of blood cholesterol. People who exercise often find they are better able to cope with stress. While these factors may not actually bring about the desired reduction in blood pressure, they still are important considerations for people with hypertension and other cardiovascular risk factors.

Alcohol

Several recent studies have suggested a relationship between alcohol consumption and hypertension. This association is independent of other factors such as obesity, salt intake, and coffee and cigarette consumption. The exact reason for the relationship is not known, but some researchers think that neurologic factors and hormonal influences may be involved. Others suggest the blood-pressure rise may be created by the physiologic effects of alcohol withdrawal. In any case, most experts recommend a limit to alcohol consumption for everyone, and especially for people with high blood pressure.

Smoking

People who smoke *and* have hypertension run a significantly higher risk not only of heart attack but also of sudden death, congestive heart failure, and stroke than those who either smoke *or* have hypertension. Smoking in and of itself may not cause hypertension, but it greatly compounds the risk of serious consequences of high blood pressure. (See page 433 earlier in this chapter and also Chapter 22 for a more detailed discussion of the effects of cigarette smoking.)

Other Dietary Factors

A continuing and growing research effort is underway to determine more effective treatments for high blood pressure. Recent investigations point to several potentially useful dietary factors. These include the following.

Potassium. Potassium is an essential element that helps maintain the balance between body cells and fluid, and it plays a key role in enabling nerves to respond to stimulation. Studies suggest that potassium-rich diets may reduce the risk of stroke among those being treated for hypertension. High potassium intake, however, does not lower normal blood pressure. This suggests that potassium intake does not alter the normal physiologic mechanisms that govern blood pressure but, rather, that it interacts with the abnormal conditions present in some hypertensive individuals.

Since potassium's role in blood pressure regulation is not entirely clear, it is not recommended that people take potassium supplements as a preventive measure against hypertension. Instead, individuals should reduce their intake of high-sodium, low-potassium processed foods and increase their intake of low-sodium, high-potassium natural foods such as fruits and vegetables. (See Table 26.7) Moreover, salt substitutes should not be used freely in place of regular salt. Such substitutes contain potassium chloride, and excessive blood potassium can induce severe muscle weakness and even cardiac arrest and death. This is particularly true in some forms of kidney disease.

Diuretics, which are frequently used to treat hypertensives, can cause potassium loss,

Table 26.7. Low-Salt, High-Potassium Foods

Food	Serving Size	Potassium (mg.)	Sodium (mg.)
Apricots	3 medium	281	1
Apricots (dried)	8 halves	490	13
Asparagus	6 spears	278	2
Avocado	½ medium	604	4
Banana	1 medium	569	1
Beans (green)	1 cup	189	5
Beans (white, cooked)	½ cup	416	7
Broccoli	1 stalk	267	10
Cantaloupe	¼ medium	251	12
Carrots	2 small	341	47
Dates	10 medium	648	1
Grapefruit	½ medium	135	1
Mushrooms	4 large	414	15
Orange	1 medium	311	2
Orange juice	1 cup	496	3
Peach	1 medium	202	1
Peanuts (plain)	2½ oz.	740	2
Potato	1 medium	504	2
Prunes (dried)	8 large	940	11
Raisins	¼ medium	271	10
Spinach	½ cup	291	45
Squash (acorn)	½ baked	749	2
Sunflower seeds	3½ oz.	920	30
Sweet potato	1 small	367	15
Tomato	1 small	244	3
Watermelon	1 slice (approx. 6½ in.)	600	6

Information derived from U.S. Department of Agriculture, Human Nutrition Information Service.

and care must be taken to assure that the proper potassium balance is maintained. Persons who take prescribed diuretics may be advised by their physicians to make sure that their daily diets include high-potassium foods. If potassium levels still remain low even after dietary alterations, potassium supplements or a diuretic that spares potassium may be prescribed.

Calcium. The possible role of dietary calcium in the development of hypertension is just beginning to be studied. There is some evidence that people with high blood pressure consume significantly less calcium than those with normal blood pressure. Although some studies have found that adding calcium to the diets of animals may counteract this problem, calcium supplements are not recommended at this time for humans who have high blood pressure. Regular intake of calcium-rich food—especially low-fat dairy products and dark green leafy vegetables—helps people maintain healthy bones, and may have other beneficial effects. It is most important in the young growing years.

Magnesium. Like calcium, magnesium contributes to the regulation of blood pressure, but it is not known whether this mineral has any relationship with high blood pressure. Some studies show that magnesium plays a major role in the control of vascular tone, which has led to the theory that low levels of magnesium may upset calcium balance and cause blood-vessel constriction and a consequent rise in blood pressure.

Adults at risk of developing hypertension should consume enough magnesium to meet the current recommended daily allowance of 300 to 350 milligrams a day. In patients undergoing diuretic therapy, magnesium may be lost, so these people should be diligent about eating adequate amounts of magnesium-rich foods. Good sources include whole grains, dark green leafy vegetables, nuts, and legumes.

Polyunsaturated fatty acids. Researchers have found that people who eat vegetarian diets have lower blood pressure than those who don't. It is not, however, known why. Some people believe that it is related to the fact that vegetarians eat more polyunsaturated fat, but significantly less total fat, saturated fat, and cholesterol than meat eaters. Linolenic acid (contained in linseed or flaxseed oil, legumes, nuts, and citrus fruits), rather than linoleic acid (from vegetable oil sources such as soybean and corn oils) may be the primary dietary polyunsaturated fatty acid related to blood pressure. More research is needed to document this, however.

Licorice. Large amounts of natural licorice may elevate blood pressure, sometimes to potentially dangerous levels. Natural licorice flavor (as opposed to the artificial flavor now used in most candy made in this country) comes from the sweet root of a plant in the pea family. It contains glycyrrhizin, a chemical that affects some people in the same way as aldosterone, a steroid hormone that can cause the body to lose potassium in the urine, and to retain sodium and chloride, causing fluid retention. People who have high blood pressure should avoid snacking on black licorice made with natural flavor, particularly if they are taking diuretics.

Dietary fiber. Epidemiologic studies have found that vegetarians and others who consume a high-fiber diet have a reduced incidence of high blood pressure. The association between fiber and blood pressure is unclear, but some researchers believe that the lowered incidence of hypertension may be due to other areas in which fiber may play a role, such as reduced blood cholesterol or lowered total weight. High-fiber fruits and vegetables are also lower in sodium and higher in potassium. (See page 450 in this chapter and also Chapter 9.)

Caffeine. Hypertensive patients are often advised to cut down on or even avoid caffeine. Just two or three cups of coffee can significantly raise a person's blood pressure for up to three hours. While it is unlikely that a cup of coffee to start the day or an occasional cola or other caffeine drink will have a significant effect on blood pressure, moderation is advised.

Diet pills and other medications. A number of common over-the-counter medications—diet pills, cold and allergy pills, and others—contain ingredients that may raise blood pressure. Always read the warning labels before taking any medication and, if in doubt, check with your doctor or pharmacist.

Behavior Modification

All of us are subjected to stress as a part of everyday life, but our individual responses to stress vary greatly. Typically, the body responds to stress by pumping out adrenal hormones, which prepare the body to defend itself (the so-called fight or flight response). In response to these hormones, the heart beats faster, blood pressure rises, circulation to the large muscles increases, blood sugar rises, and other changes take place to prepare the body to overcome the perceived danger.

Studies have found that some people are "hyper-responders": Their bodies are almost constantly poised to ward off danger. Even a minor stress will cause a transient rise in blood pressure and pulse rate. What role these hormones play in long-term high blood pressure is unknown, but some studies suggest that hyper-responders to stress have an increased incidence of high blood pressure.

Even though the role of stress in high

blood pressure is unknown, behavior modification may be of some use in its treatment. Studies have found that relaxation and biofeedback therapies (or combinations of behavior modification) may produce modest reductions in blood pressure among some people with mild hypertension. There is no good evidence, however, that the reductions are sustained or can be used as a substitute for other therapy, such as antihypertensive medication. Thus, these techniques are probably most useful when part of a comprehensive program that may include both drug and nondrug treatments. Most importantly, careful monitoring to document the treatment is the only way to be certain you are on the right course.

Hypertension in Children

Doctors are increasingly aware that youngsters may have mildly elevated blood pressure, which places them in a special high-risk category for premature heart disease and other consequences of hypertension. (Very high blood pressure in children is usually secondary to some other disorder, such as kidney disease or a tumor.) Sometimes the elevated blood pressure is transient, as in the cases of adolescents whose pressures are high for a few years and then fall back into the normal range.

Until recently, blood pressure was not usually routinely measured in young people. Now, however, pediatricians are urged to make blood-pressure measurement a part of routine pediatric checkups, beginning at an early age. Although there is continuing debate as to whether these young people with mild primary hypertension should be treated, there is no doubt that they should be watched carefully. A number of follow-up studies of youngsters with childhood high blood pressure show they will continue to "track"; that is, their blood-pressure levels will rise as they reach adulthood. (See Table 26.8 for the upper limits of normal blood pressure in children.) Some specialists urge that childhood hypertension be treated with low-dose medications that are unlikely to interfere with normal growth and development. Nondrug treatments, such as weight control and low salt intake, are recommended as commonsense preventive measures.

IN SUMMARY: A TOTAL COMMONSENSE APPROACH

Throughout this book, we stress that moderation and common sense should be the governing factors in all areas of nutrition. Since heart disease is so widespread among Americans from all backgrounds, and it seems there is a strong link between diet and heart disease, it is reasonable to say that most of us can benefit from adopting a prudent diet that is not too high in calories or saturated fat. Unfortunately, all too many of us seek out quick, easy "fixes." In a typical scenario, let's say you are diagnosed as having high blood cholesterol. Your response is likely to be an immediate, frightened grasping for whatever promises to work the fastest. This may mean

Table 26.8. Upper Limits of Normal Blood Pressure in Children

Age	Blood Pressure
6 or younger	110/75
6 to 10	120/80
11 to 14	125/85
15 to 18	135/85–90

Reprinted with permission from *Lower Your Blood Pressure and Live Longer*, Marvin Moser, M.D. (New York: Villard Books, 1989).

rushing to the nearest pharmacy or health-food store to stock up on fish-oil pills, a hasty, ill-guided attempt to adopt a restricted and boring "healthy" diet, and an equally hasty and ill-guided exercise effort, all of which may be unsafe. After a week or two, the fright wears off and before you know it, everything settles back into your previous pattern.

Ingrained lifestyle habits are difficult to change, and diet is one of the hardest. Success lies in a gradual, reasoned approach that starts with taking stock of what you are eating now and—perhaps in consultation with a qualified dietitian or a doctor schooled in the kind of sound nutrition advocated in this book—concentrates on deliberately and permanently improving those areas that are the most troublesome.

A logical starting place is to carry a pad and pen with you so that you can keep a careful food diary for a week. Eat as you normally would, and be sure to write down everything you consume during the course of a day, along with the time and circumstances (e.g., a half bag of potato chips while watching TV). Jot down what you eat at the time; it's almost impossible to reconstruct an accurate food record at the end of the day. If anyone laughs, tell them it's doctor's orders.

Common Myths and Facts About Hypertension

MYTH: Nervous tension is another name for hypertension.

FACT: No, it isn't. Hypertension refers to the elevated (hyper) pressure (tension) against the artery walls, and not to a person's emotional state. Actually, many people who are very quiet and serene have severe hypertension. However, nervous tension may temporarily elevate blood pressure.

MYTH: High blood pressure can be cured.

FACT: High blood pressure can be controlled and brought down to normal levels if prescribed treatment is followed. It can be cured only in rare instances (usually when it is secondary to another condition, such as a narrowed artery supplying blood to the kidney or a tumor that produces excessive adrenal hormones).

MYTH: Once hypertension is under control, it is possible to stop treatments, both drug and non-drug.

FACT: Sometimes an individual may be able to stop antihypertensive drugs after blood pressure has been normalized for several years, but this tends to be temporary and does not occur in all patients. In such cases, the person should be checked periodically to make sure that the blood pressure remains normal. As a general rule, hypertension is a lifelong disease that requires life-long treatment.

MYTH: High blood pressure has many symptoms.

FACT: Hypertension is a "silent" disease: Those who have it often do not know it until it is too late. Even those with dangerously elevated blood pressure can feel perfectly normal. Headaches, dizziness, and weakness sometimes may occur with high blood pressure, but more often, these symptoms are associated with other conditions or states.

MYTH: A person with high blood pressure needs to rest more, avoid tense situations, cut back on activities.

FACT: If proper treatment is followed, a person can lead a normal, active life.

MYTH: If you take hypertensive drugs, you can use all the salt you want.

FACT: No such luck. Reducing sodium often means that the drugs will be more effective in lowering blood pressure and that smaller drug doses may be prescribed, thereby reducing the potential for adverse side effects.

MYTH: Eating garlic will lower blood pressure.

FACT: In a limited number of studies, consuming large amounts of garlic has been found to inhibit blood clotting, as well as to lower blood cholesterol. However, there is as yet no objective study showing garlic is useful in treating high blood pressure.

This food diary will give you (and a nutrition counselor) an accurate picture of your present diet. Let's suppose that it turns out you are consuming 40 percent of your daily calories in fat, and 20 percent come from saturated fats—meats, butter, milk, commercial baked goods, ice cream, and so on. Instead of immediately halving the consumption of these foods—which may well be your favorites—try gradual modification and substitutions. For example, instead of immediately going from whole milk, which you may really enjoy, to skim, which you may find watery and tasteless, switch first to milk that is 2 percent fat. Chances are that you will notice very little difference, even though it contains only half the fat of regular whole milk. After a couple of weeks, switch for drinking to milk that is 1 percent fat, and use skim milk in cooking. Then try skim milk on your cereal and use milk that is half skim and half 1 percent fat for drinking (adding a teaspoon of dried skim milk to a glass of regular skim milk also will give it more body). Chances are that within a month or so you'll find that skim milk is perfectly acceptable.

You can follow a similar approach to meat, ice cream, baked goods, and other foods. Reducing portion size or concentrating on dishes in which small amounts of meat are used as condiments instead of as the main ingredient can make a big difference in fat consumption. Examples include pasta with a mushroom and tomato sauce that can either be meatless or have a small amount of well-drained lean meat; stir-fried vegetables with strips of chicken, turkey, or lean beef; hearty vegetable stews or soups with bits of lean meat. (Chapters 6 and 17 offer a number of specific tips on reducing fat and cholesterol intake.) If you begin by making gradual changes, purposefully seeking new, tasty foods that are low in fats and cholesterol, your chances of adopting a lifelong heart-healthy diet are good to excellent.

New Insights into Cholesterol *

In 1990, Dean Ornish and his associates reported some regressions of coronary artery heart disease using rigid comprehensive lifestyle changes, including a low-fat vegetarian diet, smoking cessation, stress management training, and moderate exercise. It is important to note that diet does not lower serum levels of lipoprotein (a) [Lp (a)], a newly recognized independent risk factor for the development of premature coronary heart disease. About 25% of Americans may have elevations of this factor, probably genetically determined (see Chapter 18).

In 1990, researchers in the Netherlands reported in the *New England Journal of Medicine* that not only do not all monounsaturated fatty acids act like oleic acid by reducing saturated-fat intake and thereby lower serum levels of ''bad'' low density lipoprotein (LDL) cholesterol, but unsaturated fatty acids of the ''trans'' variety (such as elaidic acid) not only raise ''bad'' LDL cholesterol but also lower ''good'' high density lipoprotein (HDL) cholesterol. Trans fatty acids are formed when vegetable and fish oils, rich in polyunsaturates, are hydrogenated to manufacture certain types of margarines, margarine-based products, shortenings, and fats used for frying. An accompanying editorial by Scott Grundy of Dallas suggest it is no longer appropriate to label saturated fat as ''bad'' and unsaturated fat as ''good,'' since stearic acid, a saturated fatty acid, does not increase serum cholesterol levels, but unsaturated fatty acids of the trans variety do.

*This section written by Victor Herbert, M.D., F.A.C.P.

27

Nutrition and Cancer

Samuel Waxman, M.D., Ludwik Gross, M.D., and Carol Schreiber

■

INTRODUCTION

Few issues in science are as controversial as the strength of the relationship between diet and cancer. Over the past few years, many groups of scientists have formulated guidelines for a diet that they believe is consistent with good nutritional practice and, at the same time, likely to reduce the risk of cancer. Most of these guidelines are still the subject of fierce debate. When experts say that fiber, certain vitamins, carotene, or selenium (to name a few recent examples) may reduce cancer risk, they also say, by implication, that they may not. The fact is that, as yet, there is no clear evidence that any diet will protect people against cancer.

Cancers are populations of cells in the body that have acquired the ability to multiply and spread without the normal restraints. In this chapter, we will examine the diet-cancer connection. We will see that predisposing factors to cancer, such as genetic predisposition, are unrelated to diet per se, but that, if the predisposing factors are there, what is in or not in the diet may determine whether or not the predisposition becomes an actual clinical cancer. It should be noted that there are both cancer-promoting and cancer-suppress-ing genes, and lack of the latter promotes cancer. We will also look at the role nutrition plays in cancer-patient care and we will offer some dietary guidelines based on recent studies.

THE DIET-CANCER CONNECTION

One of the methods used to determine risk factors for cancer is known as epidemiological research. Investigators seek to associate exposure to dietary components with the increased or decreased incidence of cancer in specific population groups. These groups may be defined according to several different criteria, such as race, gender, nationality, occupation, or age. For instance, breast cancer was not common among women in Japan, while it is one of the most common forms of cancer among women in America. It has also been shown that women who are clinically overweight and who consume a diet high in fat have a tendency to develop specific forms of cancer, including cancer of the breast. The Japanese diet, which consisted largely of rice, vegetables, and fish, was much lower in animal fat than the average American diet. The concept that diet plays a role in breast cancer is further supported by the fact that when Japanese women emigrate to the United States and adopt the American diet, their incidence of breast cancer rises.

However, a diet that is high in one component may be low in another. For example, a diet that is high in fat may be lower in complex carbohydrates such as fiber and starch. A high-carbohydrate diet may be low in protein. Fad diets may be nutritionally unbalanced and exercise levels vary from individual to individual, thereby increasing the likelihood of identifying the wrong contributing factors. For example, all the evidence that high-fiber diets reduce cancer frequency may have nothing to do with fiber per se, but rather with other things (such as some antioxidants) present in high-fiber diets, or not present (such as fat).

Laboratory methods have been used to provide information on the potential carcinogenicity of food constituents. These studies are difficult to interpret for many reasons. Some foods that are not toxic to humans are toxic to laboratory animals. It is extremely difficult to select a valid control diet in these studies, and some responses may be species-specific and have no relevance to human nutrition at all. Data obtained from laboratory tests are useful for evaluating the role of dietary factors in human cancer, but they also depend upon simple assumptions that may not be valid for humans. The projection of such data to humans without confirming evidence from epidemiological studies must be treated with caution. As a consumer, you always should be suspicious of health experts who urge changes based upon the latest scientific information, especially if that information has not been confirmed in humans or is too new to be thoroughly analyzed. The advice you get may be premature, unsound, or even unsafe.

Despite these reservations, it is currently believed that diet and cancer interact in the following three ways:

1. Certain dietary components in excess seem to raise cancer risk.
2. Certain dietary components in moderation seem to lower cancer risk.
3. In people who already have cancer, food can be used as adjunctive therapy to improve well-being, tolerance of treatment, and quality of life.

Let us examine the facts—and fallacies—of each of these areas.

Dietary Components Associated with Increased Cancer Risk

Several food constituents have been identified as possibly increasing our risk of cancer: excess fat, calories, protein, and alcohol; nitrites; nitrates; pesticides; and some preservatives and other food additives. Conversely, some preservatives may reduce cancer risk. Substantial evidence links some of these components to cancer risk, while the data concerning others is highly questionable.

Food constituents that are considered to be part of the cancer link are generally thought to promote the disease, not initiate it. During initiation, an irreversible change occurs in a cell's genetic message. This is generally a direct consequence of damage to the cell's DNA by substances known as mutagens. An example of this is radiation exposure. The change occurs rapidly and is essentially irreversible. It programs the cell to become a cancer. Promotion will produce cancer, but only if the cell has already been initiated. The results of promotion are reversible to some extent, but at this time the exact molecular biology of these events is obscure. (A simplified scheme for the steps in the induction of cancer is shown in Figure 27.1.)

If diet influences cancer risk, it does so by acting as a promoter (see Possible Tumor Promoters on page 471) by hastening the reproductive rate of the initiated cell and changing its character to that of a malignant cell. Thus, while some food components are not in themselves carcinogenic, they may intensify the damage already done by the carcinogens. To complicate matters further, the normal metabolic process creates many carcinogenic initiators. For example, the mold aflatoxin B, a contaminant found in poorly stored peanuts and corn, is a toxic compound that is normally quite stable. However, during detoxification by the liver, it becomes a highly reactive derivative that interacts with the DNA of the liver cell. Metabolic activation has one other important consequence. In some cases, a carcinogen can be partially metabolized in one tissue and then enter the bloodstream to undergo its final activation in some other distant tissue. Therefore, it is not uncommon to observe that a carcinogen that enters through the gastrointestinal tract can produce a cancer in a distant organ such as breast, brain, lung, or uterus.

The following sections briefly review some of the conflicting studies and emphasize the difficulties in establishing firm cause-effect links between diet and cancer. (For the reported relationship between dietary components and types of cancer, see Table 27.1.)

Fat, Calories, and Cancer Risk

Breast cancer. A diet resulting in high body fat has been linked to cancer of the breast, colon, and prostate. Epidemiological studies support these conclusions. These cancers are common in the United States, where, on the average, caloric intake is high, with fat comprising about 37 percent of the total calories. The incidence of these cancers is lower in Japan, where the average diet has fewer total calories, of which only 10 to 20 percent are derived from fat. (Figure 27.2 shows the fat

Figure 27.1. Mechanisms of Chemical Carcinogenesis*

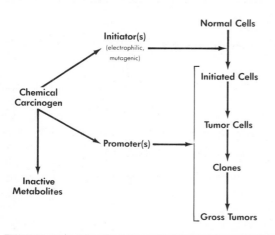

*As distinguished from genetically predisposed carcinogenesis, which may prove more important for the total population.

Reprinted with permission from E. C. Miller and G. A. Miller (*Cancer* 47:1055–1064, 1981).

Possible Tumor Promoters and/or Cocarcinogens in Man

Alcohol
Asbestos
Tobacco
High fat, protein, and calorie content of food
Vitamin deficiencies
Unnatural balance of endogenous hormones
Exogenous hormones, diethylstilbestrol (DES)
Diterpenes from plant sources (tea, etc.)
Environmental chemicals, such as hydrocarbons and chlorinated hydrocarbons
Drugs
Radiation
Viruses

content of some common foods in the American diet.)

Breast cancer risk is associated with several factors that influence the levels of circulating hormones, such as:

1. above-average height and weight

2. early onset of menarche

3. nonchildbearing, or first pregnancy after the age of 30

4. late onset of menopause

Scientists have hypothesized that a diet high in fat or high in calories that leads to increased body fat may affect the development of breast cancer by increasing the circulating levels of certain hormones, such as prolactin. Body fat contains an enzyme that increases circulating estrogen levels, and high estrogen levels promote estrogen-dependent breast cancers. It has also been suggested that dietary fat or body fat may affect the immune system in some way and make it less capable of fighting cancer cells when they arise.

Colon cancer. The relationship between colon cancer and dietary fat has also been well studied. Fat digestion requires, among other things, bile acids, which help the body absorb and utilize the fat. The higher the fat content of the diet, the more bile acids may be released. Some of these bile acids travel from the small intestine, where fat absorption occurs, to the colon, or large intestine, where they are broken down by bacteria. Some experts believe that one of these breakdown products is the carcinogen 3-methylcholathrene, which may account for part of the association of colon cancer with a high-fat diet.

Prostate cancer. The link between a high-fat diet and prostate cancer appears to be via high body fat. Some studies have shown that vegetarians, who have a low dietary fat intake,

Table 27.1. Reported Relationship Between Selected Dietary Components and Cancer

Selected Cancer Sites in Descending Order of Incidence (age-adjusted incidence, SEER, 1984)		Fat	Body Weight and Calories	Fiber	Fruits and Vegetables	Alcohol	Smoked, Salted, and Pickled Foods
Lung	(55)[a]				--	+[b]	
Breast	(51)	+	+		−	+	
Colon	(36)	+	+	−	−		
Prostate	(34)	+	+		−		
Bladder	(16)				−		
Rectum	(15)	+				+	
Endometrium	(13)	+	+				
Oral cavity	(11)				−	+	
Stomach	(8)				−		+
Kidney	(8)		+				
Cervix	(5)		+		−		
Thyroid	(4)		+				
Esophagus	(4)					+	+

Key: + = Positive association; increased intake with increased cancer.
     − = Negative association; increased intake with decreased cancer.

[a]Rate per 100,000 population, age-adjusted incidence from United States, 1984, Sondik et al., 1987.
[b]Synergistic with smoking.

Source: *The Surgeon General's Report on Nutrition and Health,* U.S. Department of Health and Human Services, 1988.

have a lower incidence of cancer of the prostate than men with a high fat intake. The same studies show that a vegetarian diet lowers circulating testosterone levels and a nonvegetarian diet raises them. Prostate cancer grows on testosterone and slows its growth when testosterone is lowered. A study of Japanese men conducted in 1977 noted that the marked increase in mortality from prostate cancer paralleled the increase in fat intake in the Japanese diet since 1950. It is

not clear whether the cancer increase relates to fat intake, or to body fat.

High caloric intake may be a factor in increasing the risk of cancer primarily by increasing body fat. The relationship between calories and cancer risk was first demonstrated in 1909, when mice on restricted diets were shown to develop fewer tumors when exposed to carcinogens than mice who ate at will. Since then, these results have been consistently duplicated. Furthermore, the tumors that do develop appear later. More recently, mice have been carefully bred to naturally develop spontaneous mammary tumors. Without any exposure to a carcinogen, these animals grow up to develop cancer and die. Studies with these mice suggest that reduced food intake was concomitant with delayed onset of tumor development.

There is a growing body of evidence that the risk of breast cancer, and possibly colon cancer as well, may have more to do with caloric intake and body weight, or both, than with fat consumption per se. The results of the animal studies described above occurred regardless of dietary fat. When rats were placed on a calorie-restricted, low-fat diet, the tumor size and occurrence declined. In a separate study, rats were permitted to eat all they wanted of the low-fat diet, while another group ate a diet restricted in calories but that contained five times the amount of fat. The rats on the high-fat, low-calorie diet developed fewer tumors than those on the low-fat, higher-calorie diet.

In humans, fat in the diet per se does not clearly increase cancer risk. In this country, cancer rates are about equally low among both Mormons and Seventh-Day Adventists. Seventh-Day Adventists follow a vegetarian diet that permits eggs and milk but little or no meat, so their cancer rate has been superficially explained on these grounds. Mormons, however, consume more fat and meat than do

Figure 27.2. Fat Content of Some Common Foods

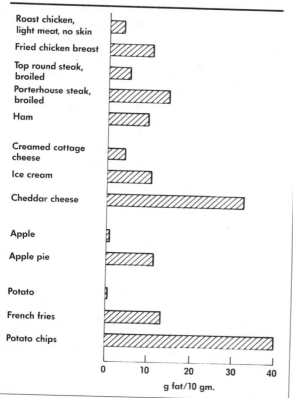

g fat/10 gm.

Note: 100 gm. = 3.5 oz.

Reprinted with permission from J. A. T. Pennington, *Food Values of Portions Commonly Used*, 15th edition (Philadelphia: J. B. Lippincott Publishing Co., 1989).

Seventh-Day Adventists and many non-Mormons, so there must be another explanation for their low cancer rates. The evidence suggests that the similar low cancer rates are due to practices common to both groups, including the fact that neither group smokes tobacco, tolerates alcoholism, or permits heavy caffeine (coffee) ingestion.

There have been several studies in humans that indicate no relationship between total fat consumption and the incidence of breast cancer. One such study, conducted at Harvard University, followed 19,000 nurses for four years. These researchers found no evidence that breast cancer incidence was related to fat intake. Citing other studies with similar results, they suggested that the factor placing some groups at greater risk may be more calories, not more fat.

It is important to consider, however, that in humans, as well as in animals, certain forms of cancer are more common in some families than in others. This is known as genetic predisposition and is particularly true for cancers of the kidney, colon, and breast. Individuals who are members of families where such a cancer history occurs should be aware of the increased danger of being overweight, should be alert to early warning signs, and should seek early medical consultation and necessary treatment. (See Chapter 18.)

Protein, Carbohydrates, and Cancer Risk

Dietary protein has often been associated with cancers of the breast, uterus, prostate, kidney, colon, and pancreas. However, since meat, the major dietary source of protein, contains a variety of other nutrients as well, the association of cancers with protein may not be direct. There have been too few studies on the effects of protein as compared to fat and the high calories of fat to draw any specific conclusions. Because of the very high correlation between fat and protein in the American diet, and because of the more consistent association of these tumors with fat intake, it seems more likely that dietary fat is the more active component.

In contrast to fats and proteins, little attention has been given to carbohydrate intake and the occurrence of cancer. The principal carbohydrates in foods are sugars, starches, and cellulose. The evidence from both laboratory and epidemiological studies is too sparse to suggest any direct role of carbohydrates (with the possible exception of fiber, which will be discussed in detail later on) on cancer risk except for the high calories associated with excessive carbohydrate consumption.

Alcohol, Tobacco, and Cancer Risk

Cancers of the head and neck, including the larynx, pharynx, mouth, and esophagus have all been linked to heavy alcohol consumption, as has cancer of the lung. Alcohol-induced cirrhosis of the liver has also been associated with some cases of liver cancer.

The combination of alcohol and tobacco (chewed as well as smoked) is especially deadly. Alcohol seems to work with tobacco to intensify cancer risk many times. Currently it is thought that moderate alcohol consumption—up to two drinks (three ounces) per day—probably will not raise the cancer risk in well-nourished people who do not smoke.

Lung cancer, which is the most prevalent form of cancer in men in technologically advanced countries, has as its prime causal factor cigarette smoking. More women now die of lung cancer (the primary promotional factor of which has been determined to be tobacco smoke) than they do of breast cancer.

Preservatives, Other Additives, and Pesticides

Currently about 15,000 direct and indirect (for example, from packaging material) additives are used in the American food supply. A few of these, namely cyclamates, the food-coloring agents such as Red No. 32, Orange No. 2, and butter yellow, and varying pesticide residues have been tested in animals for carcinogenicity. With the exception of saccharin, any food additive known to cause cancer in animals at any dose, no matter how high, has been banned by the Food and Drug Administration in any dose, no matter how low. Bruce Ames has pointed out that natural foods are loaded with thousands of natural carcinogens and anticarcinogens, which tend to balance each other out, and that a lot of the natural carcinogens serve as pesticides that protect plants from predatory insects.

Nitrates and Nitrites

Many N-nitroso compounds have been shown to be potent carcinogens in several species. Consequently, in recent years there has been much concern about the use of nitrates and nitrites as preservatives in meats and other cured products. Nitrates can be reduced to nitrites, which interact in the stomach with dietary substances such as amines and amides to form N-nitroso compounds. However, about 80 percent of the nitrates are not additives but are present in our own saliva and occur naturally in our food supply. Each day Americans consume an average of about 200 micrograms from processed meats such as ham and bologna, in addition to 200 micrograms from vegetables and 3,500 micrograms from our own saliva.

The fact is, nitrates and nitrites are unavoidable parts of our environment. The Japanese, who eat more vegetables than Americans, consume about three times more of the naturally occurring nitrites, and they experience about eight times more stomach cancer. Cancers of the esophagus and stomach are high in countries such as Iceland and China,

as well as Japan, whose inhabitants consume large daily quantities of smoked, salted, cured, or pickled meats. Since these products are the most likely source of added nitrites in the United States, it would seem reasonable to recommend that Americans attempt to decrease their intake.

In the United States, death from esophageal cancer has remained at 2 percent of all cancer deaths since 1930. Mortality from stomach cancer has decreased over the past few decades in the United States but not elsewhere in the world. This is in spite of the fact that the consumption of "smoked" and processed meat has *increased* from 42 pounds per person per year in 1930 to 61 pounds per person per year in 1980.

There are several reasons for this discrepancy. Firstly, methods of preservation differ vastly from country to country. Few American meats are as heavily salted or preserved as they are in some countries where there is little or no refrigeration. Secondly, while smoked foods have been linked to cancer risk, 85 percent of what is sold in the United States is smoke-flavored using a compound known as "liquid smoke," which has not been shown to be carcinogenic. Thirdly, the government imposes strict limits. Small quantities of nitrites may be added to foods to prevent the growth of the organism that causes botulism—a usually serious and sometimes fatal form of food poisoning. By United States law, for each part of nitrite added, five parts of ascorbate, a form of vitamin C, must be added to prevent the formation of N-nitroso compounds.

While many people associate all food preservatives and other additives with a greater cancer risk, these products have actually made our food supply safer over the years. The fact is that there is no evidence to date that American smoked or salted meats are dangerous when eaten in moderation. In the United States, nitrates and nitrite food additives do not significantly contribute to cancer risk.

Artificial Sweeteners: Cyclamate, Saccharin, and Aspartame

Artificial sweeteners have been sources of fear and confusion among consumers in recent years. Cyclamate and saccharin have been implicated as possible carcinogens as a result of data obtained from animal studies. However, epidemiological studies tend to refute this data; dose levels needed to produce tumors in these laboratory animals are far greater than even excessive consumption in humans.

Cyclamate was first approved by the Food and Drug Administration (FDA) in 1951 and was added to the Generally Recognized as Safe list in 1958. Evidence that it might cause cancer in rats first appeared in 1969, and in 1970 the FDA removed cyclamate from the market. By 1973, numerous studies had failed to confirm cyclamate's carcinogenicity. Several prestigious organizations, including the World Health Organization and the United Nations Food and Agriculture Organization, declared cyclamate safe. Today, cyclamate is used in over 40 countries. In the United States, cyclamate is periodically resubmitted for evaluation. However, the Food and Drug Administration hesitates to approve its use.

In 1972, the FDA proposed banning saccharin in response to studies indicating that enormous quantities could promote bladder tumors in rats. Congress placed a moratorium on this proposal after considerable public outcry. After several moratorium renewals, the Senate finally voted to allow the continued use of saccharin in the American food supply.

Saccharin was implicated as a carcinogen mostly on the strength of three double-generation animal studies, in which two generations of animals were exposed to saccharin. Saccharin was fed as 5 to 7.5 percent of the diet to adult rats during mating, pregnancy, and nursing. The offspring of these rats were exposed to saccharin from the time of conception (from the placental blood supply and from the milk during nursing) until death. It was equivalent to a human ingesting every day the amount of saccharin contained in 2,000 cans of diet soda. An objective analysis of the results showed that only the males from the second generation had a higher-than-expected incidence of cancer of the bladder. In single-generation studies, where rats received saccharin from weaning until death, there appeared no carcinogenic effect of saccharin—or the results were inconclusive.

Epidemiologic studies in humans suggest that saccharin use is safe. Diabetics who use nonnutritive sweeteners do not develop bladder cancer more frequently than other people. Among patients with bladder cancer, there is no evidence that they use more saccharin than anyone else. Investigators, in a study of 9,000 people, sponsored by the National Cancer Institute, found no association between saccharin consumption and the incidence of bladder cancer in either men or women.

Aspartame was first discovered in 1965 and introduced in the United States as a low-calorie sweetener in 1981. It consists of two amino acids (aspartic acid and phenylalanine) linked to a molecule of methyl alcohol, and it is 180 times sweeter than sugar. It is a potential risk only for those persons with a rare inborn metabolic error known as phenylketonuria (a liver-enzyme deficiency). Aspartame did not cause carcinogenicity in laboratory studies, but as yet there is no epidemiological data pertaining to cancer in humans. It is highly unlikely that its component parts, in the quantities one could possibly reach in each day's diet, could be carcinogenic.

Dietary Components Associated with Lowering Cancer Risk

Vitamin A and the Carotenoids

Vitamin A is the vitamin most often studied for its effect on the process of tumor growth. As part of a normal, balanced diet, vitamin A plays an important role in cell growth and differentiation, particularly of epithelial (skin) tissue. Since tumor development often involves a derangement of cell differentiation, it is thought that promoting differentiation may lower cancer risk. In animals, high doses of vitamin A decrease the number of tumors induced by some carcinogens, slow the growth of those tumors that do appear, and lead to tumor regression. Vitamin A deficiency in animals is associated with premalignant changes in the respiratory, digestive, and genitourinary tracts. Some studies in humans with malignant or premalignant changes in the skin have shown that topical applications of vitamin A may reverse these lesions.

The best food sources of vitamin A are liver, milk, and milk products such as butter. Ingested vitamin A is absorbed in the bloodstream and stored in the liver, where it is released into the tissues as needed. The liver cannot handle prolonged and excessive intake of vitamin A, and it soon reaches toxic levels and results in liver damage. In pregnant animals and humans, it also causes fetal damage.

Results from studies on vitamin A have led scientists to develop analogues of this vitamin with a greater inhibitory effect on cancer cells and less toxicity when used in higher doses. These compounds are known as the retinoids. They are not normal constituents of the diet and should not be confused with the naturally occurring vitamin A, which is also sometimes referred to as retinol. Several laboratory studies using cells from patients with a malignancy known as promyelocytic leuke-mia have confirmed that retinoids can cause these cancer cells to revert to a more normal type of cell. As a result of these studies, retinoic acid is now being used in clinical trials at several major metropolitan hospitals.

Another source of vitamin A is known as beta carotene. This is one of a group of plant pigments called carotenoids. Beta carotene is abundant in dark green and deep yellow vegetables and is converted in the body to vitamin A. While excess beta carotene is much less toxic than vitamin A, it is responsible for the yellow skin color observed in people who eat carrots to excess or who take beta-carotene tablets in large amounts. This yellow pigment is reversible. It is, however, a good indicator of excess.

All carotenoids are thought to exert similar cancer-protective effect through their action as antioxidants. They trap oxygen radicals and prevent cell damage due to oxidation, a metabolic process that renders the cell more susceptible to carcinogens.

Dr. Walter Willett and his colleagues at Harvard University reported that diets high in carrots did not protect against cancer. The carotenoids in carrots are mainly beta. Conversely, diets high in tomatoes, whose carotenoids include almost no beta carotene, were associated with some protective action. The promotion of beta-carotene pills to protect against cancer is not justifiable.

More recently, researchers at Johns Hopkins University found that people with lower than normal blood levels of carotenoids coincidentally had more lung cancer. Another study comparing people, mostly smokers, who developed cancer with those who did not found that levels of carotenoid in the blood of the cancer patients were nearly 14 percent lower than those of patients without cancer. They noted, however, that smokers will not avoid lung cancer by taking carotenoids.

A growing accumulation of epidemiological evidence indicates that an inverse relationship exists between the risk of cancer and the consumption of foods containing vitamin A (e.g., liver) or its precursor, beta carotene (e.g., green and yellow vegetables). Most of the data, however, do not show whether these effects are due to vitamin A itself, to the beta carotenes, or to some other component of these foods. Beta carotene is only one of a family of about 500 carotenoids. Of these, only about 10 percent are converted to vitamin A. The protective effects of these carotenoids may involve the carotenoids that are not converted to vitamin A, or the effects may be due to other factors entirely. For example, foods rich in beta carotene are frequently high in vitamin C and fiber, both of which have been associated with anticancer effects.

While the evidence supporting the cancer-protective effects of the vitamin A derivatives is suggestive, the toxicity of vitamin A in doses exceeding those established for optimal nutrition argues against increasing vitamin A by the use of supplements, as does the fact that the average American is already eating 120 percent of the RDA in his/her diet, and the dietary daily vitamin A intake is so high that excess stores in the liver tend to increase with every decade of life.

Vitamins C and E

Vitamins C and E both function as antioxidants and prevent the formation of N-nitroso compounds. At least five studies in humans have shown that the incidence of gastric (stomach) cancer falls as people consume more fresh vegetables and fruits, especially citrus fruits, but this may also mean that they are eating less of other things, including calories and fat. Gastric cancer has declined dramatically in the United States, perhaps partly due to our year-round consumption of fresh fruits and vegetables, and to our decreased reliance on heavily salted and preserved meats, alcohol, and tobacco.

A diet low in foods containing vitamin C has also been coincidentally associated with more cancer of the mouth, esophagus, larynx, and cervix. In one study, a precancerous condition called cervical dysplasia was high in women whose diets included fewer than 30 milligrams of vitamin C—well below the RDA.

At present, the epidemiological evidence pertaining to the effect of vitamin C on the occurrence of cancer is not extensive. The limited evidence suggests that consumption of foods rich in vitamin C is associated with a lower evidence of cancer of the stomach and esophagus. Despite what you may see in the popular press, there is no evidence that large supplements of vitamin C will either prevent or cure cancer. In fact, even though most of the excess vitamin C is either not absorbed (and therefore produces diarrhea) or is rapidly excreted in the urine, megadoses may produce a wide variety of harmful effects including diarrhea and oxalate kidney stones.

Vitamin E, because it is an antioxidant, may inhibit the formation of nitrosamine-induced tumors. The evidence is scanty, but new studies associate high blood levels of vitamin E with a decreased risk of lung cancer in smokers. Since vitamin E is widely present in foods (vegetable oils, whole-grain-cereal products, and eggs), it is difficult to identify population groups with substantially different levels of intake. In addition, a clear-cut deficiency has not been established in humans. The use of megadoses of vitamin E should be treated with caution, and a wide variety of harms from it were summarized by Charles Marshall in his book *Vitamins and Minerals: Help or Harm?* (Consumers Union, 1985).

Selenium

Selenium, an essential mineral, acts as an anti-oxidant and has therefore been postulated to lower cancer risk. The evidence for this is still very limited. A study conducted in 1973 compared the selenium levels in the blood of more than 100 cancer patients with those of 48 normal subjects. The levels in patients with cancers of the gastrointestinal tract and Hodgkin's disease were significantly lower than those in the normal subjects, but there was no difference between the normal subjects and patients with cancers in other sites, such as the breast. However, in a large joint Chinese-American study in Mainland China, it was found that the highest frequency of cancer was found in those subjects with diets that had the highest selenium content (those consisting of cereals, meat, seafood, as well as mineral-rich drinking water). Looking for an alternative explanation, the investigators claimed that this result was due to the unusually high consumption of salted fish. This study dramatically illustrates that epidemiology can teach only coincidence and not cause and effect, because so many alternative explanations are possible. Furthermore, increasing selenium intake to more than 200 micrograms per day may be toxic. Excessive selenium is highly toxic.

The Role of Fiber in Lowering Cancer Risk

Fiber has been fashionable since the publication of a popular diet book based on the findings of Dr. Denis Burkitt, who discovered that rural Africans eat much more fiber than Americans: 50 to 150 grams per day versus 10 to 20 grams per day. He observed that colon cancer among these Africans was quite low, while it is one of the leading causes of cancer death in the United States. Largely ignored was the fact that a wide variety of other factors were also different among these rural Africans as compared to Americans: i.e., lower genetic predisposition to colon cancer, no smoking, no alcohol, no industrial pollution of water or air, no lead exposure, relatively low-calorie diets, etc. These other things, which epidemiologists refer to as "confounding variables," so dilute the claim that it is fiber that produces their lower colon cancer rate as to make the claim almost nontenable.

Fiber is the modern term for *roughage*. Technically, it is the indigestible parts of grains, fruits, and vegetables. Fiber is further divided into two categories: soluble and insoluble. Most plant foods contain a mixture of both.

Soluble fiber becomes gel-like in water. It is notable for its action in the stomach, where it attracts water, adding bulk to the stomach contents and slowing down the emptying of these contents into the small intestine. Soluble fiber also tends to help lower blood-cholesterol levels, and it may slow the absorption of sugar from the small intestine. Different kinds of soluble fiber include pectins and gums. Good sources include cabbage, apples, prunes, pears, oranges, dried beans, and oat and corn bran.

The second category of fiber is insoluble fiber. It does not dissolve in water but it attracts water into the small intestine, thus adding bulk to its contents. Insoluble fiber has also been shown to decrease the time it takes for the intestinal contents to pass through and be evacuated. It may also stimulate the production of mucus, which coats the lining of the large intestine (colon). Some scientists have suggested that this makes it more difficult for carcinogens to come in contact with the tissues. Different kinds of insoluble fiber include bran forms from beans and whole grains, and some vegetables. (The list on page 480 summarizes the effects of fiber in the colon.)

Scientists have postulated several ways in which fiber may influence cancer risk. The first is through reduction in transit time. By speeding the intestinal contents through the digestive tract, the amount of time that these contents come into contact with the intestinal walls is decreased. Thus, any carcinogens present in the food or introduced during the digestive process have less time in which to affect the cells. A second way is through fiber's effect on fecal weight. Because both kinds of fiber attract more water into the digestive tract, the weight of its contents—and ultimately, the feces—is increased. This additional water dilutes the fecal contents, which, in turn, dilutes the bile acids and, at the same time, speeds them through to evacuation. The strongest evidence to date points to this process as a factor in reducing cancer risk.

Fiber has also been shown to attach to bile acids. It has been postulated that fiber may promote the breakdown of bile acids to short-chain fatty acids and their products: hydrogen, methane, and carbon dioxide. While it has been suggested that these substances inhibit colon carcinogenesis, it has never been demonstrated. Fiber is also divided into two other categories: fermentable and nonfermentable. Fermentable fiber is fermented

Effects of Dietary Fiber in the Human Colon

Increases fecal weight
Increases frequency of defecation
Decreases transit time
Dilutes colonic contents
Increases microbial growth
Alters energy metabolism
Absorbs organic and inorganic substances
Decreases dehydroxylation of bile acids
Production of hydrogen, methane, carbon
    dioxide, and short-chain fatty acids

in the lower small intestine and upper large intestine into volatile short-chain fatty acids, whose acidification of the colon wall may promote colon cancer, as studies in rats suggest.

Epidemiological studies have yielded results that both support and contradict the hypothesis that dietary fiber protects against colon cancer. Urban Danes, who eat roughly 17 grams of fiber per day, have three times the incidence of colon cancer than do rural Finns, who eat about 31 grams of fiber each day. American vegetarians, whose diets are higher in fiber than the rest of the population, have lower cancer rates, and people who are suffering from colon cancer often report having eaten less fiber than people who do not get the disease. However, colon cancer in Hong Kong and Puerto Rico was shown to be more frequent among people who ate more fiber. In another study, the rates of colon cancer in Australian women increased as they increased their intake of dietary fiber.

There is no study demonstrating that fiber in and of itself prevents human cancer. If there is any effect, other components of high-fiber foods, rather than total dietary fiber itself, are more likely to be responsible.

Currently, the best nutritional advice is that the daily intake of fiber should not be more than 35 grams (and not less than 15 grams) obtained from a variety of fruits, vegetables, cereals, breads, and pastas. There is strong evidence that more than 35 grams per day (which is slightly more than 1 ounce) may be harmful. Too much fiber too fast causes gas and intestinal discomfort. Over time, diets with excess fiber may cause interference with the absorption of zinc, iron, and calcium, and may lead to rickets in children. Too much cereal bran may cause painful intestinal obstructions that ultimately may require surgery. (For further information on dietary fiber, see Chapter 9.)

NUTRITION AS THE TREATMENT OF CANCER

Questionable Therapies

Every year, 50,000 cancer patients spend roughly $3 billion on questionable therapies for their diseases. (The definition of "questionable," adopted in 1990 by the American Cancer Society, is that the therapy fails to answer the fundamental questions: Is it more effective than a placebo? Is it safe?) Nutrition plays a large role in these therapies. These different nutritional treatments are called by such names as nutritional therapy, metabolic therapy, holistic therapy, or nontoxic therapy. Any of these terms should warn the consumer that the so-called therapy is probably not therapeutic at all: "alternative therapy" is another name for irresponsible therapy; that is, therapy without regard for efficacy.

Many tumors wax and wane, frequently with no treatment, and any "remedy" that is taken at the time the cancer becomes quiescent will get the credit as a cure, when in fact what most often occurs is a spontaneous and temporary remission. What then accounts for the popularity of these treatments?

Many cancer patients, especially those who may have been given a bleak prognosis by their physicians, may seek hope outside the "medical establishment." Many irresponsible practitioners of "alternative" therapies offer quick, guaranteed, and painless remedies for diseases such as cancer, which are often not curable and whose legitimate treatments may be traumatic. However, practitioners of unorthodox therapies who extol the virtues of their "therapy" treatments are telling the consumers only about their coincidental successes and not about their failures, which outnumber "successes" a hundredfold. All responsible therapy must be able to stand up to the scrutiny of the peer-review process of the scientific press. Remedies published only in the popular press invariably cannot meet these rigid criteria. In addition, some of the patients who are reported to have recovered from cancer may never have had the disease. Cancer can be confirmed only by a biopsy and microscopic examination of the tissues by a trained pathologist. Patients should remember that cancer takes a long time to develop and the appropriate treatment for it may also bring slow results.

Vitamin C

The claim that vitamin C (ascorbic acid) is an effective cancer therapy was based largely on studies by a particular physician in Scotland. This investigator claimed that vitamin C in daily doses of 10 grams, taken along with conventional treatment, could help every cancer patient. He claimed that vitamin C could increase the patient's appetite, strength and vitality, decrease muscle wasting, and generally improve the quality of the patient's life. These claims were demonstrated to be without basis in fact when dissected by reviewers at the National Cancer Institute.

In response to the furor created by the proponents of vitamin C, physicians at the Mayo Clinic treated advanced cancer patients with similar megadoses of vitamin C. They found that patients given such large doses deteriorated more rapidly than those patients given a placebo. Studies conducted at two other responsible institutions supported these results.

Proponents of the vitamin C hypothesis criticized these studies, however, claiming that the patients' doses were too small and not given over a long enough period of time. They also claimed that the responsible chemotherapy that these patients received suppressed their immune systems, neutralizing the vitamin's effects. However, this contradicted their original statement that vitamin C was beneficial even when combined with responsible treatment.

The Mayo Clinic doctors performed the study a second time. They chose patients with advanced colon cancer, who had never received chemotherapy, for treatment with an average of 9.5 grams of vitamin C per day. The study was randomized and double-blind, meaning that neither the doctors nor the patients knew until the conclusion of the study who received vitamins and who received placebos. The researchers administered the vitamin C until the patients' tumors had increased by at least 50 percent—or until their condition deteriorated to the point where it was no longer justifiable to withhold responsible treatment. When the code was broken at the end of the study, once again, the patients who fared the worst were the ones receiving the vitamin C.

The debate rages on between megavitamin enthusiasts and more responsible physicians. Those who advocate large vitamin doses to treat and prevent cancer rationalize away the Mayo Clinic studies. They claim that they cannot get their results published in respectable medical journals because of a conspiracy of silence meant to maintain the physicians' monopoly on treating the sick. The Mayo Clinic studies show that responsible medicine *is* willing to test any alleged treatment. Vitamin C therapy, however, does not stand up to the rigorous examination that every new form of treatment must undergo.

Laetrile

Also called amygdalin, aprikern, or vitamin B_{17}, laetrile is isolated from the pits of stone-bearing fruits, especially apricots.

Laetrile is a cyanogenetic glycoside, which means that it contains cyanide, which it generates when the pit is crushed or when eaten with other plant foods. Thus, it is a potential poison. In fact, it was used in ancient Egypt as a method of execution. Certain compounds, such as megadoses of vitamin C with which laetrile is often combined, enhance the release of cyanide into the blood and increase the danger of cyanide poisoning and death.

Several respected institutions have tested laetrile many times against cancer, with consistently negative results. It has been illegal in the United States since 1978. Nevertheless, as of 1990, about 50,000 Americans were still using laetrile. Some people have been able to obtain it from clinics in foreign countries, while others use laetrile smuggled into this country. Fortunately, as more and more people are realizing that laetrile is not only worthless but poisonous, it is beginning to lose its popularity (but is still lucrative).

Other Nutritional Therapies

Other worthless nutritional therapies for cancer have waxed and waned in popularity over the years. These include the Gerson therapy, the Kelley therapy, macrobiotics, hydrogen peroxide, and others too numerous to mention. Special diets have also been recommended for promotion of health in people undergoing other forms of irresponsible therapy, such as laetrile treatment.

These diets vary to some extent, but they do have a few things in common. Firstly, they usually exclude whole categories of food, most often animal products such as milk and meat. This makes them low in protein and vitamin B_{12}, absorbable iron, and possibly in other nutrients as well, such as calcium. Secondly, they involve bizarre rituals such as nose irrigation and coffee or enzyme enemas, which are not only worthless and uncomfortable but potentially dangerous. The proponents of these therapies say that these measures cleanse the body of toxins. However, these toxins are never named and the elimination of the alleged toxic effects has never been demonstrated. These diets also usually require the purchase of vitamin and mineral supplements, often in toxic doses, and often at huge expense.

Finally, these regimens usually involve a period of fasting, as another way to rid the body of unnamed toxins, as well as to exploit the finding in rats that low caloric intake may slow tumor growth. However, fasting should not be attempted by cancer patients, most of whom are already debilitated and need all the nutrition they can get to help them withstand treatment and fight their disease. (This debilitation is also a problem with responsible treatment and will be discussed later.) Furthermore, starvation compromises the immune system, which further compromises the patient.

Worst of all, however, is that these therapies fool people into thinking that cancer can be cured through diet—and fatally delay them from seeking effective treatment.

NUTRITION FOR THE CANCER PATIENT: RESPONSIBLE STRATEGIES

Cancer affects the patient's nutritional status in several ways. Locally, tumors may obstruct the mouth, throat, intestine, or other areas associated with digestion. As a tumor grows, the function of the organ in which it is growing may be substantially reduced or even lost, as with the pancreas or intestine.

Tumors also can have a systemic effect. For example, certain tumors may secrete hormones or other substances that can alter metabolism or lead to diarrhea and subsequent loss of water, sodium, potassium, calcium, and minerals. Certain tumor products may also alter a patient's taste perception, causing the rejection of food and complicating other therapy.

Many cancer patients also experience a problem called cachexia, a wasting of the body mass that most often occurs in patients with tumors of the liver, pancreas, and digestive tract, as well as those with widespread malignancies. Although the causes of cachexia are unclear, it is believed to result from certain tumor-induced metabolic changes, combined with a loss of appetite. Recent research has focused particularly on a substance produced in the body called cachectin-tumor necrosis factor (TNF).

These problems are exacerbated by the side effects of cancer treatment. For example, radiation and chemotherapy may cause nausea and vomiting, which contribute to nutrient loss and the patient's reluctance to eat. These treatments, as well as cancer surgery, may also leave the patient feeling weak and depressed.

Cancer treatment may affect patients in more specific ways. Radiation to the head and neck may induce changes in taste perception: Red meat may no longer be palatable; desserts may not taste sweet enough. Decreased saliva production can cause difficulties with chewing and swallowing.

The nausea and loss of appetite that is not an unusual consequence of some effective chemotherapy is due to the destruction of some of the normal cells that line the gastrointestinal tract. This is reversible upon discontinuation of treatment.

While *no* diet can prevent the more unpleasant aspects of this treatment, good nutrition is crucial for the cancer patient. Malnutrition depresses immune function; it also makes recovery from surgery and other treatments more difficult. And it may, by itself, contribute to the patient's death. In patients with some forms of cancer, such as colon cancer, extreme malnutrition suggests the terminal phase of the disease. (For tips on encouraging cancer patients to eat, see page 486.)

Patients who cannot eat enough to maintain good nutritional status may need supplements through a gastric tube. More recently, doctors have used parenteral nutrition through intravenous administration in order to improve the malnourished patient's ability to tolerate effective cancer therapy. (With parenteral nutrition, fluid, amino acids, fats, carbohydrates, vitamins, and minerals are administered by catheter directly into the bloodstream.)

NUTRITION AND CANCER: RECOMMENDATIONS

Any new discovery linking a nutrient with cancer promotion or prevention will make headlines. The advocates for these ideas can be so persistent and persuasive that even experts have mistakenly been convinced that the link between a certain nutrient and cancer is unequivocal, when, in fact, it is not.

As discussed, evidence indicates that the

The Effect of Nutrition on the Development of Cancer or Leukemia*

In most animal species thus far tested, transmissible viruses have been implicated as the actual cause of tumors and leukemia. This refers to tumors, leukemia, and lymphomas in fish, chickens, mice, rats, cats, hamsters, cattle, and nonhuman primates. From these experiments, it is assumed that tumors, leukemia, and lymphomas in humans are also caused by transmissable viruses. In fact, certain forms of leukemia and lymphomas, as well as a form of liver cancer in humans, have been demonstrated to be caused by viruses.

Studies on mice, rats, and chickens have shown that many animals carry latent oncogenic (tumor-producing) viruses that usually remain harmless but occasionally become activated to cause the development of tumors or leukemia. The activation process can be triggered by several external or internal factors, such as radiation, certain hormones, or chemicals. However, the activation of the latent, tumor-inducing viruses can be substantially delayed, or even prevented, by avoiding or reducing exposure to tumor-inducing factors, and also by *reduction of the caloric value of food*

intake. However, the reduction of food intake has no effect on the course of an already-established disease.

The following experiments support these findings.

Mammary tumors, as well as leukemia and lymphomas developing spontaneously, were studied in mice and rats, respectively, following exposure to ionizing radiation.

Recent studies showed that fractional total body X-ray or gamma irradiation of Sprague-Dawley rats (150 rads five times at weekly intervals) increased the incidence of tumors from 22 percent to 93 percent in females and from 5 percent to 59 percent in males. Fifty percent of these tumors were malignant. When the rats received a similar dose of radiation but were placed on a calorically restricted diet, the tumor incidence was reduced to 35 percent in females and to 6.7 percent in males.

In previous studies, irradiation of rats increased significantly the incidence of tumors, and occasionally also that of leukemia. In striking contrast, total body X ray or gamma irradiation of mice of certain inbred lines, such as the

*This section has been written by Ludwik Gross, M.D.

correspondence between cancer incidence and most individual nutrients is tenuous at best. By changing the diet to emphasize one particular nutrient, or taking supplements of a specific nutrient, an individual may not only be missing some essential others, but also may interfere with the body's ability to use others, and, in some cases, may actually accelerate the growth of the cancer.

Based upon recent information about possible diet-cancer links, we make the following suggestions to those who don't have cancer.

1. Choose a diet for variety, balance, and moderation. The greater the variety, the greater the assurance that whatever anti-cancer nutrients there are will be eaten. The better the balance, the better those nutrients will be able to interact. And the more moderation, the less likely something will be eaten to excess.

2. Maintain desirable weight. Of all of the alleged diet-cancer links, that between excess calories or body weight and cancer is the best established. (See the commentary by Dr. Ludwik Gross on page 484.)

3. If you don't have cancer, follow the recommended dietary guidelines on nutrition to reduce the risks of cancer; these have been formulated by six respected institutions in

---

The Effect of Nutrition on the Development of Cancer or Leukemia* *(cont.)*

C3H line, induced a high incidence of leukemia.

In a current study, mice of the C3H inbred line, known to be essentially free from spontaneous leukemia, were exposed to total body gamma irradiation. The mice were divided into two groups; animals in the first group were allowed to eat as much as they wanted. Fifty percent of these animals developed leukemia. In the second group, consisting of brothers and sisters of the first group, the animals received a restricted diet consisting of approximately half of the food consumed by the animals in the first group. Although mice in this group had the same irradiation exposure, only 4 percent of the mice on the restricted diet developed leukemia. The great majority of these animals remained healthy and active during the experiment. These studies demonstrate clearly that the development of leukemia following exposure to ionizing radiation could be inhibited by the reduction of food intake.

Leukemia in mice is caused by a virus. This virus remains harmless until activated. Radiation is a potent factor that may activate the virus and cause the development of leukemia. Nevertheless, reduction of food intake did not influence the progress of the disease once leukemia had developed.

In Humans

In human studies, statistical data confirms that the incidence of cancer and leukemia is substantially higher in men and women who are overweight than in the general population. Recently compiled statistical data reported by the American Cancer Society suggest that men and women who are overweight have an almost 50 percent higher probability of developing cancer than individuals of similar gender and age who do not exceed weight limits considered normal for their age and gender.

Similar observations were made in experiments carried out on laboratory animals, such as mice and rats, developing tumors or leukemia spontaneously or with tumors or leukemia induced by hormones or carcinogenic chemicals. Animals that were underweight had a lower incidence of tumors or leukemia, as compared with those that had an excessive weight, according to standards considered normal for a given species's gender and age.

the United States and abroad. They are: Avoid obesity; cut down on total fat intake; regularly eat fresh vegetables, including cruciferous (cabbage-type) dark green and deep yellow vegetables, and deep yellow fruits, which are high in vitamins A and C.

4. Use alcohol in moderation.

5. Stop smoking completely.

If you do have cancer, modify the above suggestions as recommended by your physician and the registered dietitian or other responsible nutrition professional who works with your doctor. They may very well suggest consuming all the calories you can handle.

Encouraging a Cancer Patient to Eat

Trying to get a cancer patient to eat can present a formidable challenge to loved ones and professionals alike. The following tips can help.

- Certain drugs, such as painkillers and those that relieve nausea, may reduce pain and nausea and allow the patient to eat a little more.

- Have the patient eat the most when he or she feels the best—usually at breakfast—and preferably in small portions.

- Serve soft, bland foods, such as scrambled eggs or milk shakes, which may be tolerated more easily.

- Keep meals small and low in fat to prevent the patient from feeling full too quickly.

- Maintain a pleasant environment; if certain odors make the patient sick, eliminate them. If the patient enjoys reading or watching television while eating, doing so might be a way to get him or her to eat a little more.

- Do not make a mealtime more stressful than it inherently is. Do not force a patient to eat more than is comfortable for him or her: Some patients fill up after only a few spoonfuls of cereal or a part of a sandwich.

Updates on Cancer *

Recent work in China, by Dr. Ran and her associates, in conjunction with Dr. Herbert at Mount Sinai, supports suggestions that deficiency of the vitamin folic acid promotes cancer of the cervix, and that deficiency of vitamin B_{12} damages the immune system. This work is reported in the Proceedings of the 1990 Congress of the International Society of Hematology in Boston.

Many experts question the usefulness of animal tests to claim chemicals at any dose, no matter how small, cause cancer in humans. Drs. Bruce Ames and Lois Gold point out that enormous doses of half of all synthetic chemicals and half of all natural chemicals cause cancer in rodents by killing or irritating cells, stimulating reactive cell proliferation that goes on to become cancer, but quantities eaten by humans do not do this, except for alcohol, salt, peppers, and some spices.

*This section written by Victor Herbert, M.D., F.A.C.P.

28

The Effects of Nutrition on Diabetes and Other Endocrine Disorders

Elliot J. Rayfield, M.D.

■

INTRODUCTION

Of all the endocrine disorders, diabetes is the most common; it also is a disease in which nutrition plays a major role in treatment. Therefore, diabetes is the major thrust of this chapter. Before discussing the specifics of diabetes and its treatment, however, we will present a brief overview of the endocrine system and how it works.

The endocrine system is made up of a network of glands and glandular tissue that secretes hormones—body chemicals that influence virtually every organ system and bodily process. Working closely with the nervous system, the endocrine system controls such diverse activities as reproduction, metabolism, growth, sleep cycles, maintenance of the body's salt, water, and chemical balance, and response to stress, among many others.

Hormones are secreted directly into the bloodstream, in response to a signal from the nervous system or blood levels of a specific substance such as glucose, sodium, water, other hormones, calcium, and so on. As hormones travel through the body, they bind to specific receptors on certain cells. Some hormones act directly on an organ. Others have no direct action of their own; instead, they prompt the manufacture and release of other hormones. (Examples of the latter include thyroid-stimulating hormone, which prompts the thyroid gland to produce its hormones, or the gonadotropins, which stimulate the production of male and female sex hormones.)

The major endocrine glands are the thyroid, pituitary, parathyroid, thymus, adrenal, pancreas, and the gonads (ovaries in women and testes in men). The pineal is also included among the endocrine glands, but its true function is unknown. A number of organs, especially the brain, kidneys, lungs, heart, and intestinal lining, also secrete hormones.

Every now and then, a new hormone is discovered, and much remains to be learned about the entire endocrine system. In fact, the endocrine system is perhaps the body's most complex. When something goes wrong with one part of it, the effects may be experienced throughout the body and in many different ways. Fortunately, most endocrine diseases are relatively uncommon, with the exception of diabetes.

DIABETES MELLITUS

It is estimated that about 10 million Americans have diabetes mellitus, but about half may not know they have the disease. For reasons that are not clearly understood, the incidence of diabetes is rising in the United States. About 40,000 Americans die from diabetes each year, but many more die from complications of the disease, such as kidney failure or vascular disease.

Types of Diabetes

Diabetes is principally a disease of disordered metabolism—the process by which the body converts food into forms that can be used for energy, growth, and other body needs—but it also adversely affects many organs and body functions. Although many people think of diabetes as being a single disease, it is actually a family of disorders related to impaired metabolism of glucose, or blood sugar. *Insulin-dependent diabetes, commonly referred to as Type I diabetes,* and also as juvenile-onset and ketosis-prone, is characterized by a failure of the pancreas to produce insulin—a hormone essential to proper metabolism. *Noninsulin-dependent diabetes, commonly called Type II diabetes,* and also referred to as adult-onset or ketosis-resistant diabetes, results from the body's inability to fully utilize insulin. (See Table 28.1.) *Gestational diabetes* occurs during pregnancy and usually disappears upon delivery (although women with this form of the disease have an increased risk of later developing Type II or, less commonly, Type I diabetes). Sometimes a person will develop temporary *stress diabetes* during an infection or after surgery. *Secondary diabetes* occurs as a result of other diseases, such as pancreatitis, or as a result of exposure to certain drugs or chemicals.

Plasma-glucose levels fluctuate within a normal fasting range of 50 to 115 milligrams of glucose per deciliter of blood. Levels rise after eating and are at their lowest following a long fast, such as before breakfast. Diabetes is diagnosed by consistently high levels of blood glucose taken after several hours of fasting or in response to a glucose challenge. Typically, a blood sample is taken early in the morning, before food is consumed (a fasting blood glucose). A diagnosis of Type I diabetes is established if two separate fasting blood-glucose tests show more than 140 milligrams per deciliter, or 7.8 millimoles, to use the newer medical terminology. In borderline cases—fasting plasma-glucose levels of 115 to 140 milligrams per deciliter—in which there are symptoms of diabetes, such as excessive thirst and urination, additional testing may be needed. These may include a glucose-tolerance test, which measures the body's response to a glucose or sugar challenge.

The causes of diabetes are unknown. In Type I diabetes, a virus or toxin may trigger the disease in a genetically susceptible individual. In Type II diabetes, a family history of diabetes is much more common than in Type I diabetes and obesity is an important risk factor.

Type II diabetes is the most common form of the disease, outnumbering Type I about 10 to 1. It usually begins in middle age; about 80 percent of Type II diabetics are over the age of 50. Most are overweight and excessive body fat is both a cause and consequence of the disease. Some Type II diabetics may require insulin, particularly younger and leaner individuals. With most patients with diabetes, the problem is not so much one of inadequate insulin as an inability of the body to use what it produces. However, it is thought that both insulin resistance and insulin deficiency, to a lesser extent, frequently coexist in the same individual. Thus, insulin resistance is a hallmark of Type II diabetes.

Type I diabetes is generally the most serious form of the disease. It usually begins in the first two decades of life; the mean age of onset is 12 years. For reasons that are not clearly understood, the body ceases to produce insulin. Type I diabetes often follows a viral infection, and many researchers believe that the onset may be related to an auto-immune response in which the immune system overreacts and, in effect, attacks some part of the body itself; in this instance, the hormone-producing portions of the pancreas. Insulin is produced by beta cells in the islets of Langerhans—clusters of hormone-producing tissue scattered throughout the pancreas. (The islets also contain alpha cells, which produce glucagon—the other major hormone that regulates the amount of glucose in the blood.)

Effects of Diabetes

Glucose is the body's major fuel, essential for proper function of the brain, muscles, red blood cells, and other tissues. Carbohydrates are readily converted to glucose; proteins and fats also can be made into glucose for energy, but not as readily as carbohydrates. Fats are stored and mobilized for energy at a later date.

When the body cannot utilize glucose, it builds up in the blood—a condition referred to as hyperglycemia. Under normal conditions, the kidneys retain glucose rather than excrete it into the urine, but when there are very high levels of blood glucose, the kidneys help lower it by letting some spill into the urine. This is called glycosuria, and it is a major symptom of diabetes.

When there is too much glucose circulating in the blood, it draws water from the cells into the blood. Consequently, when glucose spills into the urine, it takes water with it, leading to the excessive urination (polyuria) that is characteristic of diabetes. The loss of water from the cells and blood lead to excessive thirstiness—another common symptom of the disease.

Typically, diabetics also feel excessively hungry and will eat large quantities of food. Even though there may be large amounts of glucose in the blood, without insulin the cells are unable to utilize it for energy. In effect, the cells are in a state of starvation. In Type II diabetes, the body will eventually make use of the food because insulin is available. The uptake of glucose is slower and less efficient than normal. Hyperinsulinemia (excessive circulating insulin) leads to overeating. Some of the

Table 28.1. Differences Between Type I and Type II Diabetes

Characteristic	Type I	Type II
Age of onset	Usually during first three decades of life, especially during periods of rapid growth	Usually after forty, increasing with age
Precipitating factors	Altered immune response to certain viruses (?)	Obesity, pregnancy, infection, and other stresses
Endogenous insulin	Little or none	May be normal, high, or low
Fasting blood glucose	High	May be near normal
Carbohydrate intolerance	Severe	Moderate to severe
Response to fasting	High blood glucose	Blood glucose becomes normal
Response to insulin	Normal	May be resistant
Response to diet alone	Negligible	Usually marked
Response to oral hypoglycemic drugs	None	Usually good

excess glucose circulating in the blood may be excreted in the urine, but because there is insulin available, varying amounts of the excess glucose are stored as body fat—one reason why so many Type II diabetics are overweight.

In contrast, patients with poorly controlled Type I diabetes often lose weight, no matter how much they eat. Since there is no insulin to promote cellular uptake of glucose, the body responds by breaking down stored fat and protein for energy. This can result in weight loss as well as the serious disturbances in body chemistry seen in Type I diabetes. When the liver is called upon to metabolize large amounts of fat, it produces acidic substances called ketone bodies. The muscles and other tissues can use some of the ketones for energy, but the excess will build up in the blood and also spill over into the urine. (One type of ketone body, acetone, produces a fruity-smelling breath, another sign often noted in Type I diabetes.) Excessive ketones in the blood can lead to an upset in the body's normal chemical balance. If this persists, the person can lapse into a life-threatening coma.

Ketoacidosis usually does not occur in Type II diabetes, because insulin is available, even though the body does not utilize it properly. Thus, the comas that sometimes occur in Type II diabetes are generally caused by very high blood glucose and resulting dehydration.

Many people associate insulin primarily with carbohydrate metabolism. In reality, however, insulin is also needed for the proper metabolism of proteins and fats. Under normal circumstances, the pancreas increases the secretion of insulin after eating. This facilitates the metabolism and the uptake and storage of all the nutrients, which, in effect, control the levels of blood glucose.

Long-Term Consequences of Diabetes

Over time, diabetes affects many body systems. Serious complications can occur in both Types I and II diabetes but are most common in poorly controlled Type I. (The lists on page 492 give immediate symptoms of high and low blood glucose.) Long-term consequences include:

Circulatory and cardiovascular systems. People with diabetes are particularly susceptible to cardiovascular diseases, especially high blood pressure, elevated blood cholesterol, and atherosclerosis—the buildup of fatty deposits in the arteries. These cardiovascular complications result in the increased incidence of heart attacks and strokes suffered by diabetic patients. Diabetes also affects the microcirculation, or the tiny capillaries that carry

Figure 28.1.

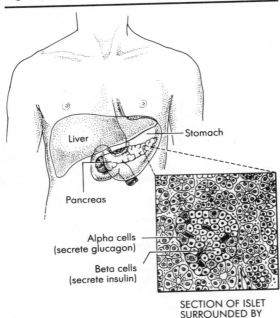

Liver

Stomach

Pancreas

Alpha cells
(secrete glucagon)

Beta cells
(secrete insulin)

SECTION OF ISLET
SURROUNDED BY
ACINAR CELLS

blood to the individual body cells. The capillary basement membranes become thickened, reducing the amount of blood (and nutrients) reaching the cells. In addition, high levels of blood glucose reduce the amount of oxygen that can be carried by the hemoglobin.

Impaired circulation in the legs and feet is a very common consequence of long-standing, poorly controlled diabetes. Reduced blood flow in the legs can lead to intermittent claudication, which is characterized by calf pain and cramping when walking for more than short distances or when climbing stairs. Seriously compromised circulation to the legs and feet can lead to chronic ulcers, numbness, and, in severe cases, gangrene, which requires amputation. In fact, diabetes is the leading cause of amputation in the United States.

Eyes. Diabetes is the leading cause of blindness among adults in this country. The disease has an adverse effect on most eye structures, particularly the retina. Diabetic patients also are more susceptible to develop cataracts, which come on at an earlier age and develop more rapidly than in the general population.

Nervous system. Diabetic neuropathy—a progressive deterioration of nerve function—is characterized by numbness or tingling sensations, especially in the fingers and toes; muscle weakness; intermittent episodes of pain; slowed reflexes; and coordination problems. In men, sexual impotence is common and may occur even before the diabetes has been diagnosed.

Kidneys. Diabetes, especially poorly controlled Type I, is one of the leading causes of kidney failure. High levels of blood glucose put an added burden on the nephrons, the kidneys' minute filtering units. In addition, high blood glucose causes membrane thickening in the nephrons, thereby reducing their fil-

Figure 28.2.

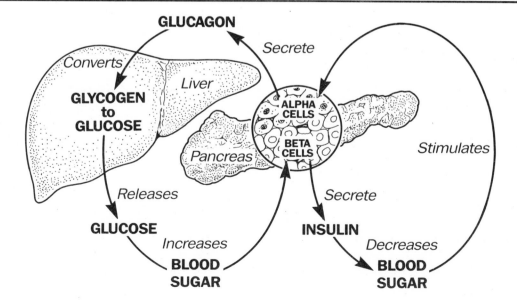

tering capacity. This results in increased glucose in the urine, as well as the loss of protein and other important nutrients via the kidneys.

Increased risk of infection. People with diabetes are particularly susceptible to infection for several reasons. High blood sugar increases vulnerability to infections of the urinary tract, respiratory tract, vagina, skin, mouth, and other structures. Not only are diabetic patients more susceptible to infections but they also heal more slowly than nondiabetics because of their impaired circulation and other factors. In addition, infection increases insulin resistance, making the diabetes more difficult to control.

Treatment of Diabetes

Numerous studies in recent years have found that many, if not all, of diabetic complications often can be prevented or mini-

mized by designing a treatment program that keeps blood glucose within a normal range. The specific approach to treatment depends upon the type of diabetes. People with Type I diabetes must take insulin injections, whereas most Type II diabetics can be treated by diet alone, or a combination of diet and drugs to improve the body's utilization of insulin. (In some instances, Type II diabetics also may require insulin injections or medication to improve insulin uptake.)

Common Misconceptions

Because diabetes is often referred to as a sugar disease, many people mistakenly think that it is caused by eating too much refined

---

Symptoms of High Blood Sugar

- Increased thirst and urination
- Loss of appetite
- Nausea and vomiting
- Weakness
- Large amounts of ketones in the urine
- Blood-sugar measurements of more than 300 milligrams per deciliter
- Breath will smell fruity (from acetones)
- Dehydration (dry mouth, skin, etc.)
- Fixed, dilated pupils, difficulty in focusing
- Heavy, labored breathing
- Loss of consciousness (diabetic coma)

Symptoms of an Insulin Reaction

- A tingling sensation in the mouth, fingers, or other parts of the body
- A cold, clammy feeling
- Paleness
- A buzzing in the ears
- Excessive sweating
- A feeling of weakness or faintness
- Headache
- Hunger
- Abdominal pain
- Irritability and change in mood or personality
- Impaired vision
- Rapid heartbeat and trembling
- Sudden drowsiness
- Sudden awakening from sleep, especially if it is accompanied by other symptoms

sugar. While it is true that sugar and other simple carbohydrates can produce a rapid rise in blood glucose in the absence of adequate insulin, they do not cause diabetes. Another common myth holds that a diabetic person cannot include sugar in his or her diet. So long as there is adequate insulin to metabolize it, a person with diabetes can have *modest* amounts of sugar. (See the section on sweeteners on page 498.)

Although diet plays an integral role in the treatment of diabetes, there is no master diabetes diet that works for all persons with the disease. (Table 28.2 outlines basic dietary approaches.) As more has been learned about effective self-management of diabetes, many of the former dietary restrictions have become more relaxed. For example, people with diabetes now routinely measure their own blood glucose and can very quickly determine the effects of specific insulin dosages, foods, exercise, stress, infections, and other factors. With proper instruction and understanding, diabetic patients can use glucose self-monitoring to adjust insulin dosages according to food intake or other factors that affect blood glucose.

Physicians and diabetes educators who use this system find that their patients often are more successful in achieving good diabetes control than are patients who are given a specific insulin regimen and a rigid dietary plan. There are a number of reasons for this: Diabetes varies considerably from patient to patient, and for any individual, the disease can even vary from day to day. (For example, a person's insulin requirements may increase during a cold or other illness, and decrease during periods of vigorous exercise.) A standardized meal also does not take into consideration individual food preferences and deep-seated cultural attitudes and traditions—both very important aspects in designing a meal plan. Trying to work with exchange lists is impractical or too complicated for many patients. Ex-

pecting an adolescent to adhere to a diet that is markedly different from that of his or her peers may be unrealistic.

In the past, there has been a tendency to blame the patient for not adhering to diet plans, with little consideration as to whether the diet was tailored to meet individual needs. Today, there is increased emphasis on patient education and understanding. Many diabetes specialists enlist the services of a dietitian or diabetes educator to work with the patient (and his or her family, if appropriate) in developing a sound and practical eating plan. As both the general public and physicians become increasingly attuned to the role of a moderate, balanced diet in maintaining overall health, we have come to recognize that the dietary principles recommended for diabetic people are very much in keeping with what all of us should be eating. Thus, it is no longer considered necessary to prepare separate dishes or meals for the diabetic family member.

This attitude represents a marked departure from past approaches, in which dozens of diabetic diets have been built on rigid restrictions, often with diametrically opposed points

Table 28.2. Comparison of Dietary Approaches in Type I and Type II Diabetes

Dietary Factor	Type I	Type II
Consistency in calorie intake	Yes	No
Consistency in meal timing	Yes	No
Need small, frequent meals	Yes	No
Consistency in balance of carbohydrates, protein, and fat	Yes	No
Adjust food intake according to blood-sugar level	Yes	No
Reduce total calories consumed	No	Yes
Adjust food intake for physical activity	Yes	No

of view. Before the discovery of insulin in 1921, dietary manipulation was the only treatment for diabetes. For Type I diabetes, diet, although important in overall control of blood glucose, is not enough to prevent a fairly rapid decline. Thus, before 1921, people with Type I diabetes typically survived only a few years, at the most.

The earliest recorded diabetic diet is in the *Papyrus Ebers*, which was written in about 1500 B.C. Those ancient physicians advocated wheat grains, fruit, and sweet beer—in other words, a high-carbohydrate diet—"to drive away the passing of too much urine." Most recorded diets over the next millennium were rich in carbohydrates. Then in the late 1700s, Dr. John Rollo, a British physician, came up with a radically different plan: a low-carbohydrate diet high in fat and animal protein. The diet—built on "blood pudding and old rancid meats"—probably was low in calories, too, because of its extreme unpalatability.

Variations of low-carbohydrate, low-calorie diets were advocated for the next 150 years or so, with a few notable exceptions, such as one that was mostly oatmeal. In the 1850s, a Paris physician suggested a diet of 125 grams of sugar candy and two portions of meat. Several of these early doctors noted that periodic fasting or calorie restriction seemed to help. In 1912, Dr. Frederick M. Allen of New York's Rockefeller Institute devised a near-starvation diet of 1,000 calories a day. Such low-calorie regimens, even though they did not allow for proper growth and resulted in extreme emaciation, may have prolonged life for a few Type I diabetics. Still, without insulin, the diabetes would grow progressively worse and the person would die.

All of this changed dramatically after two Canadian researchers, Drs. Frederick Banting and Charles Best, discovered insulin in 1921. A 13-year-old boy, Leonard Thompson, was the first patient to receive the hormone injec-

tions. He was treated with regular insulin injections for five months, and with normal blood-sugar levels, the boy was released from the hospital as cured. He was back a few months later, weighing only 60 pounds and again near death. This time, it was recognized that the injections would not provide a cure but that he could manage quite well so long as he received them daily. His diet was high in fats, moderate in protein, and relatively low in carbohydrates. Under this regimen, the boy began to grow and, until his death from pneumonia in 1935, he led a relatively normal life.

Since then, a great deal has been learned about insulin dosages and diabetes control, and over the last 50 years dietary recommendations have been revised several times. Even though insulin injections are not as precise as the body's own system of secreting the hormone in response to need, we have learned a good deal about the fine tuning of insulin dosages and matching the hormone to food intake, exercise, and other variable factors. Today's diabetes specialists and patient educators also recognize that "there is no single, specific food plan suitable for all individuals with diabetes."*

General Guidelines for Type I Diabetes

Meal Planning

Developing a workable eating pattern that fulfills the person's individual needs is the cornerstone of dietary management of diabetes. This is perhaps the most time-consuming aspect of the diabetes patient's education but also one that pays off in terms of improved

---

*Ronald A. Arky, M.D., "Nutritional Management of the Diabetic" in *Diabetes Mellitus: Theory and Practice*, third edition, edited by Max Ellenberg, M.D., and Harold Rifkin, M.D. (New York: Medical Examination Publishing Co., 1983).

health and well-being. In designing a workable meal plan, the following should be considered.

Family eating patterns. As much as possible, the diabetic person's meal plan should fit in with normal family eating habits. Timing of meals, food choices, and portion sizes all are important in achieving good control of Type I diabetes, and these factors all are influenced by family eating patterns. Some adjustments may be needed, but in most instances, a treatment program can be tailored to fit in. The greatest difficulties seem to be with adolescents, whose eating patterns tend to be erratic, and the elderly, especially those who eat alone without any specific meal patterns. (See section on Problem Solving on page 501.)

Individual food preferences and cultural background. Most of us have favorite foods, and changing preferences that have been built up over a lifetime of eating is very difficult. Our cultural and social heritage also are important dietary determinants: We are introduced to certain foods and eating patterns as children and carry these through life. Virtually every national or ethnic group has its own distinctive cuisine; for example, menu plans that may work well for someone of Italian heritage can be strange and quite unacceptable for a person of Middle Eastern, Japanese, Jewish, southern, or some other cultural background. In developing a meal plan, it is vital to build it around the individual's food preferences; otherwise, experience has shown it is unlikely to be followed over time.

Caloric requirements. Any meal plan is built around calculating total caloric needs and then picking appropriate foods to provide these calories. For the person with diabetes, maintaining a relatively constant caloric intake is important because food intake is one of the determining factors in calculating insulin

dosages. Body weight, age, gender, and activity level all should be considered in determining how many calories are needed per day. A sedentary adult will not need as many calories as one who is active; a growing child or adolescent may need many more calories than an older adult. Enough calories should be consumed to maintain ideal body weight and provide the energy needed for the individual's activity level. (See Chapter 17.)

Timing of meals. Consistency is one of the most important aspects of a workable meal plan for a Type I diabetic. The total calories should be consumed throughout the course of a day and timed according to insulin injections to avoid wide variations in blood-glucose levels. Although this sounds rather complicated, it is now much easier than in the past because the person can use blood-glucose self-testing to see how well he or she is doing. Many diabetes education programs now emphasize teaching the patient how to match insulin and food intake and to make whatever adjustments are needed to maintain normal blood-glucose levels. In the beginning, however, most patients are given a master plan that gives the times when insulin should be injected, and, based on this and the considerations outlined above, when meals and snacks should be eaten. There is no one plan that works for all patients; some do nicely on three regular meals a day; most may need to add snacks in between meals, depending upon the individual's insulin regimen. The important thing is that the plan be followed with reasonable consistency from day to day. Adjustments can be made to allow for special circumstances, but this requires understanding the principles of self-monitoring and matching food and insulin.

A workable meal plan can be developed for almost everyone, including people with erratic schedules; for example, a person on rotating work shifts. The latter may do better on an insulin pump, an automatic device that can be programmed to deliver small amounts of insulin at different times and adjusted to cover erratic meal patterns. The average person, however, usually manages well with a program worked out to meet his or her normal needs. Table 28.3 provides a sample meal program.

Distribution of Calories Among Nutrients

As noted earlier, the basic concepts of balance and moderation that apply to sound nutrition for the general public are even more important for the person with Type I diabetes. In recent decades, recommendations for how calories should be distributed among carbohydrates, fats, and protein have been revised considerably, and some experts still disagree on some points. Increasingly, however, the following guidelines are recommended.

Carbohydrates. Prior restrictions on carbohydrate intake have been eased considerably. The typical meal plan now allows for 45 to 55 or 60 percent of calories to come from carbohydrates, but there is still controversy over the proportions of complex (starches) versus simple (sugars) carbohydrates. Earlier restrictions

against simple carbohydrates have been relaxed considerably, and typical meal plans now allow up to 5 percent of calories to come from simple carbohydrates. It is well known that consuming simple carbohydrate by itself—for example, a glass of orange juice, soft drink, sugar candy, and so on—will produce a quick rise in blood glucose. When the sweet is consumed as part of a meal or in combination with fats, protein, and complex carbohydrates, however, the glycemic (glucose-producing) effect is moderated. For example, ice cream, which most people regard as a sweet, actually produces only a moderate rise in blood glucose because of its large amount of fat. Thus, a diabetic patient should avoid simple carbohydrates alone, and, instead, include them with complex carbohydrates, protein, or fats.

The method of a food preparation also affects the glycemic potential of food. Cooking starchy vegetables, for example, may alter the glycemic response. One study showed that cooking carrots reduced the glycemic rise. (Table 28.4 lists the glycemic index of a number of common foods. The higher the glycemic index, the greater and quicker the rise in blood sugar.)

Fat. In the past, high-fat diets often were recommended for diabetic patients because of their low glycemic effect. It is now known that a high-fat diet may promote high blood cholesterol, atherosclerosis, and heart disease. Since people with diabetes are especially vulnerable to these disorders, it is now recommended that they moderate their fat intake to no more than 30 percent of total calories. (An even lower fat intake may be recommended for patients with high cholesterol or coronary disease.) The types of fats consumed also are important. In general, saturated fats (i.e., the fats predominant in milk, cheese, butter, meats, and palm and coconut oil) tend to

---

28.3. Suggested Distribution of Consumed Calories in Type I Diabetes

	Preschool to Age 9 (%)	Age 10 to Adult (%)
Breakfast	20	20
Mid-morning snack	10	NA
Lunch	20	25
Afternoon snack	10	10
Dinner	30	35
Bedtime snack	10	10

Adapted from Dr. Ronald A. Arky, "Nutritional Management of the Diabetic" in *Diabetes Mellitus*, with permission from Medical Examination Publishing Co., Inc.

raise blood cholesterol. Saturated fats should be limited to 6 to 8 percent of calories, polyunsaturated fats should comprise 10 percent or less of calories, and the balance should be from monounsaturated fats.

A high-fat diet also is thought to promote cardiovascular disease and a number of other disorders (including Type II diabetes). Since fats contain more calories—nine per gram—than proteins and carbohydrates, which each contain about four per gram, a high-fat diet is likely to be high in calories. The effects of dietary cholesterol on blood cholesterol, atherosclerosis, and heart disease is well established.

Table 28.4. Glycemic Index of Different Foods

| Food | Subjects | |
	Nondiabetic	Diabetic
Glucose	100	100
Grain products		
Bread, white	69	70
Bread, whole-grain	72	70
Rice, white	72	56
Spaghetti, white	50	42
Cereals		
All-bran	51	50
Cornflakes	80	86
Oatmeal	49	69
Vegetables		
Carrots	92	NA
Corn	59	NA
Peas	51	NA
Potatoes, new	70	54
Legumes		
Beans, kidney	29	46
Lentils	29	31
Fruit		
Apples	39	NA
Bananas	62	58
Oranges	40	NA
Raisins	64	NA

Data from Jenkins, D.J.A.; Wolever, T.M.S., Taylor, R.H., Barker, H., "Glycemic Index of Foods." Reprinted with permission from the *American Journal of Clinical Nutrition* 34:362, 1981, American Society for Clinical Nutrition.

People with diabetes tend to have high blood cholesterol. A lack of insulin promotes changes in fat metabolism, including an elevation of serum triglycerides. In general, diabetes specialists recommend that dietary cholesterol be limited to about 300 milligrams a day—a recommendation in keeping with the American Heart Association and the National Cholesterol Education Program. (See Chapter 6 for a more detailed discussion.)

Protein. The balance of calories—about 12 to 20 percent of total daily intake—should come from protein. This can be from animal protein or a combination of vegetable proteins to form complete proteins. A certain amount of dietary protein can be converted to glucose and burned as energy if needed, but most is used for tissue growth and repair or other metabolic processes. Any excess is converted to fat and stored. Under some circumstances, dietary protein may be restricted; for example, in the presence of kidney disease. In general, however, diabetic patients can eat normal amounts of protein without difficulty.

Dietary fiber. The role of dietary fiber on blood glucose is still another area under considerable debate and study. Fiber is the part of plants that is not digested or absorbed by humans. There are many kinds of fiber, which fall into two general categories: the insoluble or structural fibers that make up plant-cell walls, and the soluble fibers, such as pectin, gums, and mucilages that form gels, repair injured areas, and sequester nutrients. A number of studies have found that high-fiber diets seem to improve glucose control, reduce insulin requirements, and help prevent some diabetic complications, such as high blood cholesterol and atherosclerosis. It is not known how fiber produces these effects, but a number of possibilities have been suggested. Some fibers, such as cellulose and hemicellulose, absorb water and speed gastric transit time. Pectin, guar, and other soluble fibers tend to bind with bile acids and thereby lower blood cholesterol. Fiber also alters the absorptive process and bacterial content of the digestive tract. Fiber, because of its ability to absorb water, gives a feeling of fullness and can help prevent overeating. There may be other as yet unidentified effects that alter the glycemic potential of foods or affect diabetes in other ways.

Many people mistakenly equate recommendations to increase dietary fiber intake with adding bran or other fiber supplements to the diet. This can lead to serious gastrointestinal problems as well as decreased absorption of iron, calcium, and other important minerals. However, this is not considered a serious concern, as most fiber diets are already higher in vitamins and minerals. Fiber should be eaten in its natural sources—grains, fruits, and vegetables. A balanced diet that includes a variety of whole-grain cereals, breads, oat bran, pasta, legumes, vegetables, and fruits will provide ample amounts of the different dietary fibers. It's a balance of fiber rather than any one type that is important. (See Chapter 9.)

Sweeteners

We are born with a preference for sweet-tasting foods, as has been demonstrated in studies with very young babies. Sweeteners, both artificial and natural, are added to a variety of foods, drinks, and products such as toothpaste, lipstick, and even soaps. Among the general population, about 18 percent of total calories come from table sugar and other refined or processed sugars, with another 6 percent coming from naturally occurring sugars, such as fructose.

Contrary to popular belief, sugar per se does not appear to be a major health hazard. A high sugar intake has been linked to increased dental cavities. Many sweet foods, such as candy and pastries, are high in fats and calories. Sugar provides calories (four per gram) but has little else in the way of nutrition. Thus, a high-sugar diet may be lacking in important vitamins and minerals. For years, people with diabetes have been warned to avoid sugar and other nutritive sweeteners. The restrictions have been used to promote artificial sweeteners and foods made with them as safe for diabetics. Restrictions against nutritive sweeteners in diabetic diets have been relaxed considerably in recent years, but some have questioned their long-term safety. As a result, there is considerable confusion over whether diabetic patients should have sweet foods, and, if so, what they should be. The use of refined sugars needs to be individualized and small quantities can be tolerated.

This should not be interpreted as carte blanche to indulge in large amounts of sweets without carefully calculating whether the insulin dosage is adequate to maintain normal blood-glucose levels. The ingestion of any carbohydrates, especially sugar, which is quickly metabolized to glucose, should be matched with adequate amounts of available insulin. As a practical general rule, many diabetes specialists recommend that nutritive sweeteners be limited to 5 percent or less of total calories consumed, and that they be consumed as part of a meal that contains complex carbohydrates, protein, and fat. (Sweeteners on page 500 outlines properties of nutritive and artificial sweeteners; Chapter 8 provides a more detailed discussion.)

Exchange Systems

In an effort to make meal planning easier for the diabetic, the American Diabetes Association and others have developed exchange systems. An exchange is a specific portion of food selected from one of six groups: milk, vegetables, fruit, bread, meat, and fat. There is also a list of free foods of 20 calories or fewer that are mostly condiments or flavorings.

The patient's meal plan will specify that he or she can have specific numbers of exchanges; for example, a typical lunch may allow two bread, two meat, one fat, two vegetable, and one fruit portion. By referring to a list of exchanges, the person can develop his or her own menu. The idea is that by following the exchange system, the person will automatically eat the proper amounts of foods with an appropriate distribution of carbohydrates, protein, and fats. Many diabetic patients find the exchange system convenient and workable. For others, however, it is better in theory than in actuality. For example, ethnic and convenience foods may be difficult to find on a standard exchange list. Most processed foods will have a number of different exchanges, and keeping track of them is more than many people can cope with. Some dietitians and diabetes educators stress working with exchanges; others will teach patients how to estimate percentages of carbohydrates, fats, and protein in a meal and then tailor portions to fit their overall meal plan. In either event, the meal plan should be based on a system that the patient (or person who prepares the meals) understands. It also should take into account individual food preferences and lifestyles.

Type II Diabetes

As noted earlier, the major problem with Type II diabetes is one of insulin resistance, rather than an absolute lack of insulin, as in the Type I form. Some patients with Type II diabetes do not make enough insulin, but many others produce normal or even higher than normal amounts of insulin. For reasons that are not clearly understood, their bodies are unable to make proper use of it.

Obesity is known to play a major role in Type II diabetes; more than 90 percent of patients with this form of the disease are markedly overweight. It is believed that the excess fat alters glucose metabolism. The excess weight also may affect the cells' insulin receptors, thereby increasing the body's insulin resistance.

Exercise also is a factor. Exercise not only helps burn up excess calories, it also appears to increase the body's ability to use insulin more efficiently.

Reduced calorie intake, weight loss, and increased physical activity are the most effective approaches to controlling Type II diabetes. Numerous studies have found that weight loss normalizes blood-glucose levels; thus, overweight diabetics should make every effort to lose weight. People with a family history of the disease should avoid becoming overweight.

In cases of extreme obesity and serious diabetes, physician-supervised fasting may be recommended. However, individuals should never undertake a fasting regimen—or any fad diet—on their own, because sharp changes in body chemistry may produce harm if not detected early by a physician. Even a physician-supervised fasting regimen will not produce lasting results if it is not accompanied by a sensible program to alter eating habits to provide long-term weight control.

For the majority of overweight Type II diabetics, a diet that provides 1,000 to 1,200 calories a day for women and 1,500 to 1,800 for men is generally recommended. Of these calories, about 50 to 55 percent should come from carbohydrates, 30 percent from fats, and the balance from protein. About 90 to 95 percent of Type II diabetic patients will respond favorably to such a regimen, but many if not most diabetic patients have difficulty adhering to a low-calorie diet. Extra counseling with a trained dietitian or diabetes educator often helps. Many also benefit from a group effort, such as Weight Watchers or Overeaters Anonymous. If, after six to eight weeks of faithfully

following a low-calorie diet, blood glucose is still too high, drug therapy may be prescribed. This usually entails taking either insulin or

Sweeteners (Other than Sugar)

Nutritive

Fructose (sugar found in honey, fruits, and some vegetables; used in Weight Watchers and other calorie-reduced products)

- Absorbed more slowly from the GI tract than glucose.

- Ingested fructose is metabolized in the liver in a process generally independent of insulin.

- Calories may be calculated into insulin-coverage curves.

- There is no bitter aftertaste.

- Large intake (more than 75 grams per day) can cause diarrhea.

Xylitol (a five-carbon sugar alcohol derived from wood sugar; used in sugar-free children's vitamins)

- Has least cavity-causing potential of the nutritive sweeteners.

- Does not increase blood glucose or triglyceride levels.

- Intake of more than 30 to 40 grams can cause diarrhea.

- There is a possible association with bladder stones and tumors.

Sorbitol (sugar alcohol found in many plants; used in sugar-free gums, candies, cough drops, diabetic ice cream, many toothpastes in blend with saccharin)

- After absorption by passive diffusion, it is oxidized into fructose.

- Results in slower, less steep rise in blood glucose than refined sugar.

- Calories may be calculated when figuring insulin dosages.

- Is less expensive than xylitol.

- Intake of more than 10.5 grams per day can cause diarrhea.

Artificial Sweeteners

Saccharin (used in diet soft drinks, many mouthwashes, Sweet 'n Low, Sugar Twin, Nutra-diet brand canned fruits and other calorie-reduced foods)

- Is not metabolized or stored in the body; orally administered saccharin is promptly excreted unchanged in urine.

- Is widely available at low cost.

- Is low in calories.

- Is possible carcinogen.

- Inhibits tooth decay.

- It has a bitter aftertaste.

Cyclamates (cyclohexane sulfamic acid)

- Have been banned from the United States since 1969 but available in Canada and other parts of the world.

- Partially absorbed from the intestinal tract; most of the absorbed substance is excreted unchanged in the urine.

- They are low in calories.

- Large doses cause diarrhea.

Aspartame (Nutra-Sweet; used in many soft drinks, sugar-free gelatins, cocoa mixes, gums)

- Breaks down in the intestinal tract into its component amino acids, which are absorbed and metabolized.

- Has very low nutrient and caloric value.

- Potency is affected by heat and high pH.

hypoglycemic drugs—medications that either increase insulin production or improve the body's ability to use it. Sometimes a combination of insulin and hypoglycemic drugs is used. With weight loss and improvement of the diabetes, the medications often can be reduced or even eliminated. An exercise program also is an important component of treatment. Walking, cycling, swimming, or water aerobics are generally more suitable for an overweight person than jogging, aerobic dancing, or other exercises that place excessive strain on joints and supporting tissues. A graduated exercise-conditioning program should be worked out with a physician, physical therapist, or exercise physiologist experienced in working with overweight diabetic patients. (See Chapter 17.)

Problem Solving in Special Circumstances

People with diabetes, especially Type I, must be extraordinarily attuned to their bodies. There are dozens of factors that can alter insulin requirements: Changes in the weather, emotional stress, illnesses or infections, hormonal changes related to the menstrual cycle, pregnancy, jet lag, and physical activity are but a few of these. Often, a person with diabetes can minimize the effects of these factors by prior planning. Still, there will be times when extra medical help is needed; it is far better to call your doctor early before the problem has evolved into a life-threatening emergency. Below are some of the more common circumstances that require extra problem-solving for a person with diabetes.

Coping with Infection or Illness

Any illness, even a cold, or period of unusual stress can wreak havoc with a diabetic patient's normal regimen. This is especially true with Type I diabetes; even people whose diabetes is under good control will usually experience problems during an illness. Insulin requirements usually rise. If the illness produces vomiting, nausea, or diarrhea, there is an added difficulty in matching insulin dosages to food intake. The best course is to consult your doctor at the first signs of an illness; he or she can give specific instructions as to how to adjust insulin dosages to avoid wide fluctuations in blood glucose during the illness.

Pregnancy

Before the discovery of insulin, it was virtually unheard of for a woman with Type I diabetes to have a healthy baby. Very few were even able to conceive, and if they did get pregnant, chances of survival of both the mother and baby were very slim. Today, the picture has changed dramatically. With improved diabetes treatment and techniques to maintain normal blood glucose throughout pregnancy, thousands of women with Type I diabetes are having normal, healthy babies. Still, these women must be particularly diligent about blood-glucose control and diet throughout pregnancy. Preferably, this should begin before pregnancy is even attempted. Many diabetes specialists and educators have special pregnancy-planning programs for their Type I patients. During these, the women are taught the nuances of fine-tuning blood-glucose control.

Maintaining normal blood glucose during pregnancy is important for several reasons. Early in fetal development, the baby's pancreas begins producing insulin. If the mother's blood glucose is too high, the fetus will increase insulin production. In utero, insulin also acts as a growth hormone; thus, if the fetus makes too much insulin, it will grow too big (this accounts for the high birth-weight of some babies of diabetic mothers). Poorly controlled diabetes greatly increases the risk of birth defects, stillbirths and death shortly after birth. In recent years, health-professional teams specializing in diabetic pregnancies have evolved. A typical team will include an obstetrician experienced in diabetic pregnancies or one who works closely with an endocrinologist or other diabetes specialist, a diabetes educator, a dietitian and, of course, the pregnant woman herself.

Gestational Diabetes

Gestational diabetes develops during pregnancy and then usually disappears immediately after delivery. An estimated 2 percent of all pregnant women develop gestational diabetes, and it is more common in population groups in which women tend to be obese. For example, gestational diabetes is more common in Italy and Mexico than in Japan. (See the list below for the factors that increase the risk of gestational diabetes.)

A number of factors contribute to the development of diabetes during pregnancy. The body requires more insulin during pregnancy to meet increased metabolic demands. High levels of estrogen, progesterone, and human placental lactogen—all needed to maintain the pregnancy—increase insulin resistance, and more insulin is needed to overcome it. The increased levels of the hormone cortisol during pregnancy alter glucose metabolism by speeding up the conversion of stored glycogen to glucose. Women who are predisposed to diabetes will often respond to these changes by developing chronically high levels of blood glucose. In many, the glucose is not high enough to produce noticeable symptoms, such as increased thirst or urination; thus, it can go undetected unless specific tests are done.

Gestational diabetes can have the same effects on the fetus as poorly controlled Type I diabetes if it is not aggressively treated. In the past, it often went undiagnosed, even though women may have been routinely checked for glucose in their urine throughout pregnancy. This test is not as sensitive in detecting gestational diabetes as blood-glucose measurements after a glucose challenge. (For one thing, many women fear excessive weight gain during pregnancy and their doctors' response to it. Therefore, they will fast or cut back on food for a couple of days before a routine checkup, which will bring their glucose levels down; as a result, urine tests or even routine blood tests may be normal.)

Today, women are routinely given a glucose-challenge test during the 24th to 28th week of pregnancy. (High-risk women should be tested more often, beginning at about the 12th week of pregnancy and then at the 24th to 28th week.) The woman will be asked to drink 50 grams of glucose and her blood-glucose level will be measured an hour later. If it is high (more than 140 milligrams per deciliter), a second test, in which the woman drinks 100 grams of glucose and blood sugars are measured hourly for the next three hours,

Risk Factors for Gestational Diabetes

- A family history of diabetes
- A prior history of glucose in the urine or high blood glucose
- Obesity (defined as 20 percent above desirable body weight)
- A poor obstetrical history, including miscarriages, stillbirths, congenital defects, previous large babies, toxemia, excessive amniotic fluid (polyhydramniosis) and recurrent urinary-tract infections during pregnancy

is indicated. If gestational diabetes is detected, the woman should begin a treatment program to normalize her blood glucose. The diabetes often can be controlled with diet, but about half of women with gestational diabetes will need insulin therapy. The composition of the diet should be worked out by a dietitian according to the woman's needs. Typically, 45 percent of calories will come from carbohydrates, 20 to 25 from protein, and the balance from fats. Frequent small meals and snacks may be recommended to minimize fluctuations in blood glucose. Exercise also is important to help control the diabetes, but strenuous aerobic exercise is not recommended, especially during the first trimester.

The woman will need to see her doctor more often than a nondiabetic; she also may be taught how to monitor her own blood glucose. Special precautions are taken near the end of pregnancy to make sure that all is well with the baby. Its heart will be monitored, and special stress tests may be done to determine whether the baby is reacting normally. The mother also may be asked to do periodic kick counts to make sure that the baby is still active.

Childhood and Adolescent Diabetes

Most Type I diabetes develops during childhood or adolescence. Understandably, this creates special difficulties for the entire family. There may be a tendency for parents to become overly protective, but it is vital that even a young child be taught how to manage his or her disease. No one likes to take injections, and this goes doubly for most young children. Still, children as young as 9 or 10 usually can master their own insulin injections, and even younger children can be taught to do their own ketone and blood-glucose testing.

Dietary management can pose special problems. For example, an ill-timed gym class can upset an insulin regimen. Meals served at school or friends' houses may not fit the child's diet plan, and it is often unrealistic to expect a youngster to adhere to a diet when all of his or her friends are enjoying other foods. Under the best of circumstances, an adolescent's eating habits are erratic, and favorite foods for this age group usually are not those recommended in a diabetic's diet. A proper balance is essential to ensure that the child will grow normally, keep his or her disease under control, yet at the same time enjoy a reasonably normal childhood.

From an early age, the child should be taught the principles of diabetes management, with emphasis on the positive. It means much more to teach a child that by sticking to an eating plan and taking the right amounts of insulin, he or she will grow properly and be able to participate in games with friends than to warn against dire long-term consequences, such as kidney failure or blindness. Lapses are inevitable and should be understood and accepted as such.

Many parents find that enrolling an adolescent in a peer-support group with other children of the same age with diabetes is more effective than constant parental or physician pressure. There are special camps for children and adolescents with diabetes; these not only provide an opportunity to gain a certain amount of independence from parents, they also provide important diabetes education. Organizations such as the American Diabetes Association or the Juvenile Diabetes Foundation can provide information about camps and peer-support groups; they also have free literature on dealing with a variety of problems.

The Importance of Understanding Diabetes

As emphasized throughout this discussion, diabetes is a complex disease that affects almost every facet of life. It would be a disservice to minimize the difficulty and frustrations of living with diabetes. It also should be emphasized, however, that it is a disease that can be controlled, and with good control, people with diabetes can lead productive, full lives. We can point to prominent people in almost every walk of life—sports, the arts, professions, education—who are living proof that diabetes does not preclude success and achievement.

Many factors are involved in achieving good control of diabetes, and we need better methods of improving compliance. With proper education and preplanning, the person with diabetes can enjoy eating out, traveling to the far corners of the world, participating in sports, and a wide variety of other activities. In recent years, many former concepts of treatment—including the so-called diabetic diet—have been altered. More than ever, the most important person in achieving good diabetes control is a patient who understands his or her disease and who takes charge of its treatment. On the preceding pages, we have briefly outlined the basic concepts in modern diabetes self-management. Individualized instruction should come from your medical team, which ideally will include a physician, nurse or other health professional trained in diabetes education, and a dietitian.

HYPOGLYCEMIA

In recent years, there has been a good deal of media attention to the symptoms attributed to hypoglycemia—low blood sugar, in the absence of diabetes. But whether there is a disease process involved is doubtful. In individuals without diabetes, there is a finely tuned feedback system to control levels of circulating insulin: When blood sugar falls, insulin secretion also falls, and the hormone glucagon

stimulates the liver to release and convert stored glycogen into glucose. In addition to diabetes, fasting hypoglycemia can be caused by certain medications (for example, salicylates, including aspirin), alcohol (especially large amounts consumed without food), insulin-secreting tumors, hormonal disorders (i.e., deficiencies of growth hormone or cortisol), and prolonged fasts, especially in infants.

Before a person without diabetes is treated for hypoglycemia, the American Diabetes Association stresses that all of the following conditions must be present.

- The occurrence of low blood sugar should be documented.

- The symptoms should be shown to be due to hypoglycemia.

- These symptoms should be relieved by ingestion of food or sugar.

In addition, the particular type of hypoglycemia producing the symptoms should be established. For example, some types of hypoglycemia may occur several hours after a meal (termed reactive, or fed, hypoglycemia) and other types may occur in the middle of the night or early-morning hours before breakfast (fasting hypoglycemia). Treatment depends on which pattern is observed and on the particular cause.

Temporary low blood sugar after a meal is the most common pattern. In its "Statement on Hypoglycemia," the American Diabetes Association notes that "it has been suggested that many individuals who are thin and nervous, especially females, may experience hypoglycemia following meals, which is responsible for their nervousness or other somatic complaints. The occurrence of such hypoglycemia following meals has never been adequately documented. The only evidence to suggest such a condition is based on changes in plasma glucose concentrations following oral glucose tolerance tests." The statement adds that use of this test in such a situation "does not seem appropriate since comparably low plasma glucose levels are observed in normal individuals without . . . any symptoms of hypoglycemia."

THYROID DISORDERS

Hormones produced by the thyroid gland control the body's metabolic rate; thus, a thyroid disorder can have profound effects on most body functions. Thyroid hormones stimulate growth and are essential for normal development of the nervous system; they also speed up the action of insulin and enhance the body's response to catecholamines.

In the past, iodine deficiency was a major cause of thyroid disease; in fact, there were so-called goiter belts in areas in which the diet was low in iodine. In order to produce its hormones, the thyroid gland requires small amounts of iodine, which is found in seafood and foods grown in areas where the soil is rich in iodine. To ensure against iodine deficiency, it is now added to salt and the dough stabilizers used to make bread. Therefore, iodine deficiency is now rare in the United States and other industrialized nations. Even so, it is estimated that about 10 million Americans have some form of thyroid disorder. Most of these disorders are caused by infection, immune-system disorders, hormonal imbalances, congenital or hereditary disorders, tumors, and, occasionally, exposure to excessive ionizing radiation.

Hyperactive Thyroid

A hyperactive thyroid, also referred to as Graves' disease or diffuse toxic goiter, is char-acterized by speeded-up metabolism. People with Graves' disease are often described as overly nervous or jittery. Other common symptoms include weight loss, muscular weakness, fatigue, excessive sweating, intolerance to heat, rapid heartbeat, tremor, thinning of hair, and loose, frequent stools. As the disease progresses, a goiter (neck swelling) may appear and the eyes take on a bulging or protruding appearance, which is caused by a swelling of tissue behind the eyeballs. Graves' disease, which often first appears during pregnancy, is much more common in women than in men. Even before other symptoms appear, women often notice irregularity in menstrual periods. Fertility problems also may develop.

The excessive thyroid hormone may be due to a disorder in the thyroid gland itself, resulting in overproduction of hormones. Or the problem may be caused by excessive thyroid-stimulating hormone (TSH) secreted by the pituitary gland. Inflammation of the thyroid gland also may cause hyperthyroidism, but hormone production usually returns to normal levels after the inflammation subsides. Other possible causes include overactive or "hot" thyroid nodules, overuse of thyroid pills (for example, as replacement therapy for a thyroid deficiency).

In susceptible people, overconsumption of iodine also can stimulate excessive thyroid-hormone production. For example, people who suddenly start eating large amounts of kelp may experience symptoms of hyperthyroidism.

Treatment depends upon the cause of the hyperthyroidism. If the problem rests with the thyroid gland itself, treatment is aimed at reducing hormone production. Common approaches include giving radioactive iodine to, in effect, destroy the thyroid's ability to produce hormones. After this treatment, the person must take thyroid-replacement hormone for life. In children, antithyroid drugs are often the preferred treatment. Surgical removal of all or part of the thyroid is another treatment option. If the problem is overproduction of TSH, treatment may be directed to the pituitary rather than to the thyroid itself.

Hypothyroidism

Hypothyroidism, also referred to as myxedema and an underactive thyroid gland, results in slowed-down metabolism and symptoms that are generally the opposite of those seen in hyperthyroidism. It is most serious in babies and young children. An infant born without thyroid tissue or a severe deficiency in thyroid hormone will develop a severe type of retardation called cretinism. Since this can be prevented by early diagnosis and replacement of thyroid hormone, newborns are now routinely tested for thyroid function. Older children who develop hypothyroidism may fail to grow properly. Sexual development also may be delayed.

In adults, hypothyroidism usually comes on slowly, and early symptoms may be overlooked or attributed to other causes. Sleepiness, lethargy, and muscle weakness are very common, as are intolerance to cold and constipation. The skin becomes thickened and scaly; nails also thicken and grow more slowly. Premature graying of the hair is common in young adults, along with thinning and coarsening hair.

As the disease progresses, facial features may thicken and the tongue become larger. Mental dullness and impaired memory also are common. If the progressive lack of thyroid hormone is not treated, the person can lapse into a myxedema coma.

The most common cause of hypothyroidism is removal or destruction of the thyroid gland to treat hyperthyroidism. This is treated by giving replacement thyroid hormone, but sometimes the dosage will be too small or the body may not adequately metabolize the drug. Increased dosage and/or switching to another drug will solve the problem.

Hashimoto's disease—a chronic inflammation of the thyroid gland without signs of infection—is the next most common cause of hypothyroidism. This is believed to be an auto-immune disorder with a strong hereditary tendency. Hashimoto's disease also is treated by giving replacement thyroid hormone (preferably thyroxine [T_4] alone, rather than the older desiccated thyroid, which contains both thyroxine and triiodothyronine [T_3]).

MISCELLANEOUS OTHER ENDOCRINE DISORDERS

There are a number of other hormonal imbalances that can result in metabolic disorders. For example, deficiencies in parathyroid hormone can result in a serious drop in calcium levels in the blood. Too little or too much growth hormone can cause dwarfism or gigantism, respectively. Fortunately, these disorders are relatively rare and are not directly related to nutrition. Certain appetite and eating disorders also may have a hormonal component (see Chapter 19).

29

Nutrition and Blood Disorders

Neville Colman, M.D., Ph.D.

■

INTRODUCTION

Blood is the fluid tissue of the body that is pumped by the heart and circulates through arteries, veins, and capillaries. It is the highway that carries the body's traffic to and from tissues. Its main functions are in respiration, where it delivers oxygen and removes carbon dioxide, and in nutrition, where it delivers nutritional materials to tissues and removes metabolic products destined for excretion. The total amount of blood in adults is roughly 70 milliliters per kilogram of body weight, which is a little over one fluid ounce per pound of body weight.

Blood consists of fluid plasma and the cells that are suspended in it. The plasma contains the protein coagulation factors required for clotting. The liquid that remains when these are removed is called serum. Between one-fifteenth and one-twentieth of serum weight is dissolved protein, which forms the nutritional building blocks for the most important structural and functional components of the body.

The blood cells, which are mostly made in the bone marrow, have specific functional roles. Red cells are by weight one-third hemoglobin, which delivers oxygen to tissues.

There are many different white cells. They include three types of granulocytes: neutrophils, which mount the first defenses against bacterial infections; basophils; and eosinophils. They include immune-defense cells called lymphocytes, which are responsible for more specific immune responses by both cells and antibodies directed against foreign invaders. They also include germ-eating cells called monocytes and macrophages. Another type of cell, called the platelet, is responsible for immediately plugging defects in the vessel walls and for starting the process of blood clotting to prevent bleeding. It also may initiate other processes in which formation of a clot may be the first step, such as narrowing of the coronary arteries and other vessels. In normal blood, red cells are about 20 times as numerous as platelets and platelets are 20 times as numerous as white cells.

NUTRITION AND THE BLOOD

Both blood plasma and blood cells are affected by alterations in the availability of nutritional factors. These disturbances may be due to either deficiencies or excesses of various nu-

507

trients. Deficiencies of nutrients harm many organ systems. Excesses in dietary fat intake can have striking effects on both the amount and type of fat (lipids) in blood plasma, making blood flow more sluggish, and play a role in damage to the arteries in the cardiovascular system, as do clotting factors in blood.

The nutritional disorders that primarily target blood, rather than other tissues, tend to affect red cells far more strikingly than the other blood cells or plasma. However, some of the nutritional disorders that affect red cells also have an effect on other blood cells, as will be discussed. Some nutritional disorders specifically target clotting factors. Others target serum proteins.

Red-Cell Disorders (Anemia)

Anemia is defined as a decrease in the number of circulating red cells or in the concentration of their main constituent, hemoglobin. When this is due to undernutrition, it is known as nutritional anemia.

The most common nutritional anemia is that due to iron deficiency. Iron deficiency is the world's most common nutritional disorder and also the most common cause of anemia; indeed, it is believed by many to be the most prevalent health disorder in the world. It affects as many as a third of all women in the childbearing years and an enormous number of infants and children.

The second major type of nutritional anemia, although not as common as iron deficiency, is megaloblastic anemia, which is caused by a deficiency of either vitamin B_{12} or folic acid (also called folate), two vitamins in the B group. Although many other nutrients have seemed to be involved in a variety of anemias, only in the cases of iron, B_{12}, folate, and protein has it been shown both that prolonged lack of the nutrient always will pro-

duce anemia, and then that supplying the nutrient always will correct it.

Anemia affects the individual by decreasing the amount of oxygen delivered to tissues. A number of biochemical and physical mechanisms protect the body against the early effects of this decrease, so that when anemia develops gradually, it may become quite severe before the individual feels any effects such as weakness and lack of energy. By this time, it may be obvious that the skin has become markedly pale, with a loss of the red color of hemoglobin from the area under the eyelid and in the creases of the palm. In contrast, such effects may be felt much earlier if the anemia develops rapidly.

When the effects of anemia are first felt, they may be similar to emotional-stress symptoms—for example, weakness, lack of energy, lassitude, breathlessness, and palpitations. The affected individual may have difficulty performing the same physical tasks, such as walking, that were easy before the condition developed. Left untreated, anemia can cause symptoms similar to heart and lung disease, such as swelling of the legs and difficulty with breathing while lying down. Chest pain may signal that the increased work load of pushing less blood around faster to deliver oxygen cannot be met by the heart and that there may be a significant risk of heart damage.

Iron-Deficiency Anemia

Iron balance varies and is most precarious when demands are highest: in pregnancy, infancy, or when disorders such as gastrointestinal ulcers or malignancy cause iron loss through bleeding. The main causes of iron deficiency are an increased demand for the nutrient, decreased dietary intake and absorption, and blood loss.

Iron requirement. Increased requirement is the most common cause of iron deficiency. The daily iron requirement is very high in premature infants, who must absorb one milligram a day to avert anemia (almost as much as adults many times their size). Full-term infants require only a third as much. From two years of age, the amount that must be absorbed increases again to about one milligram a day until the adolescent growth spurt, when it doubles for a limited period before settling at approximately 1.2 milligrams per day in men.

Women in the childbearing years require approximately twice as much iron as men in order to cover menstrual blood losses, with a wide range of 0.5 to 2 milligrams per day of absorbed iron based upon about one milligram of iron per milliliter of red blood cells. About 10 percent of the iron in the average American diet is absorbed, so the *dietary* iron requirement averages *ten times* the *absorbed* iron requirement.

During pregnancy, the requirement for iron increases, doubling in the second trimester and tripling in the third to supply the needs of increased blood volume, the enlarged uterus, and the developing fetus.

Iron intake and absorption. The major determinants of the amount of iron absorbed from the diet are the components of the diet and the increase in absorption that occurs when the gut senses a need for more iron. The total amount of iron eaten and the health of the gastrointestinal tract are obviously also important.

Iron derived from animal sources is generally much better absorbed than that derived from plant sources. Iron from the hemoglobin in red blood cells, such as that in red meat and liver, is absorbed far better than any other form (about 20 to 30 percent absorbable). The absorption of iron from other sources (which is all called nonheme iron) depends more on the general content of the meal eaten than on the individual food in which the iron is contained. Absorption of iron from an all-plant-food diet averages 3 to 5 percent. Nonheme iron absorption is improved if the meal contains meat, fish, or vitamin C, and is reduced by tea, coffee, wheat bran, soy, or eggs, all of which make nonheme iron almost unabsorbable. A person who eats little red meat, fish, or poultry has an increased risk of iron deficiency, especially if the main dietary iron source is a direct inhibitor of iron absorption, such as soy protein. (For a list of foods that contain iron, see Table 29.1; for dietary sources that inhibit and boost iron absorption, see listing on page 512.)

Changes in the gut may diminish iron absorption. Of these, the most common cause of iron deficiency is probably loss of gastric acid, such as occurs with removal of part or all of the stomach (partial or total gastrectomy). Gastric acid is necessary for optimal nonheme iron absorption. Nonheme iron malabsorption is common in the elderly, since about one-third of the people over 70 have lost the ability to produce adequate stomach acid.

Many medications interfere with the absorption of nonheme iron, mainly by binding the metal or by removing the acid necessary for its absorption. The antibiotic tetracycline is a strong binder of nonheme iron. Gastric acid may be counteracted by antacids or stopped by inhibitors of gastric-acid secretion such as cimetidine (Tagamet) and ranitidine (Zantac). (See drug list on page 512.)

Fortification. For Americans who significantly limit their intake of meat, fish, and poultry, the number-one source of iron comes from foods that are fortified with the mineral. Almost all processed flours, cereals, white bread and rolls, and baking mixes in the United States are enriched with iron, but absorption is poor. The consumer should read labels to be sure that the flour does contain added iron.

Many snack foods, breading products, frozen breakfast foods, and some pasta and rice are not fortified with iron. While flours labeled enriched, whole wheat, entire wheat, or cracked wheat do not have added iron, those marked unbleached wheat flour do.

Another way to increase the iron content of foods is to cook them in ironware, such as a cast-iron Dutch oven. For a detailed list of how much iron content is increased by preparing food this way, see Table 29.2.

Blood loss. Blood loss is a major cause of iron deficiency, most commonly because of increased menstrual blood losses or gastrointestinal blood losses. Gastrointestinal blood losses result from inflammation, ulcers, or malignancy, or from drugs that cause gastric and intestinal bleeding, such as aspirin, other antiinflammatory agents, anticoagulants, or alcohol.

Diagnosis of iron deficiency. Iron deficiency is diagnosed by conducting a number of different laboratory tests that reveal the amount of stored iron, the extent to which it is available to cells, and the effect of deficiency on the blood. The results of these tests allow iron status to be classified, as described below, into four sequential stages: (1) normal iron status,

Table 29.1. Iron Content of Selected Foods

Heme Iron Sources (All Well-Absorbed Iron)	Portion	Iron (mg.)
Beef, roast	3.0 oz.	6.1
Beef liver (fried)	3.5 oz.	5.7
Beef sirloin (lean, cooked)	3.5 oz.	3.4
Blood sausage	2.0 oz.	1.0
Calves' liver	3.5 oz.	14.2
Chicken, dark meat	3.5 oz.	1.3
Chicken, light meat	3.5 oz.	1.1
Chicken liver (simmered)	3.5 oz.	8.5
Clam (raw meat)	3.5 oz.	3.0
Flounder or sole (baked)	3.5 oz.	0.4
Ham (canned)	3.5 oz.	0.8
Hamburger (lean, cooked)	3.5 oz.	2.1
Lamb, leg (roasted)	3.5 oz.	2.2
Lamb chop (lean, without bone)	3.5 oz.	1.8
Liverwurst, pork	1.0 oz.	1.8
Oysters, eastern (raw meat)	3.5 oz.	6.5
Pork chop	3.5 oz.	4.5
Pork liver (braised)	3.5 oz.	17.9
Pork loin (broiled, lean)	3.5 oz.	0.9
Salmon (red, baked)	3.5 oz.	0.6
Sardines	3.5 oz.	3.0
Shrimp (cooked)	3.0 oz.	2.5
Shrimp (raw)	3.5 oz.	1.8
Tuna (light, oil-packed)	3.5 oz.	1.9
Tuna (white, water-packed)	3.5 oz.	0.7
Turkey, dark meat	3.5 oz.	2.3
Turkey, light meat	3.5 oz.	1.4
Veal cutlet	3.5 oz.	3.0

Nonheme Sources (Less Well-Absorbed Iron)	Portion	Iron (mg.)
BEANS		
Black beans	½ cup	1.4
Chick-peas	½ cup	2.4
Kidney beans	½ cup	2.8
Lentils	½ cup	2.1
Lima beans	½ cup	3.0
Pinto beans	½ cup	2.7
GRAIN PRODUCTS		
Bagel	1	1.8
Bulgur, uncooked	¼ cup	2.4
Cheerios	1 oz.	4.5
Cornflakes	1 oz.	1.8
Farina	¾ cup	0.9
Grits	¾ cup	1.2
Oatmeal (fortified)	¾ cup	6.3
Oatmeal (nonfortified)	¾ cup	1.2
Pasta, enriched	2.0 oz.	2.2
Rice, cooked enriched	½ cup	0.9
Rice, cooked brown	½ cup	0.4
Rye bread	1 slice	0.7
Saltine cracker	4	0.5
Total	1 cup	21.0
Wheat germ (plained, toasted)	1 T	0.6
White enriched bread	1 slice	0.8
Whole-wheat bread	1 slice	0.8
NUTS AND SEEDS		
Almonds (whole)	1 oz.	1.0
Cashews, oil-roasted	1 oz.	1.2

(2) depleted iron stores, (3) iron-deficient eythropoiesis or red blood cell production, and (4) iron-deficiency anemia.

The first evidence of impaired iron status is usually the development of depleted iron stores. In the past, this could be detected only by the direct examination of iron stores in bone marrow, by looking at a bone-marrow sample under a microscope. Today, however, iron stores can usually be assessed by measuring serum levels of ferritin, a circulating iron-storage protein. In general, 1 unit of serum ferritin represents 10 units of body iron stores.

Iron-deficient red blood cell formation, as a rule, only occurs after iron stores have been almost completely depleted. In this stage, there is the first evidence that the formation of early red blood cells may be occurring without sufficient iron. This can be seen in bone marrow by a decrease in the amount of iron granules present in early red cells, but it is virtually never necessary to perform a bone-marrow examination. A serum test is done instead in order to reveal the decrease in the amount of iron on the circulating iron-delivery protein, which is called transferrin; it delivers the iron to the red cells. A low serum iron alone does *not* mean that the person needs iron, because illnesses that reduce the amount of iron-delivery protein produce a low serum iron and

Table 29.1. Iron Content of Selected Foods *(cont.)*

Nonheme Sources (Less Well-Absorbed Iron)	Portion	Iron (mg.)
NUTS AND SEEDS *(cont.)*		
Cashews, dry-roasted	1 oz.	1.7
Peanut butter	1 T	0.3
Peanuts, oil-roasted	1 oz.	0.5
Peanuts, dry-roasted	1 oz.	0.9
Pistachios	1 oz.	1.9
Pumpkin seeds	1 oz.	4.2
Sesame seeds, hulled	1 T	0.6
Sunflower seeds	1 oz.	1.9
Walnuts	1 oz.	0.7
VEGETABLES		
Acorn squash (baked)	½ cup	1.0
Asparagus (fresh, cooked)	½ cup	0.6
Bean sprouts (mung), raw	½ cup	0.5
Beets (boiled)	½ cup	0.5
Beet greens (boiled)	½ cup	1.4
Broccoli (cooked, chopped)	½ cup	0.9
Brussels sprouts (cooked)	½ cup	0.9
Collard greens	1 cup	1.7
Corn (boiled)	½ cup	0.5
Corn grits	¼ cup	1.4
Green peas, frozen	½ cup	1.3
Hash-brown potatoes	½ cup	1.2
Kale (cooked)	½ cup	0.6
Mushrooms, cooked	½ cup	1.4
Mustard greens	1 cup	2.5
Parsley (raw, chopped)	½ cup	1.9
Potato (baked with skin)	1 large	2.8

Nonheme Sources (Less Well-Absorbed Iron)	Portion	Iron (mg.)
VEGETABLES *(cont.)*		
Pumpkin, canned	½ cup	0.7
Spinach	1 cup	0.8
Snow peas, boiled	½ cup	1.6
Sweet pepper, raw	½ cup	0.6
Tomato, raw	1 medium	0.6
Tomato juice	½ cup	0.7
Tomato sauce	½ cup	1.0
Turnip greens (fresh, cooked)	½ cup	0.6
Turnip greens (frozen, cooked)	½ cup	1.6
SOY PRODUCTS		
Miso	½ cup	2.4
Tofu	3½ oz.	1.8
FRUITS		
Apricots (dried)	8 halves	2.5
Avocado, California	½ fruit	1.0
Blackberries, raw	1 cup	0.8
Blackstrap molasses	1 T	5.0
Cantaloupe	½ melon	0.6
Light molasses	1 T	1.2
Orange (Valencia)	1 med.	1.0
Prune juice	½ cup	1.5
Prunes	5 fruits	1.0
Raisins	¼ cup	0.8
Raspberries, raw	1 cup	0.7

Source: U.S. Department of Agriculture.

poor iron delivery. In such instances, the solution lies in treatment of the specific disease, not in taking iron.

Another test for reduced hemoglobin production due to iron deficiency (or other causes such as lead poisoning) is known as the FEP, or *free erythrocyte protoporphyrin*. This protoporphyrin is the prehemoglobin that becomes hemoglobin on adding iron. When there is not enough iron, this precursor will accumulate. The accumulation of protoporphyrin is also promoted by lead poisoning, a disorder affecting about 5 percent of young inner-city children. For this reason, it is common to screen for both iron deficiency and lead poisoning in inner-city children by giving a simple test using a drop of blood collected onto filter paper.

In the final stage of iron deficiency, the lack of iron is so great as to produce anemia.

Studies show that the bone marrow responds to loss of red blood cells by greatly increasing its generation of new blood cells by 500 percent or more in the presence of adequate iron, whether the loss of blood cells is due to bleeding or due to rapid red cell destruction (a condition called hemolytic anemia). When the iron supply is limited, the bone marrow can increase red-cell production 200 to 300 percent when there are modest iron stores, but will be unable to increase it at all in true iron deficiency. The red cells themselves may appear normal, or they may look like iron deficiency, with very young red cells having ragged cell borders, and mature red cells being small and colorless.

Other effects of iron deficiency. Patients with iron deficiency frequently experience generalized symptoms, particularly listlessness, fatigue, and impaired muscular function, which are not due solely to anemia. A number of studies indicate these symptoms are due to the effect of iron deficiency on iron-containing enzymes in muscle tissues.

A well-known but poorly understood behavior in many iron-deficient individuals is pica, the practice of eating clay, soil, ice, and other unusual substances. This can result in damage to the lining of the gastrointestinal tract, interference with various chemicals important in the transmission of nerve signals,

Nonheme Iron Absorption

Dietary Sources That Boost Nonheme Iron Absorption
Fish
Meat
Meat products
Poultry
Shellfish
Vitamin C

Dietary Sources That Inhibit Nonheme Iron Absorption
Calcium phosphate salts
Coffee
EDTA (ethylenediamine tetra-acetic acid), a food preservative used in margarines, carbonated and malted beverages, and some foodstuffs
Egg yolks
Soy proteins
Tea
Wheat bran and other dietary fiber

Drugs That Interfere with the Absorption of Iron

Antacids
Cholestyramine
Cimetidine (Tagamet)
Pancreatin
Ranitidine (Zantac)
Tetracycline

and impairment of learning and attention span in children. Certain infections occur with increased frequency, with others being more prevalent during the treatment phase with injectable iron preparations.

Treatment of iron deficiency. The treatment of iron deficiency can almost always be accomplished by taking three pills each day, each containing 60 milligrams of iron as sulfate or gluconate. If abdominal discomfort or constipation occurs, the symptoms can be diminished by taking the pills with meals or by using delayed-release preparations. Doing either decreases both gastrointestinal symptoms and the speed of the treatment. No individual should take iron supplementation (or any supplementation therapy) for any suspected blood disorder without a doctor's diagnosis and guidance. Mild anemia can occur from iron overload just as it can from iron deficiency. Twice as many men suffer from congenital iron overload (a condition called hemochromatosis) as suffer from iron deficiency, so men taking iron on their own are twice as likely to be hurt as helped by it.

It may be necessary to resort to injectable iron if it is impossible to restore iron status to normal by the oral route. This can occur when absorption is impaired, when there is continuous blood loss due to chronic active bleeding, or when there is a need to correct a severe deficiency rapidly during pregnancy. In these circumstances, iron in the form of iron dextran may be injected into muscles or veins, in daily amounts sufficient to supply enough iron for 100 milliliters of red cells, or about 240 milliliters (a half-pint) of whole blood.

Treatment of iron deficiency must always be accompanied by a thorough search for the cause of the deficiency. One of the most common causes of unexpected iron deficiency in a man is an underlying malignancy that causes bleeding from an intestinal or other site. Because of this, every case of iron deficiency that is not of obvious cause, especially in adult men, needs to be rigorously investigated.

Megaloblastic Anemia Due to Deficiency of Vitamin B$_{12}$ or Folate (Folic Acid) or Both

Megaloblastic anemia is characterized by changes in the appearance of blood and bone-marrow cells resulting from a slowing in the synthesis of deoxyribonucleic acid (DNA). The main change in appearance is a slowing in the maturation of the cell's nucleus, which con-

Table 29.2. Increasing Iron Content by Cooking in Ironware*

Food	Iron Content (milligrams/100 grams)			Food	Iron Content (milligrams/100 grams)		
	Raw	Noniron Utensil	Iron Utensil		Raw	Noniron Utensil	Iron Utensil
Unsweetened applesauce	0.35	0.28	7.38	Fried corn tortillas	0.86	1.14	1.23
Spaghetti sauce	0.61	0.69	5.77	Spanish rice	0.87	0.83	2.25
Pancakes	0.63	0.81	1.31	Fried chicken	0.88	1.37	1.89
Stir-fried green beans	0.64	0.69	1.18	Chili with meat & beans	0.98	1.28	6.27
Beef-vegetable stew	0.66	0.81	3.40	Scrambled egg	1.49	1.79	4.76
Baked corn bread	0.67	0.83	0.86	Pan-broiled hamburger	1.49	2.00	2.29
White rice	0.67	0.86	1.97	Poached egg	1.87	1.71	2.32
Spaghetti sauce with meat	0.71	0.94	3.58	Fried egg	1.92	1.84	3.48
				Beef liver with onions	3.10	3.82	3.87

*This was standard practice more than a century ago.

From the *Journal of the American Dietetic Association*, vol. 86, no. 7, July 1986, pp. 897–901.

tains most of the DNA, as compared to the maturity of the rest of the cell. This change is also caused by anticancer drugs, which damage DNA synthesis. More than 95 percent of cases of megaloblastic anemia result from deficiencies of vitamin B_{12} or folate (folic acid) or both.

Vitamin B_{12} and folate are two B vitamins that are essential for all dividing cells. The search for these agents is one of the great stories in the history of medical research. The blood disorder of megaloblastic anemia was originally recognized in a disease called pernicious anemia, so named because affected patients followed a slow, inexorable course to death.

In the 1920s, George Minot, a hematologist in Boston, found that pernicious anemia could be cured by eating large amounts of liver, a discovery for which he and his assistant, Dr. Murphy, received the Nobel Prize. The active component in liver was discovered two decades later to be in vitamin B_{12}, the last of the eight B vitamins to be discovered. Shortly after Minot's discovery, a young member of his group, William Castle, discovered that the absorption of vitamin B_{12} required an intrinsic factor (subsequently named by others "Castle's intrinsic factor"), which was produced in the stomach. He uncovered this fact by swallowing chopped meat, letting it mix with his normal stomach juices, bringing the mixture back up via a stomach tube, and feeding this mixture to a patient who lacked stomach juices. This discovery explained why the disease pernicious anemia was found only in association with loss of stomach secretions.

Megaloblastic anemia was thought to be due to a single nutritional deficiency, of extrinsic factor (discovered in 1948 to be vitamin B_{12}). In 1931, Lucy Wills, a British nutrition scientist working in India, discovered that a form of the disease found in pregnant women with tropical sprue in that country (and in experimental animals) was not aided by the purified liver extract known to help pernicious anemia (now known to be a purified extract of vitamin B_{12}). It did respond, however, to Marmite, a yeast extract containing no extrinsic factor, which is available in the United States, Canada, and many other countries. Pursuit of her observations led to discovery in the U.S. of folic acid (folate) in spinach, named after the leaves (foliage) from which it was isolated. It was believed folic-acid deficiency occurred only if one had both dietary lack and intestinal malabsorption until Victor Herbert showed by putting himself on a strict no-folate diet that dietary lack alone would produce megaloblastic anemia in four and a half months. Working with him was Louis W. Sullivan, now U.S. Secretary of Health.

Although the blood disorder looks identical whether the cause is deficiency of vitamin B_{12} or folate, neurologic and psychiatric damage of a type marked by anatomically damaged cells is caused only by vitamin B_{12} deficiency and not by folate deficiency. This neuropsychiatric damage, sometimes presenting as subacute combined degeneration of the spinal cord, is due to deterioration of myelinated nerves. Myelinated nerves are those surrounded by a white insulation sheath called myelin, which requires vitamin B_{12}.

Interactions of vitamin B_{12} and folate. Folate requires vitamin B_{12} to be converted to a form necessary in the manufacture of the DNA required for cell division. Thus, when there is either B_{12} or folate deficiency, the anemias that result are identical. In the absence of vitamin B_{12}, folate is trapped in a nonusable form. This "folate trap hypothesis," conceived by Drs. Herbert and Zalusky, is no longer considered a hypothesis, but it is accepted as fact by most nutrition scientists.

Dietary deficiency of vitamin B₁₂. It is extremely difficult to induce vitamin B_{12} deficiency by removing it from the diet; this is true for two reasons. Firstly, vitamin B_{12} is found in almost all animal products in copious amounts, so that any diet containing meat, fish, eggs, or dairy products contains amounts in excess of requirements. (For a list of foods containing vitamin B_{12} and a listing of those which contain folate, see below.) Secondly, there is such a large body store of the vitamin that the average person will show no signs of deficiency until 6 to 12 years after removal of all sources of vitamin B_{12} from the diet. Dietary deficiencies of vitamin B_{12} occur only in people called vegans—those who eat nothing but plant products. Nothing that grows out of the ground contains vitamin B_{12}, except from contaminating microorganisms in root nodules of some Indian pulses, and attached animal fecal matter. Most American vegetarians have no B_{12} problem because they eat animal products such as milk and/or milk products and/or eggs. Those who don't eat such foods need B_{12} supplements, such as a B_{12}-spiked cereal.

Pernicious anemia and other causes of vitamin B₁₂ deficiency. Vitamin B_{12} deficiency is almost always caused by a defect in absorption. The signs of deficiency from malabsorption may appear in only 2 to 4 years, which is much less than the 15 to 20 years it takes to get B_{12} deficiency from no B_{12} in the diet. This is because defective absorption means not only failure to absorb food B_{12} but also failure to reabsorb the greater amount of B_{12} that is in the bile, which is daily discharged into the intestine from the liver via the gallbladder.

The best-known cause of vitamin B_{12} malabsorption is pernicious anemia, a specific disease in which there is a deficiency of Castle's intrinsic factor, which is necessary for the intestine to absorb dietary vitamin B_{12}. Pernicious anemia is more common with increasing age, and it was once described as being common in men of northern European descent, probably because they formed the majority of patients treated in the major academic institutions in Boston about the turn of the century, where the disease was intensively studied. We now know that pernicious anemia also occurs among young black women—probably the patients most commonly affected under the age of 40. There are also forms of the disease that affect children.

Dietary Sources of Vitamin B₁₂*

Meat
Organ meats
Cheese, yogurt, etc.
Eggs
Milk
Milk products
Fish
Shellfish

*"Anything that walks, swims, or flies contains B_{12}. Nothing that grows out of the ground contains B_{12}." (Quote from Victor Herbert, M.D.)

Dietary Sources of Folate

Barley	Oranges
Beans	Orange juice
Brewer's yeast	Peas
Endive	Rice
Fruits	Soybeans
Garbanzo beans (chick-peas)	Split peas
Green leafy vegetables	Sprouts
Lentils	Uncooked vegetable greens
Liver	Wheat
Most animal products	Wheat germ
	Whole wheat

In pernicious anemia, so-called auto-antibodies (antibodies against self) are formed against Castle's intrinsic factor, as well as against the stomach cells themselves. There also may be other auto-antibodies, most commonly directed against the thyroid gland. A similar end result occurs without antibodies when the stomach is removed, since the intrinsic factor is absent.

Absorption of vitamin B_{12} can also be defective if there is poor function in the lower half of the small intestine, called the ileum, where vitamin B_{12} is normally transported across the cells of the gut with the help of the intrinsic factor. This poor function can result from an inflammation of the ileum—called Crohn's disease (regional enteritis)—infestations of the small intestine, and a diarrheal disease called sprue, which is caused by either an inborn intolerance to a wheat protein called gluten or to a relatively common tropical disease of infectious origin. (For more information, see chapters 30 and 33.)

Causes of folate deficiency. In contrast to vitamin B_{12} deficiency, where the defect is almost always in absorption, folate deficiency can be caused by virtually any of the general mechanisms of nutritional deficiency, ranging from inadequacies of dietary intake, absorption, and utilization to increases in requirement, excretion, and destruction. In alcoholism, all six of these possible ways to get folate deficiency occur together, explaining why more than 90 percent of chronic alcoholics are folate-deficient. The most common cause of folate deficiency in the United States is probably abuse of alcohol.

Folate is in much more tenuous balance than vitamin B_{12}, and evidence of negative balance is seen in humans after only two to three weeks of dietary deprivation. A wide range of diseases affecting the absorption of many nutrients also affect folate, which, un-like vitamin B_{12}, is absorbed in the upper part of the small intestine in a manner similar to most other nutrients. Increased requirements of folate in pregnancy and lactation have led to the recommendation that all pregnant women take folate supplements (along with iron). Requirements are also increased in premature infants.

Diagnosis of megaloblastic anemia. Megaloblastic anemia can be confirmed by examination of the blood cells in the bone marrow. Just as it is essential to determine the underlying cause once iron deficiency has been diagnosed, so is it necessary to take two further steps once megaloblastic anemia is diagnosed. One is to determine whether the deficiency is of folate or vitamin B_{12} (or both); the other is to diagnose which of the six possibilities is the underlying cause of the deficiency.

Although these steps may appear obvious, their importance is often not appreciated because short-term correction of the blood problem can be achieved by treatment with both folate and vitamin B_{12}. The problem is long-term management of the patient. For practical purposes, every patient with vitamin B_{12} deficiency requires treatment for the rest of his or her life, usually with monthly intramuscular injections, to avoid the risk of irreversible nerve damage. It is important to accurately distinguish between the patients whose megaloblastic anemia is caused by a deficiency of vitamin B_{12} from those whose cause is deficiency of folate in order to avoid withholding appropriate treatment from those patients who need it and to avoid imposing it on those who do not.

Measuring the levels of vitamins in blood is the most widely used method of determining which vitamin is deficient. Although vitamin B_{12} need be measured only in serum, it is necessary to measure folate in both serum and red cells because serum folate may be low in many normal subjects who have been eating poorly for two weeks. Red-cell folate stores may be low in both folate and vitamin B_{12} deficiency, the latter through the interactions described earlier.

Once the missing vitamin has been identified and the problem is known to be poor B_{12} absorption, further evaluation is usually undertaken to identify why absorption is poor. The Schilling Test, devised in Boston by Dr. Robert Schilling, now in Madison, Wisconsin, can determine whether vitamin B_{12} deficiency is caused by disease in the stomach or in the small intestine. In this test, radioactive vitamin B_{12} is given by mouth and its absorption is determined. If absorption is subnormal, and is corrected when gastric intrinsic factor is fed with it, it suggests that the problem is in the stomach. If there is no correction, the problem is probably in the intestine. In occasional elderly subjects with vitamin B_{12} deficiency, the Schilling Test is unexpectedly normal when done in the conventional manner using vitamin B_{12}. This is because many elderly people are unable to remove vitamin B_{12} from food in their stomachs due to the fact that they lack the stomach acid and enzymes that implement this process. In these cases, one modifies the Schilling Test by mixing radioactive vitamin B_{12} with a raw egg before swallowing the B_{12}. If radioactive B_{12} bound to egg protein is not absorbed, this means the person's stomach lacks acid and enzymes. If there is fear of salmonella contamination, the egg should be beaten into an omelet before being eaten.

30

Nutrition and Gastrointestinal Disease

Mitchell Conn, M.D., and David B. Sachar, M.D.

∎

INTRODUCTION

The gastrointestinal (GI) system is responsible for the digestion and absorption of food. During the process, food is converted into energy and into other substances that are used by cells throughout the entire body. The core of the GI system is the alimentary tract, a long hollow tube that starts at the mouth, where the breakdown of food begins, and terminates at the anus, where waste products are eliminated. Along this tube, which reaches approximately 28 feet in length in an adult, are the esophagus, stomach, small intestine, and large intestine (colon). Other organs connected to this tract, such as the liver, gallbladder, and pancreas, are also intimately involved in the digestive process. In fact, the liver, which is the largest of all internal organs in the body, is the body's main biochemical factory, where most metabolic processing takes place. Its importance is such that the nutritional implications of liver disease are considered in a separate chapter.

A number of diseases can afflict the various organs of the GI system. Contrary to popular belief, however, diet plays a relatively minor role in the onset of such GI diseases. Spicy foods do not cause ulcers and fatty foods do not cause gallstones, although they may exacerbate the symptoms.

Since food is processed along the digestive tract, there is a tendency to blame the food rather than the disease when the processing is impaired and pain, nausea, or diarrhea result. Food is the culprit only when the food is contaminated or when there is a food allergy. In most cases, it is some part of the complex mechanical or chemical system itself that is malfunctioning.

Although diet has little to do with gastrointestinal disease, the diseases and their treatments often have serious nutritional consequences. The digestion, assimilation, and delivery of nutrients to the cells involve an intricate interplay among chemical, neurological, and mechanical systems. A single flaw anywhere along the pathway in any of the systems can alter many other processes; multiple flaws compound the problem. Because many of the processes involved are not yet fully understood, and since there is a wide variation of reactions among individuals with the disorders, the nutritional consequences of gastrointestinal disease and the recommendations for dietary treatment included in this chapter can be only general in nature. Specific treatment is highly individualized, with the patient and physician working closely together.

HEARTBURN

Most people will at sometime experience the discomfort of heartburn, a burning sensation behind the breastbone (sternum) that may extend up as high as the throat. When heartburn occurs on a regular basis, it is not simply the penalty for stress or overeating, as the ubiquitous antacid commercials suggest, but a symptom of a disorder called gastroesophageal reflux.

At the bottom of the esophagus (the tube that conducts food from the mouth and throat to the stomach) is a ringlike muscle called the lower esophageal sphincter (LES). This muscular ring normally opens to admit food into the stomach and then closes to prevent stomach contents from backing up. If this muscle is weakened or improperly regulated, however,

it will not stay closed when the stomach is full or under increased pressure. Food and digestive juices may then back up (or reflux) into the esophagus. Since the walls of the esophagus do not have protection from stomach acid, this reflux often causes the burning sensation we know as heartburn.

Nutritional Consequences

Most people can tolerate gastroesophageal reflux for years with no significant harm to their nutrition. Although a few foods should be avoided to control the symptoms, the dietary restrictions are not severe and nutrition is usually not impaired. Occasionally, symptoms may depress a person's appetite to such an extent that food intake is inadequate. In the rare cases when dietary and medical therapies fail, the repeated back flow of acid and other digestive substances can cause inflammation of the esophagus (esophagitis), esophageal ulcer, and ultimately scarring and narrowing of the lower esophagus. These complications may, in turn, produce dietary deficits.

Treatment

For reasons not fully understood, certain foods and drugs decrease esophageal sphincter muscle strength, while others increase it. The goal of treatment is to increase the contractile strength to prevent the stomach contents from backing up into the esophagus. The individual should also eliminate foods that might irritate an inflamed esophagus and follow a high-protein, low-fat diet. (See Table 30.1 for lists of foods and substances that one should avoid because they decrease sphincter pressure; those that one should emphasize or that might be prescribed because they increase

Figure 30.1.

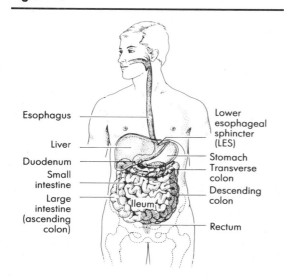

Esophagus

Liver

Duodenum
Small
intestine

Large
intestine
(ascending
colon)

Ileum

Lower
esophageal
sphincter
(LES)

Stomach

Transverse
colon

Descending
colon

Rectum

sphincter pressure; and those that increase acidity or may irritate the esophagus.) Except for avoiding alcohol, nicotine, chocolate, and coffee (whether regular or decaffeinated), only minor dietary changes such as substituting lean cuts of meat for fattier ones, skim milk for whole, baked potatoes for French fries, and so on, are required. There is no evidence that spicy foods need be avoided, with the possible exceptions of red and black pepper. Forgoing large meals and late-evening snacks may also increase comfort.

Dietary changes alone may suffice for treating mild heartburn, but additional measures may be required for more severe cases. Antacids, because they neutralize acid and increase esophageal sphincter contraction, are the mainstay of medical therapy for heartburn. Typically, those patients with recurring or resistant symptoms take antacids after meals, but in acute cases, antacids may be prescribed as often as every hour until symptoms cease.

Other recommendations may include taking care not to bend over or recline for two or three hours after meals and sleeping with the chest higher than the stomach (by raising the whole head of the bed on four- to six-inch blocks, not just by using extra pillows).

If these measures do not produce results, bethanechol chloride (Urecholine) may be prescribed to increase sphincter pressure, cimetidine (Tagamet) or other acid secretory inhibitors, including omeprazole (Losec) to reduce acid secretion, and metaclopramide (Reglan) to both increase sphincter pressure and facilitate emptying of the stomach.

Hiatal Hernia

Gastroesophageal reflux was once thought to be caused by a hiatal hernia, a condition in which a portion of the stomach protrudes through the diaphragm into the chest cavity. Forty percent of the American

Table 30.1. Heartburn and Diet

Foods and Substances That Increase Sphincter Pressure			
AUTONOMIC DRUGS	HORMONES	OTHERS	FOODS
Bethanecol	Gastrin	Histamine (H₁ receptor)	Protein
Methancholine	Pentagastrin	Serotonin	
Norepinephrine			
Phenylephrine			
Beta blockers			
Metaclopramide			

Foods and Substances That Decrease Sphincter Pressure			
AUTONOMIC DRUGS	HORMONES	OTHERS	FOODS
Nicotine (cigarettes)	Secretin	Nitroglycerine	Coffee (whether with or without caffeine)
Atropine	Cholecystokinin	Histamine (H₂ receptor)	Chocolate
Epinephrine	Glucagon		Fat
Dopamine	Progesterone		Alcohol (liquor, wine, beer)
	Estrogen		Caffeine (cola, coffee, tea)
			Peppermint and spearmint oils (candies, liqueurs)
			Tomato sauce and paste

Foods That Are Irritating or Cause Increased Acid Secretion			
Citrus juices	Tomato juice	Decaffeinated coffee	Whole milk

population have a sliding hiatal hernia, but the majority of these have no symptoms and require no treatment. The heartburn that afflicts those with this problem is more likely related to an incompetent lower esophageal sphincter than to the hernia itself.

ULCERS

Peptic ulcers can occur at any time from infancy to old age, and afflict about 1 person in 10. A peptic ulcer is a sore in the stomach or intestine that occurs when acidic digestive secretions penetrate the protective mucous lining of the gastrointestinal wall and expose the muscular layers underneath. There are two kinds of peptic ulcers: duodenal and gastric. *Duodenal ulcers* are the most common and form in the duodenum, the part of the small intestine immediately adjacent to the stomach. In some cases, they are associated with excessive amounts of acid moving from the stomach into the intestine, either because of oversecretion of acid while food is in the stomach or prolonged secretion of acid after food has passed out of the stomach. In other cases, the lining of the duodenum may be especially susceptible to damage even by normal acid levels. *Gastric ulcers* occur in the stomach when hydrochloric acid irritates and erodes the vulnerable mucosal lining.

Even though stress and spicy foods may be contributory factors, the popular image of the ulcer candidate as a tense, workaholic executive or curry-loving gourmand is not entirely accurate. Although no one knows definitively what causes the initial weakness in the mucosa, a number of factors, including smoking, use of certain drugs (e.g., aspirin and corticosteroids), bacterial colonization, and genetic characteristics, are believed to predispose individuals to ulcers.

There is no permanent cure for ulcers. Regardless of the medical therapy used, about 50 percent of ulcer patients have a recurrence, often within two years. The recurrence rate is much lower for those who undergo surgery to remove a part of the stomach or intestine, but surgical intervention has its own side effects and is considered only as a last resort.

Nutritional Consequences

Ulcers can produce loss of appetite, pain, nausea, or vomiting. To avoid discomfort, many sufferers reduce their food intake radically, some even eliminating solid foods altogether. The subsequent loss of calories and nutrients can result in severe weight loss and many nutritional deficiencies.

Various medications are prescribed to neutralize or decrease stomach acidity: antacids and/or secretory inhibitors like cimetidine reduce acidity and promote healing; sucralfate coats the lining of the ulcer crater, protecting it from acid injury and allowing the ulcer to heal; antispasmodics reduce acid secretions and delay emptying of the stomach; and tranquilizers ease tension and anxiety.

Most ulcers heal within two to six weeks no matter what kind of treatment is chosen. When healing takes place within this span of time, there are no nutritional consequences of the treatment. However, for those people with large, long-standing, or recalcitrant ulcers, treatment may have to be prolonged.

Antacids containing aluminum hydroxide and calcium carbonate can cause constipation, while those containing magnesium salts may produce diarrhea. Prolonged use of antacids containing aluminum hydroxide, alone or in combination with magnesium hydroxide, may prevent the body from properly utilizing phosphorus, a deficiency that can result in softening of the bones. Long-term treatment involves the addition of foods high in phosphorus to the diet, or a change in antacid regimen. Severe loss may require supplementation.

Prolonged use of baking soda (sodium bicarbonate) or antacids containing calcium carbonate, especially for those who consume a great deal of milk, can cause the body to accumulate an excess of calcium and alkali, which can produce symptoms of nausea, headache, and weakness, and if undetected may progress to kidney damage.

An ulcer may lead to obstruction of the stomach as a result of swelling or scarring. The poor appetite and vomiting that may accompany obstruction, and the need for continuous suction of the stomach contents, or both, can result in malnutrition, dehydration, and chemical imbalances, all of which may require hospitalization for parenteral nutrition (intravenous feeding).

The Role of Diet

Therapy for ulcer sufferers is controversial, because research indicates diet has little or no effect in treating peptic ulcers. Studies comparing a bland diet with an unrestricted diet in patients with duodenal ulcers have shown no difference in the healing rates.

Most physicians today believe that a restricted diet is unnecessary for those who have uncomplicated peptic ulcers. They recommend instead changes in dietary patterns. The issue, in other words, is not what you eat but how and when you eat. For example, late-evening snacks are discouraged because they stimulate acid secretion during sleep. Coffee drinkers are urged to limit their consumption (even of decaffeinated coffee) to one cup after meals, and those who drink alcohol are restricted to a glass or two of wine with either lunch or dinner. Milk, which can stimulate even greater acid secretion than coffee or beer, is no longer encouraged, while orange juice and other acidic beverages and foods, long considered taboo, are prohibited only if the individual is intolerant of them. Although more and more doctors embrace the unrestricted diet for patients with uncomplicated ulcers, some believe that when complications exist or the problem is persistent, there is a role for the bland diet.

Because food acts as a buffer in the stomach, frequent small meals were once advised to prevent pain. Now, because it is understood that food provokes further acid production, regular, well-spaced, moderate-sized meals are recommended. As there is no evidence that high-fiber foods irritate ulcers, they are no longer restricted in favor of the soft foods of the traditional bland diet. Depending upon individual tolerances, spices are usually allowed, with the exceptions of black pepper and chili powder. Cigarettes, on the other hand, remain on the strictly prohibited list because they inhibit acid neutralization, delay healing, and are associated with the recurrence of duodenal ulcers. Indeed, in all studies, cigarette smoking is the single worst prognostic factor in promoting resistant or recurrent ulcer disease.

Medications

Although most ulcers will eventually heal without any drug therapy, medications that inhibit acid production (Tagamet or Zantac, for example) significantly accelerate healing and are therefore often prescribed. Antacids, which neutralize stomach acidity, are also commonly utilized. These medications offer some protection against recurrence, but once they are discontinued, the ulcer will return in about 50 percent of the cases. Some recent studies suggest that eradication of colonizing bacteria may reduce this recurrence rate.

If the pain is intense and unrelenting, medication will most likely be given and the patient put on a bland diet, with gradual progression to a less restricted regimen as symptoms abate.

Surgery

Surgery may be necessary for any of the following conditions: obstruction that fails to respond to medical therapy; perforation of the stomach or intestinal wall; major hemorrhage; suspicion of stomach cancer; or repeatedly recurring ulcer attacks. How much of the stomach or intestine is removed and what reconstruction is done are determined by the size and location of the problem. The extent of the surgery and the nature of the reconstruction will affect the nutritional consequences. Some of the resulting nutritional deficits are immediate and temporary; others emerge years later as the cumulative result of subtly altered digestive processes.

Complications of Surgery

Dumping syndromes. This is a group of symptoms that occur in about 10 percent of patients after ulcer surgery. Either during or within 10 to 15 minutes after eating a meal of high-carbohydrate foods, the sufferer of early dumping syndrome experiences a feeling of fullness, flushing, sweating, weakness, rapid heartbeat, diarrhea, and sometimes fainting. Although it is not known for certain, it is suspected that the effects of gastric surgery cause food to move too quickly from the stomach to the small intestine. The sudden presence of large numbers of food particles in the small intestine attracts the liquid portion of blood or plasma into the bowel, via osmosis. The intestine becomes distended with fluid; at the same time, circulating blood volume falls. Other dumping symptoms are attributable to the release of intestinal wall hormones stimulated by the rapid entry of foodstuffs.

The treatment of early dumping syndrome is exclusively dietary: carbohydrates are limited, fats and proteins are increased, and liquids are taken separately from meals. Patients are given frequent small meals of low bulk and encouraged to lie down after eating. Some people can return rapidly to a normal diet; others must follow the low-carbohydrate, high-protein regimen for life.

Late dumping syndrome (alimentary hypoglycemia) occurs when carbohydrates are precipitously dumped into the duodenum and rapidly absorbed; glucose levels rise in the blood, draining the duodenum; and a large amount of insulin is suddenly released, causing the blood-sugar level to fall rapidly throughout the body. Patients feel faint or weak, sweat profusely, and may lose consciousness one and a half to three hours after eating. The treatment is dietary, with frequent small meals high in protein and low in sugar, although concentrated sweets are kept in case of a hypoglycemic attack.

Weight loss. The smaller stomach that remains after ulcer surgery may feel distended after a relatively small meal. To avoid these unpleasant sensations and those of dumping syndrome, the patient may eat less. Frequent, small, high-protein, high-calorie meals are advised.

Malabsorption. In one type of surgical procedure, the small intestine is rejoined to the stomach in such a way as to form a blind loop. Bacterial overgrowth may occur in this stagnant portion of the bowel, causing a variety of chemical reactions that lead to the malabsorption of fat and vitamin B_{12}. In other instances, anatomical changes affect the proper mixing of bile and enzymes with the food leaving the stomach. Treatment will depend upon the severity of the problem and might include any or all of the following: replacement of missing or deficient substances, administration of antibiotics and or antidiarrheal drugs, eating a fat-restricted and vitamin-supplemented diet, or resorting to surgical repair.

Deficiencies. Anemia sometimes occurs several years after surgery. In most cases, the type of anemia that follows gastric surgery is iron-deficiency anemia, which results from eating less and possibly from impaired iron absorption. Another fairly common postoperative anemia is vitamin B_{12}-deficiency anemia. Both of these are treated with appropriate supplements; iron by mouth, B_{12} by injection. Vitamin D deficiency and poor calcium absorption may also result from gastric surgery. After a few years, either or both of these problems can result in osteomalacia, a softening of the bones, or osteoporosis, a loss of bone substance that causes thinning of bones. Replacement therapy with vitamin D and calcium corrects the difficulty.

Postoperative diet and drug therapies. Postgastrectomy diets will vary according to the type of surgery and its nutritional consequences. Following removal of a portion or all of the stomach, fluids are usually given intravenously until clear liquids can be taken orally. Thereafter, the progression is from liquids to soft foods to solids, and from continuous or frequent small feedings to larger and less frequent meals. In some cases, special formulas are required to provide the necessary calories or nutrients at the outset, but the ultimate goal is to provide the maximum possible nutrients and calories through food. Only when normal eating cannot provide a nutrient do supplements need to be introduced.

MALABSORPTION SYNDROMES

Malabsorption is not a specific disease but is the result of any one of many diseases that prevent the small intestine from properly absorbing nutrients or minerals. Malabsorption can occur, for example, when secretory deficiencies prevent proper digestion of food, when the surface area of the bowel is reduced by surgery or intrinsic disease, or when normal mechanisms for absorbing nutrients are impaired due to disease, infection, or damage by drugs or alcohol. Any of these circumstances can hinder the integrated functioning of bile, the digestive enzymes, and the tissues of the small intestine that are all needed for proper nutrient absorption.

Many conditions can cause malabsorption (those most common to the gastrointestinal tract are discussed subsequently); some involve a single nutrient; others, a host of nutrients. Symptoms depend upon the severity of the disease and the number and type of nutrients malabsorbed. Typically, there may be weight loss, diarrhea, and abdominal distention and bloating, with accompanying discomfort, intestinal gas, and perhaps fatty, pale, bulky, malodorous stools that may float and are difficult to flush away. Those with malabsorption syndromes risk malnutrition because they eat less due to their symptoms; the nutrients that are consumed are poorly absorbed and surgery or drug therapy imposes increased nutrient needs that are difficult to meet.

When the digestive or absorptive functions break down, nutrients may be lost altogether, or they may be improperly processed and retained, often with adverse effects. Although many different consequences may result from various malabsorption syndromes, there are some that are common to most of these disorders, especially when fat is malabsorbed.

When fat is malabsorbed, it is lost in the stool. With it, calories and fat-soluble vitamins (A, D, E, and K) are lost, creating deficiencies. Caloric deficiency produces substantial weight loss. Vitamin K deficiency may result in blood-clotting disorders. A deficiency in vitamin D, which facilitates calcium absorption, can result in calcium depletion and bone disorders. Calcium and magnesium may also be lost because they form soaps with unabsorbed fatty acids. Normally, calcium binds with oxalate, a substance found in some foods. However, when calcium binds with fatty acids instead, oxalate is absorbed and excreted in excessive amounts in the urine. Too much oxalate in the urine can cause kidney stones. Vitamin C pills make this problem worse.

When fat malabsorption occurs, it is necessary to determine and, if possible, correct the underlying cause. Meanwhile, to alleviate the overload of unabsorbed fat in the bowel, which may produce uncomfortable gas and diarrhea, the patient is placed on a fat-restricted diet. In some acute cases, no fat will be allowed for several days. Usually 40 grams of fat (representing 15 percent of total calories, half the usual amount) will be allowed. When greater numbers of calories are required, a synthetic fat supplement is provided in the form of medium-chain triglycerides. These fats are more easily digested and absorbed than the usual dietary long-chain triglycerides because they do not require pancreatic enzymes or bile for digestion and because they enter the bloodstream more readily. Calcium deficiency and excess oxalate in the urine are both treated by supplementing with calcium. Foods containing oxalates (tea, cocoa, leafy green vegetables, and unbleached flour) are restricted.

Bile-salt diarrhea can occur when the lower part of the small intestine (ileum) is damaged by disease or when a significant portion is surgically removed. Bile salts normally depend for absorption on this segment of the intestine, and if they cannot be absorbed here, they are eliminated in excessive quantities in the stool. Because bile salts act as a cathartic on the colon, diarrhea results. Also, since bile salts are essential for normal fat absorption, their excess loss often leads to fat malabsorption as well.

When this type of diarrhea occurs, the bile-salt binding agent cholestyramine (Questran), is generally prescribed along with dietary treatment. When bile-salt losses are too great to be compensated for by the body's increased synthesis, however, cholestyramine may accelerate the bile salt depletion and cannot be used.

Besides fat malabsorption, another complication of bile-salt depletion is gallstones. Gallstones are formed when the concentration of bile salts is too low to keep cholesterol soluble in the gallbladder. Adequate concentrations of bile salts are dependent upon the ability of the small intestine to absorb them, keeping them in circulation. For a more complete discussion of gallstones, see Chapter 31.

Lactose Intolerance

About 75 percent of the American adult population are lactose-intolerant to some degree. This disorder is most prevalent among blacks and people of Asian origin, and least common among those of northern European extraction. The problem is caused by a lack of lactase, an enzyme on the surface of the cells lining the small intestine that is necessary for the digestion of lactose, the sugar in cow's milk. Symptoms include diarrhea, cramps, and gas following ingestion of milk or milk products. Infants or young children with this disorder may also experience weight loss or failure to thrive. Lactase deficiency is also sometimes seen as a secondary problem in association with disorders such as celiac disease and intestinal infections.

Treatment for lactose intolerance is usually entirely dietary: Babies are given formulas based on soy or other milk substitutes; children and adults are placed on a lactose-free diet that excludes milk and most milk products. Label reading becomes an important skill in order to avoid hidden offenders. Many people are able to tolerate yogurt and aged cheeses because the lactose has already been broken down in these foods. Lactase preparations that make lactose more digestible are available in powder, liquid, and capsule forms. Although some people experience relief by eliminating only milk and milk drinks, the degree of lactose intolerance varies from person to person and each individual must determine which foods cause problems and which can be safely consumed.

Cystic Fibrosis

Cystic fibrosis is an inherited disorder of the mucus-producing glands in the pancreas, bronchi, intestines, and liver. It afflicts about 1 child in 1,600. Although this disease affects many systems, the most prominent problems affect the lung and pancreas, and the latter organ is closely involved in nutrition.

In most cases of cystic fibrosis, the pancreatic enzymes necessary for the digestion of protein, carbohydrate, and especially fat are either absent or reduced. Steatorrhea (fatty stool) generally occurs. Because there is great variation in the disease, diet must be individually prescribed. Usually large doses of pancreatic enzyme extracts are given with each meal. A low-fat, high-protein, high-carbohydrate diet is employed, and it is often supplemented with medium-chain triglycerides and protein powders to provide sufficient energy. The diet must be high in calories to maintain weight and offset the nutrient loss. Multivitamin supplements are prescribed. In cases where there is no pancreatic insufficiency, no dietary changes are required. However, additional salt is needed during hot weather, with fever, and whenever sweating is excessive, because abnormal amounts of sodium and chloride are secreted in the perspiration of patients with cystic fibrosis.

Other causes of pancreatic insufficiency include those caused by nutritional deficiency in underdeveloped countries and the chronic pancreatitis of alcoholics.

Celiac Sprue

Celiac sprue, or gluten enteropathy, is an intolerance to gluten, a protein found in wheat, rye, oats, and barley. The delicate folds of the small intestinal lining (villi) are damaged when exposed to this dietary protein, preventing the absorption of many nutrients, including fat, protein, carbohydrates, and fat-soluble vitamins. It affects approximately 1 to 6 of every 10,000 Americans. Typically, the condition appears in infancy when cereals are first added to the diet, or between the ages of 20 and 30 in adults. Although there may be a remission of symptoms during adolescence, it is a lifelong condition. While the cause is not known, it is thought to be a hereditary abnormality in the immune-defense system of the intestine.

Symptoms vary, but people with celiac sprue often have abdominal bloating, cramping and distention, steatorrhea, and diarrhea, accompanied by weight loss in adults and failure to thrive in babies. Irritability is also a typical symptom. Damage caused to intestinal cells results in secondary lactose intolerance and loss of potassium and other electrolytes. Vitamin deficiencies can cause osteomalacia, rickets, muscle spasms, night blindness, impaired blood clotting, and anemia.

Treatment involves the elimination of

gluten from the diet, not an easy feat, since many processed foods contain gluten: salad dressings, ice cream, candies, gravies, meats with fillers, most baked goods and pastas, beer and ale, and others. Because of the difficulty in substituting acceptable ingredients, special recipes have been created to allow maximum variation in the diet.

Physicians sometimes have food lists and recipe resources in the office; more frequently, they refer patients to a nutritional counselor or to the nearest chapter of the American Celiac Society or Glucose Intolerance Group. The gluten-free diet is generally a lifelong requirement. The damage done to the intestine can usually be repaired within six months after gluten is eliminated. Sometimes it may be necessary to restrict fat in the diet and to avoid lactose during the period when the intestine is healing. However, once the intestine is back to normal, fat and lactose can again be included. Multivitamin supplements are generally recommended for all celiac patients.

ACUTE DIARRHEA

Acute infectious gastroenteritis is a common illness; it is estimated that there are 5 billion cases of diarrhea worldwide every year. In developing countries, as many as 10 million deaths may be attributed to it annually, especially among infants; in industrialized countries where the general population is well nourished, diarrhea is rarely fatal but it can still threaten infants, the elderly, and the infirm. Usually, it is a self-limiting disorder that lasts from two to seven days and is followed by a rapid and complete recovery. Nevertheless, in the United States it is second only to the common cold as a cause for absenteeism from work.

The rotavirus is responsible for most of the acute diarrhea seen in babies and young children. In North America, it occurs more frequently in winter months and is characterized by severe watery diarrhea that may be accompanied by vomiting, low-grade fever, and cramping. It lasts from five to eight days, with the vomiting subsiding first. Adults may be infected by this virus, but this is either a less common occurrence or affected adults are not symptomatic.

Family, school, restaurant, or camp epidemics of diarrhea are most commonly caused by the Norwalk virus or a similar viral agent. They usually arise from a common source of infection such as the water supply, poorly cooked seafood, or salad. Outbreaks last about a week; individual cases last one or two days. Watery diarrhea is the hallmark, but vomiting and fever may also be present, especially in children.

Diarrhea is experienced at one time or another by most people who travel across international borders—so-called travelers' diarrhea. Contrary to popular belief, however, it is not usually contracted by drinking the water, and it is rarely caused by a parasite. (Confining drinking water, though, to bottled water, cooled water from the hot-water tap in urban areas, or boiled water in the bush is still a good idea.) In about 75 percent of the cases, bacteria, typically *Escherichia coli*, ingested with raw unpeeled fruits and vegetables, are the most likely culprits. Travelers' diarrhea rarely lasts more than three days, and symptoms are usually confined to passing about four stools a day, with mild to moderate abdominal cramps. Rarely is there a need to consult a physician; self-medication is simple and effective.

Nutritional Consequences

For most normally healthy American children and adults, the dehydration and loss of electrolytes caused by acute diarrhea do not pose a significant threat. However, babies and very young children, the elderly, and those who might become quickly dehydrated, such as diabetics, should be treated promptly.

For years, those suffering from diarrhea were given nothing orally because it was assumed that if the number of stools increased, the diarrhea was worsening. This concept results in unnecessary and inappropriate nutritional deprivation.

Dietary Treatment

With rare exception, the treatment for diarrhea involves oral rehydration therapy; replacing fluids and electrolytes lost in frequent, watery stools by drinking liquids containing sugar (or starch) and salt. The liquids used depend upon the individual's age and his or her degree of dehydration: for children and adults with mild diarrhea, carbonated beverages, juices, tea, consommé, water, and salted crackers; for more severe cases, Gatorade, sweetened mineral water, or alternate cups of eight ounces of water plus one-quarter of a teaspoon of baking soda and eight ounces of fruit juice with a pinch of table salt and one-quarter of a teaspoon of corn syrup or honey. (The World Health Organization has a rehydration mixture available in packets to be mixed with a quart of water. This is useful for travelers, and especially for native children in developing countries.) When solid food is appealing and can be tolerated, salted crackers, bread, or rice is introduced, with the gradual addition of other carbohydrates, protein, and, finally, fats. Dairy products should be avoided because several agents that cause diarrhea also produce temporary lactase deficiency.

Breastfed babies should continue to nurse, but all babies and children should abstain from cow's milk until their symptoms have disappeared. Instead (and in addition for breastfed babies), they should be given either a commercial rehydration product or precooked rice cereal mixed with water and a half a teaspoon of salt for each pint—to the consistency of a milk shake. The home remedy of chicken soup with rice (blenderized for babies) has the additional advantage of replacing potassium (provided by the chicken). Parents should not worry about overfeeding infants and small children with diarrhea and should continue giving extra food for several days after the symptoms are gone in order to ensure that adequate nutrition is supplied.

INFLAMMATORY BOWEL DISEASE
(Ileitis and Colitis)

Crohn's Disease

In Crohn's disease, the walls of the intestine become inflamed and swollen. When the inflammation is of the ileum, or lower part of the small intestine, it is called ileitis; when the colon, or large intestine, is affected, it is referred to as Crohn's colitis. *Ileocolitis* is the term used when disease is present in both the small and large intestines. Symptoms include abdominal pain, diarrhea, fever, loss of weight, and joint pain. In young children, it can cause growth retardation.

Ulcerative Colitis

In ulcerative colitis, sores form in the lining of the colon and rectum, causing abdominal pain and diarrhea that is usually bloody. Although Crohn's disease and ulcerative colitis are different diseases that require slightly different treatment, they both cause inflammation of the intestine, tend to have similar symptoms, and frequently run in the same families. They are therefore frequently grouped together under the term *inflammatory bowel disease*, or *IBD*.

Since the cause for these disorders is unknown, there is no cure. They can usually be well controlled with proper diet and medication, and sometimes there are long periods when there are no symptoms at all. In cases where drug therapy is not effective, surgery may be required. In a sense, removal of the large intestine constitutes a cure for ulcerative colitis, since the colon is no longer present; with Crohn's disease, however, the problem can recur anywhere along the intestinal tract, so removal of one part of the intestine, while often helpful, necessary, and even lifesaving, still offers no guarantee that the disease will not reappear a few years later.

Nutritional Consequences

Inflammatory bowel disease can compromise nutrition. With a poor appetite, abdominal pain, and intestinal obstruction, the person suffering from IBD may take in too few calories and nutrients. Because the intestine has been damaged by inflammation, it no longer functions properly: Vitamins and nutrients are excreted instead of absorbed, and bacterial growth is excessive, causing chemical reactions that interfere with the absorption of fats and alter the metabolism of absorptive cells.

Treatment, too, can result in poor nutrition. Steroids are often given for severe symptoms, and sulfasalazine, a combination of a sulfa drug and an aspirinlike compound, is prescribed for milder cases and for maintenance of remission. Both medications have potentially adverse effects on nutrition. Regular use may, therefore, require supplements such as potassium and calcium in the case of steroids, and folic acid with sulfasalazine.

When large portions of the small intestine are surgically removed, the absorptive surface and the digestive secretions are reduced. As a result, nutrients pass too quickly through the remaining intestine and absorption is impaired, especially affecting bile salts and vitamin B_{12} when the ileum is removed. In some situations, bacterial overgrowth in the intestine also contributes to losses of bile salts and vitamin B_{12}. Furthermore, physicians sometimes advise unnecessarily bland or restrictive diets—no fried foods, no dairy products, no spices, and so on—leaving few choices for patients who already have trouble enjoying food and maintaining adequate nutrition. Conversely, patients sometimes blame flare-ups on whatever they have eaten, adding even more foods to their personal forbidden list.

There is no specific diet for IBD. Since maintaining adequate nutrition is so difficult, it is important that individuals eat well-balanced meals and avoid only those foods that provoke symptoms or complications. There are a few exceptions; those who have partial bowel obstruction may require a low-roughage diet, or those with kidney stones would benefit from a low-oxalate diet. See page 556 in Chapter 32 for foods high in oxalates that should be avoided. (Although there may be secondary lactase deficiency, dairy products are too often restricted for IBD patients, even when there is no physiologic reason.) Even strict adherence to a superior diet may not provide enough vitamins and minerals to make up for those lost through malabsorption or drug-nutrient interaction, so many IBD patients need multivitamin supplements, and some may require additional specific supplements such as vitamin B_{12} injections.

Those with severe disease or extensive surgery will be unable to obtain adequate nutrition through diet alone and will need to be treated with various formulas and supplements. These include supplements that serve as meal replacements, which have the composition of a normal diet; individual supplements, which are not complete feedings but supply a single nutrient; and elemental diets, which are usually low in fat and contain other nutrients in easily digested form.

Since the goal is to stay as close to normal diet patterns as possible, the use of individual supplements is preferred. When this is not adequate, elemental diets may be employed. Since most patients find these unpalatable and difficult to drink, they are frequently given by a nasogastric tube in the evening. For patients who cannot or will not eat enough, elemental or defined formula diets have proven useful. Such enteral supplements have been especially helpful for children and adolescents with growth retardation.

Under certain conditions, enteral nutrition—in which feeding is done through a tube, usually inserted into the nose and into the stomach—may not be appropriate. Patients with significant nutritional defects who need surgery may require a period of total parenteral nutrition (TPN), when all necessary nutrients are administered intravenously into the bloodstream, totally bypassing the digestive tract. TPN allows for improving nutritional status prior to surgery, and it may be useful in treating some patients with Crohn's disease who do not respond to medication, especially children with growth retardation. Until recently, this treatment was extremely costly and disruptive because of the long hospital stay required. Now TPN can be provided in the home, making it relatively less expensive and allowing patients to live a more normal lifestyle. Often patients are able to return to work or school while maintaining the TPN regimen. Unfortunately, total parenteral alimentation has not proved helpful in the treatment of ulcerative colitis.

TPN in and of itself is not a treatment for IBD. It is generally indicated only for those patients who show evidence of malnutrition. Its only use as primary therapy is in those patients who, as a result of severe Crohn's disease or extensive intestinal surgery (short bowel syndrome), cannot maintain adequate nutrition through normal eating. Moreover, nutritional management is only a small part of the overall care of patients with IBD. Potent medications are frequently required, and patients and physicians must develop a close working relationship, often aided by the educational programs of the National Foundation for Ileitis and Colitis.

IRRITABLE BOWEL SYNDROME (Spastic Colon)

Irritable bowel syndrome (IBS) is the most common medical complaint after the common cold. It is so widespread that its sufferers represent about 70 percent of the patients seen by gastroenterologists, yet it is estimated that as many as 70 percent of the sufferers never consult a doctor. IBS is made up of a group of symptoms, the most common of which are diffuse cramping, abdominal pain, constipation, daytime diarrhea, or constipation alternating with diarrhea. Other possible symptoms are bloating, a feeling of fullness in the rectum, and stomach distress. Emotional stress is closely linked to IBS, and it is thought that stress or anxiety may trigger attacks.

Although the syndrome has become better defined in recent years, the firm diagnosis of IBS still requires a process of elimination. Since all of its symptoms may also be associated with potentially serious gastrointestinal, endocrine, or reproductive diseases, these other conditions must be ruled out. When there is no fever, no weight loss, and no positive finding after appropriate tests, then IBS is a reasonable diagnosis.

While it is reassuring to know that irritable bowel syndrome is not a disease but, rather, a functional disorder, it is frustrating to know that its cause is not understood and that its treatment may alleviate symptoms but will not effect a cure. There appear to be at least three separate factors involved in IBS: disturbances in peristalsis, the innate muscular movement of the intestines; altered neurohormonal functions; and stress reactions. Sometimes food intolerances account for or coexist with some cases of IBS, but true food allergies, while frequently diagnosed, are, in fact, exceedingly rare. Therapy typically includes regulation of the diet, identification and control of stress-producing factors, and the use of combinations of drugs designed to reduce stress and alter intestinal motility.

Nutritional Consequences

Irritable bowel syndrome rarely causes any weight loss or nutritional deficiencies. Most nutritional consequences result from attempts to alleviate its symptoms. Fad diets and laxative abuse can create imbalances and fluid and electrolyte losses and can result in chronic diarrhea as well as vitamin and mineral deficiencies.

Fad diets run the gamut, but their salient characteristic is that they emphasize one thing, whether it is the exclusion of one food or substance claimed to be detrimental or the inclusion of extraordinary amounts of something purported to be beneficial. Such extreme lack of balance can be disruptive to a sensitive system. It is understandable, however, that people suffering from regular bouts of pain or erratic bowel habits might be willing to try just about anything for relief.

Notwithstanding clear medical evidence to the contrary, many are convinced that a daily bowel movement is necessary for good health and that the lack of it causes various ailments such as headaches, lethargy, bad breath, and so on. The casual use of laxatives to treat head colds, headaches, and menstrual cramps and their availability without prescription (suggesting to many that they are harmless) pose potential hazards of misuse, especially to those with recurrent bouts of constipation.

There are five different types of laxatives, each of which acts in a different way, has different side effects, and can be dangerous for people with certain medical conditions. None is safe for continuous use without monitoring by a physician. Any use other than the suggested dosage for a period of two or three days is not recommended. Overuse causes nutrient losses and attendant deficiencies and can result in dependency, a potentially serious problem.

Dietary Treatment

In our current state of ignorance, the primary means of treating the symptoms of IBS is dietary manipulation, a highly individual process that may require time and effort, as well as trial and error to achieve the best result. Most physicians prefer not to impose restrictions but to work with the patient to discover food sensitivities.

Since symptoms of lactose intolerance may mimic those of IBS, this disorder should be ruled out first. To do so, a patient should omit lactose from the diet for two weeks or take a lactose-tolerance test. Keeping a food diary and recording the response to various foods such as gas-producing vegetables, caffeinated beverages, and peppery foods is another way of determining which foods can and cannot be tolerated. (For a list of foods that cause gas, see page 532.)

A high-fiber, low-fat diet is recommended for many patients whose sensitivities have been established. In recent years, fiber has been touted as a cure for a host of digestive disorders. While many of the benefits claimed for fiber consumption have yet to be shown in controlled studies, it seems that appropriate and moderate fiber intake facilitates digestion and has protective properties in some instances. A few people cannot tolerate bran, the most common source of fiber in the American diet, and those suffering from diarrhea may respond negatively to other kinds of fiber as well. In general, however, a high-fiber diet is well tolerated (and particularly helpful for those who suffer from constipation) if the fiber content is increased gradually and the fiber source is tailored to individual sensitivities. Since fat is more difficult to digest than carbohydrate or protein, the low-fat component of the prescription is aimed primarily at reducing symptoms.

Most people can get adequate amounts of fiber from their normal diet by judicious selection. When sufficient dietary fiber cannot be obtained from the regular diet, fiber supplements are useful, but they should be chosen with the advice of a physician. (See below for a list of foods that are high in fiber.)

DIVERTICULOSIS AND DIVERTICULITIS

Diverticulosis of the colon is a condition in which saclike herniations protrude through the intestinal lining. This disorder occurs predominantly in the industrialized Western world, where it is estimated that as many as 50 percent of people over age 80 may be affected. Diets high in fat and low in fiber are believed to play a role. Although there are usually no symptoms associated with uncomplicated diverticulosis, when they do occur they resemble those of IBS and are often difficult to distinguish from them. Dietary and medical management is similar to that already discussed for IBS. Occasionally, diverticulosis leads to complications of inflammation (*diverticulitis*), obstruction, or hemorrhage; in contrast to simple diverticulosis, these complications may be serious and often require intensive medical and even surgical therapy.

Foods That Cause Gas

There is great variation in foods that cause gas in different individuals. Some of the more common offenders are listed below, but finding the specific personal culprits is a matter of trial and error.

Apples	Corn
Bananas	Cucumbers
Beans	Meringues
Broccoli	Milk
Cabbage	Oats and other
Carbonated	high-fiber foods
beverages	Onions
Cauliflower	Turnips

Foods High in Fiber

Almonds	Parsley
Apricots	Peaches
Beans	Pears
Blackberries	Pineapple
Bran	Pistachio nuts
Brussel sprouts	Popcorn
Corn	Prunes
Coconut	Raspberries
Dates	Strawberries
Figs	Walnuts
Kiwi	Whole-grain
Lentils	products

31

Nutrition and Liver and Gallbladder Disease

Charles S. Lieber, M.D.

■

INTRODUCTION

The liver is one of the body's most complex organs, playing a major role in a wide variety of body functions that range from helping with the digestion and absorption of food to producing the substances that cause blood to clot. Liver disorders can have a significant impact on diverse activities of the body, particularly on the digestion and metabolism of food. As a result, proper treatment of diseases of the liver often involves considerable attention to nutrition.

Adjacent to the liver is the gallbladder, a much smaller organ. The gallbladder stores bile, a digestive substance produced by the liver. After a meal, the gallbladder releases bile to assist with the digestion and absorption of fats. In some people, particularly as they grow older, excess bile precipitates as crystals and forms stones, which can block the duct leading from the gallbladder. This can be very painful and is usually treated by surgically removing the gallbladder and the stones, although in some cases drugs are used to dissolve gallstones. Gallbladder disease also involves nutritional considerations.

LIVER DISEASE

The liver, the body's largest internal organ and one of its most complex, is located in the upper portion of the abdominal cavity, beneath the diaphragm, and to the right of the stomach. It is one of the few organs capable of regeneration, growing new cells to replace damaged ones. Studies have found that the body can continue to function even if only one-quarter of the liver is functioning normally. There is a limit to the insults the liver can withstand, however; excess alcohol consumption over many years, for example, invariably damages it. Despite the liver's remarkable recuperative powers, liver disease is often serious, and a nonfunctional liver soon becomes fatal.

The liver is a veritable biochemical factory and a pivotal organ in nutrition. It serves as a storehouse for many essential vitamins and minerals. It produces cholesterol and triglycerides and manufactures substances that cause the blood to clot as well as prevent it from clotting. Bile is produced in the liver and sent on to the gallbladder, where it is stored and concentrated, to be released after a meal to aid in the digestion and absorption of fat.

The liver is the main organ controlling carbohydrate metabolism. It takes molecules produced by the metabolism of protein and carbohydrates and converts them to glucose, the sugar used by the body to supply energy to the cells. The liver also regulates the level of glucose in the blood by converting excess glucose into the starchlike carbohydrate glycogen, which it stores for the future. Later, when glucose levels are low and the body needs more energy, the glycogen is converted back to glucose and released slowly into the blood. The liver also produces certain amino acids, the building blocks of proteins. The amino acids are key elements in the body's ability to generate new cells and repair tissue damage. The liver converts other amino acids into energy sources.

The liver is also a cleansing and detox-ification system. Blood carrying nutrients from digested food passes through the liver and is cleansed of noxious substances such as am-monia, which is produced by protein metabo-lism. Foreign compounds in the body, such as drugs or chemicals found in the environment, are removed by the liver. Some drugs and chemicals, however, can cause severe liver damage, including work-place chemicals such as toluene, carbon tetrachloride, trichloro-ethylene, and vinyl chloride. Yellow phos-phorus, a rat poison, is also toxic to the liver, as are large amounts of alcohol. Hence, liver disease is one of the serious consequences of long-term alcohol abuse. In all, at least 100 drugs are known to alter the liver's function-ing or to harm it.

When blood passes through the liver, a number of vitamins and minerals are removed and stored there. These include vitamins A, D, and B_{12}, copper, and iron.

It is not surprising that when liver disease develops, the effects on the body's metabolic system can be widespread and sometimes sub-tle. Because of the liver's central role in glucose metabolism, problems with the breakdown of carbohydrates can develop. Glucose intol-erance is seen in some patients with various liver diseases, as is hypoglycemia or low blood sugar. Some patients have difficulty removing lactic acid from the bloodstream—another part of the carbohydrate-metabolism system. Lac-tic-acid acidosis, a condition in which lactic acid builds up in the blood, can result.

Liver disease can also upset protein metab-olism, affecting a whole sequence of important protein complexes, including the one that pro-duces the substance that makes blood clot. A test of the blood's ability to clot is an important clinical test of impaired liver function and the need for vitamin K therapy. The body's vitamin balance may also be disturbed by liver disease. Deficiencies of water-soluble vitamins such as folic and nicotinic acids, riboflavin, thiamine, and fat-soluble vitamins, such as vitamin A, are encountered in patients with liver disease.

Hepatitis

Hepatitis, an inflammation of the liver, is one of the most common liver diseases, and nutrition plays an important role in its treat-ment. Hepatitis is usually caused by viral in-fections, but alcohol and drug abuse, and some bacterial, parasitic, and fungal infections can also cause the liver inflammation. Symp-toms can vary in severity from a mild flulike illness to the much less common liver failure, coma, and death.

Several viruses are implicated in hepatitis and produce the different types of the disease. Hepatitis A virus comes from the body's intes-tinal tract and usually is spread when food has been contaminated by fecal content. An in-fected person who does not wash his or her hands properly and then handles food is proba-bly the most common route of transmission. Sometimes shellfish become contaminated with hepatitis A virus, such as in a bay con-taminated with sewage, and an epidemic of the disease can occur when people eat the shellfish.

Hepatitis B, also called serum hepatitis, is spread by direct blood contact. A screening test that can detect contaminated blood has largely eliminated blood transfusions as a source of this form of hepatitis. Use of contaminated needles by drug abusers is now a common source of the disease. Sexual contact, particularly among homosexuals, can also spread it. Some people harbor the hepatitis B virus and spread it to others but are themselves unaffected.

A third form of viral hepatitis is known as hepatitis C or sometimes non-A, non-B hepatitis. Little is known about it, except that it, too, can be transmitted through blood contact.

One of the first symptoms of hepatitis is loss of appetite, followed often by nausea, vomiting, and fever. Smokers can lose their taste for cigarettes. Joints may ache, and after a few days, the urine may turn dark. Jaundice may follow, which is caused by too much bile pigment (bilirubin) in the body. The skin and whites of the eyes and other parts of the body take on a yellowish hue.

There is no cure for hepatitis. Instead, rest and a good diet are prescribed, and the disease often resolves itself in four to six weeks. The best diet for hepatitis is a well-planned, appetizing, mixed diet. Usually, the biggest nutritional problem is loss of appetite and unwillingness to eat, just at a time when good nutrition is necessary to speed the liver's recuperation and regeneration of damaged cells.

Many people in this stage of hepatitis say they are hungry but quickly lose their appetite after eating only a few bites. Sometimes severe nausea can occur after a few bites. One way to deal with this is to serve frequent small meals. Sometimes a tasty and nutritious liquid formula, such as a liquid breakfast mixed with milk or a milk shake or eggnog between meals, can overcome the problem.

Care should be taken in the preparation of the liquid meals, since improper mixing can reduce their appeal. A blender or milk-shake mixer should be used, although a hand-held beater is satisfactory if used properly. In some patients, hepatitis may also be accompanied by a poor tolerance for fats or for milk products. In that case, the amount of milk in the liquid formulas should be cut back and water substituted. After a milk-tolerance level is found, the amount of milk often can be slowly increased without a recurrence of the intolerance.

The hepatitis patient's diet should ideally consist of a minimum of 60 grams of protein a day for an average-sized person. This amount is easily obtainable in a mixed diet. The protein should come from both animal and vegetable products. Sufficient amounts of amino acids and vitamins are provided in a mixture of protein-containing foods, such as meats, fish, eggs, dairy products, legumes, and cereals. Amino-acid supplements are unnecessary.

Fats need not be restricted for the hepatitis patient unless fat seems to cause indigestion, possibly from fewer bile salts in the intestine to aid digestion, a condition probably caused by the hepatitis itself. On the other hand, there is no need for a high-fat diet, but fat certainly can add to the palatability of a diet, particularly if lack of appetite is a continuing problem. As a general rule, fat that comes from dairy products and eggs is easier to digest than fat that comes from fried foods and fatty meats.

A balanced diet also will contain adequate amounts of carbohydrates, without the need for special supplements. In the past, doctors sometimes recommended that patients eat as much candy as they wished as a means to increase total nutritional intake and to overcome loss of appetite. This practice is now not regarded as a wise one, particularly between meals, since the sweets provide an unbalanced source of calories and disturb appetite at mealtimes.

In most cases, rest and the nutritional management outlined above will bring full recovery. In a few cases, however, the loss of appetite can become serious, particularly if it is accompanied by nausea and vomiting after eating a little food. If such problems are not quickly overcome, tube feeding or even intravenous feeding may be necessary. In such cases, the patient most likely will be hospitalized and the feeding conducted under a doctor's direct supervision. In tube feeding, a thin plastic tube is inserted down the throat and into the stomach, then special formulas are passed through the tube. If tube feeding causes vomiting, then intravenous feeding might be necessary. The goal in either case would be to end such feeding quickly and return the patient to normal eating.

Fatty Liver

Fatty liver is a condition in which molecules of fat are deposited in the liver cells. Fat collects within the liver cell and distorts it. Too much alcohol consumption—for example, six ounces a day for several weeks—can induce the condition. It can also be brought about by severe protein malnutrition known as kwashiorkor, severe calorie deficiency such as marasmus, diabetes, extreme obesity, and Reye's syndrome. The toxicity resulting from some drugs, including the antibiotic tetracycline, can also cause fatty liver.

Treatment of fatty liver consists of dealing with the underlying condition. Severe malnutrition such as kwashiorkor or marasmus is treated with a high-protein diet. If a toxic drug or alcohol is responsible, its use must be discontinued or moderated. In fatty liver relating to diabetes and obesity, a low-sugar, high-protein diet and maintenance of desirable body weight constitute the treatment.

Cirrhosis

Cirrhosis is marked by the development of extensive scar or fibrous tissue. Hepatitis can lead to cirrhosis; several other rarer bacterial, parasitic, congenital, and chemical conditions also can cause the progressive destruction of liver tissue. However, in the United States, excessive alcohol consumption—a pint or more of alcohol a day for several years—is the dominant cause of cirrhosis. Not all alcoholics develop cirrhosis, but its incidence among them is more than 10 percent. In 1975, cirrhosis was the sixth most common cause of death. It is now the fourth most common cause of death in the age group 25 to 64 in urban areas. Traditionally it has been concentrated among men over age 45, but the growing incidence of alcoholism among women has broadened the disease's base.

Even after many liver cells have died, the organ's remarkable recuperative power permits it to regenerate healthy new tissue. Nevertheless, the disease is serious and irreversible. Cirrhosis caused by hepatitis can be the most progressive. Alcoholic cirrhosis has a better prognosis if all alcohol consumption ceases. Nutrition can be very important in treating cirrhosis, and, in some stages of the disease, the patient's diet becomes critical.

Because the liver plays such a central role in keeping the body's metabolic and hormonal systems in balance, cirrhosis can have severe effects that feed back into one another in a negative way. In the person with a normal liver, the portal vein and the hepatic artery carry one and a half quarts of blood every minute through the miles of blood vessels in the organ. The portal vein delivers blood rich in nutrients to the liver, where they are processed. The hepatic artery arrives with oxygen-rich blood.

However, liver scar tissue is rigid and unyielding in the cirrhotic liver and this volume of blood encounters difficulties in making its way through the organ. Blood in the portal vein backs up and causes portal hypertension. This increased pressure forces plasma out of the liver's blood vessels and into the abdominal cavity. This fluid accumulates and the belly swells in a condition known as ascites. This, in turn, means that less blood is reaching the kidneys, which send out biochemical signals calling for more of the hormone aldosterone. This causes the body to retain sodium, which causes further retention of fluid, worsening the ascites. Excess fluid is now present throughout the body.

Since normal blood flow is restricted, the blood must seek other routes out of the liver and into the body. One route is the blood vessels that pass through the esophagus. This causes the blood vessels to bulge into the esophagus, resulting in a condition called esophageal varices. Sometimes they bleed into the esophagus, a serious condition that carries a grave risk of death. Many of the nutritional considerations in cirrhosis arise from the alterations in the blood flow through the liver and the vicious cycle that arises.

To make matters worse, the diseased liver has an impaired ability to deal with a very common but essential metabolic function: the breakdown of amino acids to provide energy or to make glucose. This process, known as deamination, produces ammonia as a by-product—the same substance used as a household cleanser. A normal liver uses some of the ammonia to synthesize proteins and combines the rest to form urea, which the kidneys remove in the urine. The diseased liver, however, cannot carry out these processes and ammonia can build up in the blood.

The ammonia is very toxic, particularly to the central nervous system. In advanced cases of cirrhosis, the increasing levels of ammonia are thought to play a role in the development of hepatic coma, a serious condition that begins with mental confusion and can lead rapidly to coma and death. The presence of the ammonia alters the biochemical system by which the brain produces energy. Investigators also believe that hepatic coma is related to ab-

normal neurotransmitters in the brain. Cirrhotic patients have an abnormal amino-acid profile: an increase in aromatic amino acids, such as phenylalanine, tyrosine, and tryptophan, and a decrease in the branched-chain amino acids, such as isoleucine, leucine, and valine. The accumulation of the aromatic amino acids may encourage formation of false neurotransmitters, which then cause the altered neurological behavior.

Doctors treating cirrhosis patients are constantly on the alert for early signs of hepatic coma: personality changes, forgetfulness, and other symptoms that progress to intellectual deterioration, confusion, and stupor.

If the cirrhosis is caused by alcoholism, as is usually the case, the first dietary consideration is abstinence from alcohol. Indeed, someone with cirrhosis should never drink alcohol again. Second, in many cases the alcoholic is malnourished because his or her diet has consisted largely of the empty calories of alcohol. The diet should therefore be balanced but robust. Like the patient with hepatitis, the cirrhotic is likely to have little appetite. Frequent small meals are preferable. Nutrition is extremely important and every possible effort should be made to ensure that the proper foods in adequate amounts are eaten.

The cirrhotic patient must receive precisely the correct amount of protein. Too much could result in excess ammonia buildup, which could risk hepatic coma. Too little would deprive the liver of what it needs in order to generate new liver cells. A typical cirrhotic patient requires about 40 grams of protein a day in a 2,000- to 3,000-calorie diet. Enough carbohydrates and fat must be provided so that the carefully apportioned protein isn't used to meet the body's energy needs instead of going toward liver repair. Recent studies have suggested that the patient with hepatic coma might benefit by receiving more branched-chain amino acids and fewer aromatic amino acids. This is usually achieved by giving a special intravenous solution, but this therapy is still the subject of debate. Some investigators have suggested that vegetable protein is better than animal protein in hepatic coma because of its higher branched-chain amino-acid content, but this question is still unresolved.

Hepatic coma patients are sometimes given lactulose and neomycin. Lactulose acidifies the intestinal contents and impedes ammonia production and absorption. Neomycin alters the digestive-tract bacteria that produce cerebral toxins.

A liver that has been long exposed to the continuous insult of alcohol cannot manufacture some of the substances necessary to handle fats. Earlier thinking was that a cirrhotic should restrict fat intake. That idea has been replaced with the belief that normal amounts of fats in the diet are permitted unless the patient develops steatorrhea, a condition in which fat cannot be digested and therefore appears in the feces.

The cirrhotic patient's diet is usually supplemented with large doses of water-soluble vitamins, often up to five times the RDA. Folate and thiamine are the most commonly decreased vitamins in cirrhotic patients; riboflavin, nicotinamide, pantothenic acid, and vitamins B_6, B_{12}, A, and D may also be low. In malnutrition, the water-soluble vitamins are among the first to be depleted in the body. They are very important as coenzymes so that the liver's many enzymes can do the necessary metabolic and repair work. If tests reveal a shortage of vitamin K, it can also be added, but it may not be very useful, since the problem is not a lack of vitamin K, but instead, poor utilization of it.

The cirrhotic diet becomes more complicated if ascites develops, since fluids and sodium must be restricted to bring the fluid accumulation under control. Depending on what the doctor determines, the amount of allowable sodium each day might range from as little as 200 to 500 milligrams. Fluid intake might range from 1,000 to 1,500 milliliters per day.

Weighing the patient as a means to monitor the body's overall fluid content becomes very important. In most cases, the daily weight is entered on a chart so trends over time can be monitored. If the patient gains weight rapidly, then the body is retaining fluid and something more may have to be done to arrest the accumulation. Weight loss means that fluid is being lost and the situation is improving. A small but steady daily weight gain may mean that the patient has begun to restore lost tissue, including, possibly, repair of the liver.

When ascites develops in the cirrhotic patient, the task of maintaining a low-salt but appetizing diet while keeping protein content at the correct level to avoid onset of hepatic coma becomes more complicated. High-protein foods such as milk, meat, and eggs naturally contain some sodium. Low-sodium supplements and dairy products will be necessary. In some cases when sodium intake must be drastically limited, less obvious sources of sodium must be reduced. They include the sodium in artificially softened water, sodium in intravenously administered blood and plasma, and the sodium in some medications.

In the most serious cases of cirrhosis when the patient has bleeding in the esophagus, there can be no feeding by mouth. Instead, nutrition must be received intravenously. When there is no esophageal bleeding, food can be taken by mouth but substances that would irritate the lining of the esophagus must be avoided. Food should be chewed thoroughly before swallowing so that no particles become caught in the esophagus.

At the first sign that the cirrhotic patient cannot take adequate quantities of food by mouth, no time should be wasted before beginning feeding by tube or, if necessary, intravenous feeding. Such treatment most likely would be carried out under the direct supervision of a doctor. Should the patient begin to show signs of impending hepatic coma, the doctor would probably sharply reduce the amount of protein in the diet—to as little as 20 grams of high-quality protein per day—and give lactulose. If coma sets in, protein is eliminated entirely. Once improvement has begun, protein can gradually be increased until a normal amount of protein in the diet is reached. When there is fear of hepatic coma, some foods that contain preformed ammonia or amino acids that are easily converted to ammonia should be avoided. They include chicken, ground beef, ham, bacon, salami, buttermilk, and gelatin.

Cirrhotic patients who are stable must be careful of their diet nevertheless. They commonly are prescribed a combination low-protein and low-sodium diet to prevent an overload of the end products of protein metabolism, to control nitrogen balance, and to reduce fluid retention. Foods of high-value protein such as meat, fish, poultry, and milk are eaten, but in limited quantities, and liberal portions of polyunsaturated fats and simple sugars are used to provide enough calories to assure proper utilization of the protein. Fruits and vegetables are served normally. A salt substitute that provides 1,000 milligrams of potassium replaces normal table salt. Since such a diet may be deficient in all the nutrients except vitamins A and C, vitamin and mineral supplements must also be taken.

Doctors and nutritionists have noted that with a restricted sodium and protein diet, it is difficult to get patients to eat enough to assure sufficient caloric intake. Meals must be interesting and palatable while at the same time maintaining the strict protein and sodium limitations. Such diets often require purchasing and preparing special foods. Frequently, the patient is a malnourished, recovering alcoholic who will have little appetite. Encouraging proper eating in such patients can be a real challenge to the doctor, nurses, nutritionists, and family members.

Although not as common as alcoholic cirrhosis, biliary cirrhosis also merits nutritional considerations. In biliary cirrhosis, there is impaired bile excretion and progressive destruction of the small bile ducts. The cause of primary biliary cirrhosis is unknown, although it may reflect a disorder in the immune system. It occurs almost exclusively in middle-aged women and is often fatal after progressing over a period of six to seven years. Secondary biliary cirrhosis occurs when the bile duct is obstructed; it is treated through the surgical removal of the obstruction. Nutritional care of biliary cirrhosis is similar to other cirrhotic diet therapy. The patient should receive a diet with adequate calories and reduction of fat to 30 to 40 grams per day. Fat-soluble vitamins are given through injections. Edema, ascites, and varices of the esophagus can also occur and are treated in the same manner as in alcoholic cirrhosis.

GALLBLADDER DISEASE

The gallbladder is sometimes described as nature's mistake, the organ that modern man apparently doesn't need. This is because the treatment of choice for gallbladder disease is removal of the pear-shaped organ that lies under the liver. In the vast majority of cases, people who have had their gallbladder removed experience no change in the functioning of their digestive system.

The gallbladder stores and concentrates bile, the enzyme that the liver produces to digest fat in the small intestine. Shortly after eating, biochemical signals from the small intestine reach the gallbladder and bile is released. With the onset of middle age, sometimes before, stones composed chiefly of cholesterol, or bilirubin and calcium, may be deposited in the gallbladder itself or in the ducts that lead from the gallbladder to the small intestine. These stones occasionally may fully obstruct the bile flow, leading to jaundice. Most gallstones are comprised of 70 to 98 percent cholesterol. Another less prevalent class of gallstone has the bile pigment bilirubin as its main constituent.

In many cases, gallstones pose no problem and go unnoticed for years. Over 60 percent of the people with gallstones will experience symptoms only once. In other cases, however, the contraction of the gallbladder after eating—to release bile—causes pain in the upper-right abdomen. The digestion of fat is interrupted. As a result, there can also be indigestion, flatulence, and vomiting. In most cases, however, the only symptom is a steady pain that can range from mild to excruciating. The preferred treatment is surgical removal of the gallbladder, which cures the disease.

In the United States, 16 million people have gallstones, 12 million women and 4 million men. Surgeons remove 500,000 gallbladders a year, making cholecystectomy—the name of the operation—the most common form of abdominal surgery. Approximately 6,000 people die from gallbladder disease or complications of its treatment annually. Four recent presidents of the United States—Hoover, Truman, Eisenhower, and Johnson—had gallbladder surgery during their terms in office.

The presence of gallstones varies with age, gender, and geographic location, but women are much more likely to develop the stones than men. Some ethnic groups apparently have a predisposition to gallstones. The Pima Indians in Arizona have a much higher incidence of the stones than Caucasians, particularly the Pima women, where the incidence is 75 percent. Blacks, particularly black men, have a lower rate, and the cholesterol gallstones common in Caucasians in the United States are rare among Orientals.

Investigators have conducted extensive studies in an attempt to identify conditions that lead to development of gallstones. Women are from two to four times more likely to develop gallstones, and studies have looked particularly carefully at this difference. A large majority of women who develop the stones have borne children. Cholesterol levels are particularly high during the last three months of pregnancy, and cholesterol levels in blood and bile increase during the postpartum period. The normal rate at which the gallbladder is emptied of bile also is slower during the third trimester of pregnancy. This has led to speculation that the high cholesterol levels lead to formation of gallstones. Other studies in animals and humans have implicated birth-control pills and the hormones progesterone and estrogen. A definitive explanation of the gender difference in the disease awaits more research.

There are indications that obese people are more likely to develop gallstones than those of normal weight, although some researchers dispute this contention. Studies to pin down this relationship often have been conflicting. One possibility is that because obese people secrete more cholesterol manufactured by the liver, their bile is more supersaturated with cholesterol than that of normal-weight people. Likewise, there is evidence that an enzyme that promotes cholesterol synthesis, HMG-CoA reductase, is increased when the level of insulin in the blood is increased, a situation that occurs in most obese people. However, studies to probe these likelihoods have been plagued with problems of inadequate sample size, disputed patient selection, and quality of dietary assessment. There remains little concrete evidence that eating a low-cholesterol diet can reduce gallstone formation. Many clinicians, however, have reported evidence that repeated weight losses from dieting followed by weight gains, or a large single weight loss, have led a patient to first begin complaining of the symptoms of gallstones.

Also unresolved are questions about whether a diet high in fiber content reduces the cholesterol saturation of bile and, presumably, the gallstone formation. One study found that gallstones were more prevalent in a group eating significantly less fiber, but the study was flawed because the amount of fiber consumed by patients was not controlled closely enough. Another major study failed to find any relationship between fiber consumption and cholesterol metabolism.

After overnight fasting, bile is lithogenic, or prone to form gallstones. This has led to suggestions that eating a good breakfast rather than skipping it is important, since the meal will cause the gallbladder to empty itself. There also have been suggestions that eating frequent meals might help prevent gallstone formation, since such a dietary habit would empty the gallbladder often. Such findings are far from clear-cut, however, and there is disagreement about the overall benefits.

Treatment of Gallbladder Disease

For years, patients suffering from gallbladder disease were instructed to eat low-fat diets because it was thought that by reducing dietary fat the gallbladder would be called upon for less bile and this would provide relief from the symptoms of the gallstones. This practice has now largely been abandoned because there is little evidence that restricting fat in the diet when gallstones are causing discomfort has a significant effect. Patients who have gallbladder disease and say they cannot tolerate fatty meals show no symptoms when

they eat foods in which the fat has been disguised. This suggests a psychological factor: If patients think they receive less fat, they may feel fewer symptoms. On the other hand, some patients with gallstones do experience discomfort when they eat certain foods. As a result, patients are generally advised to be the judge and avoid any foods that produce digestive problems, but otherwise to eat a normal diet. A further consideration is that eating a fatty meal from time to time empties the gallbladder, which some studies indicate could have a beneficial effect. In the end, it is a matter of trial and error for each person.

The standard treatment for persistent gallbladder disease is surgical removal of the gallbladder. The procedure is associated with the risks accompanying any abdominal surgery performed under general anesthesia. Afterward, however, there is no need to follow any dietary restrictions, since the liver continues to manufacture bile and this steady bile synthesis is sufficient to handle a normal diet. However, gallbladder removal does not provide complete relief of discomfort in all patients. Intermittent abdominal pain and upset may continue for reasons that are unclear.

In recent years, there has been some success treating gallbladder disease with chenodeoxycholic acid. In many cases, this bile acid can dissolve the gallstones, although it has side effects—including diarrhea—at the rather large dosage needed. Ursodeoxycholic acid, a chemical cousin, also has been used with success to dissolve cholesterol gallstones. The long-term toxicity of these drugs is unknown. In the United States, they are generally used in patients when surgery is deemed risky. Use of the drugs does not appear to solve the problem permanently, since gallstones can reappear after the drug's use has been discontinued, requiring readministration of the drug. Shock wave therapy (lithotripsy) is also used.

32

Nutrition and Kidney Disease

Sheldon Glabman, M.D.

■

INTRODUCTION

The kidneys function as master chemists, constantly assessing the body's internal environment and preserving a proper biochemical balance. They maintain fluid, electrolyte, and acid-base balance and rid the body of waste products that result as the cells use the energy produced by ingested food. The kidneys also perform other critical functions. They are the central organs in a series of complex hormonal systems that regulate blood pressure by secreting one hormone and responding to the presence of another. They are involved in the production of red blood cells and play an essential role in the reabsorption and metabolism of several minerals.

Diseases of the kidney and the urinary tract are the fourth largest health problem in the United States, the leading cause of work loss among women and the second largest cause of work loss among men under age 25. Nearly 10 million people have kidney or urinary-tract disease; another 3.5 million people are thought to have urinary tract problems of which they are unaware. In addition, childhood nephrosis, a condition in which protein is lost in the urine, resulting in swelling of the body, strikes 4,000 preschool children each year.

Long-term high blood pressure, which damages the kidney's filtering units and blood vessels, is one of the most common causes of renal failure, in which the kidneys cease to function entirely. Other causes include diabetes, infection, and trauma—for example, a major burn, complicated surgery, a serious injury in an automobile accident, or exposure to a substance toxic to the kidneys. This sudden failure of the kidneys, usually reversible, may require temporary dialysis. More serious than sudden failure, in a long-term sense, is the gradual deterioration of the kidneys. They function less and less efficiently and eventually fail, leading to serious problems that finally require long-term dialysis or kidney transplantation.

Whatever the cause, when the kidneys cease to function normally, the body's biochemical equilibrium is thrown off balance. If the malfunctioning progresses, serious consequences develop. In few other body systems does proper nutrition play such an important role as in the presence of kidney disease. The proper diet when the kidneys are malfunctioning can mean the difference between leading a relatively normal life and continuing down a road in which kidney disease inevitably worsens and necessitates renal-replacement therapy.

HOW THE KIDNEYS WORK

The body has two kidneys, which are small, reddish brown, bean-shaped organs the size of a man's fist. One kidney is located on each side of the spinal column behind the abdomen and below the last rib, and each weighs about one-quarter of a pound. This redundancy could be an indication of how important the kidneys are to overall health, since so much capacity allows for a large loss of kidney function, including the removal of an entire kidney, without any untoward consequences. Up to 90 percent of the kidneys' ability to function can fail with the kidney disease patient still maintaining reasonable health, provided he or she follows certain dietary rules.

The central unit of the kidney is the nephron; each kidney has about a million nephrons. They are sophisticated filters that each day filter three times the body's weight in water, salts, and other substances. Each nephron consists of a cup-shaped structure called a Bowman's capsule. This encloses a tuft of tiny blood vessels, called the glomerulus, and an attached tube, called the tubule. If the tubules in one kidney were placed end to end, they would make a 35-mile-long chain.

The kidneys process about 18 gallons of blood every hour, 24 hours a day, as the heart continues to beat. The blood carries nutrients that have been processed and prepared by the digestive system for the body's cells to burn as energy, as well as carrying waste products from energy production. The blood is pumped through the nephrons, and the kidney, per-

forming its chemical functions, filters out a small part of the substance it encounters, concentrates it, and then sends it to the bladder to be expelled from the body as urine. However, the vast majority of the substances that pass through the filters return to the blood and then to the body for further utilization.

The kidneys' regulatory functions involve a number of substances, such as sodium, potassium, vitamin D, calcium, phosphorus, and metabolic waste products. The kidneys control total water volume in the body and thus help to regulate blood pressure. Remarkably sensitive to the body's minute-by-minute needs, the kidneys can adjust quickly to changing demands. For example, the nephrons filter out two and a half pounds of table salt, or sodium chloride, each day, returning all but two to four ounces to the blood. However, the kidneys immediately detect a change in the level of salt intake and adjust the level of salt or water excretion or retention to maintain the correct saline level within the blood and cells.

Figure 32.1. The Kidneys

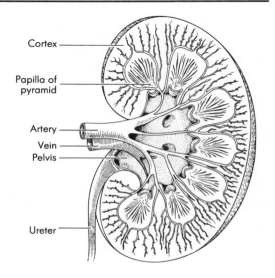

Cortex

Papilla of pyramid

Artery

Vein

Pelvis

Ureter

Maintenance of Fluid and Electrolyte Balance

A fundamental task of the kidneys is to regulate total water volume and the balance of acidity and alkalinity. Each day, the metabolic activity of the body produces an excess of metabolic products that are acidic in nature. Some of the acid can become gaseous and is excreted through the lungs. The rest is processed by the kidneys and sent in the urine to the bladder. This accounts for the fact that urine, particularly of people in Western cultures, whose diet is rich in protein, is acidic. Some of the acid is in the form of phosphates, some consists of organic acids such as citrate, the rest is ammonium.

The acidity-alkalinity relationship is a teeter-totter that can move up and down according to the body's activities. Heavy exercise, for example, increases acid. Acid levels can build up in some diabetics. Bicarbonate in the blood buffers the acid, and the kidneys, along with the lungs, control this relationship to maintain the proper balance.

The kidneys are responsible for eliminating the nitrogen-containing wastes that result from the cells' utilization of the amino acids. This nitrogen appears principally as urea. About 70 percent of the nitrogen leaves the body in the urine, the rest in the feces and through the skin.

Urine is formed in a three-step sequence consisting of filtration, selective reabsorption, and secretion. In this process, between 150 and 200 quarts of fluid are filtered through the glomeruli of the kidneys each day. The kidneys, relying on various hormonal signals, filter out to the urine only about 1 percent of this volume, depending on the body's needs. The rest is returned to the blood through selective reabsorption.

In the first step, blood is filtered through the glomeruli, leaving behind red and white blood cells, platelets, and plasma with proteins. The remaining fluid, which is similar to plasma without proteins, contains glucose, amino acids, salts, urea, uric acid, and creatinine. In the selective reabsorption process, almost all the glucose is returned to the blood. Other substances, such as salts, are returned depending on the body's needs.

The rest—urea, uric acid, creatinine, some sodium, potassium, phosphate, sulfate, and other waste products—become part of the urine, which usually consists of 90 to 95 percent water.

Overall water content of the body is controlled in part by the hormone vasopressin, which is secreted by the pituitary gland but acts upon the kidneys as the body's water content fluctuates. Vasopressin, also known as antidiuretic (anti-urinating) hormone or ADH, causes the kidneys to conserve water and send less out in the urine if water is in short supply. If water volume is high, vasopressin production is inhibited, and the kidneys send large volumes of water to the urine. In an abnormality of the pituitary gland in which vasopressin is in short supply, a person may excrete as much as two or three gallons of water a day and drink an equivalent amount to compensate. Alcohol inhibits the release of vasopressin, which explains the frequent urination while drinking and the subsequent dehydration and thirst the morning after substantial alcohol ingestion.

Aldosterone, a hormone secreted by the adrenal cortex, regulates the kidneys' retention and excretion of sodium and potassium. If the body is deprived of sodium, the kidneys drastically reduce excretion of sodium. If high levels of sodium are present, aldosterone concentrations shift and cause the kidney to excrete much larger amounts of sodium. The mechanism for controlling potassium balance is similar.

Even a slight disturbance of the delicate

balance between the supply of aldosterone and the functioning of the kidneys can upset either sodium or potassium balance and have severe consequences. Blood pressure can increase if the kidneys are unable to finely regulate sodium and water excretion. If this high blood pressure is sustained, it can damage the kidneys. The risk of stroke increases and there is some evidence that arteriosclerosis, or hardening of the arteries, is hastened. Too little sodium can produce weight loss, low blood pressure, dizziness, weakness, and impairment of kidney function.

Upsets in potassium balance also can lead to difficulties. Too much potassium can produce heart arrhythmias, and, if levels rise even higher, cardiac arrest may result. This is a rare problem that is sometimes encountered in advanced kidney disease. On the other hand, too little potassium can also cause arrhythmias as well as profound muscle weakness.

The maintenance of water, sodium, and potassium balances in the body on a minute-by-minute basis proceeds hand in glove with the kidneys' equally essential task of removing waste products from the blood and sending them to the urine. The normal activities of all cells, in which carbohydrates, fats, and proteins are broken down and then consumed as fuel to provide energy, produce waste products. If these waste products are not removed, chemical equilibrium can rapidly be disturbed.

The kidneys are critical organs in the body's complex protein-metabolism system. Protein is composed of two types of amino acids, the essential and the nonessential. The essential amino acids, of which there are nine, are called essential because they cannot be manufactured by the body and must be obtained from food. Since humans are animals, animal protein has the best balance of essential amino acids. Meat, eggs, and milk contain adequate amounts of all the nine essential amino acids, which makes these foods high-quality, or high-biological-value, protein sources. The nonessential amino acids can be manufactured by the body.

The kidneys also are a veritable hormone factory, secreting hormonal agents that are essential in several of the body's biochemical systems. For example, the kidneys help control blood pressure through a hormonal system—the RAA system—that involves renin and two other hormones, aldosterone and angiotensin.

When the healthy body needs an increase in blood pressure, the kidneys synthesize renin and secrete it to activate the RAA system. This happens in the blood when the renin encounters angiotensinogen, a hormone secreted by the liver. Through a complex series of steps, angiotensinogen becomes angiotensin. Then another agent, angiotensin-converting enzyme, known as ACE, converts angiotensin I to angiotensin II.

The angiotensin II is believed to have two effects. It causes the blood vessels to constrict, which requires higher blood pressure to pass the same volume through the cardiovascular system. It also causes the adrenal glands to secrete additional aldosterone, which reduces sodium loss through the kidneys and increases the body's water volume. This salt retention has the effect of forcing more fluid through the fixed volume of the cardiovascular system, thus causing a rise in blood pressure in a different manner. An adequate increase in pressure triggers a decrease in the renin supply.

When the kidneys malfunction, too much renin may be secreted, and result in high blood pressure. This is known as secondary hypertension.

Primary hypertension, which is high blood pressure *not* caused by abnormal kidney function, can sometimes be controlled by giving drugs that block the RAA system.

Another hormonal system involving the kidneys regulates the production of red blood cells, which are essential for carrying oxygen throughout the body. Through a complex system of hormonal messenger chemicals, possibly in response to a reduced supply of oxygen to the kidneys, the kidneys secrete erythropoietin factor, which then interacts with cells in the bone marrow to stimulate the release of additional blood cells from the bone marrow, where blood is manufactured. These cells become mature red blood cells. The additional oxygen-carrying cells presumably increase the oxygen supply to the kidneys, which, in turn, decreases the call for formation of more red blood cells—a classic example of a biofeedback control system.

Finally, the kidneys are also involved in the body's use of calcium and phosphorus, which are essential for strong, healthy bones. The balance of calcium and phosphorus in the blood functions like a seesaw. If phosphorus levels rise, calcium levels fall. When calcium is low, release of parathyroid hormone results, causing the release of calcium from the bones and increasing the excretion of phosphorus in the urine.

KIDNEY DISEASE

Causes

Considering the wide variety of activities in which the kidneys are involved in the biochemical and hormonal systems, it is not surprising that their malfunction can quickly have a dramatic impact. A number of conditions can impair kidney function.

Inflammation of the kidneys or the glomerular capillaries is one cause of renal disease. *Nephritis* is the general term used for inflammation of the kidney. Inflammation of the glomerulus is known as glomerulonephritis.

Hypertension or arteriosclerosis can eventually damage the renal vasculature, impairing blood flow in the kidneys. Such restricted blood flow and the resulting kidney disease is one of the major long-term consequences of high blood pressure. In this condition, fibrous tissue builds up in the vasculature of the kidneys and the capillary tufts of the glomeruli. Left untreated, hypertension may rapidly lead to renal disease and eventual kidney failure. Arteriosclerosis, or hardening of the blood vessels, can be a consequence of progressive cardiovascular disease, the same process that can cause stroke or heart attack. Fatty deposits build up on the walls of the renal artery, decreasing blood flow and reducing kidney function. The narrowing of the renal arteries can also cause hypertension by leading to renin release.

Kidney disease is also a consequence of diabetes, since in advanced cases capillaries in many parts of the body thicken and reduce blood flow.

Glomerulonephritis, diabetes, infections, blockage of the renal vein, and other associated disorders can lead to a condition called nephrotic syndrome. This is not a disease but a group of symptoms that results when the kidneys begin to pass excessive amounts of protein, particularly albumin, to the urine. Edema often develops, and patients are prone to infections. The levels of fats in the blood can rise substantially.

Other causes of renal disease, particularly for an older person, include conditions outside the kidneys that restrict blood flow to them, an enlarged prostate or tumor of the kidney pelvis that obstructs the passage of urine to the bladder, substances that directly poison the kidneys, such as some drugs and chemicals, and complications following surgery. Long-term use of massive dosages of analgesics, such as phenacetin, can lead to kidney damage. Several types of industrial solvents when either inhaled or swallowed can damage the kidneys. Inhaling the fumes of carbon tetrachloride can cause damage. Wood alcohol, toluene, ethylene glycol, and naphthalene can be toxic to the kidneys. Consuming excessive amounts of vitamin D also can harm them.

The process of aging itself is one of the most common causes of renal disease. From the onset of middle age, kidney capacity steadily declines. By age 80, the total number of nephrons has markedly decreased, the flow of blood to the kidneys has dropped considerably and the kidneys' ability to respond quickly to changes in blood chemistry has substantially diminished. An older person will have normal body chemistry unless he or she indulges in excesses: drinking too much or too little liquid, eating too much or too little food.

Because the body starts out with so much extra kidney capacity, diminished function as a person ages does not necessarily cause problems. There are few signs of the overall diminished kidney capacity. Some other, sudden insult to the kidneys can lead quickly to kidney malfunction, however, because of the diminished total number of nephrons; that is, the diminished reserve capacity.

The precise cause of this reduction in renal capacity with age isn't understood, but recent studies suggest that eating too much protein over the course of a lifetime may play a role. Some experts now believe that excess protein consumption provokes a hyperfiltration situation, in which excess or standby glomeruli are pressed into service to handle the increased load of metabolic by-products of the protein degradation by the cells. Repeated episodes of hyperfiltration may lead to glomerular sclerosis, or death of nephrons. For a person in good health, this poses no problem. If renal disease occurs, however, the burden can be compounded abruptly.

What Happens in Kidney Disease

When a significant number of the kidneys' 2 million nephrons become impaired, those that remain work harder to compensate. The remaining nephrons enlarge and are so efficient at continuing to manage the body's chemistry that up to 80 to 90 percent of the total number can be destroyed before renal function is seriously impaired and clear symptoms of renal failure appear.

The extent of nephron damage and renal insufficiency can be assessed through several measures, including the glomerular filtration rate, known as GFR, the blood urea nitrogen level, known as BUN, and the amount of creatinine in the blood. The GFR reflects the volume of fluid passed through the kidneys. The normal amount is 100 to 120 milliliters per minute. The symptoms of renal disease may not appear until the GFR has dropped to one-fifth the norm. Normal BUN is 5 to 25 milligrams per deciliter of blood and can rise above 100 milligrams per deciliter in the patient with renal disease. Normal creatinine levels are 0.7 to 1.4 milligrams per deciliter. The value in the renal patient varies widely, from slightly to greatly above normal.

The first stage of impending renal disease is called diminished renal reserve. The patient has no symptoms; only careful testing can detect the lessened renal capacity, which presages approaching difficulties. The test results are frequently subject to conflicting interpretation.

When kidney function fails further, the next stage, renal insufficiency, appears and the first signs of azotemia can be detected. Azotemia is a slight buildup of the nitrogen-containing waste products resulting from the cells' use of amino acids. The levels of urea, nitrogen, and creatinine in the blood may be slightly elevated at this stage. Physical symptoms may be vague. Nocturia, excessive urination during the night, may develop, an indication that the kidneys are unable to form a concentrated urine. There may be occasional swelling or edema of the legs, a mild anemia, and slight elevation in blood pressure.

As the situation worsens and the glomerular filtration rate falls and the blood urea nitrogen and creatinine values rise, the unmistakable signs of uremia appear. Lassitude, fatigue, and decreased mental alertness are the first signs of uremia. Itching and twitching movements of the limbs, particularly the legs, can develop. Worsening uremia produces an array of symptoms in virtually every body system. Symptoms can include headaches, nausea, weight loss, vomiting, and an unpleasant taste in the mouth.

The kidneys' role in various hormonal and chemical systems is disrupted. Phosphorus levels in the blood increase because of inefficient excretion in the urine. This causes calcium levels to decrease. Low calcium levels trigger release of parathyroid hormone, which works to rid the body of phosphorus and increase calcium. As renal failure worsens, however, more and more parathyroid hormone is needed, until it eventually fails to elicit a response. Calcium phosphate deposits can appear in the skin and in the joints, causing joint pain. Since calcium from the diet is not handled properly, the body may turn to the bones themselves for calcium, leading to weakening and then destruction of the bones, which may fracture. Long-term kidney failure in children can lead to growth retardation. Disturbed calcium metabolism also can manifest itself in altered absorption of nutrients in the intestines. Sodium and potassium are thrown out of equilibrium. Potassium excretion is reduced, which could, in rare instances, lead to potassium overload and cause heart arrhythmias. Retention of sodium causes edema and worsening high blood pressure. Secretion of erythropoietin is al-

tered, leading to anemia. Gastrointestinal ulcers develop; the resultant bleeding can cause iron-deficiency anemia. This is exaggerated by abnormal platelet function, impairing clotting.

Renal failure is usually a progressive disease in which kidney function declines steadily, sometimes over a period of several years. Eventually, renal insufficiency is so marked that the kidneys perform at less than 10 percent of normal. This situation, known as end-stage renal disease, requires that the patient begin receiving dialysis treatments or have a transplant. In hemodialysis, an artificial kidney machine cleanses the blood of waste products several times a week. A catheter attached to a blood vessel in the lower arm shunts blood into the device and then back into the body. An alternative for some patients is continuous ambulatory peritoneal dialysis, in which a catheter is inserted into the abdominal cavity and fluid in a portable plastic container is run into the abdomen and then back out again, removing excess wastes, fluids, and electrolytes. Continuous ambulatory peritoneal dialysis has the advantage of being machine-free and performed four to five times a day at home, allowing the patient to continue normal activities during the treatment. There also is a type of ambulatory dialysis that is done at home while the patient sleeps; this is called continuous cycling peritoneal dialysis.

Once the renal patient requires dialysis, only a kidney transplant will end the need for a lifetime of dialysis treatments. Transplants have become increasingly successful in recent years, provided a kidney from a genetically similar donor can be found. The best results are obtained when the kidney comes from a close family member, although matches can also be found outside the family circle. If the transplanted kidney is not rejected and functions normally, its capacity is usually sufficient to handle the body's needs and return the recipient to good health, although it may be necessary to take anti-transplant rejection drugs for some time. Some kidney-transplant recipients are leading relatively normal lives with a kidney received over ten years ago.

The Role of Nutrition in Kidney Disease

Nutrition plays an important role in the medical care of patients with kidney disease. The progression and severity of the symptoms of kidney disease can be decreased by the management of certain nutrients in the diet. As noted in previous chapters, the dietary recommendations for healthy Americans call for 55 percent or more calories to come from carbohydrates, with emphasis on starches; 12 to 15 percent of calories from protein; and less than 30 percent of calories from fats, mainly unsaturated. Cholesterol intake should be less than 300 milligrams per day.

In general, the person with chronic renal failure who is not being treated with dialysis should follow these guidelines, with the exception that the protein intake will be lower and the calorie intake can be maintained by increased carbohydrate intake. The same recommendations are for kidney patients who also have diabetes, except that food intake must be balanced with insulin action to maintain good blood-glucose control.

The objectives of dietary management in kidney disease are the following:

1. To achieve and maintain desirable body weight.

2. To correct signs and symptoms of under-nutrition.

3. To decrease the workload of the diseased kidney.

4. To prevent fluid and electrolyte disturbances (potassium, sodium, and phosphate).

5. To prevent uremia, which is the rise of blood urea nitrogen concentration.

To achieve these objectives, it is necessary to control the amount of protein eaten; to balance fluid intake with the amount lost in urine, perspiration, and so forth; and to regulate the foods high in potassium, sodium, and phosphate. At the same time, it is important to make sure that adequate calories are consumed, because a diet that has sufficient calories will help maintain nitrogen balance and what protein is consumed will be spared to maintain body tissues and replenish the protein stores. If the diet does not provide adequate calories, the protein will be used up to provide energy. (In general, the kidney patient should consume about 16 calories per pound of desirable body weight.)

The nutritional needs of people with chronic renal failure who are not being treated with dialysis therapy are different from the patients who are on continuous ambulatory peritoneal dialysis. Therefore, the dietary management is tailored to each patient's needs by a registered dietitian with the participation of patients and their family members.

Dietary Management in Chronic Kidney Failure

Patients who have chronic kidney failure that is not severe enough to require dialysis treatment have a combination of nutrition-related problems. These patients develop azotemia and uremia and, in the advanced stage of renal failure, the absorption, excretion, and metabolism of several important nutrients is affected, thereby causing undernutrition and wasting. Therefore, while attempting to decrease the production of toxins that damage the kidney and to stop or slow down the progression of renal failure, it is of utmost importance to maintain good nutritional status.

Urea production results when the dietary protein is broken down. The quantity of protein-containing foods recommended would depend on the glomerular filtration rate.

The protein foods that are selected by the patient should be of good quantity. They should provide complete proteins containing the essential amino acids in the right amounts to replenish the body's stores of protein. Animal-protein foods like low-fat milk and cheese, egg whites, fish and other seafood, lean, trimmed meats, chicken and turkey without skin are better in quality than plant proteins, with the exception of soybean curd (tofu). These proteins are also referred to as being of high biological value. Plant foods like legumes, grains, and vegetables contribute protein of lower biological value because they are incomplete (they are deficient in one or more of the essential amino acids). This does not mean, however, that the diet should not include bread, rice, or vegetables. These foods can be included according to the doctor's diet prescription.

High-protein foods that are low in saturated fats and cholesterol are recommended because a large number of people with chronic kidney disease, including those treated with dialysis, have high levels of blood cholesterol and triglycerides (another lipid that circulates in the blood). Good choices would include small amounts of shellfish, fish, skinless chicken and turkey, nonfat (skim) or 1 percent-fat milk, and egg whites. Red meats are generally high in saturated fats; the yolk in whole eggs also is high in saturated fat and cholesterol. In contrast, egg whites do not have fat; they are pure protein of high biological value. One ounce of lean poultry, meat,

or fish has seven grams of protein. Nine medium shrimp have the same amount of protein but have much less fat than poultry or meat.

Sodium and potassium. These two important electrolytes are measured in the blood and urine to determine how much the patient should obtain from his or her diet. For example, the amount of sodium that will be recommended depends on body weight, blood pressure, and levels of serum creatinine and the amount of sodium in the urine excreted over a 24-hour period. In the patients with chronic renal failure, sodium also is restricted to varying levels when there is edema and increased blood pressure. (See Chapter 8 for specific tips on reducing sodium intake.)

Potassium is restricted when the levels of potassium in the blood are too high, a condition called hyperkalemia. Many foods, with the exception of fats and sugars, contain varying amounts of potassium. The amount of potassium in vegetables can be decreased by cooking them in large amounts of water and then discarding the water.

Fluids. Fluid intake for the person with chronic renal failure should balance the body's output or loss. In addition to urine, this output includes water used by the gastrointestinal tract and water lost from the lungs and skin, which can amount to as much as two and a half cups (20 ounces) a day.

Phosphorus and calcium. Intakes of these two minerals are also important to monitor in kidney patients. When the level of phosphorus rises, the level of calcium falls. It is difficult to increase calcium intake from foods without increasing the intake of phosphorus. Therefore, patients are given with each meal daily supplements of 500 milligrams of calcium—a total of 1,500 milligrams of calcium to ensure adequate intake. Several foods that are high in protein and potassium are also high in phosphorus; thus, when the meat and dairy intake is reduced to lower protein intake, the phosphorus intake is also lowered. In addition to a low-phosphorus diet, phosphate binders, which prevent absorption of the minerals, may be used.

Other nutrients. Intake of other essential nutrients, such as vitamins B and C and folic-acid intake, is decreased in the diets of patients with chronic renal failure. Therefore, the physician will recommend that the patient takes these supplements daily. It is not necessary to take supplements of fat-soluble vitamins A, E, and K. Small amounts of vitamin D may also be recommended to help correct the abnormal calcium metabolism.

Nutritional Needs of Patients Treated with Dialysis

Protein intake. Dialysis treatment causes losses of protein and amino acids. Therefore, while maintaining energy needs, the protein intake for patients on hemodialysis must be increased to provide 0.45 to 0.55 grams per pound of body weight per day. For example, if the patients weighs 140 pounds, he/she will need 63 grams to 94 grams of protein per day. Patients being treated with continuous ambulatory peritoneal dialysis may need even more protein: 0.55 to 0.65 grams per pound of body weight.

Sodium and fluid. Generally, sodium and fluid intake are restricted. A patient on hemodialysis usually tolerates less sodium and fluid intake than a patient treated with continuous ambulatory peritoneal dialysis, but this is determined according to the individual patient. In a sodium-restricted diet, it is important to look for hidden sources of sodium. Remember, all foods and drinking water have varying amounts of natural sodium. Food processing that includes salt increases sodium intake.

Potassium. The potassium intake of most dialysis patients is restricted. It is difficult to make the right food choices for these patients because their protein intake is not as restricted as for a person with chronic renal failure who is not being treated with dialysis; the potassium content of several foods is related to their protein content. Some vegetables and fruits, such as citrus fruits, tomatoes, potatoes, and beverages such as coffee and tea can be restricted to lower the intake of potassium.

Phosphorus. It is important to maintain the normal level of serum phosphorus and not to let it get too high. To prevent this, foods high in phosphorus may be limited (see list below), but usually phosphate binders are also needed to control the serum-phosphorus level.

Calcium. Supplements of calcium carbonate (1,000 to 1,500 milligrams a day) are given to ensure adequate calcium intake for dialysis patients. Calcium also serves as a phosphate binder, thus helping control phosphorus levels.

Vitamins. Supplements of vitamins B_6, C, and folic acid are prescribed for all dialysis patients in RDA amounts. More C can harm.

Foods High in Phosphorus

Almonds	Peas, dried
Apricots	Phosphates in
Brazil nuts	processed foods
Cheese	and soft drinks
Eggs	Poultry
Fish	Pumpkin seeds
Meat	Sesame seeds
Milk	Soybean nuts
Milk products	Sunflower seeds
Peanuts	Walnuts

Tips to Meet Your Diet Prescription

The diet prescription that calls for 50 grams of protein, 2 grams sodium, and 2 grams potassium a day can still include favorite recipes. These recipes may need to be modified to meet your dietary prescription, however. Here are some general rules to follow in modifying recipes.

1. Recognize all the ingredients and the nutrients that recipes contain. Read food labels and make sure you understand them (see Chapter 40).

2. To reduce protein intake, decrease the amount of animal food in the recipe or make the servings smaller. Due to their high levels of sodium, avoid processed, smoked, and salted protein foods such as cold cuts, frankfurters, sausages, salted cod, and cheese.

3. In addition to choosing low-fat dairy foods, pay attention to the sodium content. For example, low-fat (1 percent-fat) cottage cheese may be preferred for its low-fat content, but remember it has twice as much sodium as regular cottage cheese made with whole milk. One ounce of cheese (cheddar, Swiss, mozzarella, ricotta) contains 150 milligrams of sodium and 40 milligrams of potassium. Cheese is also a rich source of phosphorus.

4. In selecting carbohydrate foods, remember that some complex carbohydrates such as pasta, bread, and beans and other legumes also provide protein, although it is incomplete (or of lower biological value). You can either decrease the quantity used or look for low-protein products. Low protein and pasta may be particularly important to meet the caloric needs of patients who have diabetes mellitus and must restrict simple carbohydrates (sugar).

5. Fruits and beverages contribute carbohydrates and varying amounts of protein and potassium. Choose vegetables and fruits that have less potassium. (See Table 32.1 for nutrient content.) For example, a pasta sauce can be made from onions, green peppers, squash, and herbs instead of tomato sauce, which can give an additional 500 milligrams of potassium for the same serving size.

6. Unsaturated oils such as the oils of olives, corn, safflower, sunflower, or canola are recommended in a cholesterol-lowering diet. Coconut and palm oil are highly saturated and can be found in commercially baked foods, granola, and cream substitutes. These oils need to be eliminated from the diet, as they are potent in raising blood cholesterol. Margarines made entirely from vegetable oils such as safflower, sunflower, corn, or soybean as the first ingredient are high in polyunsaturated fatty acids and may be selected in place of unsaturated oils. Choose skim or 1 percent-fat milk. Exclude milk prepared with chocolate and malt.

7. To reduce phosphorus, sodium, and potassium, eat less of the following: pumpernickel bread, bran muffins, prepared quick breads, pancake and waffle mixes, stuffing mixes, granola-type cereals.

8. There are foods that contain negligible amounts of protein, sodium, and potassium, although they do contribute calories. These are the starches from wheat, rice, and corn; sugar candy such as gumdrops, sour balls, jelly beans, and lollipops; and sugar, honey, and cranberry sauce.

9. Molasses, brown sugar, and commercial chocolate sauces and syrups should be avoided due to their high potassium content.

10. Foods that cannot be prepared with salt or tomato-containing sauces can be made interesting by using a whole variety of herbs, spices, and flavors, such as basil, chili powder, chives, cinnamon, curry powder, dill, garlic (fresh and powdered), ginger (fresh and powdered), lemon juice, mint, mustard, nutmeg, onion powder, oregano, paprika, pepper, and almond, lemon, peppermint, and vanilla extracts.

Table 32.1. Specific Nutrient Content of Selected Foods

Food Group	Amount	Protein (gm.)	Potassium (mg.)	Sodium (mg.)	Phosphorus (mg.)	Calories
MILK						
Skim	4 oz.	4.0	200	65	120	45
1% fat	4 oz.	4.0	190	65	120	60
MEAT AND OTHER PROTEIN FOODS						
Lean meat, poultry without skin, fish	1 oz.	7.0	100	30	70	55
Egg (medium)	1	6.0	62	59	50	78
Egg whites	2	6.4	86	90	10	32
Shrimp (medium)	10	7.7	39	45	84	37
Cottage cheese (1% fat)	2 oz.	7.0	48	229	75	40
BREADS, GRAINS						
Whole wheat	1 slice; 4 oz.	2.0	35	120	30	60
CEREALS						
Oatmeal	¾ C	4.5	100	NA	15	110
VEGETABLES						
Group A*	4 oz.	1.5	110	10	40	30
Group B*	4 oz.	1.5	200	25	40	30
FRUITS AND JUICES						
Group A†	4 oz.	0.5	100	5	20	60
Group B†	4 oz.	0.5	200	5	20	60
FATS AND OILS						
Margarine	1 t	NA	NA	50 (reg.)	NA	45
Corn oil, olive oil	1 t	NA	NA	NA	NA	45
BEVERAGES						
Coffee						
Brewed	4 oz.	NA	NA	44	2	NA
Instant	1 t	NA	NA	44	2	NA
Tea						
Brewed	4 oz.	NA	44	2	NA	NA
Instant	1 t	NA	NA	44	2	NA
Soda						
Regular	4 oz.	NA	2	7	NA	50
Diet	4 oz.	NA	4	15	NA	NA

*Vegetables are divided into 2 groups: A and B.

Group A vegetables include cooked eggplant, alfalfa sprouts, mung-bean sprouts, mushrooms, corn, cabbage (all kinds), watercress, lettuce (iceberg and romaine), sweet peppers, white turnips, water chestnuts, wax beans, and onions.

Group B vegetables include asparagus, beets, cooked carrots, cauliflower, celery, cucumbers, green peppers, greens (like kale, mustard greens, collard greens, turnip greens), zucchini or yellow squash, sweet potato (fresh, boiled without skin), white potato (boiled without skin), tomato (1 small).

Vegetables such as artichokes, brussels sprouts, parsnips, raw carrots and juice, peas (fresh and dried), spinach, okra, canned sweet potato, tomato sauce, juice of tomatoes, and V-8 juice have large amounts of potassium and may need to be omitted.

†Fruits are divided into 2 groups: A and B.

Group A includes apple sauce, fresh and frozen blackberries, blueberries, and boysenberries, fresh cherries, grapes, kumquats, canned peas, canned pineapple or 1 slice of fresh, fresh and frozen raspberries and strawberries, tangerines (1), watermelon, juices of apple, apricot, grape, papaya, peach, and pear.

Group B includes small apple, canned cherries, canned figs, fruit cocktail, one-half of a fresh grapefruit, canned grapefruit sections, fresh and canned peaches, fresh pear, fresh and canned plums, fresh and frozen rhubarb, juices of grapefruit, lemon, and pineapple.

Fruits that have large amounts of potassium are apricots, avocados, bananas, dried fruit, kiwi, all melons, oranges, and juices of orange, prune, and tomato. These have almost twice as much potassium as group B fruits.

Iron. Iron supplements are prescribed for patients who are iron-deficient and develop anemia.

All patients with renal failure should be seen by a registered dietitian regularly so that they can have meals tailored to their individual eating style.

Kidney Stones and Urinary-Tract Infections

Kidney Stones

Stones, or calculi, that form in the kidney or the tract leading to the bladder are responsible for more than 1 percent of all hospitalizations in the United States. The condition can be very painful and the loss of productivity and workdays is thought to be even greater than the percentage of hospitalizations implies. An estimated 12 to 14 percent of men and 5 percent of women will have suffered at least one episode of kidney-stone pain by the time they reach 70. Few other common diseases have as close a link between cause and successful treatment with nutritional considerations.

Kidney stones develop in four different compositions: calcium stones (oxalate or phosphate), uric acid, cystine, and magnesium ammonium phosphate. These latter are also known as struvite or triple-phosphate stones. The cystine stones form only in patients with inborn errors of metabolism. About 90 percent of all stones are of the calcium oxalate or calcium phosphate variety. All four types are virtually insoluble in urine.

When the concentration of any of these compounds in the urine is high, crystals form and then grow larger. The stones generally pass from the kidney into the ureter, where they may become lodged. The pain can be excruciating, occurring in the lower back and spreading to the thigh and groin. After a period of time, stones generally pass from the body in the urine, but in some cases they become lodged in the urinary tract and must be removed, either by breaking them up with sound waves (lithotripsy) or, if this technique is not available, surgically. Stones in the ureter sometimes restrict the flow of urine and irritate the tissues, causing kidney infection and blood in the urine.

The circumstances that can lead to the formation of kidney stones have been intensively studied, but the reasons for their formation and how to prevent it are still poorly understood. Many people never form kidney stones, while others are likely to have recurring episodes. Stones are prevalent in some regions of the world and virtually unknown in others. One of these "stone belts" exists in the United States, running from the Carolinas to northern Florida and across to Texas.

Nutritional factors are important in dealing with both calcium and uric-acid stones.

Calcium stones. In the past, it was thought that too much calcium in the diet was the cause of the calcium-based stones, which are the most prevalent kind. Dietary calcium was reduced to treat the condition. An increased understanding of the chemistry of calcium utilization in the body has led some scientists to question this concept, however. Instead, research suggests that the balance between calcium and oxalate is involved in some way.

Elevated levels of calcium in the urine, leading to calcium stones, may or may not be associated with elevated levels of calcium in the blood. A number of conditions can lead to elevated levels of calcium in the blood, including hyperparathyroidism, hypervitaminosis D, sarcoidosis, bone tumors, and others. When the diagnosis is established and appropriate therapy rendered, elevated blood calcium and thus the hypercalciuria return to normal.

When the calcium in the blood is not elevated, a high urinary calcium may be a consequence of excess absorption of calcium in the gut from foods. Excess urinary calcium may also be due to a "kidney leak" of calcium. This form of hypercalciuria may be aggravated by a high salt intake. The absorptive type of hypercalciuria is best treated by restricting calcium intake without depending on the high-oxalate foods usually substituted for high-calcium foods. (See page 556 for a list of high-oxalate foods.) Both the renal leak and the absorptive forms of hypercalciuria are best treated by administering a thiazide diuretic, which lowers calcium excretion.

Except in special situations, restricting calcium intake can have a detrimental effect on the body's calcium balance. A calcium-starved body can take calcium from the bones to make up the difference. This can lead to demineralization of the bones and bone disease. Patients prone to form calcium-oxalate stones should not decide on their own to restrict calcium intake sharply, since the reduction could produce long-term damages. Its value in preventing stone formation is also questionable. Overall calcium intake should be reviewed by a physician before one takes any action.

Calcium and oxalate are absorbed from the intestine by the same process. It has been suggested that as calcium levels fall because of dietary calcium restriction, more oxalate passes to the colon, where its absorption makes it available to form renal stones. Conversely, an increase of calcium in the intestine reduces oxalate absorption. This would seem to suggest that people who form calcium-oxalate stones should increase their calcium intake. The picture is believed to be far more complicated than this, however, and most doctors do not recommend increasing calcium consumption to prevent formation of calcium-oxalate stones. It has also been suggested that oxalate may rise after calcium is restricted in the diet simply because the patient switches from high-calcium foods such as milk and cheese to high-oxalate foods such as nuts, chocolate, and fruit juices. Nevertheless, the prevalent thought is that oxalate levels are responsible for stone formation and that foods high in oxalate should be restricted.

Megadoses of vitamin C also promote oxalate kidney stones. Absorbed vitamin C is converted to oxalate and increases the oxalate load on the kidneys. Because the absorbability of vitamin C is limited, excesses tend to be lost in the stool. Unfortunately, some of the unabsorbed vitamin C is also converted to oxalate in the intestine. This oxalate is absorbed and can contribute to oxalate kidney stones.

Another body of recent research has also suggested a relation between high-protein diets and kidney-stone formation. The chemistry involved is under study and the picture is far from clear. One explanation is that excessive protein can increase both calcium and oxalate excretion in the urine, leading to stone formation.

Uric acid stones. These are formed from uric acid, which is the metabolic product of the breakdown of the purine found in protein-containing foods. The acidity of the urine is considered of greater importance in the formation of these stones than the overall uric-acid content of the urine. Persistently acidic urine is a common problem for patients suffering from gout, and people with gout develop uric-acid kidney stones more often than the rest of the population. Certain blood diseases can also cause high uric-acid excretion. Dietary therapy consists of reducing protein intake and avoiding foods high in purine content. Medications might be added to alkalinize the urine or reduce uric-acid production in the body, thus lowering its excretion. (Foods high in purine are listed below).

Struvite or triple-phosphate stones. Such stones are formed when the urinary tract is infected with a bacterium that can chemically split the urea in the urine into constituents that favor formation of these stones. The condition is usually treated with antibiotics to clear up the infection and with other drugs that inhibit the biochemicals that result from the urea splitting. Frequently, struvite stones

Foods High in Oxalate

Vegetables

Baked beans canned in tomato sauce	Mustard greens
	Okra
Beets	Parsley
Carrots	Peppers, green
Celery	Rutabagas
Chard, Swiss	Sorrel
Chives	Spinach
Collards	Summer squash
Dandelion greens	Sweet potatoes
Eggplant	Tomatoes
Escarole	Turnips
Green beans	Watercress
Leeks	

Fruits

Blackberries	Lemon peel
Blueberries	Lime peel
Cranberries	Orange peel
Currants	Oranges
Dewberries	Plums
Figs	Prunes
Fruit cocktail	Raspberries
Gooseberries	Rhubarb
Grapefruit	Strawberries
Grapes, Concord	Tangerines
Grape juice	

Miscellaneous

Beer	Peanut butter
Chocolate	Pepper (more than 1 t per day)
Cocoa	
Cola drinks	Soybean crackers
Fruit cake	Soybean curd (tofu)
Gelatin	Tea
Grits	Tomato soup
Marmalade	Vegetable soup
Nuts	Wheat germ
Ovaltine	

Foods High in Purine

The following foods contain about 150 to 1,000 milligrams of purine per 100 grams.

Liver	Sardines
Sweetbreads	Fish roe
Brains	Mussels
Kidneys	Gravies
Heart	Broths
Anchovies	Beer
Herring	Wine

The following foods contain moderate amounts of purine, 50 to 150 milligrams per 100 grams, and are usually limited to one serving each day for patients who form uric-acid stones.

Meats	Lentils
Peas	Yeast
Cauliflower	Whole-grain cereals
Beans	Fowl
Asparagus	Fish (except as noted above)
Mushrooms	
Spinach	Other seafoods

The following foods contain negligible amounts of purine and are not subject to dietary limitation.

Vegetables, except as noted above	Refined cereals and cereal products
Fruits	Butter and fats in moderation
Milk	
Cheese	Sugar and sweets
Eggs	Clear vegetable soups
Spices and condiments, including salt and vinegar	Nuts

must be removed surgically. When doctors attempt to treat the stones nutritionally, they recommend restriction of phosphorus in the diet and calcium in tablet form, or a phosphate binder to reduce intestinal absorbtion of the phosphorus. (See list on page 551.) Such nutritional management has the best result when the patient rigorously adheres to the fairly rigid diet that restricting phosphate requires. As in the case of renal disease, this dietary regime should be undertaken only under a doctor's supervision.

Cystine kidney stones. These are the fourth type. They result when the patient inherits defects in the renal tubular absorption of the amino acids cystine, ornithine, arginine, and lysine. As a result of the inborn defect, concentrations of these amino acids are high and crystallize as stones. The condition is relatively unresponsive to attempts at dietary management.

Whatever type of kidney stone a patient forms or is likely to form, the best and often most effective treatment is to drink large quantities of fluids to increase the total volume of urine. The goal is to void 2,000 milli-liters (two quarts) of urine every 24 hours. The concentration of the chemicals that could precipitate as crystals and aggregate into stones is much lower in highly diluted urine. Studies have found that soldiers stationed in desert areas form kidney stones unless they force their intake of fluids. New joggers sometimes form kidney stones because they don't drink enough water and their urine becomes too concentrated. Some women have been taught that it is unladylike to urinate too often and thus they don't drink enough fluids.

Rather than thinking of glasses of water or other beverages consumed, people prone to formation of kidney stones should focus on total volume of urine voided. Six glasses of water a day for an office worker in the wintertime is sufficient, while the same volume of water during a two-week tropical vacation is inadequate. Only total urine volume is an accurate gauge of whether or not sufficient fluid is being consumed. Average total urine volume is about 1.5 to 2.5 quarts a day. If a normal adult urinates less than a quart a day, he or she may well not be drinking enough fluids.

33

Food Allergies

Stuart H. Young, M.D., and Ellen M. Buchbinder, M.D.

■

INTRODUCTION

Adverse reactions to foods have long been recognized. Hippocrates observed in the fifth century B.C. that a food could cause illness in some people even though others had no adverse reactions. He cautioned the physicians of the day to look for patients with food reactions and advised that these patients should avoid the offending foods. Interestingly, treatment of food allergy today is largely the same as in ancient times—avoidance of the offending food.

Food allergies, like other allergies, can occur at any age. In general, however, such allergies are much more common in infancy. The incidence of food allergy has been estimated at 2 percent in children. As a child grows older, food allergies often change, and an adult may be able to tolerate foods that produced symptoms in infancy. Anyone who has a tendency toward allergy has the potential of developing sensitivity to one or more different foods.

ALLERGIC FOOD REACTION

A food allergy is a type of hypersensitivity reaction that occurs when an individual's immune system reacts in an abnormal way to a protein food or protein-food ingredient.

The Immunologic Basis of Allergic Food Reactions

The immune system is a complex and vitally important network that protects against dangerous invaders such as disease-causing bacteria or viruses. An allergy is a disorder of the immune system causing the body to react to substances that are ordinarily well tolerated and harmless. The word *allergy*, in fact, is from the Greek *allos*, meaning other, and *ergon*, meaning work. The implication is that the body is working in a way other than expected, that the reaction to the stimulus is an inappropriate one.

When foreign substances (called antigens or allergens) enter the body, special proteins called antibodies form. These antibodies bind to the foreign substances to prevent them from circulating freely in the body and causing possible harm to it. Antibodies are also called immunoglobulins, and fall into five different classes: immunoglobulin A (IgA), immunoglobulin D (IgD), immunoglobulin G (IgG), immunoglobulin M (IgM) and immunoglobulin E (IgE). IgE is the primary mediator in an allergic reaction. People who are prone to food allergies may have large amounts of IgE in their bloodstreams and tissues.

An allergic reaction occurs when an allergen enters the body if an IgE antibody specific to that allergen is present. The allergen may be inhaled, penetrate the skin, or, in the case of food, be ingested. It is important to note that each antibody is precisely matched to a particular antigen and is able to interact *only* with that substance. In general, antigens attach to antibodies like a key fitting in a lock. Thus, an IgE antibody against egg-white protein will react only with egg-white protein and not with any other protein. A first exposure to the allergen usually causes production of the IgE antibodies against the specific allergen. These antibodies attach themselves to the surface of two types of cells: mast cells and basophils. When the allergen enters the body again—and it may be months and even years before it happens—the allergen binds to the IgE antibodies located on the surface of the mast cells and basophils. The new combination of the allergen and the antibody signals these cells to release chemicals, such as histamine, that can cause the various unpleasant symptoms of allergy.

Since mast cells and basophils tend to be concentrated primarily in the skin and in the lining of the gastrointestinal and respiratory tracts, many of the symptoms of an allergic reaction affect these organs. Thus, the most common symptoms of food allergy are nausea, vomiting, diarrhea, skin rash, difficulty breathing, itching, swelling, and hives. In severe cases, life-threatening shock, known as anaphylaxis, may occur. (See Symptoms of an Allergic Reaction and Signs of Extreme Sensitivity on page 560.)

Figure 33.1. An Allergic Reaction

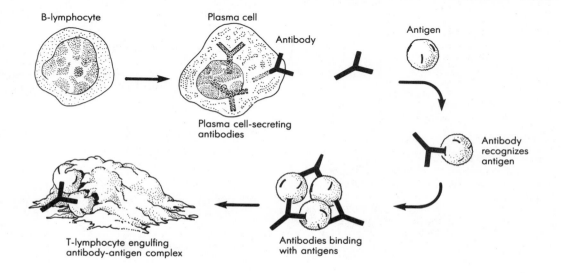

B-lymphocyte

Plasma cell

Antibody

Antigen

Plasma cell-secreting antibodies

Antibody recognizes antigen

T-lymphocyte engulfing antibody-antigen complex

Antibodies binding with antigens

Heredity

The tendency to develop allergy is inherited. A person with allergy is likely to have more first-degree relatives with allergy than might be expected on the basis of chance alone. Studies have shown that a child born to two allergic parents will be more likely to be allergic than a child born to one allergic parent. However, even if only one parent is allergic, the child's likelihood of being allergic is higher than that of the general population.

While the tendency toward allergy is inherited, the type of allergy may vary greatly. Hay fever in a parent does not necessarily predict the same allergy in a child. Nor does the presence of food allergy in a parent mean that the child will be allergic to the same foods.

The appearance of an allergy early in a child's life may suggest, however, that the allergic potential is there and that the child may develop different allergies as he or she grows older.

Immediate and Delayed Reactions

Food-allergy reactions can be categorized according to the length of time it takes for the symptoms to appear. The most common type of food allergy is *immediate*. These reactions happen within two hours of eating the offending food. Typical symptoms may occur within seconds of eating the food; sometimes even smelling the food may set off the allergic reaction.

Delayed food reactions may appear anywhere from several hours to 48 hours after the food has been eaten. In general, the symptoms of a delayed allergic reaction are less se-

---

Symptoms of an Allergic Reaction

Respiratory Symptoms
Rhinitis: a watery discharge from the mucous membrane of the nose
Nasal congestion, sneezing, tearing eyes
Asthma: breathing difficulty, wheezing

Skin Symptoms
Urticaria: hives
Eczema or dermatitis: skin rash
Flushing of the skin

Gastrointestinal Symptoms
Vomiting/nausea
Diarrhea: watery stools, usually with cramping

Other Symptoms
Angio-edema or edema: swelling on the skin and especially around the mouth and inside the throat
Headache
Anaphylactic shock: severe collapse of the respiratory system and blood vessels, which can result in death

---

Signs of Extreme Sensitivity

Extreme sensitivity should be expected if the following produce symptoms:

1. Traces of offending food appearing in other foods because of improper cleaning of utensils or incomplete removal of the offending food from mixtures.

2. Touching utensils that have come in contact with the offending food

3. Kissing the lips of a person who has eaten the offending food

4. Opening of packages containing the offending food

5. Inhalation of vapors from the cooking of the offending food

6. Exposure to food allergens via seminal fluid during intercourse

vere than those of the immediate type. Delayed food reactions may cause eczema, urticaria (hives), and asthma. Delayed food reactions are, by comparison to immediate reactions, more difficult to recognize and much less common. Most people cannot recall in more than very general terms what they had to eat in the one or two days prior to an allergic reaction. The degree of cooking also modifies the allergenicity of the food allergen. A seven-day food and symptom diary—a highly useful tool in the treatment of food allergies in general—can be invaluable to those who suffer from this.

Food-dependent, exercise-induced anaphylaxis. This is a rare phenomenon probably at least partially mediated by IgE. In this syndrome, hives or anaphylaxis, or both, occur when a person exercises directly after eating a specific food or even a whole meal. The foods most often implicated in this syndrome include celery, shrimp and other shellfish, and peaches. (See Eating in Restaurants and Commonsense Dos and Don'ts on page 562.)

NONALLERGIC FOOD REACTIONS

In contrast to the true allergic reactions discussed above, many adverse reactions to food do not involve the IgE-mediated response. These include the following.

Metabolic Abnormalities

Gluten intolerance. In this disease, also known as gluten-sensitive enteropathy, celiac sprue, nontropical sprue, idiopathic sprue, and celiac disease, there is an intolerance to wheat, rye, barley, and probably oat gluten, caused by sensitivity to a portion of the gluten protein called gliadin. Consuming any grain containing gluten results in damage to the lining of the small intestine, markedly decreasing the absorptive surface area and resulting in poor digestion and poor absorption of nutrients. Damage to the small intestine causes diarrhea, steatorrhea (fat in the stool), and nutritional deficiencies. It was once believed that children with celiac sprue would outgrow the disease eventually, but this has proved not to be the case. Children with the disease must be started on a gluten-free diet, which will continue for life. (See Chapter 30 for a more detailed discussion.)

Lactose intolerance. This disease results from the inability to produce an enzyme called lactase, which, in turn, is necessary for the digestion of lactose, a complex natural sugar found in milk. Lactase-deficient individuals become lactose-intolerant and develop symptoms that include gas, bloating, cramps, and/or diarrhea after drinking milk or eating milk products.

Lactase deficiency is generally hereditary. Population groups likely to carry the gene causing the disorder are American Indians, Asians, blacks, Mediterraneans, Ashkenazic Jews, southern and central Europeans, and Central and South Americans. In fact, it is thought that 75 percent of the world's population is lactase-deficient. But lactose intolerance can also occur as a secondary event from a physical condition. Temporary or permanent lactose intolerance sometimes occurs in persons who have had intestinal infection, gastric surgery and other intestinal problems, or who are taking certain medications, particularly antibiotics or some antiinflammatory drugs.

The dietary treatment for lactose intolerance is some degree of a lactose-reduced diet, depending on the severity of the symptoms. For the highly lactose intolerant, the diet must be strictly lactose-free. Since milk and other dairy products provide 70 to 75 percent of the dietary calcium supply, the elimination of these foods can have severe health implications. Many lactose-intolerant people can handle four to six ounces of milk, chocolate milk, ice cream, or yogurt at one sitting, but more produces symptoms. The lactose content of cheese and yogurt is low. Many health-food stores sell lactose enzymes (Lact Aid, etc.) that can be eaten with milk or added to milk to predigest lactose. Combining milk with other foods will reduce the concentration of lactose that reaches the intestine, and heating milk is sometimes advisable, since milk in that form seems to be better tolerated. Special low-lactose dairy products are now available in supermarkets in most areas. Lactose-intolerant individuals should also be aware that thousands of medications have added lactose as a "carrier."

Anaphylactoid Reactions

Some reactions mimic true anaphylaxis (an immediate severe hypersensitivity reaction) but subsequent laboratory tests fail to show evidence of an allergic reaction involving IgE, nor do they require a prior exposure to the substance. These responses are termed anaphylactoid because they resemble anaphy-

---

Eating in Restaurants

People with food allergies can safely dine out given the following guidelines:

1. Avoid ordering mixed foods, processed foods, and foods that might be prepared with a potential allergen. Order plain broiled meats, baked potatoes or rice, and steamed vegetables.

2. Ask what ingredients are in the foods you wish to order. If the waitress or waiter does not know, ask to see the chef.

3. Call beforehand to ask whether food can be specially prepared. Explain that you are allergic to certain foods; state them.

4. Do not try to remove allergenic ingredients from a mixed dish; even though the visible ingredients are gone, the entire dish is probably contaminated. Reorder a plain food.

5. Take substitutes with you, such as rice wafers as a bread substitute, or fruit for dessert.

6. Alcoholic beverages increase absorption of food from the intestine and should be avoided. Even a usually well-tolerated amount of a food may bring on an allergic reaction in the presence of alcohol.

Commonsense Dos and Don'ts

1. Read labels on the foods before buying.

2. Prepare for dinner parties by contacting the hostess or caterer to inquire about the menu and bring along some allowable foods if necessary.

3. Eat before leaving home when you are not sure what food will be available.

4. Don't overeat.

5. Don't eat too fast.

6. Don't talk while you are eating.

7. Don't hesitate to call the product manufacturer's consumer-service departments to find out its ingredients.

8. Wear a Medi-Alert bracelet if you have experienced an anaphylactic reaction to food in the past. It is also recommended that susceptible individuals carry an emergency kit that contains epinephrine (adrenaline) for the immediate treatment of respiratory distress. Antihistamines also should be carried at all times.

laxis, but they should be distinguished from the true allergic reaction.

Histamine intoxication. Some foods have the ability to release histamine directly. The most common foods are scombroid or spiny-finned fishes such as tuna and mackerel and another fish called mahi-mahi. These fish can become contaminated with certain microorganisms that cause large concentrations of histamine to form. High histamine concentrations can also form if fish are held at temperatures above the refrigeration range. A single meal that includes a fish with high histamine levels can bring on flushing of the skin, inflamed red patches, itchy eyes, gastrointestinal upset, and headaches. These symptoms may last up to a day and usually disappear without further effects.

Reactions to Food Additives

Sulfites. Severe allergylike reactions may occur after eating foods treated with a group of preservatives known as sulfiting agents. These preservatives are widely used in convenience and restaurant foods, especially shrimp, peeled and processed potatoes, and the vegetables in salad bars. They also are present in beer, wine, champagne, and dried fruits.

Five percent of people with asthma are highly sensitive to sulfites and may suffer asthma attacks or even loss of consciousness or shock if they ingest sufficient quantities of sulfites. Less severe reactions include shortness of breath, tightness of the chest or throat, coughing, diarrhea, hives, or headaches.

Packaged foods usually list sulfiting agents on the labels; shrimp and salad ingredients do not. Sulfiting agents include sulphur dioxide, potassium or sodium metabisulfite, potassium or sodium bisulfite, and sodium sulfite. Dining out can pose a particular prob-lem to the sulfite-sensitive person because restaurant staff may be unaware of whether foods used and served by them were previously treated with sulfiting agents. Recently, an over-the-counter dipstick test became available for sulfite-sensitive people to test questionable food right at the table before eating, but this test is reliable only when it gives a positive result. The FDA is working on regulating this problem further. The true mechanism of this reaction is unclear at present.

Monosodium glutamate. Commonly known as MSG and used very widely in Chinese restaurants, this substance may induce the so-called Chinese restaurant syndrome. This reaction consists of severe headache, facial flush, chest pressure, and chest pain; MSG can also induce asthma in some asthmatics. There is a marked variation in the dose required to induce an adverse effect.

Vascular Responses

Migraine headache. Several research studies suggest a relationship between food allergy and migraine headache. Therefore, some patients may benefit from an evaluation of foods in their diets if another cause cannot be found for migraines. The foods most commonly implicated are aged or strong cheese, particularly cheddar cheese, chicken livers, pickled herring, canned figs, pods or broad beans, cured meats, such as hot dogs, bacon, ham, and salami. Other possible provocative substances include monosodium glutamate (MSG) and alcohol, particularly red wines and champagne. Avoiding alcoholic beverages is extremely important.

Vasoactive-amine toxicity. These compounds, contained in foods such as cheeses, wine, beer, chocolate, bananas, and some other fruits are capable of dramatically increasing blood pressure when eaten in the presence of certain medications, such as MAO inhibitors, and can even cause death.

Methyl-xanthine toxicity. These compounds, found as caffeine and theobromine in coffee, tea, colas, chocolate, and cocoa, can cause symptoms as diverse as headache, palpitation, vomiting, panic attacks, and anxiety in sensitive individuals.

Food Toxicity and Food Poisoning

Food toxicity. Naturally occurring toxins are not often encountered in the average American's daily diet. However, naturally occurring toxins in foods growing wild are not uncommon. When people eat unusual plants, experiment with hallucinogenic plants, or harvest from nature—such as hallucinogenic or other mushrooms—they are in danger of encountering food toxins. Two books for the public on this subject, both from the George Stickley Company of Philadelphia, are *The New Honest Herbal* and *Natural Product Medicine.*

Food poisoning. Food contamination by infectious agents and their toxins may result in food poisoning. As in the case of food toxicity, the signs and symptoms are varied and include gastrointestinal complaints of nausea, vomiting, and diarrhea; cardiovascular complaints such as tightness in the chest, palpitations, and pressure; and neurological symptoms such as headache. Fever is frequently present.

DIAGNOSING FOOD ALLERGY

The diagnosis of food allergy and hypersensitivity can be a complicated task, given the enormous variety of foods available. Once a food allergy is suspected, the patient should consult a physician who has been certified by the American Board of Allergy and Immunology. This will ensure that reliable tests are used to determine whether or not the symptoms are allergic and to track down the offending foods. Accepted aids to diagnose food allergy included allergy skin testing, RAST testing, and double-blind food challenge. A reasonable approach to diagnosis of food allergies is outlined on page 565.

TREATING FOOD ALLERGIES

The best method for treating an allergy or intolerance to a food or group of foods is avoidance. At the same time, many factors must be considered in developing safe and effective avoidance diets. These include the following.

- Essential selectivity of safe foods
- The possibility of cross-reacting foods (reactions to genetically related foods, even if they have not been eaten before)
- Adequacy of labeling (government regulations are improving, but consumers must learn to recognize the important language)

The time and sometimes money that go into constructing an avoidance diet is still another consideration. The greater cost, however, must be measured in terms of nutritional deficiencies that can arise as a result of omitting major food groups from a diet. A registered dietitian is invaluable in such cases, not only to learn how to make up for nutritional shortcomings but also to help plan meals that are pleasurable *and* free of problematic foods.

Approaches to Diagnosing a Food Allergy

Step 1: A detailed patient history, paying special attention to frequency of symptomatic episodes, details of symptoms, and time relation between eating and onset of symptoms.

Step 2: A complete physical examination, with special attention to the condition of the skin, eyes, and inside the nose and mouth, and to abnormal lung sounds such as wheezing.

Step 3: Ordering an immunologic test to aid in diagnosis of the suspected food allergy. One such test is the skin test, in which an extract of a single food is placed on the skin of an arm or back and pricked or scratched on the skin. The appearance of an itchy swelling indicates a positive response. One problem with this test is that sometimes people do not show a skin reaction to foods that actually cause a problem when eaten. In addition, people can have a positive skin-test reaction to a food or foods that do not cause problems when eaten. Another test is the RAST (radioallergosorbent test), which involves mixing small samples of the patient's blood with food proteins absorbed onto a special dish in a test tube. The procedure is a sophisticated radio-immunoassay and has the advantage of being safer for someone who might react severely to a scratch test.

Step 4: Performing necessary tests to rule out bacterial infections, intoxications, or underlying diseases unrelated to food allergy.

Step 5: Asking the patient to keep a daily food and symptom diary that documents food intake and frequency of symptoms along with time notations. (See Chapter 17 for a sample Daily Food Diary).

Step 6: Eliminating suspected foods from the diet for a period of time while recording symptoms.

Step 7: If no improvement occurs, a more stringent elimination diet may be tried, omitting additional foods considered to be allergenic.

Step 8: When improvement is noted, omitted foods are introduced back into the diet *one at a time* to determine whether symptoms reappear.

Step 9: If none of the methods succeeds in turning up the source of the problem, a double-blind challenge may be tried. This should be performed in an allergist's office or in a hospital under close supervision. The challenge involves giving the patient capsules of dried food suspected of causing reactions, as well as capsules containing a nonreactive substance (a placebo). Since neither physician nor patient knows what is in the capsule at any given time, both are "blind." The appearance of symptoms after taking any of the food extracts confirms the presence of an allergy to that food. Double-blind challenges can detect (and rule out) allergies or intolerances to many foods and other substances such as additives. They can also rule out psychological factors that may have caused symptoms.

Patients with food allergy should carry medication with them prescribed by their physician in case of an accidental ingestion of a food to which they are allergic.

COMMON OFFENDERS

For the allergy-prone individual, every food has the potential for causing an allergic reaction. Researchers, however, have identified a small group of foods that appear to be the most common offenders. What complicates the problem of identifying the culprit is the fact that these foods are often hidden in other food products. It is also possible to be allergic to a food that has never been eaten previously. This is because there are families of foods that are related to each other. The seven foods most commonly implicated in food allergies, along with a listing of food products that might contain them, are listed in Table 33.1.

With diligent attention to diet, it is possible to avoid a great many allergic reactions to foods. It is also helpful to note that there are some foods that almost never cause allergic symptoms. (See list on page 567.)

QUESTIONABLE THEORIES AND TREATMENTS

In attempting to find relief from their discomfort, allergy sufferers frequently respond to the promise of tests and remedies that have never been shown accurate or effective. Here are some of the approaches that have gained a popular following in recent years. These tests are *not* considered scientifically valid and are not recommended by the American Academy of Allergy and Immunology. (See accompanying box at the end of the chapter, page 572.)

Cytotoxic Testing

This method claims to measure sensitivity to over 200 commonly eaten foods and additives. Also called Bryan's test, leucocytotoxic testing, and food-sensitivity testing, this test involves taking small samples of a person's blood, separating out the white blood cells (leukocytes), and mixing them with dried extracts of specific foods. According to the test's proponents, if the white blood cells change in shape or size, the patient is said to have a sensitivity to that food and is told to avoid it. In reality, the food we eat is completely altered by digestion before it even reaches the body's white blood cells. There is no evidence to show that the white blood cells of allergy-prone people have defects that would cause them to change in shape or size. There *is* evidence to show that the test does *not* pick up true food allergies when they do exist. (Cytotoxic testing should not be confused with the RAST, which involves a different type of reaction and is a valid way to evaluate food antibodies, but not sensitivity.)

Sublingual Provocative Tests

In this procedure, patients are given doses of suspected allergenic foods either under the tongue or in an injectable form to provoke the onset of symptoms that correspond to prior complaints. As soon as the reaction appears, a second, weaker dose is given, supposedly to neutralize the reaction. In a true food allergy, the second dose of the allergen would only exacerbate the first reaction. Moreover, there is no provision for testing for IgE levels in the blood to determine whether there is actually an immune reaction in the sublingual area.

Pulse Test

The individual's pulse is measured immediately before and 30 minutes after eating; an elevated pulse is supposed to indicate food allergy. There is no evidence that this test is reliable.

Kinesiologic Testing

This test uses small amounts of the test food under the tongue; the individual's muscle strength is measured before and after. Again, there is no evidence that it has any value. Patients relying on it have been hurt.

Yeast Hypersensitivity

This speculation contends that a yeast fungus, called *Candida*, multiplies in the body and weakens the immune system. Treatment usually involves a diet in which all yeast- and

---

Foods That Rarely Cause Allergic Reactions

The following foods are frequently found on hypoallergenic diets:

Apples	Lettuce
Artichokes	Peaches
Carrots	Pears
Gelatin	Rice
Lamb	

---

mold-containing foods, as well as fruits and milk, are temporarily avoided. Individuals must also avoid refined carbohydrates and all processed foods. However, candida normally inhabits the mouth, skin, and intestines of most healthy persons without causing problems. Even persons who do develop fungal infections on the skin and nails have never developed the vast array of symptoms blamed on yeast sensitivity. No reliable evidence supports this speculation, and patients given anticandida drugs for yeast hypersensitivity may be harmed, says the *New England Journal of Medicine*.

FOOD-ALLERGY PREVENTION

Research suggests the marked benefits of early identification of infants at high risk for developing allergic disease and the implementation of measures designed to avoid exposure to potentially sensitizing foods. Such infants are identified in two ways: first through determining whether there is a family history of allergic disease (for example, examining the parents' medical history) and, second, through measurement of blood IgE levels in the infants soon after birth.

While IgE does not cross the placenta from mother to infant, the developing fetus can develop its own IgE when exposed to antigens in the uterus. For this reason, it is recommended that during pregnancy, women carrying babies who have been identified as high risk for allergy reduce intake of certain foods such as milk, eggs, peanuts, soy, fish, and citrus particularly during the last trimester. Breastfeeding for at least six months may decrease exposure to sensitizing antigens and, possibly, reduce intestinal protein antigen absorption in the infant. (The infant's intestinal wall is permeable to dietary protein

Table 33.1. Food Most Likely to Trigger Allergic Reactions

1. Milk and Milk Products
Including:

Biscuit and biscuit mixes	Ice cream
Boiled salad dressings	Ice cream soda
Butter or cheese sauces and gravies	Luncheon meats
Cakes and cake mixes	Malted milk
Canned fish balls	Mousses
Chocolate and some hard candies	Muffins and muffin mixes
Chowders (made with milk or cream)	Noodles
Cookies and cookie mixes	Scrambled eggs or omelets
Cream soups	Seasonings containing milk solids
Custards	Sherbets
Doughnuts and doughnut mixes	Spaghetti or meats using dried milk as filler (meat loaf, hot
Hot chocolate	dogs, sausages)

Also check food labels for the following ingredients:

Calcium caseinate	Lactate solids
Casein	Milk-solid pastes
Casein hydrolysate	Sweetened condensed milk
Caseinate	Whey or whey solids
DMS (dried-milk solids) lactalbumen	

2. Eggs
Including:

Bavarian cream	Hollandaise sauce
Breaded foods	Ice cream
Cakes and cookies (unless labeled egg-free)	Mayonnaise
Chicken (if fricasseed or in broth)	Meats using egg as binder
Custard and cream pies	Pancakes
Egg broths	Salad dressings
Egg sauces	Sherbets
French toast	Waffles

Also check food labels for the following ingredients:

Albumin	Globulin
Dried egg solids	Ovomucin
Egg solids	Vitellin

3. Wheat and Wheat Products
Including:

Ale	Cheese spreads and sauces
Baked beans	Chili con carne
Beer	Chowders
Biscuits	Coffee substitutes
Bisques	Cookies
Bread	Corn bread
Bread crumbs	Crackers
Breaded or canned fish	Creamed soups
Breadings	Creamed vegetables or vegetable sauces
Cakes	Croquettes
Candies	Doughnuts and doughnut mixes
Canned soups with noodles	Dry or cooked breakfast cereal

Table 33.1. Food Most Likely to Trigger Allergic Reactions *(cont.)*

3. Wheat and Wheat Products *(cont.)*
Including:

Dry soup mixes	Pretzels
Dumplings	Processed meats using wheat
Floured meats such as Swiss steak	Puddings
Fritters	Rye products
Gin	Scalloped dishes
Gravies	Seasoning mixes
Ice cream	Some baby foods
Ice cream cones	Some bouillon cubes
Jams with wheat flour as thickener	Some soup mixes
Malted milk	Some wines
Meat loaf	Soy bread
Muffins	Stuffed poultry
Pancakes	Thickeners
Pasta	Waffles
Pastries	Whiskey
Pies	Yeast made from wheat extract
Popovers	

Also check food labels for the following ingredients:

Enriched flour	
Flour	Monosodium glutamate (MSG)
Hydrolyzed flour	Self-rising flour
Modified food starch	Sodium glutamate (if from wheat gluten)

4. Corn
Including (unless labeled corn-free):

Baby foods (with cornstarch added)	Cured or tenderized ham
Bacon	Custards
Baking mixes	Deep-fat frying mixtures or breadings
Baking powder	Doughnuts and doughnut mixes
Bologna	Frankfurters
Canned meats	French and other salad dressings
Canned or frozen string beans	Gelatin capsules
Canned peas	Graham crackers
Canned pie fillings	Harvard beets
Chili preparations	Icings
Chop suey	Luncheon ham
Commercial breads	Marshmallow creme
Commercial syrups	Marshmallows
Confectioner's or powdered sugar	Monosodium glutamate
Cooked meats with gravies	Pancakes
Cooked sausages	Pastries
Corn and frying oils	Pie crusts
Corn grits	Prepared frostings
Corn-oil margarine	Pretzels and corn chips
Cream pies	Sauces and gravies
Cream puffs	Seasoning mixes
Creamed, thickened, and vegetable soups	Some canned and frozen fruits (corn syrup)

Table 33.1. Food Most Likely to Trigger Allergic Reactions *(cont.)*

4. Corn *(cont.)*
Including (unless labeled corn-free):

Some cereals
Some cheeses
Some jellies and preserves
Some peanut butter
Some potato and rice mixes

Soybean milks
Tortillas
Vanilla pudding
Vitamin capsules
Waffles

Also check food labels for the following ingredients:

Corn solids
Cornstarch

Corn syrup
Vegetable starch

5. Legumes (dried peas, beans, peanuts, soybeans, etc.)
Including:

Baking chocolate substitutes
Baby foods
Cheese spreads
Cold cuts
Commercial one-dish meats
Flavored potato chips
Ice cream containing soy or other legume products or fillers
Imitation salad dressings
Noodles
Peanut butter and peanut spreads
Salad dressings
Salad oils
Sausages

Seasoning mixes
Seasoning sauces
Shortenings
Some breakfast cereal and pastry preparations
Some candies
Some crackers
Some potato mixes
Some soups
Spaghetti
Steak sauces
Substitute milks
Whipped nondairy toppings

Also check food labels for the following ingredients:

Hydrolyzed vegetable protein
Soya flour
Soy concentrate

TVP (textured vegetable protein) vegetable protein concentrate

Allergy to one type of legume, such as soy, does not necessarily mean allergy to all types of legumes.

6. Nuts and Seeds
Including:

Cake icings
Candies containing nuts
Cottonseed meal and oil
Ice creams

Lard substitutes
Nut crumbs on cakes and cookies
Oils from nuts

7. Seafood
Including:

Bisques
Broths
Caviar
Fish and shellfish stews
Fish-liver oils and concentrates in vitamin preparations

Fresh, canned, smoked, or pickled fish and shellfish
Hor d'oeuvres made from fish
Salads
Soups

Also avoid licking labels that may be made with fish glue. The shellfish category is unique in that if you are allergic to one type of shellfish, you are probably allergic to all.

Questionable Practices and Theories in Dealing with Allergies*

Two out of five Americans believe that they have had adverse reactions to certain foods, yet when properly tested, less than 2 percent of the American population have true food allergies. Among adults who are properly tested, only 5 percent who think they have food allergies turn out to be correct.

In recent years, a number of myths have been promoted about food and food ingredients. Here are a few of them. None are true.

- Foods with artificial colors and flavors and with added sugar cause hyperactivity and other behavioral problems in children.

- Some forms of schizophrenia, manic depression, or chronic tension and chronic fatigue are actually "cerebral allergies," and result from eating common foods.

- Some people with chronic mental disorders actually have "masked food allergy," a condition in which certain foods bring about a feeling of well-being at first and then a type of hangover.

- Premenstrual syndrome (PMS), cystitis, and bed-wetting are caused by certain foods, including those containing amino acids.

- Compulsive overeating and obesity are a result of food allergies.

The belief that different foods are responsible for a myriad of neurological and behavioral problems can be traced at least as far back as the 1930s when certain ill-defined disorders, such as paralysis, epilepsy, itching, headache, insomnia, fatigue, and abnormalities of mental performance and behavior were reported to be caused by an allergy to food.

This speculation, popularly known as clinical ecology, is still being promoted today. Many of the symptoms clinical ecologists have attributed to a reaction to food are the same as those caused by neuroses. However, scientific studies have revealed that true food allergies do not present themselves as psychiatric or behavioral problems.

In 1973, Dr. Benjamin Feingold contended that hyperactivity and attention-deficit disorders in children might be a reaction to natural salicylates and food additives. (Natural salicylates are found in some foods, such as bananas, green peas, licorice, and blueberries.) In a book written on the subject, he promoted the Feingold Diet, in which he maintained that the removal of foods containing natural salicylates, preservatives, and colors produced improvement in half of the children affected by these problems. Subsequent studies have not supported Dr. Feingold's conclusion. Some parents have put their hyperactive children on his diet instead of giving them medication and have observed improvement. This is coincidence masquerading as cause and effect, since secretly additive-spiked diets also work. (See Chapter 38.)

There is no denying that for some people the simple act of eating a food to which they are allergic can provoke frightening and even life-threatening allergic responses. It is equally true, however, that not all adverse reactions are allergic ones and that blaming innocent foods can lead to adopting a diet that is not nutritionally balanced. It is important to know the difference between allergic and nonallergic reactions to foods.

Clinical Ecology

This speculation holds that a limitless list of complaints—including dizziness, headaches, insomnia, fatigue, tension, itching, weight gain, confusion, irritability, crying, learning disorders, and water retention—are caused by damage to a person's immune system by polluted air, food, and water. Aside from the fact that the approach does not meet accepted requirements for diagnosing and treating illness, it also focuses on vague symptoms that are related to a number of physical and emotional illnesses. Studies have also shown that many patients treated by clinical ecologists simply exchange old for new symptoms.

Immune-Power Diets

This approach claims to revitalize an immune system that has been allegedly weakened and destroyed by improper foods and inadequate sup-

Questionable Practices and Theories in Dealing with Allergies* *(cont.)*

plements. To correct the alleged (and undemonstrated) condition, proponents offer two remedies. First is an elimination diet, which removes common foods that are accused of damaging the immune system. Second is a program of megadose vitamin, mineral, and amino-acid supplements, which is alleged (but again, not demonstrated) to rebuild the patient's supposedly damaged immune system.

What proponents of the theory do not reveal is that few individuals in developed countries suffer from the severe chronic malnutrition that might conceivably damage the immune system. Furthermore, the supplement level recommended far exceeds the Recommended Dietary Allowances of the National Academy of Sciences or the Reference Daily Intakes (RDIs) of the Food and Drug Administration. These high levels may be dangerous in some instances.

No evidence supports claims that these so-called immune-power diets have any value. The questionable practices of Dr. Stuart Berger, a New York City "diet doctor" and leading proponent of immune-power diets (who also sells supplements in his office), were exposed by an investigative reporter with a hidden camera on the NBC-TV show "Inside Edition" in 1990. Dr. Berger had obtained from a federal judge a restraining order against showing the film, but the Supreme Court overturned this order.

Steps to Protect Yourself

To avoid the questionable practices outlined in this section, plus myriad others that are constantly being developed, I advise consumers to steer clear of:

- Anyone who diagnoses and/or treats "candidiasis hypersensitivity syndrome."

- Anyone who suggests cytotoxicity testing to "diagnose" food allergy.

- Anyone who diagnoses "chronic Epstein-Barr virus syndrome."

- Anyone who promotes immune-power diets.

- Anyone who diagnoses "chronic fatigue syndrome" without having done a thorough psychiatric examination as part of evaluating the patient.

- Anyone who calls him- or herself a "clinical ecologist."

- Anyone who says that everyone needs vitamin supplements to make sure they get enough. (As stressed throughout this book, most people get all the vitamins and minerals they need by eating a varied and balanced diet.)

- Anyone who treats "chronic fatigue syndrome" with allergy and/or nutritional supplements.

- Anyone who suggests that most diseases, including allergies, are caused by faulty nutrition.

- Anyone who suggests that large doses of vitamins are effective against a large number of diseases and conditions.

- Anyone who suggests hair analysis as a basis for determining the body's nutritional state or for recommending vitamins and minerals. Hair analysis is not reliable for this purpose.

- Anyone who uses a computer-scored questionnaire for diagnosing "nutrient deficiencies." Computers used for such tests are invariably programmed to recommend supplements for virtually everyone.

- Anyone who uses "chelation therapy" to treat heart disease.

- Any practitioner, licensed or not, who sells vitamins in his or her office. Scientific nutritionists do not sell vitamins. Unscientific practitioners often do—at two or three times their usual cost.

*This section written by Victor Herbert, M.D., F.A.C.P.

during the first few months of life, after which time it gradually "seals.") Consult your physician for a restricted, hypoallergenic diet recommended for the entire breastfeeding period, and for the latest information on this changing subject.

If supplemental feeding is necessary, a low-allergenic formula (no cows' milk or soy formula) is recommended. After six months, foods with low allergenic potential are gradually added to the diet.

FUTURE RESEARCH

Research advances depend on refining knowledge and developing tools necessary to measure allergic response and to identify potential allergens.

Manned space flights have yielded much information that is important to the study of food allergy. The chemical diet developed for astronauts in flight included all essential nutrients—vitamins, minerals, amino acids, and carbohydrates—in a form that could not cause allergic symptoms. This diet has been used successfully in small groups of patients whose allergies required hospitalization.

In other research areas, scientists are working to isolate the active fraction in food extracts so that more reliable results can be obtained by skin testing. This may also make specific food proteins easier to avoid.

34

Nutrition and Bone Disorders

Donald Bergman, M.D.

■

INTRODUCTION

The adult human body has more than 200 bones that form the skeleton. To most people, the best-known function of the skeleton is to provide a framework for the body, giving it shape and strength while protecting the vital organs. In concert with muscles, which are connected to the bones by tendons, bones enable the body to move. In addition to this role, bones also serve as the body's storehouse for minerals, particularly calcium and phosphorus. About 98 percent of the body's calcium is stored in the bones, and approximately 1 percent of that amount can be moved rapidly into the circulating blood.

Despite its solid, rocklike appearance, bone is metabolically active organic tissue that is constantly being perfused by blood. For example, small amounts of calcium are required by all body cells to function normally. The blood constantly carries this calcium to the cells. When the blood's calcium level falls below a certain point, the bones release some of their stored calcium into the bloodstream.

Another important function of bone tissue is the manufacture of blood cells, which takes place in the marrow found within certain types of bones.

BONE STRUCTURE AND GROWTH

The average bone is composed of two-thirds mineral, primarily a calcium-phosphate-hydroxide compound known as hydroxyapatite. The remaining one-third is made up of organic matrix, which is mostly collagen. The hydroxyapatite gives the bone rigidity and the collagen matrix provides resilience.

Within each bone are two types of tissues: compact, or dense, bone and spongy, more porous tissue, known as trabecular bone for the trabeculae, or little beams of bone, present. Compact bone makes up the smooth outer layer, or cortex, and trabecular bone, which is more readily influenced by changes in metabolism, fills the interior. The ratio of those two bone types varies throughout the body. The long bones of the arms and legs, for example, are 90 percent or more cortex. In contrast, the vertebrae are overwhelmingly trabecular. Covering the outside of the compact bone is the periosteum, a connective-tissue layer containing the bone-forming cells known as osteoblasts.

As with all other aspects of prenatal development, the fetus relies on maternal nutrients for skeletal growth. Both pregnant and lactating women absorb more calcium than usual, which enables them to protect their own skeletal integrity at the same time as supplying calcium to the fetus, and, later, the newborn baby if they breastfeed. The demand for calcium is highest in the last two or three months of pregnancy, when the fetal skeleton is developing. (See Chapter 12 for a discussion of the nutritional needs of pregnancy.)

The fetal skeleton is composed primarily of cartilage, the fibrous connective tissue that serves as a model for bone development. Following birth, breastfeeding will require that the mother maintain her calcium stores to meet the needs of making milk. As during pregnancy, the woman's body is more efficient in absorbing dietary calcium while breastfeeding.

After birth, an infant's bones grow rapidly. Growth takes place outward from bony centers, the developing units of bone, which undergo ossification (depositing of minerals) and fusion with other bony centers. The growth of long bones occurs principally at the epiphysis, the enlarged end of the bone shaft. At the bony center, inorganic calcium salts are deposited on the cartilage, which serves as a template for bone growth. Gradually, the cartilage is replaced by trabecular bone overlaid by cortical bone. The increase in diameter results primarily from the layer of bone tissue added around the cartilage. Over time, the innermost bone layers are resorbed, leaving a hollow, tube-like center.

Once the ends of each bony unit have been transformed from cartilage into epiphyseal tissue, the only remaining growth in long bones takes place at the epiphyseal disk, a thin cartilaginous plate sandwiched between the bone shaft and the epiphysis.

The Skeleton Throughout Life

The infant skeleton. The shaft of an infant's bone is filled with a porous matrix that responds readily to consumed nutrients present in milk. Calcium in the infant accounts for about 1 percent of total body weight, and the greatest increase in calcium content relative to body size occurs in the first year of life.

Childhood. The condition of the bones in a child affects the skeleton he or she will have as an adult. Thus, calcium intake between ages 1 and 10 years affects the peak bone mass of adulthood; however, due to the more gradual rate of growth during early childhood, the body does not retain as much calcium as it did in infancy. The long bones begin to hollow, leaving spongy, trabecular bone only at the bone ends. Up to about the age of six, a child's hollow bone spaces are filled with red marrow, which produces blood elements such as red blood cells. After the age of six, the marrow in the long bones changes from red to yellow and no longer takes part in the manufacture of blood elements. Marrow in the flat bones of the ribs, pelvis, vertebrae, and skull, however, continues to supply blood components.

Adolescence. From the age of 10 to about 18, the body needs more calcium than at other times in life. About 45 percent of the adult skeletal mass forms in adolescence. Once the bones have achieved their full size, they continue to increase in density and thickness for a few more years.

Adulthood. Bone growth is completed when the cartilage that forms the epiphyseal disks near the ends of the long bones turns to bone itself. The last bone to unite its shaft and epiphysis is the clavicle, or collarbone; the end that is attached to the breastbone fuses between the ages of 25 and 28. The peak skeletal mass is attained and bone consolidation takes place into the thirties. Thereafter, bones begin to lose varying amounts of their mass. The amount of bone tissue that is lost is influenced by many factors, including gender, weight, pregnancy, hormonal status, and level of physical activity, among others.

Old age. Increased bone loss is common among the elderly, due to a number of causes. For example, there is decreased absorption of calcium and availability of vitamin D (needed in order for the body to absorb calcium) with age, and this can gradually lead to a thinning of bones (osteoporosis). Hormonal changes that occur with age—especially the lack of estrogen in postmenopausal women—also lead to bone loss. Bones require a certain amount of stress from physical activity to maintain their strength. Thus the reduced physical activity that occurs with age speeds bone loss. The use of certain medications (for example, high-fiber laxatives) can interfere with calcium absorption.

The elderly are particularly susceptible to bone fractures for a number of reasons. As bones weaken with advancing age, tiny fractures that are not noticed at the time may occur. These fractures further weaken bones and increase the risk of major fractures, such as a broken hip or leg. The changes in equilibrium, use of medications with sedating side effects, and poor vision that may occur with aging also contribute to falls and the increased risk of fractures.

DIET AND BONE MAINTENANCE

Calcium

The major nutritional building block of bone is calcium. (For a list of some of the functions of calcium, see below.) Between 1.5 percent and 2 percent of an adult's weight is comprised of calcium. About 99 percent of the calcium is found in bones and teeth.

In recent years, calcium has gained considerable media attention as a nutrient that is not found in adequate amounts in the diets of many Americans, particularly women who shun milk and cheese. (The RDAs for calcium from age 25 in both sexes and children 1 to 10 are 800 milligrams; for ages 11–24 and pregnant or lactating women, they are 1200 milligrams.)

Large numbers of women are now taking calcium supplements as a result of the many media reports linking osteoporosis with calcium deficiency. However, unless supplements are specifically recommended by a physician, it is better to get calcium from the diet than from pills. Many foods contain varying amounts of calcium, but by far, the best sources are milk or milk products or foods

Functions of Calcium

- Serves as the major mineral composing bone and teeth.
- Regulates muscle contraction and relaxation, including that of heart muscle.
- Activates enzymes important in various metabolic pathways.
- Aids in blood clotting.
- Enhances cell adhesion.

such as canned sardines or salmon with the softened bones. (See Table 34.1 and Table 34.2.)

There are different types of calcium supplements, each with its own disadvantages and advantages. Although side effects are usually not common, calcium chloride and calcium carbonate may irritate the stomach and cause bloating and gas. In addition, calcium-carbonate supplements may cause constipation, which is a common complaint of older individuals who often take the supplements. Switching to calcium lactate or calcium gluconate may remedy the problem. (Calcium gluconate can occasionally cause diarrhea, however.) Antacids that contain aluminum can cause losses of calcium, especially in those who have a diet low in calcium, and therefore should not be taken. Bone meal and dolomite supplements may contain trace amounts of metal contaminants, such as arsenic, lead, mercury, and cadmium, and should be avoided.

In susceptible persons, excessive supplementation of calcium (over 1,000 to 1,500 milligrams per day) may cause kidney damage. Individuals with a personal or family history of kidney stones should take calcium supplements only with a doctor's guidance—and with plenty of water.

There can also be difficulties with absorption of calcium from supplements. When calcium is consumed in the diet in milk, vitamin D is also supplied, which aids in the absorption of calcium. However, supplements supply only calcium. Calcium carbonate, for example, contains the greatest amounts of calcium of the supplements, but it is not easily absorbed by individuals who lack sufficient stomach acid, a condition common in those over 60. For this reason, it is recommended that when supplements are taken by those who have impaired gastric acidity, they should be taken with meals, because the acid

generated by food permits better absorption. The absorption can also be enhanced if the supplements are taken with milk or yogurt, both of which contain vitamin D and lactose. Because the intestines can absorb only a certain amount of calcium at one time, calcium supplements should be taken in small amounts more frequently.

Excessive amounts of calcium can also interefere with the absorption of other minerals—zinc, copper, iron, and magnesium.

Research at the University of Texas Health Science Center at Dallas found that of the supplements, calcium citrate was most efficiently absorbed by the body, contributed less to kidney-stone formation, and had the fewest gastrointestinal side effects.

In addition to the diet, a small amount of calcium is supplied by the body itself, from secretions of sloughed-off cells. Ingested calcium is absorbed into the bloodstream from the intestine.

Hormonal Regulation of Calcium Balance

The intricate mechanisms of the body are designed to keep a delicate balance in all systems. When food containing calcium is ingested, varying amounts are absorbed in the intestine and taken up by the circulating blood. The calcium that is not immediately used is stored in the trabecular meshwork at the ends of the long bones; any excess calcium is excreted in the urine or feces.

A number of substances affect the absorption of calcium and its level in the blood. Parathormone, also known as parathyroid hormone, is secreted by the four parathyroid glands, which are located near the base of the neck. When the amount of calcium in the blood falls below a certain level, these glands release parathormone, which activates bone cells known as osteoclasts in order to break down bone. Parathormone also triggers the kidneys to convert an inactive form of vitamin D (calcidiol) into the active one (calcitriol). By enhancing calcium absorption from the intestine and reducing excretion of phosphorus in the urine, calcitriol counteracts the loss of minerals while increasing levels in the blood.

When the blood-calcium level goes above a certain point, the thyroid gland secretes the hormone calcitonin, which blocks the action of the parathormone, preventing release of calcium from bone.

Other Factors Affecting Calcium Absorption

Estrogen. This female sex hormone (present in small amounts in males) slows the break-down, or resorption, of bone by countering parathormone's stimulation of bone-destroying osteoclasts and increasing the amount of this hormone required to break down calcium. Estrogen also stimulates the thyroid gland to secrete calcitonin, which works against bone resorption.

After estrogen production falls at menopause, bone resorption exceeds bone production, increasing a woman's susceptibility for osteoporosis. Caucasian women lose as much as 10 percent of their trabecular bone each year for the first few years after menopause and about 1 percent of their cortical bone each year. Hormone-replacement therapy helps prevent or slow this bone loss, and many physicians now recommend hormone

Table 34.1. Dietary Sources of Calcium

Food	Serving Size	Calcium (mg.)	Food	Serving Size	Calcium (mg.)
MILK AND MILK PRODUCTS			**FRUIT**		
Milk (skim, whole, etc.)	8 oz.	300	Figs, dried	5 medium	126
Ice cream, vanilla	8 oz.	208	Orange	1 medium	65
Ice milk, vanilla	8 oz.	283	Prunes, dried	10 large	51
Nonfat dry milk	1 T	57	**NUTS/SEEDS**		
Yogurt, whole milk	8 oz.	275	Almonds or hazelnuts	12–15	38
Yogurt, skim with nonfat-milk solids	8 oz.	452	Sesame seeds*	1 oz.	28
			Sunflower seeds	1 oz.	34
Cheese			**VEGETABLES**		
American	1 oz.	195	Bean curd (tofu)	3½ oz.	128
Cheddar	1 oz.	211	Beans, garbanzo	½ cup	80
Cottage, creamed	8 oz.	211	Beans, pinto	½ cup	135
Cottage, low-fat, dry	8 oz.	138	Beans, red kidney	½ cup	110
Cream cheese	1 oz.	23	Broccoli, cooked	⅔ cup	88
Parmesan, grated	1 T	69	Chard, cooked*	½ cup	61
Swiss	1 oz.	259	Collard greens, cooked*	½ cup	152
FISH/SEAFOOD			Fennel, raw	3½ oz.	100
Mussels (meat only)	3½ oz.	88	Kale, cooked	½ cup	134
Oysters	5–8 medium	94	Lettuce, romaine	3½ oz.	68
Salmon, canned with bones	3½ oz.	198	Mustard greens, cooked*	½ cup	145
			Rutabaga, cooked	½ cup	59
Sardines, canned with bones	3½ oz.	449	Seaweed, agar, raw	3½ oz.	567
			Seaweed, kelp, raw	3½ oz.	1,093
Shrimp	3½ oz.	63	Squash, acorn	½ medium baked	61

*Foods high in oxalic acid, which hinders absorption.

Source: U.S. Department of Agriculture, Human Nutrition Information Service.

Nutrition and Bone Disorders ■ 579

therapy for women at high risk for osteoporosis. (See Risk Factors for Developing Osteoporosis on page 581.)

Phosphorus. About 85 percent of the mineral phosphorus in the body is combined with calcium as hydroxyapatite in bones and teeth. When combined with calcitonin, phosphorus stimulates production of trabecular bone tissue. Phosphorus also decreases the amount of calcium lost in the urine and increases the mineralization of bone.

The body requires phosphorus and calcium in about the same amounts, and foods such as milk contain good amounts of both minerals. Phosphorus is also found in ample amounts in meats, soft drinks, and other popular foods that do not contain calcium. Thus, the average American diet provides more phosphorus than calcium, and this excess tends to decrease the amount of calcium absorbed in the intestine and increase that lost in the feces. It was once thought that high phosphorus intake depleted calcium from bone. However, recent research does not support this.

Vitamin D. This vitamin works with calcium to maintain muscle function and enhance bone formation and maintenance. The inactive form of vitamin D, known as vitamin D_3, is found both in food and synthesized in the skin in the presence of ultraviolet rays absorbed from sunlight. (See Getting Vitamin D from the Sun, below.) Vitamin D is ubiquitous in the body but is stored primarily in the liver. It is also metabolized in the skin and

Table 34.2. Sample High-Calcium Menus

The following menus provide well over 1,000 milligrams of calcium per day and also meet requirements for other essential nutrients.

Food	Approximate Calcium (mg.)
Breakfast	
Sliced orange (1 medium)	65
Cooked oat cereal (instant)	170
½ cup skim milk	75
Beverage	
Lunch	
Turkey sandwich with 1 oz.	
Swiss cheese	260
on whole-wheat bread	50
Apple	10
1 cup skim milk	300
Snack	
8 oz. fruit yogurt (low-fat with	
nonfat-milk solids)	450
Dinner	
Chicken-mushroom soup	30
Green salad with vinegar	
dressing	10
Flounder fillet (3 oz.)	25
Broccoli (½ cup)	90
Baked potato	20
Stewed pear	20
Total Calcium	1575

Getting Vitamin D from the Sun

For those who do not get enough of this vitamin from foods such as fortified milk or other rich sources, judicious sun exposure can make up for the deficiency. The amount of vitamin D manufactured depends on time of year and day, presence of air pollution, clouds, and geographic location. Window glass blocks the ultraviolet light rays needed for manufacture.

• For most people, 5 to 15 minutes of exposure twice weekly to the summer noontime sun will provide an adequate supply of vitamin D to prevent deficiency in the winter. People who burn easily need less exposure than the elderly, whose skin does not convert vitamin D as easily.

• People who are at high risk for skin cancer should check with a dermatologist before using sun exposure as a way to provide vitamin D. Dietary sources such as vitamin D-enriched milk may be a better alternative for them.

kidneys. The active form, calcitriol, which is produced in the kidney, acts much like a hormone. Adequate amounts of Vitamin D can be obtained from milk that has been vitamin D–fortified, or from a few minutes of exposure to the sun. Other good sources include egg yolks, liver, and some dark-fleshed fish such as tuna, herring, sardines, and salmon. Oils from cod liver and other cold-water fish also are good sources and are sometimes used as vitamin D supplements. Care must be taken in using supplements, however, since excessive vitamin D is toxic.

Vitamin D deficiency, which is now rare in this country, still may occur in some elderly people who spend most of their time indoors or who do not consume dietary sources. Even among older people who get adequate sun or dietary sources, some research indicates that they may be unable to utilize it easily, which can conceivably result in deficiency problems.

Lactose. Lactose is the natural sugar in dairy products that helps to improve calcium absorption. In order for the body to use it, though, it must be broken down by the enzyme lactase into glucose and galactose. A lactase deficiency, often seen in adults who are not of northern European heritage, prevents the breakdown of lactose, but this can be corrected by taking commercially available lactase. In addition, lastose-reduced foods or lactose-free dairy products are available.

Protein. Meat, fish, eggs, and dairy products supply the greatest amounts of protein to the diet. Purified amino acids may cause a negative calcium balance, with increased loss of calcium through the urine and feces, but studies have shown this does not happen with intact protein, such as that found in foods.

Fiber. Some studies have implicated dietary fiber, especially bran and other forms of cel-lulose, as decreasing the amount of calcium that is absorbed. The amounts of fiber consumed in those studies were, however, far in excess of normal. A balanced diet that contains moderate amounts of a variety of fibers probably will not affect calcium absorption.

Oxalic acid. This substance is found in spinach, chard, beet greens—all rich in calcium—and other foods, such as rhubarb. Large amounts of oxalic acid inhibit the absorption of calcium.

Caffeine and other drugs. Caffeine, the stimulant found in coffee, tea, chocolate, colas, and a number of over-the-counter medications, increases the amount of calcium lost in both urine and feces. Those who consume a large amount of caffeine can offset this loss by increasing calcium intake. (For information on other medications, see Table 34.3.)

Table 34.3. Medications Affecting Calcium

Medication	Effect
ANTACIDS CONTAINING ALUMINUM	
Maalox, Mylanta, Amphojel, and others	Increased calcium excretion
ANTIBIOTICS	
Tetracycline	Decreased absorption of calcium
Erythromycin	
Isoniazid (used to treat tuberculosis)	
ANTICOAGULANTS	
Heparin	Increased calcium excretion
CHOLESTEROL-REDUCING DRUGS	
Cholestyramine	Increased calcium excretion
DIURETICS	
Furosemide	Increased calcium excretion in urine
Thiacide group	Decreased calcium excretion in urine
HORMONE PREPARATIONS	
Corticosteroids	Increased trabecular bone loss
Thyroid hormone	Increased bone loss

Alcohol. Alcohol has been shown to be directly toxic to bone cells. Heavy alcohol consumption can also cause bone loss by creating abnormalities in calcium and vitamin D absorption. In addition, chronic alcohol abusers often consume a poor diet and may not get enough calcium and vitamin D from foods.

Smoking. The nicotine in tobacco reduces the body's ability to use calcium. In addition, women who smoke tend to have lower estrogen levels and reduced bone mass. It has been suggested that in smokers estrogen breaks down faster in the liver and as a result is unable to stimulate the secretion of sufficient calcitonin to prevent excess bone breakdown.

Effects of Excess Calcium

When the calcium level greatly exceeds the body's requirement—unlikely in an otherwise healthy individual with normal dietary intake—a number of problems can result. Some of these, including abdominal gas, flatulence, and constipation, often resolve as the body adjusts to the increased calcium intake. More serious consequences of high blood calcium, or hypercalcemia, include kidney stones and kidney damage if the condition remains untreated. Hypercalcemia is generally a consequence of disease, for example, hyperparathyroidism (overactivity of the parathyroid glands) or certain kinds of cancer. High calcium levels can be detected in the blood.

Osteoporosis

As noted earlier, osteoporosis—the abnormal loss of bone density—had been in the media spotlight for the past few years. Osteoporosis is responsible for more than a million fractures each year, and is particularly common among older women of northern European extraction. After peak bone mass has been reached during the thirties, the rate of bone breakdown or resorption normally exceeds that of bone deposition. In osteoporosis, however, bone deposition lags even further behind resorption, resulting in an exaggerated loss.

Two types of osteoporosis have been identified. The incidence of both types increases with age but differs between the sexes. Type I osteoporosis occurs in postmenopausal women and in younger women whose ovaries have been removed surgically or those with ovarian disorders. (The best means of preserving bone mass after menopause is through estrogen-replacement therapy.) Type I osteoporosis results in a disproportionate loss of trabecular bone over cortical bone, and it is characterized by a low rate of bone turnover. Recent interest in osteoporosis has focused primarily on Type I.

Type II osteoporosis, also known as senile osteoporosis, occurs in both men and women over the age of 75 at nearly equal rates. Bone loss tends to affect both trabecular and cortical bone to a similar degree.

Risk Factors for Developing Osteoporosis

Factors that increase the risk of Type I osteoporosis include the following.

Gender-related influences. In addition to bone loss following the drop in estrogen levels after menopause, women tend to have a lower peak bone mass than men. They also tend to consume less milk and other calcium-rich foods, and they are not as physically active as men (although this is changing). Women today also tend to live longer than in the past, thus their postmenopausal years are increasing in number.

Weight. Heavier women are less likely to develop osteoporosis. As a rule, thin individuals who often have a lower bone mass have a greater chance of fracture because they have less trabecular bone to provide tensile strength. In addition, fat tissue becomes a major source of estrogen, needed to regulate bone resorption.

Childbearing status. Pregnancy brings about a rise in the body's calcium levels. Although breastfeeding, particularly if prolonged, may deplete some of the excess calcium stores, repeated pregnancies can actually create a calcium surplus. Women who have never been pregnant are at a greater risk for osteoporosis.

Ethnic and race background. Women of northern European and Oriental ancestry are at greatest risk for developing osteoporosis; the lowest risk among Caucasian women is found among those of Mediterranean heritage. Because of their greater peak bone mass, on average, blacks are less likely to develop osteoporosis.

Physical activity. Those who take part in weight-bearing exercises such as running and walking on a regular basis lose less skeletal mass than do sedentary individuals. Some who exercise extensively can develop more cortical bone in their limbs. However, women who exercise so much that menstruation stops or its onset is delayed (for example, ballet dancers or long-distance runners) may have an increased risk of developing osteoporosis because of depressed estrogen levels.

Heredity. Women whose mothers, sisters, or other female relatives have osteoporosis are at greater risk for developing the condition. How important a role genes play in the development of osteoporosis has not been firmly established because it is difficult to isolate heredity from all other risk factors.

Disease factors. Certain digestive disorders can cause increased risk for osteoporosis. In some cases, the cause is a sensitivity or allergy to important nutrients, such as lactose intolerance. In others, the problem lies in the body's inability to absorb properly the nutrients consumed. For example, with advancing age, the level of hydrochloric acid in the stomach declines, slowing the digestion of nutrients. If the presence of a disease limits calcium intake or physical activity, the risk for osteoporosis increases. Diabetes and rheumatoid arthritis (which also causes decalcification of bony areas around joints) are among the diseases that may increase the risk.

The Role of Diet in Preventing Osteoporosis

Because osteoporosis usually progresses to an advanced state before its effects are obvious, prevention of bone loss appears to be the single best way to avoid the potential for fracture and the resulting disability. Although increasing calcium in the diet is one of the strategies most often suggested, many studies have failed to find any clear-cut relationship between dietary intake of this mineral and bone density. Consuming calcium- and vitamin D–rich foods is probably more important in the years of bone growth before peak mass is reached rather than later in adulthood.

Dairy products account for more than 70 percent of the calcium in the typical American diet. Their calcium is readily absorbed because they contain lactose and some are fortified with vitamin D.

Vegetarians who avoid all animal food products can still obtain calcium from soy milk, tofu (soybean curd) processed with calcium sulfate, grain (particularly unprocessed or slightly processed), some green leafy vegetables (kale, turnip greens), beans, and nuts. (See also Chapter 25.) Some currently popular mineral waters and tap water also contain calcium, the quantity of calcium varying with the source.

Because of the widespread—and questionable—publicity linking dietary calcium to osteoporosis, the mineral has been added to a number of products, including orange juice, soda, and cereal. Calcium supplements have also become popular, but their value as a source of calcium remains in dispute. Supplements vary considerably in absorbability and many people take them improperly. For example, until recently, calcium supplements were in the form of large, hard-to-take pills. Supplement manufacturers have reduced the size of the tablet for easier swallowing, but in doing so they may have compressed the pill so much that it will not dissolve in the stomach, instead passing through the gastrointestinal system intact.

Calcium supplements vary according to the percentage of mineral in each dose, and in its effects on the body. Among the most frequently used calcium compounds are calcium carbonate (Tums, Os-Cal, and others) and calcium citrate (Citrical and others). Calcium carbonate is highest at 40 percent pure calcium per pill. It reacts with the hydrochloric acid in the stomach to form calcium chloride, a highly soluble, readily available compound.

Undesirable effects of large amounts of calcium carbonate include bloating, nausea, and constipation. Excessive supplementation may also produce excess stomach acid due to the stimulation of gastric secretions, and it has also been implicated in the development of kidney stones. Calcium carbonate can reduce the absorption of such medications as aspirin, tetracycline, the antihypertensive atenolol (Tenormin), and iron sulfate if the supplement and the medication are consumed together. Antacids containing both calcium carbonate and aluminum will actually block calcium absorption.

Calcium citrate contains a smaller percentage of calcium, about 24 percent. The compound does not require hydrochloric acid for dissolution, making it more suitable for those lacking this component of gastric juice. This condition, known as achlorhydria, is relatively common in the elderly.

In addition to their potential for causing gastrointestinal problems, other evidence makes the use of calcium supplements of questionable value. Supplements alone appear to have little effect in reversing postmenopausal bone-mineral loss. They may slow the loss of compact bone but are ineffective in staving off trabecular bone loss. In addition, preparations that also contain vitamin D can cause a toxic buildup of this fat-soluble vitamin if taken in excess. Bone meal and dolomite—both of which contain calcium and are relatively inexpensive—may contain toxins such as lead, and they should be avoided.

Exercise and Osteoporosis

Although no direct evidence exists to show that regular exercise can reduce the risk of osteoporosis-related fractures, vigorous physical activity is the only way to strengthen bones without medication once growth has stopped. Weight-bearing exercise, including running, walking, and tennis, creates stress on bones and tends to make them stronger. Exercise also stimulates the production of hormones that help protect bones, and it generates electrical currents within bone to stimulate growth and repair. In addition, exercise increases the flow of blood to the bones.

Drug Therapy

Estrogen-replacement therapy (ERT). After the onset of menopause, estrogen-replacement therapy has been shown to help prevent bone loss. The estrogen dose necessary to forestall osteoporosis, control hot flashes, and prevent other symptoms associated with menopause is low—much less than that used in birth-control pills, for example. In the past, there has been concern that estrogen replacement increased the risk of endometrial and other cancers, but new approaches to giving the estrogen in combination with progesterone reduce this risk.

Fluoride. This mineral, which is added to drinking water to help prevent dental disease, gives teeth and bones hardness. Some researchers believe that fluoride supplements can help improve skeletal integrity, and clinical studies have found that giving oral sodium fluoride with calcium has brought about some increase in bone mass. However, in large doses, fluoride can cause joint pain, swelling, and digestive problems. In addition, fluoride stimulates the formulation of abnormal bone, which may be prone to stress fracturing. Moderation is the key to fluoride use.

Calcitonin. Calcitonin is a drug that decreases the resorption of bone and enhances calcium retention by the body. It must be taken by injection and is expensive.

Detecting Osteoporosis

There are many methods for detecting osteoporosis, but most are not conclusive until considerable bone thinning has taken place. Most signs of osteoporosis appear so gradually that they are hardly noticeable; others, such as fractures, occur suddenly and usually indicate advanced disease.

The most basic detection method is self-observation. For example, a change in the fit of clothing, especially from one season to the next, may reflect changes in the spine. Reduced height, due to collapsed vertebrae, is a common sign of osteoporosis. Sometimes women lose as much as six to eight inches in a relatively short time.

A number of tests may be used to detect osteoporosis. These include the following.

Blood and urine tests. Blood tests given to people with osteoporosis will usually show normal levels of calcium, phosphorus, and alkaline phosphatase (an enzyme that reflects bone repair and that rises in conditions of rapid bone turnover). The urine-calcium level is usually normal, but it may be increased if there is very rapid bone turnover. Excretion of calcium can occur even though the skeletal needs have not been met.

X rays. Standard X rays are ineffective in detecting early osteoporosis: Bones appear relatively normal on X rays until 25 to 40 percent of their calcium is lost. However, more sophisticated testing employing radiation may provide earlier indication of loss in bone density, reflecting loss of mineral content. Tests that measure only cortical bone density or do not differentiate cortical from trabecular bone loss are generally felt to be less accurate than those that measure both cortical and trabecular bone. The following bone-density studies vary in cost, amount of radiation to which the patient is exposed, and precision of readings.

Single-photon absorptiometry uses a radioactive beam to detect only cortical bone loss in the wrist end of the radius bone of the forearm and in the heel bone. The presence of little tissue near the bone helps maintain accuracy in the readings. The cost of the test ranges from about $40 to $120.

The accuracy of evaluating bone integrity increases with *dual-energy absorptiometry,* which better distinguishes calcium from adjacent soft tissue. This technique measures the bone density of the spine and the thighbone near the hip joint but does not distinguish cortical from trabecular. Radiation exposure is greater than for single-photon absorptiometry but is still less than for a chest X ray. The cost, between $75 and $200, and limited availability prevents its widespread use.

Quantitative computed tomography provides a more accurate picture of trabecular bone density and is probably the most accurate measure of bone mineralization currently available. The technique provides a computerized image of a cross-section of bone. However, the procedure involves the greatest radiation exposure, costs from $150 to $300, and is not widely available.

X-ray densitometry is a new technique that should make osteoporosis screening more available. It is very accurate and relatively easy to perform.

Bone biopsy. The bone biopsy for osteoporosis is one of the few new techniques for analyzing bone integrity. Although effective, the equipment and competently trained personnel needed are few in number, so the test is not yet widely available.

Sites Commonly Affected by Osteoporosis

Osteoporosis usually appears at one of four sites, three of which result in bone fractures. The combination of less bone density and greater frequency of falls among the elderly makes osteoporosis a particularly serious condition. (Poor eyesight and medications that disturb balance, cause dizziness, or affect depth perception contribute to falls.)

Hip joint. The National Osteoporosis Foundation estimates that osteoporosis is responsible for 185,000 hip fractures each year. Studies show that about 15 percent more hip-fracture patients die within one year of injury than would be expected for the same age group as a whole. This is partially due to the consequences of immobility following surgery, which include pneumonia, development of blood clots that may travel to the lungs, and bedsores. (Awareness of the dangers of immobility has resulted in physicians getting hospitalized patients out of bed as soon as possible.)

Vertebrae. Occurring more frequently in women, vertebral fractures are common because the spine is primarily trabecular bone with only a thin outer cortical layer. The vertebrae most often affected are those corresponding to the level of the lower chest, waist, and upper hip. A fracture can occur spontaneously, or may even be provoked by a sneeze, and usually little discomfort follows the initial sharp pain. With repeated fracturing, the vertebrae collapse and become compressed, resulting in a shortened stature, curvature of the spine, and pronounced rounding of the back, known as "dowager's hump." If the fractures lead to pain during breathing, the individual may avoid normal deep breathing or coughing, and thereby may develop a lung infection. When the vertebrae in the abdominal region fracture, constipation and bloating can result.

Wrist. Fractures of the end of the radius just above the wrist (Colles' fracture) occasionally result in long-term inability to perform household tasks, perform hygiene, and other activities of daily living.

Jaw. Early signs of osteoporosis are loosening of teeth and a need for frequent replacement of dentures, due to bone loss and receding of the jawbone.

Rickets

Rickets is a metabolic disease of growing children, caused by defective calcification of the bones. Three types of rickets have been identified. The first, nutritional rickets, which can occur at any age, is caused by a diet deficient in vitamin D. Due to improved nutrition in general and vitamin D—fortified dairy products in particular, nutritional rickets has nearly disappeared from the United States. In developing countries, where nutrition is poor and children are often confined indoors to escape the sun and heat, it is more common. Children who are breastfed long after birth without nutritional supplementation or who have been fed a strict vegetarian diet are also at greater risk for developing nutritional rickets.

The second type, vitamin D—dependent rickets, is caused by a metabolic abnormality that prevents the body's use of calcitriol, the active form of vitamin D. The third type, vitamin D—resistant rickets, appears to be genetically transmitted, as well. The defect has been traced to the tubules of the kidneys, where phosphorus is wasted, preventing the body from using calcium to lay down mineral and bone.

In children with rickets, cartilage of the epiphyses enlarges because new cartilage cells continue to be produced but do not become calcified. Additional unmineralized bone accumulates around the bone shaft. The excess growth of cartilage also occurs at the epiphyseal disk.

Symptoms of Rickets

Children with rickets show the characteristic enlarged epiphyses, especially knobby, enlarged knees. They begin walking at a later-than-normal age, and may experience pain, bowed legs, and knock-knees if the disease is severe. The effects on the spinal column can cause rounding of the back and displacement of the spine from the center of the back.

Infants with rickets have abnormally soft skulls, are restless, and have poor sleeping patterns. In later infancy, sitting up and crawling are delayed. The fontanelles (open spaces at the top of the skull to allow for brain growth) are slow in closing, and the skull itself protrudes forward. Beadlike swellings of each rib and its cartilaginous end appear along the breastbone, known as rachitic rosary.

Diagnosis and Treatment

Blood and urine testing can detect rickets before symptoms become acute. People with nutritional or vitamin D—dependent rickets have decreased blood calcium and phosphorus. Treatment with vitamin D therapy can bring about improvement in as little as two days. Calcification begins, a normal blood supply is established, and unmineralized bone ceases to accumulate around the bone shaft. With long-term nutritional therapy, the child can develop a nearly normal skeleton.

Vitamin D—resistant rickets is characterized by low blood phosphorus and decreased reabsorption of phosphate in the kidneys. The calcium level is normal in the blood. Large doses of phosphate and calcitriol supplementation are given as therapy.

Osteomalacia

Osteomalacia, the adult form of rickets, is an abnormality in the mineralization of the bones and it decreases bone density. The spine, pelvis, and lower limbs are most often affected, leading to bone pain and difficulty in walking. Over time, the long bones may bow, the vertebrae may shorten vertically, and the pubic bones can flatten. Osteomalacia may be caused directly by a deficiency of vitamin D in the diet (or lack of exposure to sunlight), or indirectly by conditions interfering with vitamin D absorption or use. Diseases affecting fat absorption (vitamin D is fat-soluble) and liver and kidney disease that interfere with the conversion of the vitamin to its active form are some of the causes.

In osteomalacia, low blood levels of calcium and phosphate (calcium may be normal in some cases) result in a failure of the osteoblasts to calcify bone. Because the process of bone turnover continues to remove already-formed bone, the skeleton softens.

Correcting osteomalacia usually requires far more than a balanced diet. Vitamin D therapy is the most common method of treatment, but it is effective only if the calcium and phosphorus intake is adequate and normal. If the production of calcitriol in the kidneys or calcidiol in the liver is impaired, synthetic forms of these compounds may be prescribed to ensure adequate calcium reabsorption.

35

Nutrition and Arthritis

Harry Spiera, M.D., Leslie D. Kerr, M.D., and Ts'ai-fan Yu, M.D.

■

INTRODUCTION

About one in every seven Americans has arthritis, one of the most widely misunderstood of ailments. Arthritis means joint inflammation (from the Greek *arth*, meaning joint, and *itis*, meaning inflammation). Contrary to popular belief, arthritis is not a single disease; rather, it is a characteristic of over 100 disorders that are lumped together as rheumatic diseases. Besides the joints, these diseases may affect the skin, the tissue surrounding the joints, the muscles, and, in some forms of arthritis, almost every organ in the body.

Although there are many different kinds of arthritis, most forms are characterized by inflamed joints that become painful, stiff, swollen, red, and hot to the touch. In some kinds of arthritis, however, patients may experience pain in the joints without noticeable inflammation and may simply feel weak and run-down.

Most forms of arthritis are intermittent. Symptoms may appear and disappear spontaneously without warning. Symptomatic periods are called flare-ups; asymptomatic ones are called remissions. Both may last for days, months, or even years.

In most rheumatic diseases, one or more joints are affected. A joint is any place where bones meet. The ends of bones are covered by cartilage, a tough elastic tissue that reduces friction between the bones. The joint is contained in a saclike structure with an inner membrane called the synovial lining, which produces the synovial fluid that lubricates the joint.

INFLAMMATION

Inflammation accompanies many disorders in addition to arthritis. The inflammatory process normally occurs to protect and repair tissue damaged by sports injuries, infections, wounds, and other assaults. Once the cause is resolved, inflammation generally subsides.

In most forms of arthritis, however, the inflammatory process goes out of control, leading to further tissue damage rather than repair. No one knows what events trigger and perpetuate the inflammation caused by most forms of arthritis.

Inflammation is caused by the accumulation of fluid and cells in response to a triggering stimulus. In an inflammatory reaction, white blood cells rush from the bloodstream into the affected tissue, releasing enzymes and other chemicals that affect the nearby cells and modify blood flow in the area. Some of the chemicals secreted by white blood cells are toxic, intended to kill bacteria in the event of an infection. However, they can also harm nearby cells. Other chemicals released by the white blood cells, which include prostaglandins and leukotrienes, stimulate cells in the vicinity to release destructive enzymes and other substances into the inflamed area. They also increase the flow of fluids and white blood cells from small blood vessels into the area surrounding the inflammation, attracting new white blood cells to the inflamed area, which release most prostaglandins and leukotrienes in a vicious circle.

Much research is being done on inflammation and, in particular, the role prostaglandins and leukotrienes play. Studies have shown that some kinds of prostaglandins and leukotrienes intensify the inflammatory process, while others slow it down. Future treatment may, therefore, involve a procedure that would promote the production of the less inflammatory prostaglandins and leukotrienes.

DIET AND ARTHRITIS

The possible association between diet and arthritis is still another area of nutrition in which there is considerable controversy. In most forms of the disease, there is very little evidence to support claims that following a special diet can either cure the disease or alleviate its painful symptoms. Nevertheless, each year Americans spend hundreds of millions of dollars on questionable treatments—including diets—for arthritis. Without exception, these diets, often alleged to cure arthritis, are questionable. In fact, some are dangerous because they exclude necessary nutrients.

Among the many forms of arthritis, scientists have established very tentative links between diet and only three kinds of arthritis: rheumatoid arthritis, osteoarthritis, and gout. Gout is the only one of these diseases for which a special diet is occasionally recommended.

The Placebo Effect

Although research has not established a dietary treatment for arthritis, there are nu-

Figure 35.1.   Joint with Rheumatoid Arthritis

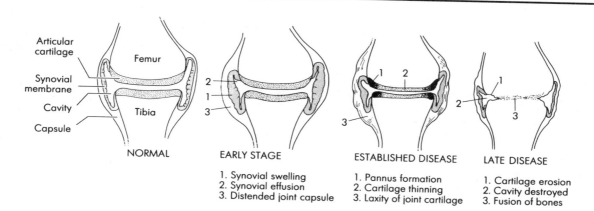

Articular cartilage
Synovial membrane
Cavity
Capsule
Femur
Tibia

NORMAL

EARLY STAGE
1. Synovial swelling
2. Synovial effusion
3. Distended joint capsule

ESTABLISHED DISEASE
1. Pannus formation
2. Cartilage thinning
3. Laxity of joint cartilage

LATE DISEASE
1. Cartilage erosion
2. Cavity destroyed
3. Fusion of bones

merous patients and practitioners alike who claim that diet is helpful. In fact, most of us have encountered patients who claim that their disease improved after eliminating a particular food or following a specific diet. Many factors may account for an individual's perceived improvement after following a popular diet, with the placebo effect being one of the most common and best documented. A placebo is a sham treatment that brings about improvement.

Similarly, a certain number of patients given a sugar pill or other placebo treatment will experience improvement of their medical conditions. This has been repeatedly demonstrated in controlled scientific studies comparing various approaches to treatment. Typically, the study volunteers are divided randomly into treatment and placebo groups. The patients are not told whether they are receiving a medication or a placebo (the researchers generally do not know either, until the code is broken at the end of the study). Invariably, people in the placebo group will show some improvement. The treatment is not considered effective unless there is more improvement in the medication group than in the placebo group.

In this regard, several popular arthritis diets have been studied. In one study, for example, patients were given a widely publicized diet, consisting of little meat except fish and occasional poultry, no fruit, dairy products, alcoholic beverages, additives, preservatives, herbs, or spices. Another set of patients served as the control group and received a placebo diet (i.e., disguised meat, fruit, etc). Neither the patients nor the researchers knew who was on which diet. Differences in improvement between the two sets of patients were negligible, thereby demonstrating that modifying the diet had no discernible effect on the patients' symptoms.

We know why people respond to placebos. The patient's belief that a pill or diet will help sets in motion a psychological response with very real physical consequences. A patient will often feel better even though intrinsically the treatment has no therapeutic value.

The natural intermittent nature of many forms of arthritis also may give false credence to worthless arthritis remedies. If the treatment is administered at about the same time that the disease is going into a remission period, the improvement may mistakenly be attributed to the therapy rather than to the natural course of the arthritis. Coincidence is misperceived as cause and effect.

In some instances, the person who attributes an arthritis cure to a particular diet or other therapy may never have had arthritis at all, but instead may have had a strain, sprain, or other temporary problem. Should the problem and its subsequent disappearance coincide with a dietary treatment, the person would likely attribute the cure to the diet rather than to the natural healing process.

Arthritis, unfortunately, lends itself to the kind of commercial quackery that abounds. Since there is no cure for arthritis, and the prognosis patients get from their doctors is uncertain, many become desperate in their search for a magical cure. Patients, often in extreme pain, suspend their critical judgment and seek what are touted as panaceas. A major danger in resorting to panaceas is that they can delay prompt medical evaluation and initiation of responsible treatment to ease symptoms and prevent deformities and other consequences of arthritis. (See How to Spot Questionable Remedies on page 592, as well as Chapter 3.)

COMMON TYPES OF ARTHRITIS

Rheumatoid Arthritis

Rheumatoid arthritis afflicts over 2 million Americans, approximately two-thirds of them women. It is one of the more severe forms of arthritis, often resulting in permanent joint damage and disability in addition to pain, stiffness, and swelling. Unlike osteoarthritis, rheumatoid arthritis is a systemic disease that can affect many parts of the body in addition to the joints. The disease usually begins in midlife, although children can develop a form known as juvenile rheumatoid arthritis.

Scientists have not yet determined whether rheumatoid arthritis is a single, unique disease or a syndrome reflecting a number of causes that produce similar symptoms. Heredity, abnormal immune response, and environmental factors may all play a role.

The primary sign of rheumatoid arthritis is inflammation, usually beginning in the synovial membrane of the joints. A tongue of inflammatory cells, known as a pannus, forms at junctions of the cartilage and the membrane. This pannus eventually extends between the two cartilage surfaces of the joint and erodes the cartilage and the underlying bone. The supporting tendons and ligaments often become weakened, making the joint unstable. The resulting dislocation can lead to deformity, which makes movement difficult.

Most people with rheumatoid arthritis experience tenderness, morning stiffness, fatigue, and achiness. Muscle stiffness occurs usually after long periods of resting or sitting. The affected joints—most often those of the hands, knees, and feet—become swollen, warm, and painful, usually in a symmetrical pattern. Thus, if the finger joints of one hand are affected, the same joints on the other hand usually will become diseased, too. The inflammation may spread to tissues in other parts of the body, causing a wide variety of symptoms. Patients commonly feel fatigued and lose their appetites and, consequently, some weight. Anemia and low-grade fever also may be present.

The Role of Diet

Most of the experiments to determine whether there are any links between diet and rheumatoid arthritis have yielded negative results, establishing no real links, or inconsistent ones at best. However, lately there have been some promising discoveries.

Fish oil. A few preliminary, short-term studies have shown that the fish-oil equivalent to that found in approximately one-half pound of fish a day may alleviate some of the symptoms of rheumatoid arthritis. In one study, researchers compared rheumatoid-arthritis patients following a diet high in polyunsaturated fats and including a supplement of 10 fish-oil capsules daily to another group on a diet high in saturated fats and including a placebo-capsule supplement. Both groups were also taking medication to relieve symptoms. Compared to the control group, those taking the fish-oil capsules showed a significant decrease in morning stiffness and joint tenderness during the 12-week study. The effects were transient, however, and symptoms returned to prestudy levels when the patients went off the experimental diet. Other studies comparing patients receiving fish oil to those following their customary diets also showed significant improvements in the groups taking fish oil.

It is not clear how fish oil works in relieving inflammation, but there is evidence it is related to the formation of prostaglandins and other body chemicals that play a role in inflammation. Fatty acids are used to form prostaglandins, and fish oil is particularly rich in a fatty acid known as EPA. Researchers theorize that EPA may lead to production of forms of prostaglandins and other body chemicals that

are less active in inflammation than those produced from either polyunsaturated or saturated fats.

How to Spot Questionable Remedies*

The following list compiled by the Arthritis Foundation gives tips to spot questionable arthritis remedies. You can spot a questionable remedy by looking for answers to the three questions listed here. If you check one or more of the items listed beneath each of the questions, you should suspect a questionable remedy. Before trying a remedy, check with your doctor or the local Arthritis Foundation.

1. Is it likely to work for me? Fake treatment:

- WORKS FOR ALL TYPES OF ARTHRITIS. There are over 100 types of arthritis and treatments vary for each kind. If you hear about a treatment that works for arthritis, ask what kind of arthritis the people in the study had. If it ''works for all,'' don't believe it.

- USES CASE HISTORIES AND TESTIMONIALS. Scientists use large numbers of people for studies, repeat these studies, and use statistical tests to show that the results are not due to chance or to the placebo effect. Ethical scientists do not reveal the names of people involved in any test of a treatment.

- CITES ONLY ONE STUDY. Usually, a number of scientists must repeat the same study and get similar results in order to prove that the treatment works.

- CITES A STUDY WITHOUT A CONTROL GROUP. The use of control groups—a group of people compared to the experimental group receiving the new treatment—helps show that the results of a test are due to the new treatment and not to some other factor.

2. How safe is it? What are the side effects?

- COMES WITHOUT DIRECTIONS FOR USE.

- DOES NOT LIST CONTENTS. The list of contents should be on the label.

- HAS NO WARNINGS ABOUT SIDE EFFECTS. There should be warnings on the label or instructions stating who should *not* use the treatment.

- DESCRIBED AS HARMLESS OR NATURAL. Natural does not always mean harmless; for example, snake venom is natural but can be harmful.

3. How is it promoted?

Promoters of fake remedies often use the media—television and radio news or talk shows, newspapers, and magazines—books, direct mail, and franchised and door-to-door sales. They make oral claims.

- BASED ON A SECRET FORMULA. Scientists share their discoveries so that other experts can review and question their results. A claim that only its inventor knows about a new discovery signals a fake remedy.

- CLAIMS IT CURES ARTHRITIS. There are many different types of arthritis and it's unlikely that one treatment will help them all. If there's a major new advance in treating arthritis, many people, including your doctor, will know about it.

- AVAILABLE ONLY FROM ONE SOURCE. Treatments for arthritis are available from many different providers of medical care, not just a single person or company.

- PROMOTED ONLY IN THE MEDIA, BOOKS, OR BY MAIL ORDER. Research on new treatments will appear first in medical journals that are read by experts in arthritis care.

*Adapted with permission from the Arthritis Foundation.

It should be noted that the benefits of fish oil are not yet unequivocally demonstrated and the use of supplements is not recommended unless they are taken under a doctor's supervision. Some supplements are high in cholesterol and vitamins A, D, and K, which may accumulate to toxic levels when taken in large amounts. (See chapters 6 and 7.) Large amounts of fish oil also can thin the blood and promote bleeding problems, including an increased risk of hemorrhagic stroke in susceptible people.

Until more is clear, the best advice regarding fish oil and arthritis would be the same as for people with heart disease or artherosclerosis: Include two or three servings of fish—especially salmon, cod, and other fatty cold-water fish—in the diet each week, but do not take supplements unless specifically prescribed by a doctor.

Elimination diets. Advocates of elimination diets allege that rheumatoid arthritis can be treated by avoiding certain foods in the diet. Such diets entail fasting for as long as 10 days, after which time foods are added to the diet one at a time to determine which *may* have an effect on the disease. Although studies show that there are no foods that consistently precipitate arthritis, there are a few patients whose symptoms appear to worsen in relation to certain foods. Contrary to media reports that have indicted specific foods—for example, tomatoes, broccoli, and certain other vegetables—studies have failed to identify any pattern or consistency in the foods or types of foods that may provoke a flare-up of symptoms.

Rheumatoid arthritis is not completely understood and researchers speculate that those few patients whose symptoms are relieved when certain foods are avoided may actually have an "allergic" arthritis that is different from rheumatoid arthritis. Because of the unpredictable flare-ups and remissions of arthritis, patients may mistakenly attribute worsening—or improvement—to a purely coincidental change in diet. If consuming a particular food or class of foods is invariably followed by a worsening of symptoms, it makes sense to eliminate these items from the diet. Common sense is needed, however, when it comes to eliminating foods. There is little danger in eliminating only one kind of food from a diet. When broad categories of food, such as all dairy products or grains are eliminated, however, dietary imbalances may result. Therefore, elimination diets should be structured only with the help of a dietition or physician knowledgeable about nutrition.

Anemia and Rheumatoid Arthritis

In the past, iron supplements often were recommended to treat the anemia that frequently occurs in any chronic inflammatory disease. However, anemia may have many causes besides iron deficiency. While it is not clear what causes the anemia of rheumatoid arthritis, there is evidence that there is a defect in the release of iron from cells that transport it in the blood. This kind of anemia can be remedied only by directly treating the inflammatory disease. Injectable iron supplements should be avoided because they may actually worsen the symptoms. Studies have shown that an increase in symptoms often began one day after supplementation and lasted for up to seven days. Because of these findings, anyone suffering from rheumatoid arthritis should consult a physician before taking injectable iron supplements. Iron-rich foods or oral iron supplements, consumed in moderation, pose no problem for some, but do for others.

Patients who are taking large doses of aspirin or other anti-inflammatory drugs may have bleeding from the gastrointestinal tract as a side effect. Since the blood loss creates a true iron-deficiency anemia, supplements may be prescribed for these individuals.

Osteoporosis and Rheumatoid Arthritis

Several factors increase the risk of osteoporosis—the thinning of bones commonly seen among older people, especially women—for patients with rheumatoid arthritis. Some of the drugs used to treat inflammation, particularly corticosteroids, contribute to bone loss. Regular exercise, especially bearing a weight on weight-bearing bones, is important in maintaining strong bones—and people with rheumatoid arthritis may become sedentary because of their disease. (See Chapter 34.)

Osteoarthritis

Osteoarthritis, also known as degenerative joint disease, is the most common form of arthritis. It involves a breakdown of the joint cartilage. It is often associated with aging, but in reality, it frequently begins at an early age. The causes are unknown, but there is evidence that it has a hereditary component.

Although osteoarthritis can cause joint pain and stiffness, for the majority of patients, the symptoms are not severe enough to cause disability. Frequently, osteoarthritis is related to stress and strain. Weight-bearing joints—the knees, hips, and ankles—are commonly affected. As might be expected, people who are overweight are particularly vulnerable to arthritis in these joints. Golfers, tennis players, and baseball players often develop arthritis in their shoulders or elbows. Typists and pianists may develop arthritis in their fingers. (This should not be confused with Heberden's nodes—a type of osteoarthritis that develops in the last finger joint, forming knobs that start out inflamed and painful, then become painless, although they persist.

Generally, the symptoms of osteoarthritis are not severe enough to seriously limit activity. Typically, joint pain and stiffness increase with use; for example, a person may have little difficulty moving around early in the day but will have more pain as the day progresses.

In addition to joint cartilage, osteoarthritis affects the bone and joint or synovium. Initially, the smooth cartilage surface softens, then becomes pitted and thinned. The cartilage loses its elasticity and is more vulnerable to stress. The destruction of cartilage leaves bone ends exposed, increasing wear and tear on the joint. In response, new and irregular bony tissue known as spurs, or osteophytes, forms. Movement becomes painful in the joint as the normal gliding surfaces erode, and loose pieces of bone and cartilage irritate the joint lining (synovium) and cause inflammation.

Traditionally, osteoarthritis was believed to be a result of normal stress on joints. In fact, there is evidence that some people are born with defective cartilage, or with slight defects in the way their joints fit together or move. However, studies also indicate that many people whose joints align properly and who have not been exposed to excessive stress also develop osteoarthritis.

A possible aggravating factor may be obesity. The more weight the joints have to carry, the greater the physical stress on them. Those who are overweight should follow a low-calorie diet until desirable weight, or as close as possible, is reached. (See Chapter 17.)

The Special Case of Gout *

Gouty arthritis is an inherited metabolic disorder characterized by a buildup of uric acid. Less commonly, gout may be caused by

*This section on gout was written by Ts'ai-fan Yu, M.D.

medications, especially some of the drugs used to treat high blood pressure.

As a waste product derived from the breakdown of purines and proteins, uric acid is excreted chiefly through the kidneys. When the body produces more uric acid than it excretes, it accumulates in the blood, a condition known as hyperuricemia. (A person can have hyperuricemia with no gout, but the reverse rarely occurs.) The excess uric acid cannot be completely dissolved in the blood and is deposited as uric acid crystals around the joints, causing acute inflammation or forming deposits called tophi. These crystals are visible under a microscope; they stick into tissue, causing the pain of gout. People with gout may produce too much purine or have another impairment of the metabolism. Purines in food are only one source; uric acid is also produced by the body.

Gout usually develops first in only one joint, typically the base of the big toe (the first metatarso-phalangeal joint). This condition is called podagra. At later attacks, it may also affect other joints of the foot, as well as the knee, elbow, wrist, and fingers. It rarely affects the spine or the pelvis.

Gout has been known for years as the rich man's disease. The disease most commonly affects men, who usually develop a first attack between the ages of 40 and 50. Women, who account for fewer than 10 percent of gout patients, rarely develop the disease before menopause.

The acute symptoms of gout are easily recognizable: swelling of the joint, warmth, and a shiny red or purple appearance of the skin around the joint. The pain can be excruciating; even the pressure of a sheet on the joint can cause extreme pain. Wearing a regular shoe can be impossible; many gout sufferers resort to cutting away the portion that fits over the affected joint or wearing open-toed sandals during an attack.

Attacks usually occur suddenly, without any warning, and may last for several days. Initially, attacks are sporadic and patients have no symptoms during periods of remission. If the disease is not controlled through diet or medication, the attacks may eventually occur more frequently and last longer. Excessive alcohol consumption, foods high in purines, an extreme low-calorie diet, injury to a joint, stress, or surgery may trigger an attack of gout.

In addition to periodic acute attacks of gout, uric-acid crystals may accumulate and form lumps under the skin, usually on the outer edge of the ear, over the elbow, or in the affected joints and the surrounding tissue. If these lumps, known as tophi, are not treated, they may break through the skin and become infected. Tophi usually do not appear until gout has been present for several years. However, in gout, secondary to blood dis-

Foods Gout Patients Should Avoid

1. Liver, sweetbreads, brains, kidneys, anchovies, sardines

2. Smoked, pickled, cured, canned, or frozen meat and fish

3. All meat extracts, gravies, and broths

4. Dried beans (lima, kidney, navy), lentils, peas, asparagus, and frozen and canned vegetables

5. Alcoholic beverages

6. Dry cereals, except puffed rice, puffed wheat, and shredded wheat

7. Dried fruits, except prunes

8. Pastries, cookies, and cakes made with salt and baking powder

9. Salt, sauces, gravies, mustard, pickles, condiments, olives, catsup, and salted foods

eases, tophi may be found during or even prior to the first gouty attack. Gout patients who excrete very acid urine or pass large amounts of uric acid in small volume may develop uric-acid kidney stones.

Unlike most other forms of arthritis, gout can be controlled completely with the proper treatment. Through the use of drugs and diet, the swelling and pain associated with the disease will disappear. Before the development

Table 35.1. The Mount Sinai Hospital Modified Gout Diet (Low-Sodium)*

Include in Each Day's Diet:

Milk	1 pint or less
Meat†	4 ounces
Cheese	1 ounce of salt-free pot cheese only
Egg	1 only
Bread	6 slices or less of salt-free or matzoh only
Cereal	½ cup or less
Potato or substitute	1 portion
Vegetable	3 portions or more
Fruit or fruit juices	As desired
Jam or sugar	4 teaspoons or less
Butter	2 teaspoons or less of sweet butter only
Coffee or tea	As desired

Meat Portions (4 ounces) Selected from the Following:

Chicken	1 medium breast or leg
Roast beef	1 medium slice
Roast veal	1 medium slice
Roast lamb	1 medium slice
Chops:	
Lamb	2 medium rib or 1 shoulder
Veal	1 loin (½" thick)
Veal cutlet	1 piece 5" × 2½" × ½"

Nutrient and Calorie Content of Gout Diet

Food	Amount	Carbohydrate (grams)	Protein (grams)	Fat (grams)	Calories
Skim milk	2 glasses	26	18	0	176
Meat or fish	3–4 oz.	0	28	12	220
Egg or	1	0	6	6	78
cottage cheese	1 oz.	4	20	1	105
Bread	3 slices	50	9	3	263
Cereal	1½ oz.	38	6	1	185
Vegetables, raw or cooked with	3 portions	25	0	0	100
vegetable oil	1 oz.	0	0	30	270
Fruits, fresh	3 portions	75	0	0	300
Fruit juice	3 portions	75	0	0	300
Margarine	⅓ oz.	0	0	10	90
Coffee or tea	2 cups	0	0	0	0
Sugar	1 t	4	0	0	16

*This diet gives approximately 1,900 to 2,000 calories, carbohydrates 58 percent, protein 14 to 16 percent, and fat 26 to 28 percent.
†Meat, fish, and fowl are interchangeable.

Reprinted with permission from the *Mount Sinai Medical Center Diet Manual*, 9th edition, 1988.

of medications to treat gout, a restrictive diet was the principal form of treatment. Today, diet often serves as an important supplemental therapy and as an alternative form of treatment for those who have problems with medications.

Some patients may, at times, have hypersensitive reactions to antigout drugs, such as rash and itching and peeling of the skin, as well as gastric-intestinal upset with nausea or vomiting. Toxic effects from medication are most likely to occur in patients with kidney disease because of the decreased excretion of these medications. Under such circumstances, diet serves as an important form of therapy.

Although medications have reduced dietary limitations, all gout patients should eat only a moderate amount of protein and avoid high-purine foods—which include organ meats such as kidneys, liver, and sweetbreads, as well as sardines, anchovies, shrimp, mackerel, dried legumes, and meat extracts.

The consumption of caffeinated beverages is no longer restricted. (At one time, caffeine was erroneously thought to break down to uric acid.) Excessive alcohol consumption results in the accumulation of lactic acid, which inhibits renal secretion of uric acid and may precipitate acute attacks of gouty arthritis. Therefore, alcohol should be avoided or used only in moderation. (For a list of foods for gout patients to avoid, see page 595.)

When gout is associated with other conditions—obesity, hypertension, coronary heart disease, or high blood lipids—it may require a change in diet. Weight reduction is recommended for obese gout patients to ensure satisfactory control of hyperuricemia and other complications such as high blood lipids or high blood sugar. It is important that weight loss be slow and steady, because a rapid drop in weight can cause the accumulation of ketones, which results in increased uric acid in the blood.

If gout is associated with hypertension or coronary disease, a diet low in calories, cholesterol, saturated fats, and sodium is indicated. The degree of restriction depends on the severity of these complications. If diabetes is present, more attention should be directed to reducing the number of calories and the amount of fat and cholesterol in the diet. When an individual has kidney disease, more emphasis should be placed on consuming large quantities of vegetables and on reducing salt intake. (See Table 35.1 for the Mount Sinai Hospital Modified Gout Diet.)

Gout patients should drink at least two quarts of fluid each day. A large fluid intake helps dilute the uric acid in urine, thus preventing kidney stones. Certain vegetables and fruits may have an alkalinizing effect on the urine, which also helps to avoid the formation of uric acid stones.

In summary, an appropriate diet for gout should be relatively low in purines and fat, with moderate amounts of proteins. Since excessive caloric food intake raises the uric-acid level in the blood, the total daily intake should not exceed 30 calories per kilogram (2.2 pounds) of body weight. About 10 to 15 percent of the total calories should be supplied by proteins, 30 percent or less by fat, and the remainder by carbohydrates. (See Foods Gout Patients Should Avoid, page 595, and Table 35.1.)

LIVING WITH ARTHRITIS

As stressed earlier in this chapter, arthritis is a chronic disease that usually can be controlled but not cured. Living with arthritis can be trying, especially during periods when the disease is active. Rest and exercise are important in the overall management of the disease. There also are a number of medications that

Food Preparation Made Easier for People with Arthritis

Simple activities such as preparing and eating food can be both painful and difficult for those who suffer from arthritis. Different methods of food organization and special devices can minimize the pain. While preparing food, an individual should do the following.

Work and eat while seated. Standing puts great stress on the hips, legs, and feet.

Place ingredients within easy reach, and use special implements to avoid additional bending and stretching. Tongs can be used to obtain a plate from a shelf, an oven shovel to retrieve a dish from the oven, and long barbecue matches to light a gas oven.

Sit in a chair with good back and arm supports. This helps relieve stress on the back, elbows, and forearms; the arm supports also makes it easier to get up from the chair.

Use chairs with leg extenders or gliders. Chairs that have large caster rollers and push-down brakes minimize stress on the hips and knees when getting into and out of a chair. Extenders, which can be fitted to almost any type of furniture, often have wheels that facilitate moving around while seated.

Those who have arthritis in the arms or hands can help relieve stress by following these tips.

- Use large joints such as the wrists, instead of small joints such as the fingers to lift pans and other heavy objects.

- Use appliances, such as a can opener or a portable electric mixer, instead of muscles.

- Hold objects for as short a time as possible. Cookbooks can be placed on a stand.

- Stretch the fingers frequently to relax them.

- Secure food by placing it on a wooden cutting board into which nails have been pounded rather than by bracing it with the hands.

- Use both hands and arms when possible so that the weight is not concentrated on any one appendage.

- Slide or roll carts and other objects rather than lift them.

- Use lightweight utensils made of plastic and aluminum.

- Grasp objects by wrapping fingers completely around the handle, with the thumb extended to meet the fingers. If the fingers are bent or utensils slip between the fingers, stress is placed on the portion of the hand that is the weakest—that which contains the little finger.

Devices to Assist Eating

HOLDERS. When the grasp is weak or absent but the hand-to-mouth action is functional, eating utensils may be placed in a holder fitted to the hand. Good holders include a large elastic band that fits around the hand with a pocket in the palm piece or a slot made by sewing together two pieces of leather in which a fork or spoon handle can be inserted. Utensil holders that fit around two or more fingers may be helpful for grasp problems and allow eating in the thumbs-up position.

THICKENED HANDLES. For individuals who have difficulty grasping objects, the handle of a utensil can be thickened in various ways: by wrapping foam-rubber strips around it; by inserting the handle into the center space of large-sized foam rubber or plastic hair curlers; by attaching a file handle, for thickness as well as length.

LENGTHENED HANDLES. The handles of utensils may be lengthened and the direction of the tines of a fork or the bowl of a spoon can be altered for those with limited range of motion. Some long-handled utensils are collapsible; others have swivels that allow the individual with limited forearm rotation to keep the bowl of the spoon level.

PLATE GUARDS. Plate guards that attach to the side of the plate or scooped dishes and spoons allow food to be cornered rather than slipping around the dish. Plates can be secured on a table with a suction cup, adhesive tape, a wet washcloth, or by making a tray with cutout

can relieve symptoms and prevent deformity. Surgical repair and replacement of diseased joints with artificial ones are other treatment options.

In controlling a chronic disease such as arthritis, it is important to find a physician with whom you feel comfortable and who can give guidance both in treating the symptoms and in managing the practical aspects of day-to-day living. Sometimes a treatment team—a physician, physical therapist, dietitian, and perhaps a surgeon or other medical specialist—will be needed. Still, the primary physician and the patient are cocaptains of such a team and should be prepared to make decisions regarding the overall management of the disease. The material on pages 598–599 offers practical suggestions for day-to-day activities such as food preparation and eating. The Arthritis Foundation offers a number of pamphlets that discuss the different kinds of arthritis and give practical tips concerning them. At times, living with arthritis can be discouraging, but patients should remember that there are numerous approaches to treatment, as well as sources of help.

Food Preparation Made Easier for People with Arthritis (cont.)

or rimmed-in sections in which a plate can fit.

STRAWS. The grasping and lifting of glasses can be eliminated by using straws. The straw can be secured with a "bulldog clip": The straw fits through the clip, which is clamped to the glass.

LIGHTWEIGHT CONTAINERS. Special cups with large handles, as well as coasters and jackets that fit over cups or glasses, help patients who are able to grip a container. The surfaces of these jackets often have straw matting or some other rough surface that is free of moisture—to allow for a more secure grip.

36

The Effects of Nutrition on Skin and Hair

Susan Bershad, M.D.

■

INTRODUCTION

Skin, hair, and nails: Each can be a mirror of good health or, conversely, illness—and an outside marker of internal processes. Nutritional deficiency, disease, or stress may first be reflected here.

Skin is the largest organ of the body. Each square inch of the skin (the average person has between 17 and 20 square feet) contains blood vessels, sweat glands, and nerve endings that measure temperature, pain, touch, and pressure.

The skin has a number of vital functions. It protects underlying tissues from invasion by bacteria and other microorganisms, the sun's harmful rays, and toxic substances in the environment. In addition to keeping undesirable things out, skin keeps in moisture and chemicals needed for myriad reactions. Through nerve impulses transmitted to the brain, the skin protects the body from injury, as well as transmitting pleasurable sensation. In the presence of sunlight, skin plays an important role in the production of vitamin D. Skin is vital in regulating body temperature, its capillaries constricting in cold weather to conserve heat and dilating in warm weather to release

it. Perspiration evaporates, further cooling the body.

Like all organs of the body, the skin and its appendages, the hair and nails, receive their nutrition via the bloodstream from nutrients absorbed in the gastrointestinal tract. (The skin receives up to one-third of the blood circulating in the body.) Contrary to expensive advertising campaigns, skin must be nourished from the inside. Popularly touted skin "nutrients" such as the proteins collagen and elastin, oily materials, and most vitamins are not absorbed into cells of the skin. (Exceptions include some topical medications; for example, cortisone-type creams and a derivative of vitamin A called retinoic acid.)

SKIN STRUCTURE

The skin is made up of three layers: the epidermis, the dermis, and the subcutaneous layer, also called adipose tissue.

The epidermis. This is the outermost layer, which itself is composed of many layers. The deepest is the basal layer, where new cells are constantly being produced. As these move toward the surface and away from their source of nourishment—the blood vessels of the dermis—they become smaller and flatter. They reach the topmost layer—the stratum corneum—as dead protein (keratin), play a protective function for a short time, and are shed, usually imperceptibly. The whole process, which is known as keratinization, takes three to four weeks.

The basal layer also contains cells known as melanocytes, which produce melanin, the main pigment in the skin.

The dermis. It lies just beneath the epidermis and is the site of the production of collagen and elastin, protein fibers that give the skin its strength and flexibility and are made from amino acids supplied by the bloodstream. The dermis contains a rich network of blood vessels, many nerve endings, and three structures unique to the skin: the hair follicles, the sebaceous glands, and the sweat glands. The hair follicles manufacture another keratin substance: hair. The sebaceous glands are attached to the hair follicles and secrete through them an oily material (sebum) that lubricates

Figure 36.1. Structure/Layers of Skin

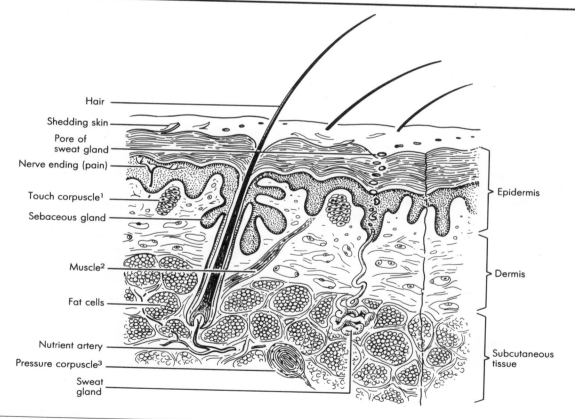

Notes: [1]Meissner; [2]Arrector pili muscle; [3]Racinian.

and protects both hair and skin. The sweat glands—distributed over the entire body, though more plentiful in some areas than in others—provide for temperature regulation through perspiration, made up of water, sodium chloride, potassium, and other substances also found in blood.

The subcutaneous layer. This consists largely of fat cells bound together by fibrous tissues. Fat protects and insulates the body. In addition, it can be converted into energy whenever the need for calories exceeds that supplied by the diet.

MALNUTRITION AND THE SKIN

The cells that produce skin and hair receive their nutrients from the underlying blood supply. A diet that is varied and well balanced will provide all the nutrients necessary for health and growth. Dietary supplementation is useful only when there is a deficiency of one or more essential nutrients.

Often the first signs of malnutrition are abnormalities of the skin, because deficiencies undermine its protective role or prevent synthesis of substances needed for normal growth and function. Where there is a major decrease in food intake or absorption—for example, because of food shortage, malabsorptive disease, or debilitating illness—many nutrients will be lacking and the skin will show signs of malnutrition. As well as revealing nutrient deficiencies, changes in the skin may be responsible for significant loss of nutrients. Severe burns and chronic diseases characterized by extensive scaling or blistering of the skin can result in loss of water, nitrogen, protein, magnesium, and other minerals.

NUTRITIONAL DEFICIENCIES AND THE SKIN

Specific skin problems are associated with severe deficiencies of the following nutrients.

Vitamin C (ascorbic acid). Perhaps the most familiar of all vitamin deficiencies is scurvy. It was first recognized in the mid-eighteenth century when British sailors were cured by the addition of oranges and limes, rich in vitamin C, to their diets. Scurvy causes a wide variety of symptoms. As it affects the skin, scurvy is characterized by poor wound healing and small purplish spots called petechiae, indicating bleeding below the surface. Scurvy also causes excess keratin in hair follicles, producing roughened bumps containing coiled hairs on the arms and legs. Inflammation of the gums is also found.

Vitamin B$_3$ (niacin). Pellagra, characterized by rough, scaly brown skin in areas of the body exposed to the sun, is the result of a niacin deficiency. Pellagra is uncommon today in this country, except among chronic alcoholics, who often suffer from multiple nutrient deficiencies. (Some forms of chemotherapy and a number of drugs—including certain antibiotics, anticonvulsants, and antidepressants—can interfere with niacin metabolism and may cause pellagra-like symptoms.) In addition to skin, the deficiency also affects mucous membranes, which become swollen and painful. The tongue becomes bright red and sometimes so sore that eating is difficult.

Vitamin A. Dietary deficiency of vitamin A is rare in industrialized countries, but digestive diseases or extensive gastrointestinal surgery can result in impaired absorption of this vitamin. Deficiency leads to reduced sebum production, clogged hair follicles, and excess keratin buildup, giving the skin a dry, rough, and scaly appearance.

Vitamin B₂ (riboflavin). Scaly, greasy red skin around the nose and mouth and on the ears and eyelids can be caused by a deficiency of this vitamin. Sebaceous material builds up in the hair follicles, giving the skin a roughened look. The tongue may be magenta-colored and the lips red and cracked.

Vitamin B₁₂. Deficiency is usually due to poor absorption of the vitamin as a result of diseases of the stomach or intestinal tract. In pernicious anemia, the lack of intrinsic factor needed for vitamin B_{12} absorption produces deficiency. With the exception of strict vegetarian diets containing no animal products, most diets contain adequate amounts of this nutrient. Deficiency causes the skin on the face, hands, and feet to turn a mottled brown, or a pale lemon yellow in pernicious anemia. The tongue may be bright red and painful.

Biotin. A deficiency of biotin produces scaling skin in both children and adults and hair loss in children. Uncooked egg whites contain a substance that prevents absorption of biotin and thus should be avoided.

Essential fatty acids. Deficiency of the three essential fatty acids is rare in people eating a normal diet. However, an extremely low-fat diet or long-term intravenous feeding lacking in these substances can cause scaly skin and hair loss. Supplementation with linoleic acid, found in vegetable oils, corrects the deficiency.

Protein. Extreme protein deficiency results in a condition called kwashiorkor. Seen mostly in children in underdeveloped countries, it is characterized by dry, wrinkly, flaky skin (sometimes called "enamel paint" dermatosis), hair thinning and loss of hair color in a bandlike pattern. A vicious cycle sets in: The protein deficiency produces scaly skin, and the loss of skin protein through scaling aggravates the deficiency.

Iron. Brittle nails with a flattened spoon shape are an early sign of iron deficiency, often preceding the pale skin associated with iron-deficiency anemia. Cracks may develop at the corners of the mouth and hair growth may be affected. Iron deficiency shows in blood tests long before symptoms of anemia develop. (See Chapter 29.)

Zinc. Severe zinc deficiency results in widespread peeling skin lesions—especially in skin creases and on the fingertips—and increasingly severe hair loss. In less extreme cases, the signs are subtle: dry skin, a scaly scalp, and hair loss so slight that it may go unnoticed.

NUTRITIONAL EXCESSES

Because vitamin deficiencies are proven to have harmful effects on the skin, it might seem to follow that vitamin supplements would be helpful in achieving or maintaining a healthy skin. However, except in cases of actual vitamin deficiency or in some rare inherited disorders, supplements of vitamins have no benefit. In fact, extra vitamins may be harmful to the skin as well as to other body systems. Excess vitamin A, for example, results in cracked lips and dry, scaly, itching skin—as well as headache, dizziness, double vision, and possible liver damage. Too much beta carotene (a precursor of vitamin A found in carrots and other orange and yellow fruits and vegetables) produces a generalized yellowing of the skin. An excess of nicotinic acid, which is a form of the vitamin niacin (sometimes prescribed to lower cholesterol), may cause chronic itching, facial flushing, and warmth; vitamin E can produce an allergic rash. Overdoses of vitamin D may result in intense itching as well as nausea, vomiting, and calcium deposits in the kidneys and other organs.

Overdoses of minerals likewise can be toxic, although symptoms often appear in organs other than the skin. Selenium, sometimes promoted by health-food faddists as a cancer preventive, can cause hair loss and fingernail abnormalities, and worse in megadoses.

SKIN PROBLEMS

Acne

Acne may appear in its mildest form—blackheads resulting from the blockage of sebaceous glands—or it may cover the face, back, and chest with inflamed pustules and cysts. The chief cause of acne is hereditary, but it is promoted by the rise in the levels of male hormones, known as androgens, that occurs in adolescents of both sexes. These hormones increase the size and secretory activity of the sebaceous glands. Although found primarily in teenagers, acne may appear later in life during times of hormonal upheaval such as pregnancy or stress. The use of oily cosmetics and moisturizers can aggravate the condition.

Although past medical—and popular—thinking held that chocolate, dairy products, and greasy foods played a role in the development or worsening of acne, research has not been able to demonstrate any clear cause-and-effect relationship between diet and acne. In studies on high school students, those who ate "junk" food did not have any higher incidence of acne than those who ate a more balanced diet. Attempts to establish a connection between chocolate and acne flare-ups have also failed. A possible explanation for the flare-ups that some acne sufferers may experi-

ence after eating certain foods is that stress is causing both a rise in hormone levels and the food craving. Despite the lack of scientific evidence of a diet/acne link, those who notice a worsening of the condition after eating certain foods might wish to avoid them.

Claims that skin conditions such as acne, hives, or eczema improve after certain dietary restrictions or additions are difficult to substantiate. Many skin conditions improve without treatment; it is difficult, therefore, to know whether or not dietary changes are beneficial.

One example of a rare diet/acne link is "kelp acne," an acnelike eruption precipitated by eating foods that are high in iodine—notably kelp, a type of seaweed sold in health-food stores as a dietary supplement.

Acne Treatments

In addition to gentle skin cleansing and topical application of products containing antibiotics or benzoyl peroxide, acne patients are sometimes treated with the oral antibiotic tetracycline. Because dairy products interfere with absorption of this medication, patients may be told to restrict intake. However, two or three glasses of milk may be taken daily if properly timed between doses of tetracycline.

Although there is no proof that dietary deficiencies of vitamin A or zinc cause acne, both nutrients have long been promoted as remedies. Although following the RDA for vitamin A will not help acne and megadoses are dangerous, derivatives of vitamin A are now being used successfully both topically and orally to treat severe cases of acne. Retinoic acid, or tretinoin (Retin-A), the topical form, seems to decrease the cohesiveness of the cells lining the follicles, thus making it less likely that they will become clogged. A common side effect of tretinoin is irritated, red, swollen skin. Animal studies have shown an increased risk of skin cancer from ultraviolet radiation combined with tretinoin, so those using the drug should limit their exposure to the sun.

Oral isotretinoin (Accutane), another vitamin A derivative, is effective in the majority of cases of severe acne. This medication may have potentially serious side effects, including liver abnormalities, visual problems, muscle and joint pain, and mildly increased cholesterol levels. These effects are reversible, usually disappearing within about three weeks after the drug is stopped. However, one study notes that prolonged use, which is not necessary for acne but that may be considered for certain rare and debilitating skin conditions, will, in some patients, cause a rise in LDL, or bad, cholesterol, and a decrease in HDL, or good, cholesterol, increasing the risk of heart disease. Accutane also causes birth defects and must never be used by pregnant women. Women should avoid attempting to become pregnant until at least one month after completing therapy.

Eczema

Eczema is an all-encompassing term, sometimes used synonymously with *dermatitis*, to describe inflamed, scaly, itching skin that may be due to any number of causes. Within this large group, individuals with atopic dermatitis, a condition that runs in families, may sometimes notice a worsening of the skin after eating certain foods, such as eggs or milk. Although skin testing using various foods may produce a reaction, this is not considered specific enough to establish any one element as a cause. Recent reports suggest a possible connection between atopic dermatitis and impairment in the skin's metabolism of the essential fatty acid linolenic acid. Patients with atopic dermatitis improved

when given supplements of evening-primrose oil, a rich source of gamma-linolenic acid. However, these results have not yet been confirmed in larger studies and are considered experimental. Vitamin and mineral supplements have not proven effective in treating atopic dermatitis.

Psoriasis

This common chronic skin condition is characterized by rapid turnover of epidermal cells. Keratinization may take as few as three days instead of the normal three to four weeks. The skin becomes thickened, red, and scaly, especially on the elbows, knees, and scalp.

The cause of this condition is unclear, but it is known that heredity plays a role. Factors such as stress, skin injury or irritation, or reactions to drugs may trigger eruptions. Because of occasional reports linking flare-ups of psoriasis to high protein intake, some patients have tried eliminating protein-rich foods, such as meat, fish, and eggs, from their diets. In general, this is ineffective; it simply deprives other tissues of needed protein. Diets high in zinc, lecithin, and a number of different vitamins have been promoted as remedies but are still questionable. Recent studies have shown high doses of a form of vitamin D to be effective in the treatment of psoriasis. However, this therapy is considered experimental, and individuals should not attempt self-treatment with vitamin D megadoses. At least one researcher has noted an improvement of psoriasis when fruits, milk, and coffee were eliminated from the diet. At this point, however, there are no studies to support such claims, and the elimination of food groups puts the individual at risk for nutrient deficiencies, with no clear benefit.

Psoriasis, like other conditions characterized by scaling skin, is helped by medications that are related to vitamin A. One of these, etretinate (Tegison), has been approved for the treatment of psoriasis. This medication must be given on a long-term basis and has similar side effects to those of isotretinoin.

Doctors may treat severe psoriasis not helped by other means with methotrexate, an anticancer drug, or exposure to ultraviolet radiation with or without the drug psoralens. Methotrexate, which slows down cell reproduction by depriving the cells of folic acid, may cause liver damage and lowered production of all blood cells. Ultraviolet-radiation therapy carries an increased risk of skin cancer.

Rosacea

This chronic hereditary condition is found primarily in people over thirty and is characterized by dilation of the facial capillaries, acnelike pimples, and, sometimes, thickened skin on the nose. Certain foods—such as tea, coffee, alcohol, and those that are spicy—are associated with worsening of rosacea. A recent study suggests that the heat in coffee or tea may be responsible. In addition to avoiding offending foods, tetracycline may be prescribed for skin eruptions. Topical antibiotics, particularly a gel containing the antiparasitic medication metronidazole (Metragel), are often effective in the treatment of rosacea.

Urticaria (Hives)

One out of five Americans is occasionally plagued by hives, medically known as urticaria, itchy welts resembling mosquito bites. Although a single hive may be due to an insect sting, multiple swellings often represent an allergic reaction to certain foods, food additives, or drugs. Stress, which leads to increased histamine release, can exacerbate hives. In response to the allergen, a chemical known as histamine is released and results in the swelling and itching. (Histamine is also responsible for hay-fever symptoms and a wide range of allergic reactions.)

Foods often associated with hives include eggs, wheat, nuts, chocolate, citrus fruits, tomatoes, strawberries, corn, shellfish, and pork. Some people react to the naturally occurring salicylates in almonds, apples, potatoes, or to the food dye tartrazine (yellow dye No. 5), found in some cheese-flavored snacks, artificial fruit drinks, and in the coating of some pills and vitamin supplements. Salicylates are also found in all aspirin-containing preparations.

Those who suspect food sensitivity as a cause of an outbreak of hives should keep a diary of what and when food is eaten and any reaction. If dietary changes are required, these should be planned with the assistance of a physician or dietitian in order to avoid nutrient deficiencies. (See Chapter 33).

Herpes

Cold sores and genital herpes are caused by the herpes simplex virus, although sun exposure, stress, or fever may precipitate attacks. Although the amino acid lysine has been touted as a treatment for herpes infections, there have been no controlled scientific studies supporting its efficacy. Today, treatment for herpes is either the oral or topical form of of the medication acyclovir (Zovirax). Vitamin C treatment appears both worthless and harmful.

THE HAIR AND NUTRITION

Hair Loss (Alopecia)

American society's emphasis on looking youthful leads many men with thinning hair to try everything from tonics or vitamins to hair transplants in an attempt to reverse the condition. With age, most men (and many women) experience some loss of hair on the temples and the crown of the head, the extent of which is determined by heredity. Although the cause is unknown, testosterone, the hormone responsible for the pattern of hair distribution in men, as well as other secondary sex characteristics, plays a role in male-pattern baldness, as it is termed. Hair loss in women usually accelerates after menopause due to a decrease in estrogen, giving testosterone a relatively more influential role. Nutritional deficiencies account for fewer than 1 percent of the cases of hair loss.

In those few cases that *do* involve nutrition, dietary deficiencies, for example iron, biotin, zinc, or protein, or excess vitamin A may be responsible. Starvation and crash dieting also occasionally cause shedding of the hair. Correction of the nutritional inadequacy, or excess, will usually result in regrowth in these cases. Topically applied nutrients, however, are ineffective in the treatment of balding, whether the cause is nutritionally related or not, since nutrients applied to the hair or scalp cannot penetrate to the hair root in the dermis.

To date, the only proven treatment for male-pattern baldness is Rogaine, a topical form of the drug minoxidil, which is used to treat high blood pressure. Some patients taking oral minoxidil have experienced new hair growth as a side effect—albeit, a desirable one in balding men. However, hair regrowth is seen in fewer than half of patients applying Rogaine to their scalps. Furthermore, once the drug is discontinued, the new hair falls out.

The vitamins and minerals found in brewer's yeast and other nutritional supplements will not prevent hair from falling out.

More generalized hair loss is sometimes related to trauma to the scalp or body. It may be the result of a chronic condition such as diabetes or a thyroid disorder or may be related to short-term illness.

Telogen Effluvium (Hair Shedding)

Any kind of shock to the body—high fever, certain medications, major surgery, starvation, or extreme stress, for example—may cause an increased number of hairs to enter the resting (telogen) phase at the same time. Due to hormonal shifts, 20 to 30 percent of women have some degree of hair loss after childbirth. Two to four months after the hairs have entered the telogen phase, they all will be shed more or less simultaneously, a condition known as telogen effluvium. After this loss, new hairs promptly replace those shed, provided that the underlying cause is resolved.

Other than restoring adequate calories and protein in the case of a starvation diet, there is no nutritional cause or treatment for telogen effluvium. However, nutritional common sense dictates that individuals take special care to eat a well-balanced diet during illness or before surgery or other anticipated stress.

Dandruff

Dandruff, the flaking of dead scalp cells, is a form of seborrheic dermatitis, a scaling condition that in more severe cases affects the skin around the nose, behind the ears, in the genital region, and in the underarms, as well as the scalp. The cause is not known, but there is a hereditary predisposition. It is not thought to be related to one's nutrition. Frequent shampooing, as often as every day if necessary, will usually keep dandruff under control. Modest scalp scaling is normal.

Many dandruff shampoos contain selenium or zinc. When incorporated into a shampoo, these minerals do not act as nutrients but as exfoliants, to promote the shedding of dead scalp cells. For this reason, a dandruff shampoo will at first appear to worsen the condition.

NUTRITION AND THE SKIN, HAIR, AND NAILS: SOME FALLACIES

Nutrient-based cosmetics can prevent skin aging. Oatmeal, vitamin E, cocoa butter, amino acids, collagen, placenta extract, and other substances formulated as creams or lotions have been advertised as having anti-aging properties. Aging of the skin, however, is an inevitable and irreversible result of the passage of time, aggravated by damage from sunlight and artificial sources of ultraviolet radiation, such as tanning parlors. After age 25, collagen fibers in the dermis begin to break down, subcutaneous fat begins to disappear, skin becomes drier and holds less water, and cumulative years of the pull of gravity lead to sagging and wrinkling. No topically applied "nutrient," with the possible exception of tretinoin (Retin-A), can retard or stall this process.

Tretinoin, the prescription medication used for acne, has recently been shown to have an "anti-aging" effect—specifically, reversing some of the effects of chronic sun exposure on the skin, known as photoaging. Researchers have found that topically applied tretinoin may lead to new collagen production in the dermis, the development of new blood vessels, creating increased circulation to the skin, and a decrease in the dead-cell layer that covers the epidermis. However, the best treatment for sun-aged skin is prevention of overexposure in the first place.

Collagen has been promoted as a supposed rejuvenator of the skin. However, when applied to the skin, the collagen molecules cannot penetrate to the important second layer, the dermis. Rather, they bind water to the stratum corneum, the outermost layer of the epidermis, which may "plump" the skin and temporarily make it look and feel younger. Injections of collagen directly into wrinkles even out the skin's surface, in effect temporarily removing the wrinkles. Treatments may have to be repeated every 6 to 18 months. Many ask: Is it worth it?

Lanolin is a fat derived from the oil glands of sheep. Like any other oil-based product—for example, petroleum jelly, cocoa butter, and mineral oil—lanolin helps the skin retain moisture, making the surface smoother as wrinkles appear to fill out. None of these preparations retards aging of the skin, however. In addition, about 2 percent of the population are allergic to lanolin.

Topical vitamin E has not been shown to retard the aging of skin. Taken orally or applied topically, it may have an anti-scarring effect that can help to prevent a raised (keloid) scar, but it is not appropriate treatment for a depressed scar.

Vitamins can reduce cellulite. The term *cellulite* was coined to describe the dimpled fatty tissue most commonly seen on the thighs or buttocks of women. It has been alleged that cellulite is a special kind of fat, a combination of fat, water, and toxic materials that have not been properly eliminated from the body. However, studies have been unable to find any difference between ordinary fat cells and so-called cellulite. The dimpled appearance seems to be due to a bulging of the fat cells between the bands of fibrous tissue that hold the subcutaneous layers to underlying tissue. Both heredity and sex-related patterns of fat distribution and fat-cell structure influence the appearance of this tissue.

Expensive vitamin and mineral supplements, as well as hormone or enzyme injections, are among the worthless remedies suggested to remove cellulite. Although weight loss and exercise are helpful, the decrease in skin elasticity and the thinning of the dermis with age inevitably make these cells more noticeable.

Nutrients can prevent graying of the hair. Gray hair is an inevitable result of heredity acting on the declining pigment production that accompanies aging. Certain rare nutrient deficiencies, or the metabolic disorder phenylketonuria—a liver enzyme disorder—can result in loss of hair color, among other symptoms.

Para-amino-benzoic acid (PABA), a component of the B vitamin folic acid, has been touted as preventing normal graying of the hair. If taken as a supplement in normal doses, PABA has not been found to have any effect on hair color; massive doses of this supplement may cause nausea, vomiting, and other problems. In lotion, it is a sunscreen.

Protein repairs damaged hair. Protein is often advertised as being a hair-repair substance. Shampoos and conditioners containing protein may make the hair seem silkier because they coat the hair shaft, but this effect will wash out with the next shampoo. Hair is not a living substance and cannot absorb protein or any other nutrient. Protein-based shampoos do not alter or strengthen hair, nor do they have any effect on its growth.

Hair analysis reveals nutritional status. Hucksters claim that laboratory analysis of samples of hair for mineral content can reveal imbalances in body chemistry and serve as a guide to reversing the aging process. Not coincidentally, some labs that perform these analyses may also sell supplements to reverse these so-called deficiencies. Apart from the fact that hair analyses of identical samples may vary from one laboratory to the next or even within the same lab, there are many reasons why this procedure, by and large, is not accepted as a valid diagnostic technique. Hair grows very slowly, so even samples taken from close to the scalp may not reflect present bodily conditions. Moreover, different laboratories reach different conclusions about the same hair samples; a normal range for minerals in the hair has not been established. Nor is

Facts About Hair

- Hair grows at the rate of about half an inch a month.

- Hair falls out at the rate of 50 to 150 strands a day.

- Thinning is not noticeable until about 40 percent of the hairs have been lost.

- Scalp hairs grow for two to five years, then rest for two to three months. At the end of the resting period, the hair is shed. Between 10 and 15 percent of the hairs are in the resting phase at any given time.

- The shape of the hair follicle determines the type of hair. Round follicles grow straight hair; oval follicles grow wavy hair; flat follicles grow curly hair.

- A healthy head of hair has between 80,000 and 150,000 hairs.

- Blonds have more hair—140,000 hairs, compared with 115,000 for brunettes and 80,000 for redheads.

it clearly understood how mineral content of the hair relates to mineral concentration in the blood and other tissues. Mineral content may vary according to age, gender, hair color, and the location from which the sample was taken, as well as with relation to outside factors, including the type of shampoo, use of bleaches or dyes, the season of the year, and the presence of air pollutants.

Hair analysis is useful only when there is a suspicion that an individual may have been exposed to a toxic element such as arsenic, chromium, or lead. Even then, shampoos or hair dyes can distort test results. (See Facts About Hair on page 609.)

Gelatin promotes nail strength. Since nails are composed mainly of protein—albeit, dead protein (keratin)—gelatin has been promoted as a dietary supplement to increase their strength. Compared to other food sources, however, gelatin is not a complete protein and is deficient in the sulfur-containing amino acids that give strength to nails.

Calcium increases nail hardness. Calcium supplements have been promoted to increase the hardness of the nails. In fact, there are only very small amounts of calcium in nails and this mineral is not responsible for strengthening the nail substance. Brittle or splitting nails are usually due to dehydration of the nails and are more common with aging. The application of moisturizing hand cream after each washing may help with this problem.

Deficiencies in calcium and zinc are wrongly blamed for the appearance of white spots on the nails. The most common cause of these marks is trauma to the nail, such as a sharp blow or overvigorous manicuring.

A well-balanced diet adequate in protein supports the growth of healthy nails. Supplements are unnecessary and cannot increase the rate at which the nails grow. Nail growth may be slowed, however, as a result of starvation, illness, and the normal aging process. (See Facts About Nails, below.)

Facts About Nails

- The matrix of the nail is at its base. It is the living part of the nail, where growth takes place.

- The lunula, the white half-moon at the base of the nail, is the visible part of the matrix.

- The cuticle is skin, protecting the matrix.

- Nails are made up of layers of hard keratinous tissue.

- Nails grow at a rate of about one-eighth of an inch a month. They may grow more rapidly in hot weather than in cold.

- An entirely new nail takes about four months to grow out.

37

Nutrition and Dental Disease

Andrew Kaplan, D.M.D., and David V. Valauri, D.D.S.*

∎

INTRODUCTION

Dental disease is one of our most prevalent health problems. Only 2 percent of all Americans can say that they have never experienced a tooth problem, and half of all two-year-olds already have at least one cavity.

Of course, dental disease is nothing new—even prehistoric human skulls show signs of gum (periodontal) disease and cavities (caries)—but prevention and treatment are. In early times, any pain associated with tooth decay was attributed to the "tooth worm" sent by the angry gods to punish. In 1986, a green tooth containing the oldest known dental filling—a piece of wire—was discovered in the skull of a Nabatean warrior who was buried in a mass grave 2,200 years ago. Archaeologists believe that the soldier thought that this wire would stop the tooth worms from entering his tooth and that it would alleviate his toothache. They also believe that the soldier was duped into thinking that he was receiving a gold wire. This is probably the earliest recorded instance of dental health fraud. Later, more sophisticated Greek and Roman physicians caught on to the fact that diet was re-

*With the advice of John Dodes, D.D.S., director, New York chapter, National Council Against Health Fraud.

sponsible for tooth problems. Aristotle even singled out figs as the main culprit.

In the nineteenth century, a more generalized theory was reached, and it was decided that sugars caused "black teeth." Yet it wasn't until the twentieth century that the connection between fermentable carbohydrates (not necessarily only sugars but starches as well) and dental decay was proved. In 1929, a group of children in an orphanage was studied. Their diets were nutritionally poor and yet they had a very low rate of cavities. Researchers were able to connect this to the fact that the children did not eat table sugar or candies. When the researchers allowed the children to eat three pounds of candy a week, they saw a dramatic increase in caries development.

In the 1940s, a study done in Sweden proved that the form as well as the frequency of sugar and starch intake were important. Sticky foods were shown to be more cavity-producing (cariogenic) than nongooey sugars.

Although many people still believe that cavities, lost teeth, and eventual dentures are inevitable, the fact is, most dental problems can be prevented with proper oral hygiene and other commonsense health practices. The addition of fluoride to the water supply ranks as one of the major tools in cavity prevention. A recent study found that 49.9 percent of all children in the United States have no decay in their permanent teeth. Public-health officials attribute this remarkable improvement to the widespread use of fluoride and high levels of dental care and say this could mean the virtual end of dental disease as a major public-health problem. Also high on the list of preventive measures is proper nutrition, which can significantly reduce the number of cavities a person gets, lower the chance of gum disease, and help to prevent tooth loss.

Most people know about the relationship of sugars and other sweets and tooth problems, but a number of other, less well-known nutritional factors also play a role. For example, researchers are conducting studies aimed at relating what we eat (and how often we eat it) with the rate of cavities and incidence of gum disease. At the same time, other foods are being examined for the ways in which they may be able to prevent cavities.

Good oral hygiene should be a lifelong undertaking, beginning before birth. Although we still do not fully understand all of the complex relationships between nutrition and dental health, enough is known to say that most dental problems can now be prevented.

FETAL TOOTH DEVELOPMENT

Even though a baby's first teeth, or primary teeth, do not appear until around six months of age, calcification of the primary teeth begins at about four months' gestation. The buds of these teeth usually start to develop during the seventh week of pregnancy.

The effects of a mother's diet on her unborn child's developing teeth are unknown, for the most part, but it is generally agreed that a balanced, nutritious diet, including adequate calcium and vitamins D, C, A, and B, should lead to healthier babies and stronger teeth. During pregnancy, additional calories are needed to ensure proper nutrition for the mother and developing fetus. Generally, a woman is advised to eat 200 to 300 additional calories a day, but the mother must be sure these come from nutrient-rich foods and not things such as candy, cookies, and other so-called empty calories.

Calcium, another important part of a pregnant woman's diet, is used by the developing fetus to form its tooth buds. About a quart of milk a day, or 1,200 milligrams of calcium, should be adequate. The diet also must include adequate vitamin D, which is essential for the proper absorption of calcium. The old wives' tale that "the baby took the calcium out of my teeth when I was pregnant, so I lost them" is entirely false. If the mother's diet is deficient in calcium, the embryo will fulfill its requirements by taking calcium from the mother's bones, not from her teeth.

Protein, the building block of every organ, including the teeth, is a must during pregnancy. Most Americans consume more than the recommended amounts of protein (about 63 grams for an adult man and 50 grams for a woman). During pregnancy, a woman should increase her protein intake by 10 grams above this recommended level (see Chapter 12). Animal studies have indicated that if the mother's diet is deficient in protein, her baby may have an increased risk of late eruption of teeth, as well as a higher incidence of dental caries.

There also are certain substances a woman should avoid during pregnancy because of their effects on fetal tooth development. One of the most notable is tetracycline, which can cause permanent discoloration of the baby's teeth. Tetracycline can also cause severe discoloration of the permanent teeth if given to children during the time such teeth are forming (3 to 12 years of age).

Various prenatal nutritional deficiencies, if severe, have been linked to increased incidence of cleft lip, cleft palate, and slower development of the salivary glands, among other problems.

There is at least some evidence that suggests that the ability of teeth and gums to resist cavities and disease may be inherited, making some people more at risk for dental problems than others. There are many other important factors that contribute to dental disease, however, and the link between genetics and tooth decay is considered a weak one. Statistics noting low cavity rates in undeveloped areas contrasted with high rates in industrialized countries led to an investigation of possible genetic resistance in certain races. However, when refined sugars and other cavity-causing foods were introduced to these populations by the industrialized world, the incidence of caries rose, leading researchers to conclude that what we eat is far more important than the type of teeth inherited.

CARE OF PRIMARY TEETH

The deciduous or baby teeth are the building blocks of later dental development. These primary teeth enable the child to chew and help to form the jaw to accommodate the second, or permanent, teeth. If these primary teeth are lost prematurely, the remaining teeth may drift, blocking the path of the permanent teeth. Furthermore, the child will experience pain from tooth decay, possible speech problems, and altered appearance. Many children develop cavities even before age two and may lose their teeth due to decay. First teeth are not immune to dental decay.

Although pediatricians agree that breast milk provides superior nutrition for the newborn, it does not necessarily follow that it will guarantee stronger teeth and gums. For example, the stronger sucking action required for breastfeeding can be simulated with commercial nipples. However, a breastfed baby is much less likely to develop tooth decay caused by a pooling of milk in the mouth, a common occurrence among babies who fall asleep sucking a bottle. An exception might be the baby who is allowed to sleep with the mother and nurses on and off all night at will.

Babies do like to suckle themselves to sleep, but the practice of giving bottles of formula or juice on a regular basis leads to a likelihood of severe tooth decay, even tooth loss. It is far better to put the baby to bed with a pacifier or a bottle of water. The sugar in the formula or juice is fermented by the bacteria that grow and multiply on it, giving the teeth an acid bath. Usually, liquids sweep quickly over the teeth and will not have time to do much harm. A baby who falls asleep with a bottle in his mouth, however, is not actively sucking and swallowing. The usual saliva flow that helps to pass the liquid by the teeth is diminished as the child falls asleep and so sugar remains pooled in the child's mouth, beginning its fermentation into acid and causing the inevitable breakdown of tooth enamel. Even during the day, if the child is not actively swallowing, the same process can occur and the bottle should be taken away.

Parents should avoid giving drinks that contain refined sugar—sucrose. Fruit juices with no added sugar may be less harmful because they contain the possibly less damaging fruit sugar, fructose, instead of sucrose; even so, they should not be used in the bedtime bottle. Formula and breast milk contain galactose, another simple sugar, which also will break down the tooth enamel, but the process takes longer than with sucrose.

The practice of giving a child sugar water

or glucose water is also not recommended. Plain water is the only liquid that does not promote cavity formation. Parents are advised never to dip a pacifier into honey. (The official recommendation is that children under the age of one should never be given honey in any form, since it can cause a form of infant botulism.) Pacifiers should be rinsed in clear water only.

Choosing Bottle Nipples

Orthodontically, the breast is considered to be better than the bottle for the baby. The sucking action necessary for breast feeding helps keep teeth aligned. Recent studies by researchers at Johns Hopkins University confirmed that breastfed babies are less likely to need later orthodontic treatment than those who are bottle-fed. There are commericial nipples available, however, which are marked as orthodontic and are acceptable alternatives to the breast. Parents should not attempt to enlarge the hole in these bottle nipples to make the liquid flow faster. The small size of the holes is designed to force the infant to suck rather than simply swallow.

Figure 37.1. Anatomy of a Tooth

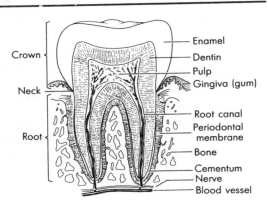

Teaching Good Nutrition

We are literally born with a sweet tooth. Studies have found that even before birth, the fetus has a preference for sweet-tasting substances. In one experiment, a glucose solution was introduced into the amnionic fluid, while the fetus was monitored by sonography. The researchers observed the fetus turning its head toward the sweet substance and making sucking motions to drink it in. Anthropologists believe that our natural preference for sweets dates to prehistoric times and the primitive realization that sweet-tasting fruits and plants were less likely to be poisonous than bitter ones.

In formulating a child's diet, common sense and moderation should prevail. On one hand, denying a child all sweets is likely to lead to later rebellion and sneaking sweets. On the other hand, pandering to a child's natural preference for sweets can be even more harmful.

The trick is to find an acceptable middle ground by planning meals that include something sweet—perhaps a fruit tart, milk pudding, or other such dessert—while limiting snacks to nonsweets, such as crackers or vegetable sticks. By providing the sweets in a meal and encouraging brushing afterward, you are limiting the child's exposure to cavity-causing substances. Sweets (or any other food, for that matter) should not be used to reward good behavior or as an incentive to do a certain task. Some sweets are more likely to damage teeth than others; hard candies that are sucked, for example, are much more damaging than a small chocolate that is quickly eaten and swallowed, which may do no harm at all. A sweet at the end of a meal, followed by rinsing the mouth or brushing the teeth, is preferable to a between-meal sweet snack. Natural fruit juice is more nutritious and less harmful to the teeth than colas or other sugary drinks. (See Chapter 13 for more suggestions on instilling good eating habits at an early age.)

There is considerable confusion over which foods are harmful to teeth and which are not. Snacks such as raw vegetables, fruits, or cheese and crackers, for example, are good choices for children. The artificial sweeteners aspartame and saccharin don't cause cavities; in contrast, sorbitol may if taken in large amounts. Parents also should be aware of foods that appeal to young children and are promoted as healthy but aren't; for example, granola bars, fruit snacks, and some breakfast cereals are high in sugar and should be avoided or eaten only in small amounts. Always read the labels on packages (especially cereal boxes) to determine the amount of sugars in the product, which is reflected by how early they appear in the ingredient list. However, some very low-sugar cereals may list sugar as early as the fourth ingredient and in this case the percentage of sugar gives a more accurate picture than the position.

Fresh fruits are not especially harmful to the teeth, even though they contain fruit sugars, because they promote the flow of saliva, which protects against cavities. However, the same is not true of most dried fruits, which are higher in fructose than fresh fruits and have the added liability of being sticky; they stay on the teeth longer and therefore have more time to cause decay.

Of course, the emphasis in feeding a child should be on the positive aspects of what should be eaten instead of what should be avoided. Children need plenty of calcium and phosphorus for growing teeth and bones and they should be encouraged to consume adequate milk and milk products, as well as other foods high in these minerals. Diets severely deficient in calcium and vitamin D can cause dental problems, such as the hypocalcification of teeth or defective enamel formation.

Parents should brush the child's teeth until the child can do a thorough job without help (usually by the age of seven or eight) and parents should also make sure that their children start seeing a dentist regularly by the age of three.

MECHANICS OF TOOTH DECAY

The mechanics of tooth decay are relatively simple. As emphasized earlier, any fermentable carbohydrate that sticks to the teeth or is in frequent contact with them (i.e., sugar and sodas) will promote the development of cavities. This is what happens:

1. Food is eaten.

2. Some of this food remains in the mouth, leading to the formation of plaque, a sticky substance, on the tooth.

3. The plaque provides a favorable environment for multiplication of the bacteria that normally exist in the mouth.

4. Sugar is fermented by the bacteria in plaque to form acid.

5. The acid causes the protective tooth enamel to break down, enabling bacteria to invade the tooth.

The greatest damage is done within the first twenty minutes of eating sweets, when acid levels are at their highest. In some cases, though, the acid levels in the mouth do not return to normal until two to four hours after eating.

Although sugars may be the most cariogenic subtances, they are by no means alone; starches also can promote tooth decay. Until recently, it was believed that starches, complex carbohydrates, were safe for teeth.

Although starches are less cariogenic than other sugars, they are not entirely innocuous. Starch turns into a readily fermentable and cavity-causing substance when it mixes with amylase, an enzyme in the saliva. According to a 1986 study published by the American Dental Association, certain starches can adhere to teeth and raise the acidity in the mouth. This study found that the consumption of high-sugar foods results in a shorter "acid bath" than that caused by eating starchy foods. When tested, it was found that starches such as breadsticks, cornflakes, and croissants actually lingered in the mouth longer than sweets and lowered the pH levels (raised the acidity) for a longer time, making the teeth more susceptible to decay.

OTHER INFLUENCES

Some foods, such as cheddar cheese, can actually help to prevent cavities. An anticariogenic food can be described as one that does not cause the acidity of the saliva to rise to a point where tooth decay can occur. Many attempts have been made to arrive at a list of cavity-causing and cavity-preventing foods. Unfortunately, so many factors influence the likelihood of caries that ranking or listing cariogenic or noncariogenic foods is difficult. Frequency, composition, and sequence of food intake all play a part in the cavity-causing nature of foods. In addition, some foods have both cavity-causing and protective components. For example, chocolate contains tannins and cocoa, which actually help reduce the impact of its cavity-causing sugar on teeth.

It has been demonstrated, though, that certain types of nutrients—proteins, fats, and fluoride—have a protective effect on teeth and may help to prevent cavities. A number of cheeses, including blue, Brie, cheddar, Gouda, mozzarella, Monterey Jack, and Swiss, as well as meat and nuts have minimal acid-causing potential and are currently thought to be safe for teeth. Furthermore, cheddar cheese, Mon-

Figure 37.2.   Mechanics of Tooth Decay

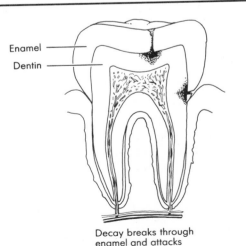

Enamel

Dentin

Decay breaks through enamel and attacks dentin.

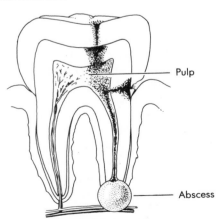

Pulp

Abscess

Pulp is attacked, destroyed, and abscess forms.

terey Jack, and Swiss have been found to work as a type of protective barrier against caries development when eaten before or after a sugary snack. This is because the cheeses seem to prevent dips in the mouth's pH, making the area around the teeth more acid resistant. They also increase the production of saliva, which "cleans" the teeth. (Any decrease in saliva due to the side effects of radiation or chemotherapy treatments for cancer or those of certain drugs, including some commonly prescribed for depression and hypertension, tend to cause an increase in caries, especially at the tooth roots.)

More research on foods that promote or protect against cavities may uncover other clues, showing how certain foods can be used to prevent acid production and reduce caries. The precise cavity-causing potential of foods is still hard to determine accurately at this time. Current knowledge, however, suggests that foods high in protein and with a moderate amount of fat, such as lean meats, are best. Fat may reduce sugar's impact and also helps to decrease stickiness so that food is not retained on the teeth. (See chapters 4 and 6 for sources and content.) Hard and fibrous foods, such as celery, cucumber, and lettuce, also help cleanse the tooth surface, removing some plaque and retarding calculus, or tartar, formation.

In planning a diet, you obviously need to consider total needs and not just the impact of foods on the teeth. As stressed throughout this book, moderation and variety should be the guiding factors. Concentrating too much on foods that protect against cavities may not be in the best interest of total health. For example, meat and cheddar cheese may protect against cavities, but eaten in excess, they may promote weight gain, elevated cholesterol, and other problems linked to a high-fat, high-calorie diet.

Frequency of Food Consumption

It was formerly thought that only what a person ate or drank influenced the development of decay. It is now known that how often a person eats or drinks is also a factor in the prevention of dental disease. The potential for tooth decay rises when there is not enough time between snacks or meals for the acid levels in the mouth to return to normal. Frequent slow sipping of a drink or constant snacking allows acid levels to remain at a peak. Similarly, a pound of candy eaten in one sitting is less harmful to the teeth than the same amount eaten off and on over the course of a day. This was documented in a study done at the National Institute of Dental Research, in which rats fed chocolate cookies once an hour had 50 percent fewer cavities than those fed once every ten minutes, even though the actual amount consumed was the same.

The form of the foods eaten can also affect dental caries formation. Obviously, foods that are sticky or chewy are worse for the teeth than less adherent alternatives. Caramels or raisins, for example, spend more time in contact with the teeth than a liquid that passes by the teeth relatively quickly. Regular chewing gum is particularly damaging due to the prolonged effect on acidity of the saliva. Sugarless gums offer no clear benefits regarding cavity prevention, other than the obvious fact that they don't contain sugar.

The sequence of food intake also influences its cavity-causing potential. A cariogenic food eaten alone does more damage to the teeth than when eaten in conjunction with noncariogenic foods. The "safe" foods eaten in conjunction with the harmful foods work to clear away the latter by chewing action and increasing debris-clearing saliva, leaving the teeth cleaner. A sweet followed by some nuts or cheese, for example, would be better for teeth than the sweet eaten alone. Some foods, such as cheese, actually minimize the acid levels and decrease the potential for cavities when eaten before or after a sugary item. Sugary foods or beverages are less cariogenic when consumed during a meal when saliva flow is at its peak and the "neutral" foods can mitigate their effects.

Fluoride

It is well known that fluoride, a mineral that occurs naturally in water in many parts of the country and that now is added to drinking water in most areas, heightens resistance to cavities. The accidental discovery of fluoride's protective nature has led to sweeping changes in the nation's caries rate. Fluoride is incorporated into tooth enamel, making it less susceptible to decay. It also strengthens bone, including the jawbone.

As far back as 1938, studies of 21 different cities were published showing that the rate of caries decreased dramatically where there were increased amounts of fluoride occurring naturally in the water. We now know that tooth decay can be reduced by as much as 60 percent when fluoride is used, either in the drinking water or administered via a tablet in unfluoridated areas. It also is added to toothpastes; in fact, about 80 percent of toothpastes sold in the United States now contain fluoride. In areas where there are high natural concentrations of fluoride in the water, it may cause staining of teeth, but this is not harmful.

Drinking fluoridated water is most beneficial to young children whose teeth are just developing. In fact, in communities where the water is not fluoridated, some pediatricians now prescribe fluoride supplements for babies, expecially those who are breastfed. The benefits are not limited to children, however; it may also help to reduce tooth decay among adults. Yet in spite of its effectiveness, there is still some resistance to fluoridation of water supplies. Claims that the mineral causes everything from cancer to allergies have been shown to be unfounded and the fluoridation of water is widely accepted by health officials. The campaign against fluoridation is often backed by the vitamin and health-food manufacturers and dealers in an attempt to substitute their products, which are useless in preventing decay, for the extremely safe, effective, and inexpensive process of water fluoridation. In 1980, the Centers for Disease Control estimated that the average cost of fluoridation is 35 cents per person per year.

Fluoride also appears naturally in certain fish and teas. Natural fluoride levels in water can range from a very low concentration of 0.05 parts per million to as high as 8 in some parts of the Southwest. It was, in fact, in Colorado, where natural fluoridation of the water is high, that its benefits were first discovered. Any foods produced in areas that have naturally occurring fluoride in the water also contain fluoride.

Brushing and Flossing

Diet alone will not prevent cavities; regular brushing and flossing of the teeth also are essential. Proper brushing and flossing help to remove plaque buildup. (The proper technique is illustrated in Figure 37.3.) Parents should help young children with brushing and teach them how to do it at an early age. Everyone should brush at least twice a day—morning and night—and more often if cavity-prone. Teeth should be flossed once a day, preferably in the evening.

When brushing, use a soft-bristle toothbrush. It should be held at a 45-degree angle to the teeth and moved in a back-and-forth motion for about ten seconds before going on to the next group of teeth. Pay particular attention to the area where the tooth meets the gums, as bacteria tend to be more plentiful there. Make sure that every surface of every

Figure 37.3. Proper Technique for Flossing

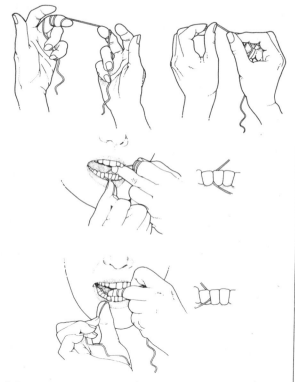

1. Break off a piece of dental floss. The piece should be about 18 inches long. Wind each end around the middle fingers of each hand, reserving a one-inch piece hanging between your hands.
2. Move your thumb to the ball of your middle finger to anchor the floss between your thumb and middle finger on each hand. Position your hands so that one is in front of the other.
3. Slip the floss between two teeth and move it down until you feel its pressure on the gum at the base of the teeth. Curve the floss slightly around one tooth. Slide the floss gently up and down.
4. Without removing the floss, curve it around the adjacent tooth. Slide it up and down again, so as to clean both sides of the area between the teeth.

tooth is cleaned. Toothbrushes should be replaced every three to four months for maximum effectiveness.

Flossing should also be done every evening to remove food particles and plaque that lodge between the teeth and cannot be reached by brushing alone. Use about 18 inches of floss (waxed or unwaxed). Wrap the ends around the middle fingers and gently guide it between the teeth to the gum line. Never snap it into place and avoid using a sawing motion on the periodontal tissue of teeth. Scrape the floss against the side of the tooth and then remove the floss. (See Figure 37.3.)

In addition to regular brushing and flossing, an effective dental-hygiene program also should include periodic dental checkups. Even with the most meticulous home care, a certain amount of tartar will build up on the teeth, and it should be removed by a professional. Regular dental examinations also discover caries or gum disorders in an early, more treatable stage. Such preventive care preserves the teeth and markedly reduces dental bills.

PERIODONTAL DISEASE

Although most people consider cavities their biggest dental problem, in reality gum disease accounts for more tooth loss than caries. According to the American Dental Association, 75 percent of all Americans will suffer from some form of periodontal disease in their lifetimes, and after age 35, periodontal disease is the major cause of tooth loss. The term *periodontal disease* covers gingivitis (inflammation of the gums) and periodontitis (inflammation and destruction of the underlying supportive structure). Gingivitis affects only the gums, and at this stage, the disease can still be stopped. If left untreated, however, gingivitis can lead to periodontitis, a more serious disease that may result in tooth loss.

Periodontal disease is caused by bacteria-containing plaque and a buildup of calculus along the gum line of the teeth. The by-products of the bacteria irritate the periodontal tissues, causing the gums to bleed and swell. This process can be exacerbated by unfilled cavities (which collect food and bacteria) and poorly fitting or contoured dental restorations.

As the irritants in plaque begin to destroy the gum tissue, small pockets form around the teeth that can harbor even more bacteria. The supporting tissue becomes inflamed, and eventually, the bone that supports the teeth is also destroyed. Calculus cannot be removed by simple brushing; this must be done with a professional cleaning by a dentist or dental hygienist. Professional cleaning is recommended every six months, or more often if the patient has periodontal disease. (See Risk Factors, below.)

Although the immediate cause of gum disease is the bacteria in plaque, nutritional factors may play an important role in its prevention or aggravation. In experiments with animals, vitamin C deficiency was associated with periodontal disease, but this has not been found to occur in humans. Diets deficient in protein, vitamin A, and the B vitamins have been linked to periodontal disease in humans. For healthy teeth and gums, the diet also should include the recommended daily amounts of vitamin A, calcium, phosphorus, and iron. (See Chapter 7 for table of RDAs.) Many studies have been done attempting to discover the precise relationship between nutrition and periodontal disease, but much still remains unclear. At present, it appears that certain foods and nutrients can have both a direct and indirect influence on a person's ability to resist periodontal disease. Sugary foods that promote plaque buildup have a direct influence and should be avoided.

A well-balanced diet indirectly helps to prevent periodontal disease by keeping oral tissues healthy and therefore more resistant to decay. A soft diet will tend to produce more bacterial plaque than a diet that requires chewing. To prevent periodontal disease, the American Dental Association suggests that you: (1) brush and floss at least once a day; (2) eat a well-balanced diet; and (3) visit a dentist regularly to have teeth professionally cleaned and to detect early signs of gum disease.

If periodontal disease does develop, it is important that it be treated in its early stages. There are now a number of treatments that can reverse the destructive process and save the teeth. These range from undergoing gum treatments, taking antibiotics, and having the gum pockets surgically removed to a rigorous home program of flossing, brushing, and using chlorhexidene rinses to control the disease-causing bacteria. Researchers are also working to develop a vaccine that can prevent the disease, but it may be years before this is available for the general public.

Outlook for the Future

A vaccine to prevent tooth decay may one day be a reality. An anticavity vaccine is

Risk Factors for Periodontal Disease

Calculus buildup	Soft diets
Faulty nutrition	Parathyroid-gland
Faulty restorative	disorders
dentistry	Blood (hematological)
Diabetes	disorders
Estrogen imbalances	Lack of saliva
Gingivitis left	Radiation therapy
untreated	

being researched and there is now hope for an injection that will protect teeth against dental decay. Preliminary tests have been conducted on both animals and humans and it is hoped that the vaccine will be available to the public by the turn of the century. (Both Forsyth Dental Center in Boston and the National Institute of Dental Research in Bethesda, Maryland, are working on vaccines.) However, the development of a vaccine does not mean a license to forget all nutritional restraints; no vaccine can protect against cavities if fermentable carbohydrates are consumed in excess.

Sealants are a thin plastic film that a dentist can paint over deep fissures and grooves on the chewing surfaces of the molars and premolars (the teeth right in front of the molars). Sealants can be used not only for decay-free teeth—to seal out decay—but also can be effective for sealing in small cavities—to prevent their spread. The National Institute of Dental Research would like the sealants to be used by a greater number of children than they currently are. Sealants are a safe, effective, and cost-conscious way to prevent decay.

The antitartar toothpastes and mouthwashes that are now for sale offer little for the patient with periodontal disease, because they fight tartar only above the gum. Toothpastes that contain *Sanguinaria canadensis* (bloodroot) have been shown in controlled studies to be effective in controlling plaque. Chlorhexidene is a prescription mouthwash that has been shown to be an effective aid in the treatment of gum problems. It can stain the teeth and may cause a loss of taste. These side effects are temporary, but it must be remembered that chlorhexidene is not a cure for gum disease, only an aid in its control.

AGING AND DENTAL HEALTH

Contrary to popular belief, the loss of teeth is not a natural consequence of aging. An estimated 22.6 million Americans, at least half of them over 65, have lost all their teeth. As noted earlier, periodontal disease accounts for most tooth loss among older people.

Tooth loss among older people tends to be a progressive process, starting with one or two teeth. Missing teeth, sore and bleeding gums, painful teeth, or poorly fitting dentistry often lead to dietary changes as the person begins to choose soft, easy-to-chew foods instead of things such as raw fruits and vegetables. This can lead to a vicious cycle of more gum disease, tooth decay, and tooth loss.

Some factors that promote tooth loss are more common in the elderly. For example, after age 30, the flow of saliva diminishes, slowing the natural cleansing action of the mouth and making thorough oral hygiene more important. Medications more frequently taken by older people, such as those for high blood pressure or certain tranquilizers, also may reduce saliva. There are artificial saliva substitutes available to assist with this problem. In dry-mouth syndrome, a hard-to-chew diet may scrape the gums and cause gum sores. In such a case, a softer diet may be prescribed to make eating more comfortable.

People who have difficulty chewing can still consume a well-balanced diet; soft foods can be nutritious if care is taken to include all the food groups. However, the limited financial resources of many elderly, coupled with lost teeth, may lead to an unbalanced diet, deficient in more expensive, harder-to-chew foods such as meats and fresh vegetables. Others try to eat these foods as they did before and end up swallowing without really chewing the food, causing gastrointestinal problems and possibly increasing the risk of choking.

Difficult-to-chew foods such as raw vegetables or nuts can be made acceptable by chopping them finely. Meats can be ground. Many raw fruits are soft enough to eat as is: bananas, oranges, grapefruit, berries, ripe pears and peaches, to name a few. Harder-to-chew fruits such as apples and pineapples can be diced.

If extreme difficulty or pain is associated with chewing, a dentist should be seen immediately.

RESTORATIVE DENTISTRY

Modern dentistry has many options available to the patient who is missing teeth. Dentures, crowns (or caps), and bridges are the most commonly used. A bridge is a relatively long-lasting replacement, consisting of two crowns with a pontic (false tooth) in the middle. Dental implants, artificial root replacements that are placed in the jawbone, can be used alone or in conjunction with dentures, crowns, and fixed bridges.

DIET AFTER ORAL SURGERY

Good nutrition is an essential, although often overlooked, component in recovery from oral surgery or other problems such as an oral infection or fractured jaw. In addition to eating a well-balanced diet, caloric needs may be increased moderately during the postoperative period to provide the extra energy needed for healing.

During the first 24 to 72 hours following oral surgery, a patient should expect to consume a clear liquid diet of fruit juices, water, and other beverages. Hot beverages should be avoided the first day because they encourage bleeding. The second day, a high-protein liquid diet is usually started, which may include a commercial dietary supplement.

Patients recovering from major oral surgery or who have had their jaws wired together for healing may be placed on a pureed diet for a week or more. Most solid foods can be liquefied in a blender or food processor so that the patient can eat preferred foods. Six to nine feedings may be needed to get an adequate amount of calories and nutrients. Although a patient might lose weight during the first few days, weight should return to normal and can be maintained with an adequate amount of calories and nutrients daily.

Care should be taken that the patient receives all the necessary nutrients—protein, carbohydrates, fats, vitamins, minerals, and water. A patient who has had excessive bleeding may require extra iron-rich foods to reduce the risk of anemia. (See Chapter 23 for a more detailed discussion.)

TEMPOROMANDIBULAR JOINT DISORDER

Temporomandibular joint (TMJ) disorders are a group of problems related to the jaw joint and the muscles that control the jaw. These disorders are often associated with psychological stress and are usually exacerbated by grinding and clenching of the teeth during the day or night. Other roots of the problem may stem from trauma to the jaw, such as an injury sustained in a car accident or fall. Symptoms can include muscular or joint pain, clicking, headaches, and/or restriction of the jaw opening (less than two fingers as a general guideline).

There is no objective evidence that temporomandibular disorders have a nutritional basis. Although it is important to maintain a balanced diet, therapies that consist only of dietary modification or vitamin supplements are unlikely to be helpful, other than for their psychological effect. As with any disease, a balanced diet is part of a speedy recovery.

Severe pain from movement of the jaw in temporomandibular joint disorders often necessitates that the patient be placed on a soft diet. This is done in order to give the jaw a rest, in much the same way as a patient is given a cane to take the weight off a sprained ankle. Other responsible approaches to temporomandibular disorders include relaxation training, biofeedback, splint therapy (a plastic device worn over the teeth), muscle relaxants, and antiinflammatory medications. In a very few cases, surgery, with the resulting postoperative soft diet, may be necessary. However, conservative, noninvasive, reversible therapies should be used at the start of treatment. TMJ is overdiagnosed by some.

ORAL MANIFESTATIONS OF NUTRITION DEFICIENCY AND EXCESS

Protein-Calorie Malnutrition

Protein-calorie malnutrition is usually not found in the United States, but it may appear in alcoholics, the homebound elderly, and the severely impoverished. The most severe effects are on children born of malnourished mothers. In animal studies, protein-calorie malnutrition has led to significantly smaller molars, increased susceptibility to caries, decreases in the volume, protein content, and amylase and aminopeptide activity of the sali-

vary glands, and retardation in the development of the mandible. In adults, it may lead to enlargement of the parotid glands. This variability may be due to secondary nutritional deficiencies that often accompany protein-calorie malnutrition.

Vitamin C (Ascorbic Acid)

Scurvy is the disease caused by severe vitamin C deficiency. Orally, its symptoms are reddened, inflamed, bleeding gums, with an extremely dry mouth and teeth that become loose and eventually fall out. This is probably related to the well-documented role of ascorbic acid in collagen metabolism.

People who take large doses of vitamin C run the risk of developing rebound scurvy if they stop the vitamin too quickly. Chewing vitamin C tablets can dissolve enamel. Doses of one gram or more can produce diarrhea. The promotion of megadoses of vitamin C to AIDS patients is particularly harmful, since it superimposes vitamin C diarrhea on AIDS diarrhea, and can lead to shock.

Vitamin B Complex

Angular cheilitis—inflammation of the corners of the lips (where the upper and lower lips come together)—and glossitis—inflammation of the tongue—are the two most common symptoms associated with deficiencies of folic acid, niacin (B_3), riboflavin (B_2), and B_{12}.

Pellagra is the disease that is caused by niacin deficiency. It is characterized by the three D's—dermatitis, diarrhea, and dementia. The dermatitis affects mainly the parts of the body exposed to sunlight, and inflammation of the mouth may be so severe that the victim refuses to eat.

Although some of the B vitamins (B$_6$, B$_1$, niacin) can be dangerous in high doses, there are no oral manifestations of overdosing.

Vitamin D

Enamel hypoplasia (incomplete or defective development of tooth enamel) can result from severe vitamin D deficiency. Excessive intake of vitamin D can lead to serious and life-threatening conditions because it causes loss of appetite, headaches, nausea, excessive urination, diarrhea or constipation, fatigue, high blood pressure, and many other more dangerous side effects.

Vitamin A

Vitamin A deficiency leads to changes in the salivary gland cells, which can cause xerostomia (dry mouth). In experimental animals, vitamin A deficiency has led to enamel hypoplasia and defective dentin formation. This may not be true for humans, but it is known that vitamin A has a significant influence on bone calcification.

Large amounts of vitamin A are toxic, leading to serious side effects such as weight loss, loss of hair, extreme drying and thickening of the skin, cracking of the lips, mouth ulcers, and birth defects if taken during pregnancy.

Vitamin E (Tocopherol)

Vitamin E is an antioxidant and has a number of important functions in humans. Deficiency is extremely rare, but there are a number of possible harmful side effects from taking very high doses of vitamin E. Some people advocate using vitamin E on cold sores, but there is no objective evidence that it is effective.

Vitamin K

Vitamin K is primarily involved with the blood-clotting mechanism. Deficiency is extremely rare but can occur. Sprue is a malabsorptive disease in which atrophy of the tongue is an important symptom, and supplementation with vitamin K is often indicated. There do not seem to be any reported cases of toxic overdoses or adverse side effects from vitamin K.

Iron

Iron deficiency is characterized by anemia (microcytic hypochromic anemia), angular cheilitis, glossitis, and fatigue. It is usually caused by blood loss or fad diets (vegetarians are particularly susceptible). The tongue has a characteristic loss of the threadlike elevations that cover its surface (filiform papillae) and appears shiny and smooth.

Overdoses caused by children taking adult therapeutic doses of iron result in hundreds of reported poisonings each year.

Zinc

Acrodermatitis enteropathica is a disease linked to altered zinc metabolism. Its symptoms include small blisters (vesicle formations) and a thickening (hyperkeratotic plaques) on the skin and in the oral cavity. One of the common features of zinc deficiency is loss of taste.

There is a wide margin of safety, but huge doses of 1,000 to 2,000 milligrams of zinc sulfate can cause acute toxicity.

Bulimia

Bulimia is an eating disorder characterized by eating binges followed by self-induced purging (usually vomiting) and periods of starvation. The vomiting leads to a characteristic loss of tooth enamel, and since bulimics often keep a nearly ideal body weight, dentists may be the first to diagnose this serious disease.

Anorexia Nervosa

This life-threatening eating disorder is characterized by severe weight loss resulting from starvation, the use of laxatives, and self-induced vomiting. Thus a patient with anorexia may also show signs of severe enamel erosion caused by vomiting.

ORAL CHANGES INDUCED BY CANCER THERAPY

Treatment of cancer can often lead to digestive and nutritional problems. Cancer patients are often placed on liquid diets. The alteration in food consistency may lead to dental problems, although the benefits of a hard, fibrous diet over a soft, liquid one have not been adequately established. Patients receiving head and neck irradiation often develop inflammation of the mouth and tongue (stomatitis) and rampant dental decay, due to the destruction of the salivary glands and changes in the oral bacterial flora. These patients need especially close dental supervision.

In America, oral cancer accounts for 2 to 3 percent of total malignant neoplasms. Smoking and chewing tobacco are major causes of oral cancer. This is especially sad because so many young athletes seem to be addicted to chewing tobacco.

DENTAL QUACKERY

Some dentists go beyond the scope of dentistry in an attempt to treat the whole body, a practice that is often referred to as holistic dentistry. Not all holistic dentists are quacks. Furthermore, most responsible dentists incorporate some holistic advice in their practices, such as the scientific findings regarding nutrition and dental disease.

There are some dentists, however, who use questionable, sometimes dangerous, and often costly approaches to dental problems. If there is any question as to the nature or quality of treatment, seek a second opinion. (Some states have begun to discipline dentists who use questionable techniques or who practice outside the realm of their license.) Some of the dental quackery being touted includes the following.

- Expensive "organic" or "natural" vitamins and mineral supplements. These are often not only prescribed but also sold by quack dentists. Megadoses of vitamins—which may actually be harmful; see Chapter 7—are falsely claimed to cure everything from cancer to temporomandibular disorders. No one has shown "natural" vitamins to be any different from "synthetic" ones.

- Hair analysis. This is fraudulently used to detect levels of trace minerals in the body. There is no reproducible correlation of mineral levels in hair and body. Hair analysis is also falsely advertised as a test for vitamin deficiency. Hair contains no vitamins.

- Homeopathic drugs such as the Bach flower remedies. Made from the essences of 38 flowering plants and trees, it is supposedly used to calm the nerves, reduce inflammation of the periodontal tissue, and relieve pain. This is not shown and may not only be harmful but also may encourage patients to stop using other, needed, prescription drugs or to postpone seeing a legitimate dentist for a problem that needs attention.

- Removal of silver-amalgam fillings. Some dentists fraudulently claim that a patient is suffering from an allergy to his silver fillings or a mercury intoxication. Various tests are used to "detect" this: hair analysis, urine and blood tests, and skin-patch tests. These dentists usually misrepresent the results of these tests. Furthermore, mercury allergy occurs in less than 1 percent of the population. Claiming that mercury leaks are the cause of a variety of diseases, these dentists replace the silver fillings with plastic or more costly gold ones. These materials are not safer than silver-amalgam, and the lucrative procedure possibly can result in damage to the tooth.

- Blood tests to determine vitamin and mineral deficiencies. The blood test itself may be normal, but the interpretation may be fraudulent. Results are used to sell worthless vitamin and mineral supplements to patients.

38

The Effects of Nutrition on the Brain, Nervous System, and Behavior

Kenneth Davis, M.D.

■

INTRODUCTION

The brain is the body's most complex organ as well as the center of thought and emotion, qualities that make man unique. It is also the organ about which medical science knows the least. Since what we eat has such a wide-ranging effect on many of the body's organs, it seems only logical that our diets to some extent might also affect the brain and, as a consequence, perhaps even our behavior and emotions. This tantalizing idea is at the core of substantial current brain research. While there is no doubt that what a person ingests can have an effect on the chemistry of the brain itself, possible links between diet, behavior, and emotion remain sketchy.

QUESTIONABLE CLAIMS AND REMEDIES

The vast network of nerves within the brain and the body can be likened to a network of highways along which messages are sent at lightning speed by biochemical messengers called neurotransmitters. There is evidence that most antidepressant and antipsychotic drugs function by altering the activity of particular neurotransmitters. In a chemical sense, these neurotransmitters are "first cousins" to some of the common components of a normal diet. This is because the body manufactures neurotransmitters and other brain chemicals from nutrients, and to do this requires certain vitamins—for example, C, B_6 and B_{12}. Can dietary manipulation or adding nutrient supplements to the diet alter the synthesis, release, and ultimate action of specific neurotransmitters? So far, the answer is sometimes yes, sometimes no. There is evidence that some nutrients may have the ability to alter levels of neurotransmitters, but exactly what the resulting action for overall help or harm on the brain and central nervous system might be is unknown at this time.

In general, it is possible to say that some nutrients have a transitory influence, but evidence that dietary manipulation or supplementation can alter behavior over a long period of time is weak. Nevertheless, scientists who have devoted their lives to understanding the brain suggest that the tiniest nerve impulses, which are virtually impossible to measure with even the most sophisticated modern equipment, perhaps have the ability to cause major changes in the brain's activities. Thus, they say, some effects of diet on the brain may be present but too subtle to measure with current technology.

Diet has been blamed for all manner of emotional and behavioral changes. Similarly, a number of questionable dietary remedies are promoted to counter emotional and behavioral problems. To date, there is little or no scientific evidence to back many of these claims. It has been alleged with no sound evidence that some criminal behavior stems from diets loaded with refined sugar and that this accounts for antisocial behavior. It has also been alleged, despite double-blind controlled studies to the contrary, that food additives account for hyperactivity in children. Still others allege with no sound evidence that food allergies are at the root of emotional and behavioral changes.

Large numbers of people are following questionable dietary treatments for nervous-system disorders. Large doses of amino-acid supplements are promoted—without objective evidence—as a way to increase the levels of certain neurotransmitters in the brain and thus affect such wide-ranging behaviors as alertness, aggression, and depression. One highly questionable practice is the use of restrictive diets to treat hyperactive children. Megadoses of specific vitamins, sometimes at dangerously high levels, are promoted with specious representations that they will increase neurotransmitter production and enhance one's memory or improve behavior. In fact, a highly profitable enterprise called orthomolecular therapy has grown up around the use of high doses of vitamins to treat behavioral disorders. It has been found to be without efficacy by a task force report of the American Psychiatric Association.

Some of the proposed food/brain connections may have semblances of validity, but still be dangerous. For example, there is some evidence that the amino acid tryptophan can help induce sleep. Tryptophan is a building block for the neurotransmitter serotonin, and thus could play a role in treating certain types of depression.

In the late 1980s, L-tryptophan supplements were widely promoted as sleep aids for insomnia sufferers, and many psychiatristis also prescribed it to treat depression. Then in 1989, there came a rash of reports of a rare muscle disorder, eosinophilia myalgia syndrome (EMS). By early 1990, several thousand cases had been reported and some 20 deaths. As of this writing, it is not known whether the eosinophilia was caused by tryptophan, a contaminant introduced in manufacturing the supplements, or both. The Food and Drug Administration barred further sales; Canada did so years ago and had no EMS problem.

Alzheimer's disease, a form of dementia that strikes older people, involves both a loss of active neurons and an inadequate supply of the neurotransmitter acetylcholine. Considerable research has focused on whether or not supplementation with lecithin, the dietary precursor of choline, can increase blood levels of acetylcholine and thereby delay or prevent the appearance of or halt the progression of Alzheimer's disease. So far, there is no evidence to support claims for taking lecithin to treat Alzheimer's.

Parkinson's disease, another central nervous system affliction often seen in late middle age and the elderly, has been alleged to respond to special diets. To date, the only diet that has shown any promise in moderately diminishing symptoms is one in which the level of protein intake is controlled and is limited to late in the day; and even here, the evidence is very sketchy. (See the discussion on Parkinson's disease on page 639.)

After years of research, what can be said about the relationship between diet, emotion, and behavior is that the relationship is very moderate and highly *indirect*. Future research will undoubtedly have a significant impact on overall knowledge in this area.

THE RELATIONSHIP BETWEEN BRAIN CHEMICALS AND NUTRIENTS

The basic brain cell is the neuron. Neurons send signals to one another using neurotransmitters. Close to 50 different compounds that act as neurotransmitters have been discovered. Each is released by very different neurons involved in a wide variety of brain activities. The ability of some neurons to synthesize a specific neurotransmitter depends upon the availability of precursor compounds in the diet. (See Table 38.1.)

Studies have shown that the synthesis and release of neurotransmitters can be altered to some extent by certain foods. As a general rule, amino acids are the precursors of the neurotransmitters. Thus, theoretically, the diet can have behavioral consequences, although any specific cause and effect is difficult to define precisely.

The four neurotransmitters that have been studied the most—and which have the closest relationship to amino acids from dietary protein—are serotonin, dopamine, epinephrine, and norepinephrine. However, while these very specific relationships are becoming better understood, the extent to which dietary changes can predictably alter neurotransmitter levels and change how a person acts and feels is still unclear.

Tryptophan and Serotonin

Probably the most widely studied of these dietary precursor molecules is the amino acid tryptophan, the precursor of the neurotransmitter serotonin. Tryptophan is an essential (it must be provided by the diet) amino acid and is found in all high-quality proteins, such as meat, milk, and eggs. Serotonin is needed to regulate sleep, secrete pituitary hormones, and perceive pain.

The levels of serotonin in the brain can be altered by ingestion of tryptophan. Tryptophan, which is in the blood after a high-protein meal is eaten, must compete with other amino acids such as tyrosine, phenylalanine, leucine, isoleucine, and valine for entry into the brain. As a result, only a small amount of tryptophan makes it to the brain and is converted to serotonin. After a carbohydrate-rich meal, on the other hand, insulin causes these competing amino acids to leave the blood and enter muscle tissue. With fewer amino acids vying for entry, more tryptophan enters the brain, is converted to serotonin, and results in drowsiness. Several research studies have borne out this finding, showing that people who eat a high-carbohydrate lunch are less alert following the meal than people who eat a small, high-protein lunch.

Table 38.1.	Three Important Nutrient-Neurotransmitter (Precursor-Product) Connections
Nutrient (Precursor)	**Neurotransmitter (Product)**
1. Tryptophan	1. Serotonin
2. Lecithin, choline	2. Acetylcholine
3. Tyrosine	3. Dopamine, norepinephrine, epinephrine

Lecithin, Choline, and Acetylcholine

The effect that the nutrient choline has on the neurotransmitter acetylcholine is less dramatic than that in the tryptophan-serotonin connection. Choline in the diet is derived mostly from lecithin in eggs, liver, soybeans, and as a food additive in some processed foods such as mayonnaise and chocolate. When animals are injected with choline, acetylcholine in their brains increases. The resulting levels of acetylcholine are relatively smaller than in the tryptophan-serotonin reaction, however. Scientists have theorized that this is due to the fact that transport of choline from the blood into the brain and the subsequent synthesis of acetylcholine are more complex than the comparable tryptophan-serotonin system.

Attempts have been made to treat neuropsychiatric disorders with choline and lecithin (which contains choline) with mixed results. Choline supplementation has produced some promising results in treating tardive dyskinesia, a disorder distinguished by involuntary facial muscle movements, often resulting from high doses of antipsychotic drugs. Choline has a bitter taste and causes an objectionable fishy body odor in people who take it, however, making it an unpleasant treatment. Some investigators have given lecithin instead and had similar success in treating tardive dyskinesia without the same drawbacks, because choline is released from the lecithin. Pure lecithin is, however, a bulky, waxy substance that must be taken in large amounts (up to 20 to 30 grams or about three-quarters to one ounce) to be effective; and it adds an unneeded nine calories a gram to a person's diet. In addition, commercial lechithin supplements from health-food stores are generally only about 3 percent pure lecithin, although purer proportions are available. As a result, huge amounts and many calories must be consumed to get the same 20 to 30 grams of lecithin used in experiments.

Choline and lecithin also have been tested for value in treating other neurological diseases such as Huntington's chorea, cerebellar ataxias, and Gilles de la Tourette's syndrome, as well as schizophrenia, mania, and depression. While a few studies have shown some minor alleged benefit in treating certain psychiatric illnesses, the number of patients studied was small and the substances were often given in conjunction with other medications, so any actual benefit is unknown. Since people with Alzheimer's disease tend, among other things, to be deficient in acetylcholine, choline and lecithin supplementation have been extensively studied as having possible value. Results have not been dramatic but they have left some scientists encouraged enough to continue the study of choline and lecithin as possibly of some use.

Tyrosine and the Catecholamines

The complex relationships between the amino acid tyrosine and a large class of neurotransmitters known as catecholamines, which includes norepinephrine, epinephrine, and dopamine, have also been extensively studied.

Eating a high-protein meal increases the amount of tyrosine in the blood, causing tyrosine levels in the brain to increase slightly. A more effective means of increasing tyrosine levels in the brain, however, is ingestion of a pure tyrosine supplement with carbohydrates. The carbohydrate stimulates insulin secretion, which reduces the levels of other competing amino acids, and allows easy entry of tyrosine into the brain. The increase in brain tyrosine will, in turn, increase the levels of catecholamines, particularly dopamine. This strategy has a potential benefit for patients suffering from Parkinson's disease, which is characterized by a deficiency of dopamine. Increasing dopamine levels by administering the amino acid precursor of dopamine, levodopa, relieves some of the disease's central nervous system effects, and there is evidence that tyrosine has a similar effect.

Tyrosine has also been used, with limited success, to treat depression, probably by increasing levels of the catecholamine norepinephrine, which is often low in people with depression. Still, research into the links among diet, catecholamines, and other neurotransmitters is in its infancy.

Tyrosine has not been approved by the FDA for use as a drug. However, like tryptophan, publicity has created a market for tyrosine—available in drugstores and health-food stores—and there is a risk that consumers suffering from various neuropsychiatric diseases may be misled into believing that they can be helped by taking amino-acid supplements. In addition, some amino-acid supplements sold over the counter have poor quality control, resulting in inconsistent and unpredictable blood levels. In addition, little is known about the possible harm of long-term use at high-dosage levels.

Vitamins

Half a century ago, more than one-third of the beds in mental hospitals in the southern United States were occupied by victims of pellagra, a disease that has both physical and psychiatric symptoms, including apathy, depression, anxiety, delirium, memory deficits, and psychosis. Pellagra was also common among institutionalized people—in prisons, orphanages, state hospitals, and other institutions. The disease had been known for three centuries, but only in the 1920s was its cause—a nutritional deficiency—and treatment—eating yeast, liver, or any high-quality protein—discovered. Finally, in 1937, the deficient nutrient was discovered to be vitamin B_3 (niacin).

A national policy of fortifying foods such as bread and cereals with niacin has relegated pellagra to the status of a medical curiosity in the United States. Pellagra, with its behavioral and other serious symptoms, however, provides a graphic illustration of the significant neurological and physical problems that a profound vitamin deficiency can produce.

Serious deficiencies of thiamin, vitamin B_6, vitamin B_{12}, vitamin C, and folic acid can also provoke psychiatric symptoms, although the physical symptoms vary. A thiamine deficiency, most often seen in alcoholics, can cause Korsakoff's psychosis, a condition that affects recent memory and causes emotional changes; it can also cause Wernicke's syndrome, a condition that reduces blood flow to the brain and can lead to coma and eventually death. A deficiency of vitamin B_6 (pyridoxine) can cause mental retardation in infants, though such conditions are rare in the United States. In adults, B_6 deficiency can result from taking the drug isoniazid, used to treat tuberculosis, and can result in mood changes and, in some cases, psychosis.

Vitamin B_{12} (cyanocobalamin) deficiency causes pernicious (megaloblastic) anemia and neurologic damage, which, in turn, damages mental function. This may occur among elderly and institutionalized people and can sometimes mimic Alzheimer's disease. The B_{12} deficiency is usually due to defective absorption, so treatment is usually with injections of B_{12}, not dietary B_{12}. Deficiencies of folic acid can also cause megaloblastic anemia, a condition that is sometimes preceded or accompanied by mental disturbances, including irritability, mood swings, and paranoid behavior. Vitamin C (ascorbic acid) deficiencies cause scurvy, whose symptoms may include depression and hypochondriasis.

Aside from these severe but mostly rare nutrient deficiencies, there is no concrete evidence that any other psychiatric illnesses are caused by nutritional deficiencies or that such illnesses can be treated with diet. The situation is different, however, in some Third World countries with widespread malnutrition among infants and children. There, nutritional deficiencies can contribute to mental retardation and behavioral disturbances.

It has been alleged that mild vitamin deficiencies might cause some impairment of brain function. For example, it has been hoped that older, poorly nourished people who have lessened brain function, which is now blamed on old age, are really suffering the effects of a vitamin deficiency. Tests have shown that people over age 60 with low blood levels of vitamin B_{12} or vitamin C score lower on cognitive ability tests than other subjects with normal vitamin levels. Such findings are open to conflicting interpretation, however. One might consider these results as meaning the vitamin deficiencies caused the lower scores on the cognitive-function tests. An equally valid explanation is that poor cognitive function led to inadequate dietary intake, which subsequently caused the low vitamin levels in the blood. Still, proponents of vitamin therapy are quick to claim a direct cause-and-effect relationship, even if the data is not adequately supportive and there are other explanations for it. In contrast, nutrition scientists are more cautious and require adequate evidence before reaching a definite conclusion.

Trace Minerals

There has been considerable research into the role of trace minerals in brain and nerve function. A deficiency of *iodine*, for example, can have a profound effect on brain maturation and neuropsychological function during fetal development. Iodine is needed in the manufacture of thyroid hormones. Thus, a severe iodine deficiency can lead to thyroid deficiency. In an infant, this can result in cretinism, which is characterized by mental retardation and other serious problems in growth and development. In some parts of the world (for example the Alps and around the Great Lakes in the United States), the soil is lacking in iodine. Thus, the mineral is lacking in foods raised in those areas. To ensure against iodine deficiency, it is added to foods, specifically iodized table salt and certain ingredients used in commercial bread. As a result, true iodine deficiencies are rare in the United States (although there still may be thyroid deficiencies from other causes).

Iron deficiency is believed to impair neuropsychological function in children, manifesting itself in part as lack of attention and alertness in school. Since iron is essential to proper oxygen transport in the body, the problems could be attributed in part to inadequate oxygen reaching the brain. In addition, research has indicated that iron is involved in the synthesis and release of the catecholamine dopamine, and a lack of this substance also can produce symptoms.

Zinc is another mineral that is essential in a number of major biochemical processes that affect brain function. *Copper* is also essential to normal functioning of the central nervous system. In humans, genetic conditions that upset copper balance cause nervous-system disorders. Menkes' disease, for example, is a hereditary abnormality characterized by inadequate intestinal absorption of copper. Affected infants suffer a gradual degeneration of the brain and growth retardation. Wilson's disease, on the other hand, is the result of gradual accumulation of copper in the body tissues, including the brain. The result, over time, is a deterioration of mental function. Both these conditions are rare.

Studies involving rats and guinea pigs suggest that the mineral *manganese* is essential for normal brain function. It appears to be involved in the conversion of levodopa to dopamine in the brain. Deficiencies of manganese causing behavioral abnormalities in humans, however, have not been documented. Excesses of manganese are better known. An accumulation of the mineral in the brain is found in Parkinson's disease and some forms of dementia. However, it is not yet known whether excess manganese plays any role in the development of these conditions.

Lead and *mercury* are notoriously toxic if large amounts are consumed. When blood levels become excessively high, the result is central nervous system abnormalities that can cause profound damage, including personality changes, irritability, and sleep disturbances. If blood levels are not lowered, death can result. The toxicity of lead has been known since ancient times. Today, it is most common among inner-city children who live in old homes and who inhale lead-laden dust or ingest it by eating chips of lead-based paint flaking from walls, and who inhale air full of the exhaust from vehicles using leaded gasoline. Recent studies have also found high lead levels in drinking water that flows through deteriorating pipes that contain lead. Children with lead poisoning suffer a variety of learning disabilities such as attention deficits and lowered IQ.

The phrase *mad as a hatter* reflects a nineteenth-century occupational hazard: the psychosis caused by inhalation of mercury vapors used in making felt hats. More recent mercury-poisoning cases have occurred when people ate fish contaminated with high levels of mercury from waters polluted with industrial wastes.

Recent research also has shown that *calcium* and *magnesium*, which work together in the body, play a role in some brain functions. Calcium, for example, is essential for the normal functioning of neurons. Insufficient dietary calcium and a lack of vitamin D can cause hypocalcemia, which can produce mental aberrations. Some patients with mood disorders who receive the drug lithium carbonate excrete less calcium in their urine after beginning to take the drug and show increased calcium levels in their blood after long-term lithium use.

ORTHOMOLECULAR AND MEGAVITAMIN THERAPY

In the late 1950s, a small group of psychiatrists began giving large doses of niacin to patients suffering from schizophrenia. They speculated that a biochemical defect was the cause of the disease and that niacin would correct it. The vitamin was given in conjunction with other treatments, such as barbiturates and electroconvulsive therapy. In subsequent years, other psychotropic drugs were added to the treatment regimen, along with large doses of other water-soluble vitamins. Today, the treatment, now known as orthomolecular therapy, includes not only niacin but large doses of vitamin C, vitamin B_6, folic acid, vitamin B_{12}, minerals, hormones, diets that reduce blood-glucose levels, and diets free of foods alleged to cause allergies.

Questionable since its inception, orthomolecular therapy's fundamental tenets have shifted with time, as have the concepts of the biochemical defects its followers allege to be the cause of schizophrenia. Linus Pauling, the Nobel Prize–winning chemist, coined the term *orthomolecular* in 1968, defining it as the "treatment of mental disease by the provision of the optimum molecular environment for the mind, especially the optimum concentration of substances normally present in the human body." This definition is operationally worthless, since it is unknown what the word *optimum* means in this context. "Optimum" levels in orthomolecular therapy appears to be a synonym for megadoses of vitamins, far above what the body needs for sound nutrition, and often at harmfully high levels.

In 1973, the American Psychiatric Association (APA) convened a task force to study orthomolecular therapy. This group found no evidence to support the practice of it, and characterized the underlying therapy as superficial, inconsistent, and contradictory. Not surprisingly, orthomolecular therapists attacked the task-force report, alleging flaws in the studies used, and argued that it did not take into account the use of electroconvulsive shock therapy and other treatment modalities often used in conjunction with megadoses of vitamins.

Nonetheless, the lucrative practice has continued into the 1990s, despite the fact that numerous well-conducted studies have failed to demonstrate that mentally ill patients fare better under orthomolecular treatment. Neither is there evidence that adult schizophrenics differ from the normal population in their need for niacin or any other vitamin. Although large doses of some of the vitamins used in the therapy are not as harmful as others, there is clear evidence that large doses of vitamin B_6, for example, can cause permanent neurological damage. Although some psychiatrists and psychologists around the country are believed to be engaged in orthomolecular therapy or some version of it, the therapy remains well outside the mainstream of modern psychiatry and is a lucrative sideshow.

Another highly questionable treatment involves giving large doses of several vitamins including A, E, C, niacin, and B_6 as a treatment for children with Down's syndrome. First proposed in 1981 after a study of 16 retarded children claimed an improvement in their intellectual functioning, the study was regarded as meritless in a formal position paper by the American Academy of Pediatrics.

Most claims that large doses of vitamins are useful in treating brain-function disorders lack support from controlled studies. Preliminary research alleges that large doses of vitamin B_6 might be beneficial in treating some autistic children. In two studies of autistic children—one in which the parents knew whether their child was receiving the vitamin or a placebo; the other in which they did not—improvement was seen with administration of vitamin B_6. Further tests are needed, however, before large doses of vitamin B_6 can be recommended as treatment. They can harm.

DIET AND BEHAVIOR

Since the beginning of modern nutritional research, there have been attempts to connect abnormal behavior directly to a person's diet. Such behavior includes hyperactivity of children, the antisocial behavior of criminals, and the impaired learning ability of some children, as well as sleep disturbances and mood swings. Numerous superficial investigations have been performed, ignoring basic requirements for securing valid evidence. Based on such investigations, sweeping and ill-founded claims have been made about diet and behavior, primarily by people with no legitimate credentials as health professionals.

After decades of research, diet has not been shown to be the cause of criminality, hyperactivity, psychosis, or depression. Nevertheless, such notions persist and reappear, sometimes disguised as new concepts in order to fill the need to believe in simple solutions to complex problems. For example, substantial numbers of parents continue to subscribe to the belief that food additives and diet underlie hyperactivity in children. In recent years, there has been considerable publicity falsely blaming the antisocial behavior of convicted felons on too much sugar in the diet (the so-called "Twinkie defense" used as an excuse by a San Francisco murderer), on reactive hypoglycemia, and on alleged food allergies or excesses or deficiencies of vitamins and minerals. This hype has fed on irrelevant unrelated research linking diet to children's school performances, some of which has focused on iron deficiency and the effects of the common practice of skipping breakfast. Even sorting out this legitimate research is often difficult because so many variables other than diet are involved.

Diet and Criminal Behavior

The notion that diet and criminal behavior are linked gained popularity in the 1980s with faddist claims that certain nutrients could trigger feelings of anger or hostility. The substance most commonly attacked by food faddists was, and is, sugar—either too much or too little. A number of correctional institutions, acting on anecdotes and testimonials by nonhealth professionals, modified prisoners' diets, providing them with vitamin and mineral supplements, and "tested" them for low blood-glucose levels, nutrient imbalances, and food allergies. The "testing" methods used were largely worthless, but the results were promoted as legitimate.

One study of juvenile offenders claimed that reducing the sugar in their diet decreased antisocial behavior. Critics who attacked the work as flawed in experimental design and statistical analysis pointed out that the experimenter was incorrect in claiming that replacing sugar in the diet with honey or replacing soft drinks with fruit juice would reduce total dietary sugar. In fact, there is no metabolic difference between natural sugars such as honey and regular processed sugar. (See Chapter 9.)

At the other end of the spectrum are claims that hypoglycemia (low blood sugar), a relatively rare condition, is responsible for aggressive behavior and is more prevalent in violent offenders and juvenile delinquents. This contention grew from scientifically worthless studies in which it was claimed that 90 percent of criminals suffered from the condition. These claims were based on highly questionable investigational techniques. In some cases, populations of prisoners were merely given questionnaires in which they listed physical and psychological complaints or diagnosed themselves. In other cases, there were unwarranted conclusions from oral glucose-tolerance tests, taken to determine blood-sugar levels, says the American Diabetes Association.

Hypoglycemia is a condition that is frequently claimed but seldom confirmed when the patient is subjected to appropriate testing. In one study, a research team tested 135 patients suspected of being hypoglycemic and could confirm the condition in only 4 cases. Scientists critical of the speculation connecting hypoglycemia and violence point out that the symptoms of hypoglycemia are headache, confusion, and motor weakness, not aggression and violence.

As with sugar, claims that food allergies are linked to criminal behavior have no legitimate basis; and like hypoglycemia, the incidence of real food allergies tends to be overestimated. Food allergies are best studied using double-blind research techniques in which neither subjects nor researchers know which patients are receiving the alleged allergenic food. To date, no such studies have been done to demonstrate any connection between allergies and behavior, and there is no reliable evidence to link food allergies with criminal behavior.

It is equally difficult to find any evidence to support claims that vitamin and mineral deficiencies or excesses are related to criminal behavior. Megavitamin therapies have been proposed for juvenile delinquents and convicted felons, despite the lack of any sound evidence behind such therapy. Experts who question the use of megavitamin therapy have also warned that large doses of vitamins or minerals can be harmful, particularly such nutrients as vitamins A, D, and B_6 and the mineral iron.

In an effort to deal with the fad connecting diet and criminal behavior, a panel of experts was convened by several professional groups. After reviewing the evidence, the panel concluded that no link existed between the two and that there was no need to change public policy regarding the accountability of offenders for their actions. The National Council Against Health Fraud also issued a position paper on diet and criminal behavior, which was subsequently endorsed by the American Dietetic Association. No evidence was found to support claims that diet and hypoglycemia are associated with criminal behavior or that dietary changes or megavitamin therapy are beneficial to prisoners.

Hyperactivity in Children

The use of diet therapy to treat hyperactive children has always been questionable, with its proponents staunchly defending the practice and its critics contending there is no evidence to support it. Formally known as attention-deficit disorder, the syndrome is characterized by excessive motor activity, impulsiveness, inattentiveness, distractibility, anxiety, and poor tolerance for frustration. Teachers in elementary schools are often the first to spot it, although parents not infrequently bring their child's abnormally high activity levels to the attention of a doctor. The cause of hyperactivity remains unknown, although both genetic and environmental factors appear to be implicated.

The Feingold diet. The idea that diet is the cause of hyperactivity came to the forefront in 1973 when Benjamin Feingold, a California pediatric allergist, proposed that salicylates (the major ingredient in aspirin; also present in tomatoes and some other foods), artificial food colors, and artificial flavors caused hyperactivity. He claimed that a diet free of those substances significantly improved behavior in hyperactive children he had treated. He wrote two popular books, and the mass media extensively promoted his claims. Large numbers of parents of hyperactive children followed his recommendations and many of them reported significant improvements in their children's behavior. The Feingold diet soon had a loyal following, many of whom continue to adhere to it today after more than 15 years. The Feingold diet works, but the success has nothing to do with the diet itself.

Under Feingold's dietary restrictions, common foods that are generally children's favorites are almost completely eliminated. Most processed baked goods are forbidden, as are luncheon meats, ice cream, powdered puddings, candies, soft drinks, and packaged and prepared foods. Tea and coffee and most condiments purchased from grocery-store shelves are not allowed. The Feingold diet also eliminates many other items that contain colors or additives, such as mouthwash, toothpaste, vitamins, and some over-the-counter and prescription drugs.

Dr. Feingold published a list of fruits and vegetables that he said contained salicylate, and he recommended that these not be eaten. Parents who strictly adhere to the Feingold plan and eliminate most fruits and vegetables from their child's diet must be careful that it contains enough vitamins and minerals to meet the child's needs. The nine artificial food colors that the diet eliminates are easily identified by product labels. Many more artificial flavors that are forbidden are difficult to identify because their constituents are also found naturally in foods. Chemically, natural flavorings are no different from artificial ones. Critics of the Feingold diet have pointed out the irrationality of banning the artificial flavors without also addressing the natural flavors. Dr. Feingold later added to his forbidden list BHA and BHT, antioxidant food preservatives used in packaged foods.

Dr. Feingold's claims of success in treating hyperactive children were anecdotal. Double-blind scientific studies gathered at considerable expense over the years have been unable to substantiate his claims. These studies clearly showed that the *belief* a Feingold diet was being used was what worked. This was done by secretly adding to a Feingold diet for the study subjects and secretly removing all additives from a normal diet for them. One test did find that huge doses of food colors given to children with more severe symptoms of hyperactivity caused a deterioration in the behavior of a very small subgroup of the children. The findings have been widely challenged, however, and questions have been raised about the relevance of behavior changes when children received doses far greater than they would ever consume in a typical American diet.

Despite mostly negative findings, the Feingold diet, or variations of it, continue to attract devoted followers among parents who are at a loss to deal with their child's hyperactivity. The thrust of the evidence is that the claims of success are due to what psychiatrists call positive reinforcement; that is, telling the child, "We love you so much we are going to extra special hardship to see that you get only selected foods." In addition to the emphasis on meal preparation, increased parental attention to the hyperactive child and the idea that food—not the child—is to blame for the behavioral problems are likely to foster a positive response.

Megavitamins. Can vitamin megadoses reduce hyperactivity? Responsible scientific studies have failed to find any relation between vitamin therapy and lessened hyperactivity, and some have found that children receiving large doses of vitamins actually became more hyperactive, compared to children receiving a placebo. In addition, megadoses of niacin, vitamin C, and the B vitamin pantothenate have also been given to hyperactive children, but no beneficial effect has been seen. The children in these studies frequently experienced diarrhea, and there was additional evidence that the large doses of the vitamins were toxic to their livers. Several health-professional groups have warned against giving megadoses of vitamins to hyperactive children because of the dangers from toxicity and from adverse interactions among nutrients.

Sugar and hyperactivity. Both excessive sugar in the diet and hypoglycemia (low blood sugar) have been alleged as causes of hyperactivity. A 1980 study at the University of South Carolina reported that the more sugar a group of hyperactive children consumed, the more destructive, restless, and aggressive they were. A control group of normal children did not act this way when given sugar. However, critics of the study quickly pointed out that there was no evidence that sugar caused the behavioral changes. Several other studies have shown the opposite: that sugar actually can have a calming effect on children. For example, in one study, children were given orange drinks sweetened with either sugar or the artificial sweetener aspartame. The children drinking the sugar-sweetened drinks experienced reduced activity levels, whereas children receiving the artificial sweetener did not. This study was carried out at the National Institute of Mental Health and was highly credible. Since consuming sugar directly enhances serotonin production, it is more logical that sugar would have a calming effect than that it would produce aggression. (See Chapter 8.)

Caffeine. There have also been claims that caffeine, which many children consume in significant quantities in soft drinks, causes hyperactivity. Although this is unlikely, what is true is that studies have shown that caffeine causes increased motor activity and fidgetiness in pre-adolescent boys, although individuals vary widely in their responses. In one carefully designed study, boys receiving the highest doses of caffeine showed a greater response than boys who received a small dose or a placebo. Other studies have indicated that hyperactive children or children who tend to be unusually impulsive in their behavior will select a diet with a higher caffeine content when given a choice. Such findings illustrate the necessity for further research, particularly regarding the long-term moderate doses that are typical of daily consumption of soft drinks.

Malnutrition and Behavior

While most links between diet and behavior are weak, there is no question that severe malnutrition can have a significant impact on behavior, particularly in children. The very young are most vulnerable, since brain development takes place not only in the womb but during the first two years of life.

The number of brain cells continues to change during the first year after birth, and the myelin sheaths that encase all nerve fibers continue to form during the first years of life. Numerous studies in animals, and autopsies of children who died of malnutrition, have shown that severe nutritional deficiencies retard these vital processes. Children who died of marasmus, a severe form of protein and calorie malnutrition, had fewer brain cells than normal children of the same age. Children who died of the protein-deficiency disease kwashiorkor had a normal number of brain cells, but the cells were smaller than normal.

Malnourished children tend to have difficulties in learning to speak, in adaptive and motivational behavior, interpersonal relationships, and development of motor skills. There have been suggestions that iron deficiency can also impede cognitive function and adversely affect the behavior of schoolchildren.

Numerous studies have shown that a past episode of malnutrition can affect a child's I.Q. and behavior in school. Children who have been malnourished are especially likely to be restless, inattentive, and have poor social skills and emotional instability in school settings. Studying such effects is usually difficult, since formerly malnourished children often come from poor socioeconomic backgrounds where other variables such as home environment could be responsible for the findings. Some researchers, however, have shown that malnourished children can be helped to overcome their behavioral handicaps if they are provided with a stimulating environment.

Breakfast and School Performance

Far more subtle are the learning difficulties that may or may not relate to fasting in schoolchildren. In most situations, fasting consists of skipping breakfast, sometimes because of lower socioeconomic background and in other cases because of poor dietary habits on the part of parents and children. The belief that children who go to school hungry do not perform well led in 1966 to passage of the Child Nutrition Act, part of the Great Society legislation of the Lyndon Johnson era.

Many studies focused on children 9 to 11 years old. In general, it was found that children who ate breakfast performed better through the morning on different measures of cognitive performance than those who skipped it. The optimal breakfast was one that was balanced in protein, carbohydrates, and fats. Although important, breakfast alone will not necessarily improve school performance. Other variables, including the time of the meal, its size, the ratio of carbohydrate to protein, and the complexity of the tasks that measure cognitive performance, also are important.

Food Allergies and Behavior

Allergic reactions to specific foods are believed by many people to cause behavioral abnormalities, but objective clinical trials have failed to show that they do so, or that they can account for neurological or psychiatric problems. An allergic reaction to food occurs when the body's immune system treats the food (protein) molecule as a foreign invader and mounts an attack, producing antibodies, histamines, and other defensive substances. The body may then, from that point on, respond with a similar allergic reaction each time the food is encountered.

Responsible immunologists and allergists generally find that true food allergies are uncommon, and behavioral problems caused by allergies are exceptionally rare. Several studies of people who claimed that food allergies were causing such symptoms as lethargy, depression, mood swings, irritability, poor concentration, anxiety, and sleeplessness found that only a small percentage suffered from genuine food allergies. For the rest of the patients, psychiatric problems rather than allergic reactions to food seemed to be responsible. (See Chapter 33.)

DIET, BEHAVIOR, AND SPECIFIC DISEASES

Parkinson's Disease

Magazines and popular books have frequently led victims of Parkinson's disease to believe that diet plays a curative role in their disorder and that following special diets could result in improvement. This is not true. No known nutritional deficiency is responsible for parkinsonism and there is no special food, nutrient, vitamin, or mineral that can cure the disease. Dietary modification, however, may improve some symptoms.

Parkinson's disease occurs most often in late middle age. It is an incurable degenerative disease of the central nervous system that causes slowness of movement, difficulty initiating movement, muscle weakness, and uncontrollable trembling movements. Many patients have difficulty in closing their mouths, biting, chewing, or swallowing. The administration of the amino acid levodopa, the precursor of dopamine, can dramatically improve symptoms. Protein in the diet tends to reduce its absorption, since it must compete with other amino acids for entry into the brain. Reducing protein in the diet to about seven grams during the day and consuming normal amounts of protein at the evening meal have reduced daytime symptoms in some patients. However, adding extra levodopa to compensate for a diet that is higher in protein has the same therapeutic effect. As a result, it is important that meals be consistent. They should be served at regular times and excesses should be avoided. A hearty steak dinner can be expected to reduce the effectiveness of the levodopa dosage until the body has cleared this protein load. Moderate alcohol consumption is not thought to have an affect on symptoms.

Over the years, various therapies involving special foods or vitamins have been proposed, but there is no evidence that any are effective.

Alzheimer's Disease

For several years it has been known that people with Alzheimer's disease—a progressive form of dementia that leads to significant behavioral abnormalities in about 7 percent of the population over age 65—have abnormally low levels of the enzyme choline acetyltransferase (CAT). CAT, in turn, is necessary for the production of the neurotransmitter acetylcholine in the brain. As noted earlier, acetylcholine has an as yet unclearly defined role in memory and learning. In Alzheimer's disease, there is also a selective degeneration of neurons that respond to acetylcholine.

Considerable effort has been expended on research in order better to understand the brain chemistry involved and to learn whether manipulating enzymes and neurotransmitters might alleviate Alzheimer's disease. Much of this research has focused on using the drug choline chloride. Results with choline and lecithin have not been promising; researchers report that they are still far from understanding the role of the brain chemicals involved, and that drugs that increase brain activity at neurons containing acetylcholine may be effective in some patients with Alzheimer's disease. (See the earlier discussion of lecithin, choline, and acetylcholine on page 630.)

Multiple Sclerosis

There are no known dietary changes or vitamin or mineral supplementation regimens that can improve the condition of a person suffering from multiple sclerosis, although MS victims over the years often have been offered false hope by various dietary claims. In this disease, the myelin sheaths that surround nerves become abnormal and interfere with the nerve's ability to function. The severity of the disease depends upon which nerves are affected and to what extent the myelin has degenerated. Many patients go into spontaneous remissions for long periods of time, sometimes permanently. Whatever diet is coincidentally being followed at the time the remission occurs is often erroneously credited by the patient with having caused the remission.

One of the most well-known MS diets is very low in fat, especially saturated fats. Industrialized countries with a high animal-fat intake have a higher incidence of MS, but whether this is a coincidence or a cause-and-effect relationship is impossible to determine, because there are so many other coincidental differences between countries with high and low rates of MS. Since MS is a disease in which the patient can undergo periodic remissions, the remissions often occur while the patient, desperate for some form of relief, has been experimenting with diet or other lifestyle changes. This has led to false claims that certain special dietary practices are useful. Attempts to lessen MS symptoms by altering diet in carefully controlled clinical trials have failed to produce results explainable by anything other than random remission variability.

Few doctors who are expert in the disease endorse any special dietary practices. The National Multiple Sclerosis Society says flatly that diet has no effect. Specialists who treat MS advise their patients to eat a balanced and nutritious diet to keep themselves as healthy as possible.

IN SUMMARY

Although there are numerous claims linking brain and nervous function and behavior to various nutritional factors, there is little real evidence that dietary therapy has any significant impact, and some of the practices are harmful in one way or another. Certainly there is no justification for taking megadoses of vitamins and minerals in the belief that this will improve intellect or mental function or prevent disorders such as Alzheimer's or Parkinson's diseases. Furthermore, megadoses have produced a wide variety of harms. Similarly, there is no scientific evidence that a restrictive diet will improve hyperactivity or behavior problems in children. A balanced and varied diet will provide all of the nutrients needed for proper brain and nerve function. In unusual cases of deficiency-related disorders, nutrition therapy may be of value, but these are the exceptions rather than the rule, and diagnosis by measuring blood-nutrient levels must precede therapy to assure the therapy will do more good than harm.

Part VI

Making Good Nutrition
Part of Your Daily Life

■

39

Restaurant Eating for the Calorie- and Nutrition-Conscious

Fran C. Grossman, R.D., M.S., Elyse Sosin, R.D., M.A.,
and Rosalinda Lawson, R.D.

■

INTRODUCTION

Dining out was once reserved for special occasions when concerns about calories and nutrition were set aside. However, restaurant eating now has become an everyday event, with Americans eating one out of every three meals outside the home. This change in eating habits coincides with a burgeoning interest in the role of diet in health in general and in the prevention of disease. Although some restaurants have made low-calorie additions to their menus to reflect the wishes of consumers who are calorie- and fat-conscious, most—even those that pride themselves on inventive cuisine—still serve foods that are high in fats, cholesterol, sugar, and salt. Butter and cream are often present in large quantities; meats are frequently prime cuts (higher in fats) and often sautéed or fried; vegetables are sauced or sometimes moussed; desserts are rich and elaborate.

Despite this, it is possible for those with special health concerns to have—and enjoy—an appropriate meal in virtually any restaurant, even in those that do not attempt to control ingredients or to modify methods of preparation. To do so, diners need to know how to select a restaurant and, once there, how to choose among the myriad items offered on the menu.

The key to balancing a dining experience with nutrition is planning. The type of cuisine served can make a difference in the selections offered. For example, it's easier to order a low-fat meal in a Japanese or seafood restaurant than at a fast-food counter serving fried chicken. Diners who patronize a few restaurants regularly will be able to preselect what they will order. Choosing the menu ahead of time removes one of the major pitfalls of restaurant eating—ordering on a whim. Those on restricted diets should select a restaurant that can accommodate special requests. A phone call will help determine what a restaurant offers, as well as the management's attitude toward fulfilling special requests. Restaurants that cook to order will have the most flexibility and are usually the most accommodating (see Special Requests on page 647).

The majority of people do not follow strict dietary regimens. Therefore, for most people dining out, it is important to know how to select foods that offer good nutritional value for the calories and how to avoid overindulging. Within those guidelines, most restaurants provide appealing choices.

Diners who need to prevent overindulging should avoid complete dinners (they usually include several unwanted courses), "all you can eat" deals, and price-fixed multi-course dinners. Eating à la carte (even if it costs more) will give a diner more control over portions eaten and remove the temptation to overeat.

All meals eaten out should be selected in relationship to other meals consumed during that day. If lunch was elaborate, dinner should be simple and light; if breakfast or lunch was a high-protein meal, dinner should include less protein and more complex carbohydrate. Those who dine out frequently—for example, on business—will need to be vigilant about this and should make every effort to balance nutrition. One way to balance nutritional needs while also controlling calories is to make trade-offs: a glass of wine before dinner instead of dessert—or vice versa; a hot dinner roll instead of a potato; or dressing on a salad instead of butter on a roll.

COCKTAILS AND BEVERAGES

Liquor is often a source of hidden calories for restaurant diners. A glass of wine or beer, or one ounce of gin, vodka, or whiskey, each has about 100 calories. To reduce calories in alcoholic beverages, diners should choose a wine spritzer or light beer; in mixed drinks, seltzer can be substituted for tonic and sugary mixes. For some people, alcohol may stimulate the appetite and lower resolve about overeating. To avoid this, a diner should decide beforehand how much he or she will drink.

Those who drink nonalcoholic beverages can also reduce calories by diluting fruit juices (which have a relatively high sugar content) with water or seltzer. Vegetable juices are lower in calories than fruit juices but may be high in salt.

THE MENU

A diner should obtain menus before dining out at a chosen restaurant, if possible. This way it can be determined ahead of time what meal will be the best choice. By ordering your meal first, one will not be "persuaded" to change a well-planned meal by the tempting suggestions of others.

To help prevent overeating, diners should, as already mentioned, order à la carte. Asking the waiter to remove the bread basket after everyone has made a selection will help avoid one of the greatest temptations for hungry diners. Having a leisurely broth-based soup, a glass of tomato juice, or a green salad before ordering the rest of the meal will help curb the appetite. Pacing a meal also helps to avoid overindulging. Certain foods by their nature take time and effort to eat—for example, artichokes, whole steamed fish, unshelled shrimp, corn-on-the-cob, or a raw vegetable salad. Whatever the selection, it should be eaten slowly with pauses between courses to enjoy the company of fellow diners.

Appetizers and Starters

The purpose of an appetizer is to take the edge off hunger and to provide something delectable while waiting for the entrée to arrive. An appetizer should nutritionally complement the entrée. If, for instance, the entrée is high in carbohydrates—for example, a pasta or rice and vegetable dish—a high-protein appetizer such as clams, oysters, or poached fish would be a good choice.

Green salads make low-calorie appetizers. Instead of thick and creamy or oil-based salad dressings, lemon or a small amount of oil and vinegar can be added. Whenever salad dressing is used, it should be served on the side, and then used in modest amounts.

For those watching calorie and cholesterol intake, appetizers such as mussels or clams poached in their own broth or in a tomato and wine sauce, raw vegetables, shrimp or crab cocktail with cocktail sauce rather than tartar sauce (which is mostly mayonnaise), and any type of melon or other fresh fruit are wise choices.

For those not on sodium-restricted diets, broth- or tomato-based soups are acceptable. However, creamed soups and onion soup (which is usually made with butter and topped with a heavy layer of cheese) are high in fat and cholesterol and, as with many appetizers, often too filling to be eaten in addition to a main meal. Grain-type soups—barley, chick-pea, bean—although also filling and generally high in calories, are higher in fiber and often vitamins, and lower in fat.

Special Requests

Patrons of restaurants have a right to request that some modifications be made in how their food is prepared, keeping in mind that a restaurant is not a private kitchen, nor is the chef a personal employee of each customer.

Restaurants that cook to order will find it easier to satisfy customer requests. Some dishes, however, can't be made without specific ingredients; for example, hollandaise sauce cannot be made without the eggs. Therefore, even in restaurants where every dish is individually prepared, there are limitations to meeting customer requests. Restaurants that serve foods mostly prepared in advance (many do little more than heat and serve), will find it more difficult to alter the contents of dishes. Even here, though, all sauces and salad dressings usually can be served on the side at the customer's request.

Patrons who make special requests should do the following.

Enlist the assistance of the waiter or waitress. Be courteous when inquiring about the menu and preparation of the food. Special requests are more likely to be accommodated when the restaurant is not busy and the waiter is not rushed. Questions should be confined to dishes being considered. Waiters may know little about food preparation or nutrition. A salad dressing that the waiter says isn't made with any oil at all may contain sour cream and mayonnaise. Waiters in ethnic restaurants may not speak English and may have difficulty explaining how dishes are prepared.

Learn about cooking basics. Béchamel, béarnaise, and hollandaise sauces and Thousand Island and creamy Italian salad dressings are made of high-cholesterol ingredients whether they're made at home or in a restaurant. Sautéed always means cooked in butter. All fried food, no matter what fat or oil in which it's fried, is high in calories.

Make requests clear, specific, and easy to follow. Requests should be precise, and not interrogative. Instead of asking whether the chef uses butter on the broiled fish, a customer should make statements such as, "I'd like the fish broiled dry, without butter or margarine," or, "I'd like a green salad with the dressing on the side." Sometimes when a customer requests that one ingredient be eliminated from a dish, the chef adds another to compensate for the loss; for example, margarine may be substituted for butter, or soy sauce may be substituted for monosodium glutamate. If a customer does not want a substitution, he or she should say so; for example, "No butter or margarine; a little lemon or herbs is all right."

When requests are clearly and politely made and yet instructions are not followed, the customer should send the food back.

An alternative to ordering an entrée is to share one in restaurants known for oversized portions, or to order two appetizers and a salad instead. A hearty soup along with a second appetizer or salad can comprise a complete dinner for many people.

There are a number of appetizers some may need to avoid. Smoked or pickled foods are usually high in sodium and should not be eaten by anyone on a sodium-restricted diet. Because a diet high in salt-cured and genuinely smoked foods (but not smoke-flavored foods) has been linked to an increased risk of stomach cancer, they should be eaten only in moderation.

Assorted or house-specialty appetizers offered by Polynesian, Chinese, and some Mexican restaurants are often deep-fried and therefore high in calories. In French restaurants, the house appetizer is likely to be a pâté, usually high in fat and cholesterol. Unless diners know the contents and preparation of house appetizers, it is usually better to order something else if high calories are a concern.

Entrées

Entrées that are lower in calories and fat include dishes whose main ingredients are skinless chicken or turkey, low-fat fish, grains, or vegetables. When ordering meat and poultry, calorie-conscious diners should avoid:

- goose and duck (which are high in fat)
- fatty cuts of beef, pork, and lamb (which are high in saturated fats and cholesterol)
- prime meats with marbling (fat)
- chopped steak made from ground chuck (which has a high fat content)
- ground lamb patties (They are high in fat; most lamb choices such as chops, leg of lamb, and shoulder roast have a medium-high fat content.)
- spareribs, ground pork, and pork sausages

When ordering red meat, choose (in moderate amounts):

- lean cuts such as London broil, sirloin, flank steak, and tenderloin
- veal chops and roast veal (veal cutlets and ground veal are not as lean)
- pork chops, loin roast, butt, and cutlets
- fresh or cured ham, Canadian bacon, or pork-tenderloin roast

All visible fat should be trimmed from any meat selection.

Preparation is often the key to any food's overall calorie and fat rating. Cream sauces, hollandaise, béarnaise, béchamel, gratin, cheese sauces, butter sauces, and generic gravy are all high in fat and cholesterol. Any food that is fried, creamed, pan-fried, crispy, or sautéed is high in calories, fat, and cholesterol. Restaurant-made casseroles, hashes, and potpies are also likely to have elevated levels of fat, cholesterol, and sodium. Vegetable casseroles may also be loaded with cheese or cream, which are high in fat and cholesterol.

As a general rule, the simpler the preparation—broiled (dry, or with lemon or wine), poached, baked, steamed, roasted, or braised—the fewer calories and less fat it has. These designations do not necessarily mean that no butter or oil is used (a special request should be made if butter, oil, or salt needs to be eliminated entirely). Tomato and wine-based sauces also may be made with some butter or oil, but these sauces are almost always much lower in fat than cream-based ones.

By pausing after each bite, a diner is better able to satisfy the appetite with fewer calories. When the diner is no longer hungry, he or she should stop eating and signal for the waiter to remove the plate. Almost every restaurant will provide a "doggie" bag. The leftovers can make an exotic and nutritious meal the following day.

Appetizers for the Calorie and Fat-Conscious

Best Choices:	Avoid:
Salads: 　Lettuce	Mayonnaise dressings
Legume (e.g., 　　chick-peas)	Creamy dressings
Tomato 　Spinach	
Raw or steamed 　vegetables	Fried vegetables
Melon	Hard cheeses
Berries and other 　fruit	Sour-cream dips
Seafood cocktails 　(especially crab)	Tartar sauce
Steamed fish Steamed clams	Mousses
Oysters or clams 　on half-shell	Pâté
Broth- or tomato- 　based soups 　with noodles or 　vegetables	Creamed soups French onion soup
Gazpacho Minestrone	
Clam chowder 　(Manhattan 　style)	Assorted appetizers 　Fried dumplings 　Fried noodles 　Tortilla chips 　Nachos, etc.
Lentil soup	
Other legume or 　pasta soups 　(occasionally)	
Tomato juice	

Low-Calorie and Low-Fat Entrées

Best Choices:	Avoid:
Fish, all varieties, 　broiled or 　poached	Fish prepared with 　butter or margarine
Poultry, without 　fat or skin	
Chicken	Duck
Turkey	Goose
Cornish hen	
Red meat	
Lean cuts, 　　broiled beef, 　　lamb, pork, 　　veal	Prime cuts Prime rib Ground beef or lamb Liver Sweetbreads Spareribs Corned beef Breaded coatings Gravies
Vegetables, all 　kinds, plain, 　including 　baked 　potatoes, 　beans, peas	Butter, oil, and cheese 　sauces on 　vegetables
Pastas and grains, 　all kinds, 　with tomato 　sauces, wine 　sauces, fish 　and seafood 　sauces, 　vegetable 　sauces	Alfredo sauce Other cream and cheese 　sauces on 　pastas/grains
Bread	
Breadsticks	Biscuits
Hard rolls	Croissants
Plain French 　　and Italian 　　bread	Commercially prepared 　bran, corn, and 　blueberry muffins
Pita bread	
Toasts	Butter rolls

Desserts

For many people, dessert is the best part about dining out. Many restaurants capitalize on this and offer a wide array of delectable concoctions.

It is possible for a calorie-conscious diner to satisfy his or her sweet tooth while at the same time avoiding excessive amounts of calories, fat, and cholesterol. Sherbet or sorbet, although sugary, does not usually contain fat, and therefore is a better choice than pudding, cake, or pie. Angel food cake and fresh fruit (without the cream or zabaglione sauce) are low in fat and calories. A calorie-conscious diner who cannot resist a rich dessert should consider sharing it or requesting a smaller portion. If an after-dinner liqueur or Irish coffee with whipped cream is ordered, it should replace a dessert.

SMORGASBORDS AND BUFFETS

For many people a smorgasbord or buffet—where the diner can choose as much as he or she wishes from among a large array of dishes—is the ultimate challenge. While such cornucopias of food can tempt almost anyone to overeat, they can also provide the opportunity for a diner to be selective. Seafood, fresh salads, freshly carved roast turkey, and exotic fruits can provide the main fare, while a spoonful, rather than an entire portion, of dishes that are high in calories can be sampled.

Most large buffets are divided into three broad selections: salads and fruits; main dishes comprised of carved meats and casserole entrées with various sauces; and desserts. Diners are expected to make separate trips to the table for each course and to return for refills as many times as desired.

Before making any selection, a diner should look over the whole buffet to decide which dishes are most appealing and offer the highest nutritional value for the calories. A good plan of action is to eat a generous serving of salad or fruit first to satisfy initial hunger pangs and to follow this with small servings of entrée selections and a fresh fruit for dessert.

BREAKFAST OUT

Studies have shown that starting the day with a healthy meal promotes a feeling of well-being and can control hunger later in the day. This may help prevent overeating at lunch or dinner.

Between 1978 and 1982, the number of people who ate breakfast out increased to a dramatic 32 percent. One factor responsible for the rise was the growing number of working mothers.

Calorie and Fat-Conscious Desserts

Best Choices:	Avoid:
Berries	Zabaglione
Fresh fruit	Sweet cream
Angel food cake	Layer cake
Gelatins	Pies
Sherbets	Frostings
Sorbets	Ice cream
Frozen-fruit ices	Whipped cream
Low-fat dairy products	Puddings
Fruit salad or compote	Custards
Apple or pear crisps with low-fat toppings	Nondairy milk substitutes

Fast-food restaurants were quick to capitalize on this trend. Unfortunately, the breakfasts offered and heavily advertised by these chains tended to be excessive in fat, sodium, and cholesterol. A McDonald's biscuit with sausage and egg, for example, contains more than 500 calories (mostly from fat) and about 1,250 milligrams of sodium. Other chains—Hardee's, Jack in the Box, Arby's, Roy Rogers, and Burger King—offer similar fare. For those who need to restrict calories, there are just too many in the croissants or biscuits topped with eggs, sausages, ham, or bacon that most fast-food chains serve. A breakfast that is low in calories and fat—one that includes a complex carbohydrate, a small amount of protein, and some fiber—can seldom be found at fast-food restaurants, except those that have a fresh-fruit bar. These chains are now cutting calories.

Most coffee shops offer lower-calorie and more extensive breakfast selections. Hot and cold cereals, oatmeal, Cream of Wheat, unsugared bran or shredded-wheat cereals topped with fresh fruit (which contains more fiber than juice) and skim milk provide balanced nutrition but are also low in fat and calories. Other choices that are low in calories and fat, such as fresh fruits, cottage cheese, and yogurt, might be listed under appetizers, side dishes, and desserts.

Some breads, including whole-grain breads, English muffins, and bagels (ordered dry, or with butter or margarine on the side and used in moderate amounts) are good breakfast selections. However, larger muffins, including bran and oat bran, are often loaded with sugar and fat. Pancakes, waffles, and French toast are reasonable breakfast choices if the amounts of butter and syrup are limited. If prepared on a lightly greased griddle or pan, they are all fairly low in fat and cholesterol, although the batter may contain eggs. (Sometimes, French toast is deep-fried; ask before ordering.)

Because of the high cholesterol content of the yolk, people with elevated serum cholesterol should limit their intake of eggs. Poaching or soft-boiling, which eliminates the fat of frying or scrambling, are the preferred methods of cooking for these people. Omelets should be made with two eggs and cooked in only a small amount of butter or margarine. When the menu lists a three-egg omelet, such diners should request that it be

Guidelines for Calorie and Fat-Conscious Dining Out

- Plan ahead.
- Read the whole menu.
- The simpler the preparation, the less fat it will usually contain.
- Choose broiled, steamed, braised, roasted, and stir-fried foods (rather than sautéed, fried, creamed).
- Mix and match appetizers, entrées, and side dishes.
- Make requests specific and to the point.
- Order à la carte.

- Select primarily fish, poultry, veal, pasta, and vegetables.
- Request sauces and dressings served on the side and use sparingly.
- Control portions (don't over-order; don't feel guilty about leaving food on the plate).
- Cut away visible fat from meats and poultry.
- Make trade-offs.
- Pace the meal.

made with one whole egg and two additional egg whites. For them, omelets should be filled with vegetables—mushrooms, peppers, broccoli, and asparagus—rather than cheeses and meats.

The only lean breakfast meats are ham and Canadian-style bacon, both of which are high in salt. Bacon and sausage are both fatty and salty and should be avoided by the overweight and the hypertension-prone.

LUNCH

Lunch is the meal most often eaten in restaurants; however, because time is short and choices often limited, it is the most challenging for weight- and calorie-conscious consumers. To circumvent this, diners who frequently eat lunch out should keep handy the menus of nearby restaurants that offer foods made to order. Although fast-food restaurants offer convenience and speed, selections are limited for those watching calories, cholesterol, and sodium (see discussion of fast foods on page 654). Plain, nongreasy burgers,

Table 39.1.   Fat and Sodium Content of Selected Fast Foods

Foods	Calories	Fat (gm.)	Fat (% calories)	Sodium (mg.)
MCDONALD'S				
Hotcakes with butter and syrup*	500	10.0	19	1,070
Scrambled eggs	180	13.0	65	205
Biscuit with sausage	467	31.0	60	1,145
Hamburger	263	11.0	39	506
Mc D.L.T.	680	44.0	58	1,030
Big Mac	570	35.0	55	979
French fries, regular	220	12.0	47	109
Chicken McNuggets (6)	323	20.0	56	512
ROY ROGERS				
Plain potato*	211	0	0	65
Potato with taco beef and cheese	463	22.0	42	726
Potato with broccoli and cheese	376	18.0	43	523
Roast beef sandwich*	317	10.0	29	785
Crescent roll	287	18.0	56	547
Crescent sandwich with ham	557	42.0	67	1,192
WENDY'S				
Pasta salad (½ cup)	134	6.0	40	400
Taco salad	390	18.0	40	1,100
Broccoli and cheese potato	500	25.0	45	430
Cheese potato	590	34.0	52	450
Plain baked potato*	250	2.0	7	60
Pick-up-window Side Salad	110	6.0	50	540
Multigrain wheat bun*	135	3.0	20	220
Chicken sandwich on wheat bun*	320	10.0	28	500
Hamburger on wheat bun	340	17.0	45	290
Double hamburger on white bun	560	34.0	54	575
ARBY'S				
Roast chicken breast (no bun)*	254	7.0	25	930
Chicken breast sandwich (fried)	592	27.0	41	1,340

lean roast beef, coleslaw, low-fat milk, and the salad bar are among the best offerings.

Cafeterias should be approached with the same cautious optimism as a buffet or smorgasbord: Possibilities should be surveyed and choices made *before* getting in line. Dessert should not be chosen until after the meal, and shared with a friend, if possible.

Sandwiches and salads, American luncheon standards, offer a wide variety of good choices. White-meat turkey or chicken, fish, or lean roast beef should be eaten instead of fatty cold cuts (bologna, salami, corned beef, pastrami), cheese, or cream cheese and jelly.

Sandwiches should be served in a pita pocket or on whole-grain bread with low-calorie fillers such as lettuce and tomatoes. (Note: Condiments such as chili sauce, catsup, mustard, and pickles are generally low in calories but may be high in sodium.)

For the calorie- and fat-conscious, fruit or lettuce and vegetable salads are preferable to salads that are made with mayonnaise and thus high in calories and cholesterol, such as macaroni or potato salad or coleslaw. Low-fat cottage cheese or low-fat yogurt topped with fresh fruit is a good choice for lunch. Frozen and fruit yogurts may be loaded with sugar.

Table 39.1.   Fat and Sodium Content of Selected Fast Foods *(cont.)*

Foods	Calories	Fat (gm.)	Fat (% calories)	Sodium (mg.)
Junior roast beef	218	8.0	33	345
Regular roast beef	353	15.0	38	590
Baked potato deluxe	648	38.0	53	475
LONG JOHN SILVER'S				
Baked fish with sauce*	151	2.0	12	361
Fish with batter (2)	404	24.0	53	1,346
Breaded clams	526	31.0	53	1,170
Chicken plank (1 piece)	152	8.0	47	515
Ocean chef salad	229	8.0	31	986
Coleslaw	182	15.0	74	367
BURGER KING				
Hamburger	275	12.0	39	509
Bacon double cheeseburger	510	31.0	55	728
Specialty chicken sandwich	688	40.0	52	1,423
Chicken tenders (6)	204	10.0	44	636
JACK IN THE BOX				
Shrimp salad (no dressing)*	115	1.3	8	460
Taco salad	377	24.0	56	1,436
Club pita*	284	8.0	27	953
KENTUCKY FRIED CHICKEN				
Original-recipe drumstick	147	9.0	54	269
Original-recipe breast	276	17.0	56	654
Extra-crispy thigh	371	26.0	64	766
Kentucky nuggets (6)	276	17.0	57	840
Corn on the cob*	176	3.0	16	10
Mashed potatoes*	59	1.0	9	228

*Denotes foods that are relatively moderate in fat (defined as less than 30 percent of calories).

Reprinted with permission from the American Council on Science and Health, 1989. It should be noted that many fast-food chains are reducing the amounts of fat and sodium in their foods. More current food values may be obtained directly from the food chains.

The nutritive quality of frozen yogurt can be improved by adding fresh fruit instead of coconut, nuts, or chocolate chips.

FAST FOODS

In response to consumer concern over calories, many fast-food chains now offer salad bars, baked potatoes, baked fish, roasted chicken, low-cal salad dressings, and other light fare. While some of the offerings provide lower calories and fat—for example, baked fish, available at some chains, has 151 calories, about half the number in fried fish and only a fraction of the sodium—the benefits of others are limited. A roasted chicken sandwich, for example, may contain large quantities of sodium added in preparation.

Despite the debut of selected items, many items at fast-food chains remain laden with calories, fat, cholesterol, and sodium; for example, a ham and Swiss cheese burger has about 750 calories and 1,200 milligrams of sodium. At some establishments, unseasoned burgers are available on request, and many chains are making an effort to reduce the sodium and fat contents of their foods. Still, for the most part, those who must restrict salt intake should eat elsewhere. (See Table 39.1 for a list of the fat and sodium content of selected fast foods.)

The best rule for fast food is to keep things simple. Oversize burgers ("jumbo," "whopper," and "double" versions) often contain extra mayonnaise-type dressings, pickles, enormous buns, and substantial amounts of fatty meat. The fat and calorie content of these extravaganzas may be more than double the levels of a regular hamburger. Cheese and bacon toppings add to the fat, salt, and calories.

Roast beef contains less fat than hamburger (assuming it is not overstuffed, super, or deluxe and has no cheese, sauces, or condiments). If a hamburger is ordered, it should be plain. Lettuce, tomato, and other items from the salad bar can increase the nutritional content. Catsup, mustard, and especially pickles contain an excessive amount of salt, so they should be used sparingly by those concerned about their sodium intake.

Most consumers are under the impression that the chicken and fish dishes at fast-food establishments are lower in calories and fat than burgers. This is true only when the chicken or fish is roasted, baked, or broiled. However, most fast-food chicken and fish is battered or breaded, then fried (often, as with French fries, in saturated beef fat). The extra-crispy fried chicken is higher in fat and calories than the regular variety. To lower the sodium and fat content, the skin or crust on all chicken should be removed. Single pieces are preferable to whole dinners or combos. Chicken sandwiches are usually battered and fried, with sauce added. As a rule, these should not be eaten by those limiting calories and fat. If "nuggets" are ordered, the accompanying sauces should be used sparingly.

Fried fish often has more fat and salt and twice the calories of baked. Like chicken sandwiches, fish sandwiches make poor choices for the calorie-conscious. Diners who insist on ordering fried fish can make modifications to reduce the calories somewhat by ordering scallops and shrimp instead of fried clams (the former usually have a little less breading), and by using lemon or vinegar, if available. Otherwise, catsup or cocktail sauce (although both are somewhat high in sodium) are preferable to tartar sauce, which contains mostly mayonnaise and is high in fat and calories.

Even if all other foods are cooked in vegetable oil, many fast-food establishments fry their French fries in beef fat. The result is a product extremely high in calories and cholesterol, and, when sprinkled with salt, as they invariably are, high in sodium. (A small, three-ounce order adds up to between 200 and 300 calories.) Those who find French fries irresistible should order only a small portion or share one large portion with others.

A 10-ounce vanilla shake at a fast-food

Salad Bars

Many restaurants, delicatessens, and other take-out establishments offer salad bars where customers can choose from a variety of greens, relishes, and condiments. Salads are an excellent source of fiber and vitamins A and C. A salad complements any meal or can be a low-calorie meal in itself. However, adding liberal amounts of dressing, croutons, prepared salads (potato, three-bean, pasta), bacon bits, chick-peas, avocado, cheese, and hard-boiled eggs can boost calories, fat, sodium, and cholesterol to levels that exceed those in a jumbo cheeseburger. Many salad bar items, while high in nutrients, are also high in calories. An example is an avocado, which has approximately 335 calories, 87 percent of which come from fat.

Many items at salad bars are high in sodium, fat, and calories and should be eaten in moderation. Salt and usually sugar are involved in the pickling process. Therefore, those who need to restrict sodium should not eat pickled items. Olives also contain fat and green olives are especially high in sodium.

Potato salad, macaroni salad, and coleslaw are made with mayonnaise, which is high in calories and fat. Because of its mayonnaise content, coleslaw, for example, while not a bad choice in moderation, contains approximately six times the calories in plain cabbage. Three-bean salads are lower in fat but are usually made with sugar and salt.

The choices that are lower in calories and fat at salad bars include the following.

- Leafy greens and lettuces, especially the darker greens, such as spinach and romaine lettuce, which are higher in vitamins and other nutrients than iceberg lettuce.
- All fresh vegetables: asparagus, bean sprouts, broccoli, carrots, cauliflower, celery, cucumbers, green beans, mushrooms, onions and scallions, peas, peppers, radishes, red cabbage, and tomatoes—because they are high in fiber and vitamins, low in calories.
- Turkey or lean beef for protein.
- A small scoop of cottage cheese, which provides calcium and protein, are two nutrients lacking in most vegetables. However, the cottage cheese served at most salad bars is the whole-milk variety and therefore has a relatively higher fat content, as compared to a favorable low-fat brand. (See Table 39.2 for the calorie and sodium content of items from salad bars.)

Salad Dressings

The dressings offered at most salad bars are creamy blue cheese, Thousand Island, or Italian. These bottled and prepared salad dressings tend to be very high in calories, fat, and sodium. Even diet dressings may have as many as 30 to 50 calories per tablespoon; a ladleful can add several hundred calories. To conserve calories, salads should not be dressed at the salad bar. Instead, dressing should be spooned into a small side dish and taken to the table, where it can be added sparingly. Tossing the salad thoroughly ensures that only a small amount is needed. If dressing is to be used, the best way to keep calories, sodium, and fat to a minimum is to sprinkle a small amount of oil and vinegar directly onto the salad.

Prepacked Salads. Some fast-food restaurants offer chef's salads, chicken salads, and fresh green salads already combined and packed in plastic containers with a variety of dressings in separate squeeze packs. Prepacked salad dressings are as high in calories as those offered at the salad bar (about 180 calories per serving or ladleful), but there is usually one low-calorie variety that has about 25 calories per serving.

chain contains about 320 calories. Its sugar content is equivalent to a can of cola and it contains as much fat as a glass of milk. A 20-ounce chocolate shake adds up to a hefty 700 calories. On the positive side, shakes are a good source of calcium and not necessarily a bad choice if one small shake is substituted for both beverage and dessert. Low-fat milk, coffee, tea, and fruit juice are lower in fat and have fewer calories.

Table 39.2. Calories and Sodium at the American Salad Bar

Food	Calories (per 100 gm. or 3½ oz.)	Sodium (mg./100 gm.)
Bacon bits (imitation)	530	3,065
Bean sprouts	40	5
Broccoli	25	12
Carrots	40	33
Cauliflower	20	9
Celery	15	88
Chick-peas	118	120
Chopped egg	160	120
Coleslaw	145	120
Cottage cheese	105	250
Croutons	390	735
Cucumber	10	6
Green onions	40	10
Lettuce, iceberg	13	9
Lettuce, romaine	18	9
Mushrooms	29	15
Olives, black	150	230
Olives, green	95	680
Peppers, hot red	21	4
Onions	36	7
Peppers, sweet green	20	13
Pickled beets	60	335
Pickles	65	1,970
Potato salad	145	480
Radishes	13	18
Red cabbage	28	26
Shredded cheese (American)	380	1,125
Spinach	22	50
Tomatoes	20	4

Source: U.S. Department of Agriculture, Human Nutrition Information Service.

SPECIALTY RESTAURANTS

Chinese Restaurants

By emphasizing quick cooking methods, vegetables in Chinese cuisine retain both their crunch and their vitamins. Seafood also can be a wonderful dining choice for the nutritionally minded gourmet. The possible minuses include salt, which is usually in the form of soy sauce, and monosodium gluta- (MSG), and quantities of cooking oil that are sometimes too large for the calorie- and fat-conscious. Fried foods such as egg rolls, dumplings, or wontons have a heavy fat content. Szechuan-style dishes frequently have more oil than other styles of Chinese cooking; however, unsaturated oils such as soybean are often used in Chinese restaurants, and therefore fried or stir-fried foods do not carry the same blood-cholesterol hazard for those with elevated cholesterol as regular restaurant fare cooked in saturated fats. Most Chinese restaurants will omit MSG on request, but it's a good idea to ask what, if anything, they substitute in its place. Some dishes—egg-drop soup, egg foo yung, and moo-shu pork or chicken—contain eggs and, therefore, cholesterol.

The best choices for those who are concerned with calories and fat are any chicken or fish dishes mixed with vegetables that are steamed, boiled, or lightly stir-fried; for example, moo goo gai pan (chicken with mushrooms and assorted vegetables) and almond gai ding (diced chicken with almonds and vegetables). Bean curd or tofu dishes deliver protein without cholesterol but, depending upon the method of preparation, may not be low in fat. In general, pork and beef dishes are fattier and more caloric than other selections. A beef and vegetable dish is likely to have fewer calories than lo mein, a noodle dish that contains more oil. Steamed white rice is lower in calories and salt than fried rice, which has extra fat and soy sauce.

Japanese Restaurants

Japanese cuisine is ideally suited for low-fat regimens; however, because of the sodium content, it may not be suited for those on sodium-restricted diets. Sashimi (raw fish) is low in fat and calories, although the soy sauce the fish is dipped in is high in sodium. Sushi (raw fish and rice) and teriyaki dishes, marinated and broiled, are other low-calorie choices, although some sugar and soy sauce may be added. Soups, sukiyaki, and most noodle dishes will also contain some sodium, but in an amount acceptable for most people. With their high-fat content, batter-fried items such as tempura should be avoided by those who need to cut calories.

Baked Potatoes

Baked potatoes are one of nature's great foods; they are nourishing, filling, and virtually fat- and sodium-free. When eaten with the skin, they provide vitamin C, fiber, iron, potassium, and certain B vitamins. Depending on its size, a plain baked potato has between 90 and 150 calories. Plain baked potatoes served hot from the oven are delicious. But those served in restaurants are often left in foil jackets all evening, which gives them a steamed quality; or they are reheated, which obliterates flavor and freshness. To compensate for the loss of flavor, baked potatoes in restaurants are usually served with scoops of butter or sour cream; in fast-food restaurants, they are topped with cheese, bacon, sour cream, or chili, all of which add quantities of fat and salt and greatly increase the caloric level.

Fortunately, there are many creative ways to enhance the flavor of a baked potato without adding large amounts of fat and salt: chopped chives, low-fat yogurt or cottage cheese, a dash of Worcestershire sauce, chopped spinach, or a tablespoon of grated Parmesan, Swiss, or cheddar cheese.

Pizza

Pizza is not only tasty, economical, and convenient but highly nutritious, as long as certain toppings are kept in moderation. Additions of meatballs, ground beef, sausage, ham, extra cheese, and pepperoni can multiply the calories, fat, and cholesterol. Pizza should not be eaten by those on low-sodium regimens, because some pizza parlors add extra salt or garlic salt. Also the tomato sauce and mozzarella cheese used in preparation are both relatively high in sodium.

Ordered plain, the combination of cheese (some pizza parlors offer part skim-milk mozzarella), crust, and tomato sauce delivers significant amounts of calcium, protein, riboflavin, thiamin, niacin, iron (if fortified), and vitamin A. Fresh vegetable toppings such as red and green peppers, onions, and mushrooms add vitamin C and fiber. One average-size slice of pizza has 300 to 400 calories and can provide a moderate and nutritious meal. If ordering a pie made to your specifications, request thin crusts, whole wheat if possible, with minimal oil. (For a list of nutrients and calories in toppings for pizza, see Table 39.3.)

Mexican Restaurants

Cornmeal and legumes are staples of Mexican food, which, like many ethnic cuisines, fits into any reduced-fat eating plan. The addition of ingredients such as cheese, avocados, refried beans, and sour cream can make many Mexican dishes high in calories and fat. By omitting or lightly eating cheese and cheese-topped nachos (700 calories an order), guacamole, sour cream, fried tortilla chips, and by adding tomatoes, salsa sauce, and lettuce, dining in a Mexican restaurant can be both festive and compatible with special nutritional needs. However, to accomplish this, as with other alternatives, for reduced calories and fat, this may require a special request, such as asking for soft corn tortillas instead of fried tortilla chips. When eaten with salsa, these provide less fat without compromising taste.

As in any other restaurant, chicken and fish dishes—broiled, baked, or Veracruzana (tomatoes, peppers, and olives)—are the entrées lower in calories and fat. Of the standard dishes, the best choices are tacos, tamales, and tostados. Although tostados are usually made with fried tortillas, they are lower in calories that burritos or enchaladas. Chicken filling is preferable to cheese or beef. When beans are prepared without lard (ask first), a diner can request that a side order be combined with rice, but without melted cheese.

SUMMING UP

Dining out should be an enjoyable and special experience, even for those who do it every

Table 39.3. Pizza Toppings

When You Add These Ingredients to Your Pizza	You Add These Calories and Nutrients†
Extra cheese (¼ lb. part skim-milk mozzarella)	320 calories; protein, vitamin A, riboflavin, and calcium
Green pepper (1 medium-sized raw)*	15 calories; vitamin C
Red pepper (1 medium-sized raw)*	15 calories; vitamins A and C
Onion (1 small)*	65 calories
Mushrooms (¼ lb. raw or canned)*	60 calories
Ground beef or meatballs (½ lb.)	630 calories; protein, riboflavin, niacin, and iron
Sausage (½ lb.)	480 calories; protein and thiamin
Ham (¼ lb.)	325 calories; protein and thiamin
Canadian bacon (¼ lb.)	160 calories; protein and thiamin
Pepperoni (½ lb.)	1,100 calories; protein (data on other nutrients not available)

*The calorie counts will be substantially higher if these vegetables are fried in oil before being added to the pizza.
†The amount of topping added to one pizza provides at least one-quarter of the U.S. RDA of the nutrients listed. Smaller amounts of other nutrients are also present.

Reprinted with permission from the American Council on Science and Health *News and Views*, January/February 1985.

Chinese Restaurants for the Calorie- and Fat-Conscious

Best Choices:	Avoid:
Chicken and vegetables, all selections	Egg foo yung
Selected fish dishes	Moo-shu pork or chicken
Whole steamed fish	Spareribs
Bean curd or tofu dishes	Lobster sauce
Beef and vegetables, all selections	Fried dumplings or wontons
Soups, all kinds	Egg rolls
Steamed rice	Fried rice
Steamed dumplings (dim sum) especially with fish and vegetable stuffings	Cold noodles with sesame sauce

day. Those who are conscious of calories and fat and wish to make sure they do not compromise their nutritional well-being should always request low-fat dairy products and foods prepared without fats (or salt, if hypertension-prone). Even if a particular restaurant is unable to oblige a special request, it is important for dining establishments to understand that diners are interested not only in how a food tastes but how healthy it is for them. By making their desires known, diners can—and do—influence what restaurants offer; for example, not long ago few restaurants served brewed decaffeinated coffee, but today diners can find it almost everywhere. The more often diners ask, the more likely it is that low-fat, low-cholesterol, low-sodium foods will begin to appear regularly on restaurant menus—to the benefit of many.

40

Food Shopping and Labeling

Elyse Sosin, R.D., M.A., Fran C. Grossman, R.D., M.S., and Rosalinda Lawson, R.D.

■

INTRODUCTION

Planning is the key to being a smart shopper. Deciding what foods to buy and where and when to buy them are the first steps toward economical and nutritious food shopping.

PREPARING TO SHOP

The best choices in the supermarket are usually made by those who are aware of the importance of reading labels and challenged by the prospect of improving nutrition. While many people enjoy shopping for food, others do not. A reappraisal of the family's shopping habits will determine who takes the most pleasure in the activity and whether that person has enough time for it. Regardless of who does the shopping, however, each member should know what products his or her family uses and why.

It is most efficient to shop for food once a week. This may not be possible for people with limited storage space who live in cities or those with erratic schedules. However, good organization is important for everyone, be-

cause the fewer trips made to the store, the fewer temptations there are for impulse buying.

Preparations for shopping should be made at home: The week's menus should be planned with enough flexibility to allow for store specials, newspaper ads to be scanned, and coupons to be clipped and organized. A running shopping list can be posted on the refrigerator and items added to it after the week's menus have been planned and whenever supplies are running low. The list should be organized according to categories—dairy products, meats, produce, and so on—that match the physical layout of the store and the shopping route planned so that cold and frozen items are picked up last.

Shoppers have consistently shown that if hungry, they are more likely to purchase unnecessary and nonnutritious food. Shopping during hours when the stores are least crowded will minimize long waits at the checkout counter. Although shopping can educate children about nutrition and consumerism, and hone their arithmetic and reading skills, it may not be worth the inevitable distractions. Nutrition is seldom the first priority with children, who are likely to badger for sweets and other goodies they have seen advertised on television. Children should be made aware of tactics advertisers use to entice buyers. They should also be taught, for example, why oatmeal and fruit are more nutritious than high-sugar cereals and snacks. Such advice should be part of ongoing family conversation and not given only as a preshopping pep talk. Anyone who finds it hard to say no firmly—and stick to it—may be better off, if possible, leaving children at home.

WHERE TO SHOP

The best shopping combines convenience, variety, quality, and competitive pricing. Suburban and rural residents have the benefit of large full-service supermarkets that provide convenient one-stop shopping. City shoppers can usually choose from a range of all-purpose and specialty stores where they can purchase produce, fish, meat, baked goods, bulk foods, and staples. In less affluent neighborhoods where food selection is often limited and prices tend to be higher on certain items, it may be worthwhile to arrange a car pool or to take a bus or other means of public transportation and shop elsewhere.

A food store should not only be an appealing place to shop but should conform to basic health and safety standards. Frozen foods should be solidly frozen, eggs and dairy products should be in refrigerator cases kept below 42° F., and produce should look fresh, not wilted, dirty, or poorly trimmed. Cans that are dented or bulging or have rusty or leaky seams should not be sold even at a discount. Prices per unit should be clearly posted and most items should be individually priced, even if scanning devices are used at the checkout.

While single items might be cheaper at different stores, it is more convenient and quicker to shop at one store for most purchases than to go from market to market. In choosing the best store, the consumer should compare the prices of 10 regular purchases at several area markets with comparable quality and selection.

Alternative Food Stores

Products sold in health-food stores are almost always more expensive and not usually more healthful than those found in conventional stores. For example, honey and molasses are still sugars, sea salt is mostly sodium, and many granolas contain a high level of fats and sweeteners. The product categories in which health-food stores do excel in terms of price and selection are those sold in bulk, such as bran, brown rice, grains, and cereals, because the consumer avoids paying for packaging. In addition, the price of beans, grains, cereal, dried fruit, nuts, oils, and spices may be competitive with larger commercial stores.

Health Foods at the Supermarket

Bulgur	Nonfat dry milk
Corn, safflower, olive, and sunflower oils	Oatmeal
	Pearled barley
Dried fruits	Popping corn
Dried peas and beans	Rice and shredded-
Dry-roasted, unsalted nuts	and puffed-wheat cereals
Fresh and frozen vegetables	Rolled oats
	Unsweetened whole-
Fresh fruits	grain granolas
Fruit juices	Water-packed tuna
Fruit-sweetened jams and jellies	and salmon
	Whole-grain flours
Lean meat	Whole-wheat bread
Low-fat and skim milk	Wild and brown rice
Low-fat cottage cheese	Yogurt
Natural cheese	

Health-food stores usually offer only limited selections of produce, fish, meat, and dairy goods and often at prices two or three times that of supermarkets.

All food (not just that sold in health-food stores) is organic, meaning it contains carbon compounds and is derived from living organisms. What purveyors of health foods mean when they claim a food is organic is that it is grown in soil that is fertilized with manure or compost and is free from chemical fertilizers, pesticides, additives, and preservatives. Since the Food and Drug Administration has set no legal definitions for *organic* or *organically grown* food, there is no regulation of such claims. Several studies, including one by Simon Gourdine, New York City Commissioner of Consumer Affairs, have found pesticide residues in organic products. The Gourdine study compared organically grown foods purchased in health-food stores with similar conventionally grown foods from supermarkets. Six different products—apples, zucchini, carrots, wheat flour, dried red beans, and cabbage—were tested for residues of 16 commonly used pesticides. The analyses were done by two different independent laboratories. Residues of two pesticides were found in the organically grown zucchini, while residues of a single pesticide were found in the conventionally grown carrots. In both instances, the residues were well below the maximum allowable levels and were considered quite safe. "Health food" usually only means costly.

In a 1983 paper published in the *Journal of the American Dietetic Association*, Mr. Gourdine emphasized that there was no difference between the conventionally grown produce and the organic products so far as quality and safety were concerned. There was, however, a considerable difference in cost, with the organic products costing more than twice as much in some instances.

Even if a farmer was to grow his produce without pesticides or artificial fertilizers, there is no guarantee they would be free of chemical residues, because pesticides can remain in the soil for years or can drift, with rain, from nearby farms. In addition, research has consistently found no difference in nutrition, taste, or safety between foods grown organically and those grown in chemically fertilized soil.

BULK FOODS

Warehouse or "box" stores often sell canned and boxed products at significant discounts, usually 10 to 30 percent below supermarket prices. In these no-frill stores, cartons are usually stacked on the floor with their tops ripped off, prices are displayed on large centrally located signs, customers bag their own food, and checks are rarely accepted.

Produce stores often have the best buys on fruits and vegetables, and a local butcher or delicatessen may have top-quality meat at reasonable prices. These and other specialty food stores usually offer good quality and price for their specialty, but they are both likely to charge a lot more for any staples that they carry. So-called convenience stores—small, local markets that generally keep late hours—are fine for last-minute emergencies but are generally expensive.

Food cooperatives or buying clubs are usually owned and run by members who purchase large quantities of food at wholesale prices and divide the savings among participants. Many food co-ops place orders with wholesalers on a weekly basis and assign members the tasks of picking up, dividing, and distributing food. Some of the largest co-ops have store fronts that are open both to members and nonmembers, but members who work a certain number of hours in the store are entitled to purchase food at a discount.

LABELING

Foods are produced, packaged, and distributed under various federal controls. The Food and Drug Administration (FDA), the United States Department of Agriculture (USDA), and the Federal Trade Commission (FTC) are all involved in setting standards for labeling, grading, and selling various foods. While the roles of these agencies overlap to some extent, in general, the FDA is responsi- ble for all food labeling except on meat and poultry (which is governed by the USDA) and the FTC is the watchdog on advertising. Information concerning labeling, grading, and advertising is frequently confusing, inconsistent, and sometimes misleading. Nevertheless, Americans can be reasonably assured that foods that appear on supermarket shelves have been produced under sanitary conditions and are relatively safe. And when problems are found, such as spoilage or contamination,

How to Save Food Dollars

An educated consumer reads labels, understands how to get the most nutrition per food dollar, comparison shops, and understands the concepts of unit pricing and open dating, which are covered in this chapter. Below are other money-saving hints.

- *Take advantage of sales.* Pay attention to advertised specials and double coupon days—when a store doubles the value of manufacturers' coupons. Check the newspaper for sales and coupons *before* making the shopping list. Avoid purchasing unnecessary items or food just for the potential savings.

- *Be flexible.* Many menus can be adjusted to take advantage of bargains a store may offer.

- *Experiment with generic products and store brands.* Store and generic brands are products supermarkets have purchased from wholesalers and packaged at reduced prices. National brands may be of a more consistent quality, but the choice is largely one of personal preference. Generic products and store brands may not always be cheaper, especially when other products are on sale. When the generic is of lesser quality or strength, such as two-ply paper napkins instead of three-ply, or cleaners with less ammonia, it can be more expensive because it takes more of the product to do the same job. Generics and store brands are not interchangeable; the only way to judge differences in quality between national, store, and generics is to try and then compare.

- *Be aware of marketing ploys.* To increase profits, supermarkets deliberately tempt shoppers with impulse items: Sweets are stacked at checkout counters; special displays are set up at the end of aisles, where shoppers slow down; and some items are strategically located out of place, such as sweet rolls in the coffee department. The more expensive products are deliberately placed at eye level, with bargains on top and bottom shelves.

- *Ask for a rain check.* According to Federal Trade Commission regulations, supermarkets must make a genuine effort to keep advertised specials in stock and must clearly indicate branch stores that are *not* participating in advertised sales. Many stores offer rain checks to enable consumers to purchase a sale item that has been sold out at the reduced price when it comes back in stock.

- *Buy in quantity when appropriate.* Stock up on nonperishable sale items if adequate storage space is available. Limit purchases of fresh produce or other foods that cannot be frozen or stored.

- *Limit purchases of convenience food.* Many highly processed and packaged foods have less nutritive value at a higher price.

Government Food Programs for Low-Income Families

The federal government has several food programs to assist low-income families in obtaining good nutrition.

- *Food Stamps.* Qualified families can stretch limited funds with food stamps, which are given to eligible families at no charge. Most markets accept food stamps, which can be used to purchase most foods for human consumption. (Food and Nutrition Service, 3101 Park Center Drive, Room 510, Alexandria, VA 22302; telephone: 202–756–3054)

- *National School Lunch Program.* Since 1947, the federal government has subsidized school lunches, which must provide one-third of the day's recommended nutrients. The lunches are free to school-age children from low-income families and available at reduced cost to others. To augment the Lunch Act, a Special Milk Program was implemented in 1954, and in 1966 the Child Nutrition Act launched the School Breakfast Programs. (Food and Nutrition Service, 3101 Park Center Drive, Room 510, Alexandria, VA 22302; telephone: 202–756–3054)

- *Child Care Food Program.* This program is similar to the National School Lunch Program. Depending on eligibility, it provides for reduced or free meals for children in day-care centers and family day-care homes. The maximum reimbursement is for three meals, one of which must be a snack. (Food and Nutrition Service, 3101 Park Center Drive, Room 517, Alexandria, VA 22302; telephone: 202–756–3590)

- *The Supplemental Food Program for Women, Infants, and Children (WIC) Program.* This Special Supplemental Food Program, operated under the auspices of the U.S. Department of Agriculture, provides foods to meet anticipated dietary deficiencies in infants, children under age five, and pregnant and lactating women. To be eligible, recipients must meet financial criteria and be considered at nutritional risk. WIC serves more than 3.3 million participants each month, one-quarter of them women, one-quarter infants under one year, and the other half children between the ages of one and five. The Commodity Supplemental Food Program, similar to WIC, is available in 12 states and the District of Columbia. This program also administers the Elderly Feeding Program. (Food and Nutrition Service, 3101 Park Center Drive, Room 1017, Alexandria, VA 22302; telephone: 202–756–3746)

- *Meals-on-Wheels* and *Congregate Meals Programs.* Both programs strive to improve the nutrition of the elderly population within the context of their physical limitations and social needs. Meals-on-Wheels brings prepared meals directly to the homes of participants, while the Congregate Meals Programs provides nourishing meals in social settings to more mobile elderly adults. (Health and Human Services, 204 East Street, NE, Washington, D.C. 20005; telephone: 202–724–5626)

- *The Temporary Emergency Food Assistance Program (TEFAP).* Since 1981, The Department of Agriculture has donated food to low-income families. (An individual is considered a family of one.) The food is free but is limited to surplus commodities in government warehouses. The majority of foods distributed are dairy products; cheese, nonfat dry milk, and butter. Flour, rice, cornmeal, and honey are other commodities regularly distributed under TEFAP. Each state receives an allocation of the surplus food, which is then delivered to eligible families by nonprofit organizations. Eligibility is determined by need: Anyone qualified for other government food programs—for example, food stamps—automatically qualifies for TEFAP. (Food Distribution, 3101 Park Center Drive, Room 502, Alexandria, VA 22302; telephone: 202–756–3680)

most manufacturers will readily remove the product or the government will issue a recall notice.

Although nutrition labeling appears on 55 percent of the packaged foods regulated by the FDA (and is used by an estimated two-thirds of shoppers), it still falls short of consumer needs. For example, less than 45 percent of meat and poultry products are regulated by the USDA. For those products that do carry nutrition labels, it is difficult to tell the nutritive value, calories, fat, cholesterol, and sodium.

As of this writing, the FDA, USDA, and other government agencies are working on new nutrition labels to provide more complete and useful information. But even with present labeling, an alert consumer can find out a great deal about the contents and nutritional value of a product by carefully reading its label. In order to do this, a shopper must know the legal meaning of commonly used nutritional phrases, the limitations on health claims, and the use of food grades, food standards, and unit pricing.

What All Labels Must Contain

Food and Drug Administration regulations require manufacturers to include the following information on food labels.

- Name of the product.

- Its style and variety.

- Any special dietary properties, such as fortified or low salt.

- Net contents or net weight, including packing fluid.

- Name and address of packer, manufacturer, or distributor.

- List of ingredients in descending order by weight. The label does not have to indicate how much of any particular ingredient the product contains. Additives, including preservatives, must be specifically named, but color, flavors, and spices need only be described as "artificial color," "artificial flavor," or "natural flavor," meaning a flavor that normally would be found in the product. For example, vanilla does not need to be listed among the ingredients of vanilla ice cream. (Mandatory ingredients are not required to be listed on foods with a standard of identity, but optional ones are. See the section on Standards of Identity on page 667.)

- If the package label includes a picture, it must resemble the contents.

- Whenever a nutrient is added or the manufacturer claims particular nutritional value for a product, the food must contain a nutrition label.

Nutrition Labeling

A little more than half of the processed foods currently on the market contain nutritional information. When a nutrient has been added to a food or a nutrition claim is made, FDA regulations stipulate it must carry a nutrition label. Many manufacturers, in response to consumer demand, also voluntarily provide nutrition labels. Nutrition information on food labels can help consumers choose foods with lower sodium, fat, cholesterol, and calories, but label reading also involves product comparison. (See page 668 for definition of terms used on labels.)

There is no standard serving size from brand to brand or product to product, so it is necessary to compare labels carefully to match up serving sizes with the number of calories and nutrients in similar products. Some manufacturers have reduced the serving size—and sometimes the size of the package—by a few ounces to make it appear that the product has fewer calories, fat, or sodium. In addition, an error of plus or minus 20 percent is permitted in calorie designation, so that a 130-calorie serving could contain anywhere between 104 and 156 calories.

A nutrition label must contain the following information.

- Serving size, based on what an average adult male engaged in light physical activity ordinarily consumes as part of a meal.

- Number of servings per package.

- Number of calories per serving.

- Number of grams of protein, carbohydrates, and fat.

- Sodium content in milligrams per serving.

- Per serving percentages of U.S. Recommended Daily Allowances for protein, vitamin A, vitamin C, thiamine, riboflavin, niacin, calcium, and iron. (Listing of other nutrients is optional.)

- Other optional information includes compositions of saturated and unsaturated fats, and the sugar, starch, and fiber of carbohydrates. When two foods are commonly eaten together, such as cereal with milk, nutritional information for the combination may also be included. The FDA has proposed regulations that would define cholesterol and fatty-acid labeling terms. Optional information about fats, sugars, carbohydrates, and cho-

lesterol may be the information the consumer is seeking, yet it is not legally required. Individuals who need such detailed information must search out products that voluntarily provide it. RDIs will soon replace U.S. RDAs.

◆

Health Claims and Misleading Advertising

Federal regulations bar manufacturers from making certain misleading health claims for their food products. For example, it is illegal to say that a particular food or ingredient will prevent, treat, or cure a disease, or that a natural vitamin is superior to a synthetic one. Existing federal regulations, however, do not protect consumers from misleading but factually accurate labeling. For example, one manufacturer boasts that an imitation breakfast drink contains as much vitamin C as orange juice. While this is true, consumers may not realize that the imitation product does not contain the other nutrients found in orange juice, such as potassium, folate, thiamine, and vitamin A. Products have claimed to provide "more iron than milk," without noting that milk actually contains very little iron; or boasted "no preservatives added" on a package of raisins, without noting that raisins do not need preservatives.

In the early 1990s, the Food and Drug Administration was in the process of changing the regulations for health-related statements on foods and dietary supplements. Under the proposed regulations, product claims should be educational about nutrition and health and founded on accepted scientific research; they would have to stress the importance of the entire diet (and not exaggerate benefits of one product) and include full nutrition labeling. Literal truths conveying false messages will stop.

The Federal Trade Commission's standards for deceptive advertising are more relaxed than FDA labeling standards. FTC regulations allow a manufacturer to make health claims as long as they are substantiated by one or two scientific studies—even if other equally or more convincing studies contradict the claim. Additionally, FTC prosecution of offenders rarely punishes them to any significant degree.

Inspection Stamps and Food Grades

Inspection stamps. USDA inspection stamps indicate that a food is wholesome and was slaughtered, packed, or processed under sanitary conditions. Meat, poultry, and packaged or processed meat products must carry inspection stamps before they can be sold to consumers.

Food grades. The U.S. Department of Agriculture's grading system measures the quality of some meat, poultry, eggs, dairy products, and fresh and canned produce. USDA grade assignments are often called "beauty contests" because they are assigned primarily on the basis of appearance, uniformity, texture, and sometimes taste but have no bearing on nutritive value. It is not always necessary to purchase the more costly, higher grades of food. For example, if vegetables are to be cooked in a stew, uniform size is not a concern.

Unlike inspection stamps, which attest that food was processed safely, the USDA grading system is entirely voluntary and some food manufacturers opt instead to establish their own rating systems. Because the same grades have different meanings on different foods, USDA grades can be confusing. For example, top-choice poultry is called Grade A, but the best eggs are graded AA; Grade A eggs are only second best. Details about USDA grades are included in USDA Standards for the Meat Group, page 672.

Food Standards

Both the FDA and the USDA issue regulations to assure uniformity and quality among certain food products.

Standards of identity. Under FDA law and regulations, some 300 foods do not require listing of mandatory ingredients on their labels. Optional ingredients must be listed, however, including optional forms of mandatory ingredients; therefore, all of the ingredients of most standardized foods are listed. Examples include margarine, macaroni and noodle products, canned and frozen fish, cheese and cheese products, and bakery goods. The purpose of these standards is to assure consumers that certain standard foods, such as mayonnaise or catsup, will be very close, if not identical, to the products with which they are familiar. Even though listing of mandatory ingredients is not required, many manufacturers supply the information. (A complete list of standards of identity is contained in Title 21 of the Code of Federal Regulations, available from the U.S. Government Printing Office, Washington, D.C. 20402.)

Minimum standards of quality. These mandatory FDA standards pertain to the color, tenderness, and allowable freedom from defects that are permitted for many canned fruits and vegetables. Any component of the food that is below standard must be noted on the label. FDA minimum standards are usually comparable to the USDA Grade C rating, which is the department's lowest.

Standards of fill of the container. In order to prevent deceptive packaging, as when unreasonable quantities of air or water are added, the FDA specifies the minimum quantity of food that can be contained in a given-size package.

Standards of composition. The USDA defines the minimum amounts of meat and poultry that must be contained in certain foods. For example, a can labeled *chile con carne* must be at least 40 percent meat; *chile con carne with beans* needs to contain a minimum of 25 percent meat; *poultry chili* must be 28 percent poultry; and *poultry chili with beans* must be at least 17 percent poultry.

A complete list of standards of composition is available from Consumer Information, U.S. Department of Agriculture, Pueblo, CO 81002.

Defining the Terms

A number of words that commonly appear on food labels have strict legal definitions.

Imitation foods. A product that contains less protein and fewer vitamins or minerals than federally specified for its standard counterpart must be labeled *imitation*. (Foods lower in calories, fat, sodium, or cholesterol are not considered imitation.) Dairy foods, juices, and processed meats are the three categories of food where imitations are likely to be found. Imitations are often cheaper than the regular product but usually are nutritionally inferior.

Substitute foods. Foods nutritionally equivalent to a usual product may be called *substitutes* or may be given a name that suggests the similarity. Egg Beaters, for example, contain no egg yolks but are made from egg whites, and therefore use this fanciful trademark instead of the label *imitation eggs*.

Enriched or fortified. When nutrients, such as vitamins, minerals, or proteins, are added to food, a product can be labeled *enriched* or *fortified*. The product must have labeling regarding nutrition, and added nutrients must be listed in the ingredient list. In a standardized food, *enriched* may simply indicate that some of the nutrients lost in processing have been returned; enriched white flour, for example, does not contain all the nutrients of the whole grain.

Low-calorie. Only food that contains no more than 40 calories per serving and not more than 0.4 calories per gram of a product can be termed *low-calorie*. This designation cannot be given to foods naturally low in calories. *Low-calorie celery*, for example, is not allowed, but *celery, a low-calorie food* is permitted.

Reduced-calorie. Food that contains one third fewer calories than the standard product may be called *reduced-calorie*. If so, the label must include comparative information on both products. *Reduced-calorie* does not necessarily mean that a product has less of any particular nutrient—for example, cholesterol or sodium. Reduced-calorie mayonnaise, for example, which has about half the calories per tablespoon as regular mayonnaise, contains exactly the same amount of cholesterol, and even more sodium, as the regular product.

Dietetic. There are two very different uses for this claim. Manufacturers can label low- or reduced-calorie products as *dietetic* or the term can be used when an item is appropriate for restricted diets, such as low-sodium regimens. Dietetic cookies, for example, may be low only in sodium, not in calories. The label must indicate what is dietetic about a product.

Sugar-free or sugarless. A food called *sugar-free* contains no sugars such as sucrose (table sugar) or dextrose (corn sweeteners). A food labeled *sugar-free* must also be low or reduced in calories; otherwise, the label must state that the product is "not a reduced calorie food," "not for weight control," or "useful only in not promoting tooth decay."

Natural. There is no official federal regulation governing the use of the term *natural*, except when it is used for meat or poultry products that are governed by the USDA. These can be labeled *natural* only if they contain no preservatives or artificial flavors or colors and are minimally processed.

Organic. No regulations restrict the use of this term, either, although it is commonly used to describe foods grown in soil in which nonchemical fertilizers or pesticides have been used. The USDA does not allow meat or poultry products to be described as organic.

Unit Pricing

Unit pricing is a technique for comparing prices, regardless of packaging or manufacturer. While the package price tells a consumer what the total cost of an item is, the unit price gives costs per ounce, fluid ounce, pound, pint, quart, gallon, square foot, or the number of individual items packaged together. Given equal quality, the best buy is always the one with the least expensive per-unit price.

Per-unit prices are generally stamped on packages of produce, poultry, and meats and

---

Defining the Terms (cont.)

No preservatives. Preservatives are one type of food additive, most often used to retard spoilage. Many other types of additives may be used in foods labeled *no preservatives*, including sweeteners, flavorings, coloring, emulsifiers, stabilizers, and thickeners.

Light or lite. There is no consistent definition for these words, which are used variously to mean that a food contains fewer calories, less fat, less sodium, or simply has a lighter color. Nor does spelling (light versus lite) carry any special connotation. To learn the components and relative value of a light or lite food, consumers must read the label and compare the product with a regular one. For a few products, *light* does have a specific meaning.

- Light cream must contain between 18 and 30 percent milk fat.

- Canned fruit in light syrup is made with less sugar, and the syrup is generally less dense than regular syrup.

- Beer identified as light on the label usually contains about one-third fewer calories than the standard version from the same brewery.

- In lite salt, potassium has replaced some of the sodium.

- Light meat and poultry products must contain 25 percent less fat than typical meat; or at least 25 percent less fat, sodium, breading, or fewer calories than the conventional product. The label must indicate where the reduction can be found.

High in polyunsaturates. The label does not have to provide the ratio of polyunsaturated to saturated fats, but products with such claims may list the amount of saturated and polyunsaturated fat per serving. Therefore, the term *high in polyunsaturates* is reliable only when most of the oil in a food is corn, cottonseed, safflower, soybean, or a combination of these.

No cholesterol. All products made with vegetable oil have no cholesterol. While the tropical oils coconut and palm-kernel oil contain no cholesterol, both are high in saturated fats.

Sodium claims. Labeling claims by manufacturers on foods regulated by the FDA must meet the following FDA definitions.

- *Sodium-free:* Less than 5 milligrams of sodium per serving.

- *Very low sodium:* 35 milligrams or less per serving.

- *Low-sodium:* 140 milligrams or less per serving.

- *Reduced-sodium:* Usual level of sodium has been reduced at least 75 percent.

- *Unsalted, No salt added, Without added salt:* No salt added to a product that is normally processed with salt.

- Products not reduced in sodium by 75 percent or more may simply state comparisons; for example, contains × (percent) less sodium than the usual or regular product.

- *Lower* or *Less sodium:* Used only by the USDA for meats that have 25 percent less sodium than normal. (The USDA also requires the above FDA phrasing on processed meats and poultry when manufacturers advertise the sodium content of a product.)

appear on shelf cards below most other items. The style of the shelf cards may vary but the basic information remains the same.

Different manufacturers often pack foods in different sizes and the larger sizes often make the most economical purchase, with some exceptions. If an item is likely to spoil quickly, if storage space is tight, or if the package will be consumed very slowly, the saving needs to be significant enough to justify a large-sized purchase. Consumers also need to be sure they are comparing unit prices on foods that are identical, not merely similar.

Although most big supermarkets provide unit pricing as a service to consumers, only a few cities, counties, and states actually require it. No federal laws mandate unit pricing.

Open Dating

Open dating, also known as freshness dating, refers to several systems in which conventional calendar dates are stamped on per-ishable products to enable the consumer to determine their freshness readily. Closed dating systems, by contrast, are virtually indecipherable alpha-numeric production codes used by manufacturers to assure quality and monitor distribution. Federal regulators have no policies on open dating, but some cities and states require it and many stores find it a useful means of maintaining quality control.

Manufacturers and retailers most commonly stamp *use by* or *best if used by* dates on their packages; pack and expiration dates are less commonly used.

Items, usually baked goods, may carry a shelf date for the day they are placed on the shelf. These products are often put on sale as *day old* and can be good buys, since most people will keep the product on the shelf at home for several days, anyway.

Sell by (or *Pull*) date represents the last day a product should be sold, assuming that it will be stored properly at home for a reasonable period of time before use. On particularly perishable foods, such as bakery products, only the day of the week is given; the month or even the year will be included on items with a longer shelf life. Dairy products, meats, and fresh fruit juices often carry a *sell by* date.

Used most often on such shelf-stable items as cereals and snacks, and on cheese, *best if used by* lists the last recommended date for using a product. Because of their long shelf life, the year is often included in the date. *Best if used by* dates do not allow additional time for home storage.

A pack date is used on frozen or canned items, and occasionally on perishable foods, to indicate when the food was processed, manufactured, or packaged. A calendar date often appears on the label without the words *pack date*. Frozen foods are best used within a few months of the pack date; canned goods should be used within a year.

Hidden Sources of Sodium

Sodium exists in foods where many consumers scarcely expect to find it. At least 70 sodium compounds are regularly used in processed foods. Watch the label for the words *soda* and *sodium* and the symbol *Na*. Examples are:

Salt (sodium chloride)	Sodium nitrate
Monosodium glutamate (MSG)	Sodium propionate
	Sodium citrate
Baking soda (sodium bicarbonate)	Sodium saccharin
	Disodium inosinate
Baking powder	Sodium ascorbate
Disodium phosphate	Sodium caseinate
Sodium alginate	Brine (salt and water)
Sodium benzoate	
Sodium hydroxide	

Expiration date is the last date by which a product should be used. It is most commonly used on drugs, packaged yeasts, refrigerated dough, and baby formulas.

SELECTING FOODS

The range of fresh, frozen, and canned products available to the American consumer is staggering. The average market sells tens of thousands of products containing a wide variety of foods from the four basic food groups—meats, fruits and vegetables, breads and cereals, and dairy products—plus an enormous variety of condiments, snacks, sweets, and fats. Following are suggestions on how to get the best value for your food dollar.

Choosing Foods in the Meat Group

Beef. Until recently, the "better"—and more expensive—grades of beef were those that are richly marbled with saturated fat. Grading of beef has been changed to recognize that leaner beef cuts, now graded as "choice," are equal to the fatter "prime" cuts. Choice cuts actually provide less fat and fewer calories and are the best food value. Such cuts have fine flavor once they have been tenderized or cooked slowly in moist heat.

Pork. The tenderloin strip, center-cut leg ham, and loin chops are the least fatty cuts of pork, but they still contain moderate amounts. Most fatty are the rib roast, bacon, feet hocks, shoulder, and shoulder butt. Pork cooked to a "medium" doneness is generally the most flavorful.

Poultry. Chicken and turkey are lower in fat than game hens; duck and goose, however, are high in fat. Birds are young and tender when their legs and wings spring back into place after being pulled back. While skin color does not affect taste, rough, dry, or bruised skin on a chicken or a turkey should be avoided because it may indicate that the bird was over- or too roughly handled. Buying whole chicken is almost always less expensive than purchasing chicken already cut into parts.

Seafood. There is no mandatory inspection of all fish or seafood by the federal government. Thus, the single most-important criterion for selecting fish is freshness, which is revealed by bright skin with a good color, clear and bulging eyes, tight scales, and flesh that is firm to the touch. When purchasing mussels, clams, or oysters, be certain that the shells are tightly closed.

Beans, nuts, and seeds. Beans are among the most versatile and economical sources of protein. Most supermarkets stock several varieties. The flavors and textures of each kind of bean may be very different, but nutritive values are roughly equal. Some varieties can be used interchangeably in recipes: pinto, pink, red, cranberry, and kidney beans; Great Northern, small whites, navy, and pea beans; mung beans and split peas. Black beans, lima beans, black-eyed peas, garbanzo beans, and soybeans each have a distinctive flavor. Selection is largely a matter of personal preference and availability.

Nuts and seeds are also excellent protein alternatives to meat. Most varieties are good sources of iron and B vitamins. Peanuts, sunflower seeds, and soy nuts are excellent snack foods, although their oil content makes them high in calories. The difference in fat content between oil-roasted and dry-roasted nuts is negligible.

Soy products. Soy-based products, including tofu, tempeh, and tamari, are excellent sources of protein. Tofu (soft cakes made from curdled soy milk) is highly perishable and should be purchased vacuum-packed or floating in water. Tempeh (cakes made from fermented soybeans), which is usually found only in health-food stores, is also highly perishable. Although it is as high in sodium as soy sauce, tamari can be substituted for soy sauce, which may have caramel coloring and preservatives added.

Eggs. Eggs are sized by weight per dozen from peewee to jumbo, with extra large, large, and medium-sized eggs most commonly found in supermarkets. Shell color—brown, white, or cream—does not affect flavor or nutritive value; the only difference is that they are produced by different breeds of hen. Likewise, fertilized eggs sold in health-food stores have no better nutritional value than unfertilized eggs sold in supermarkets. In fact, those sold in the supermarket are almost always adequately fresh and are likely to keep longer than fertilized eggs, whose yolk may begin to develop, bringing on quicker deterioration.

Prices vary by size and grade. Larger sizes usually cost more per dozen than smaller sizes of the same grade but are sometimes cheaper by weight. A rule of thumb for buying eggs: Purchase the smaller size if the next largest is more than eight cents higher in price.

Choosing Fruits and Vegetables

Although fresh fruits and vegetables generally have the highest nutrient levels, frozen and canned produce are not far behind. Freezing is actually one of the least destructive methods of food preservation available. Nutrient loss in canned produce is only slightly

USDA Standards for the Meat Group

- *Beef, veal, lamb:* graded prime, choice, or select. Since ranking is largely determined by how well marbled the meat is, prime is usually the most fatty, although it is also the most flavorful and the most expensive. Choice meats, which are also tender and juicy, are the most common.

- *Pork:* graded no. 1, no. 2, and no. 3. Grades are seldom used at the retail level.

- *Poultry:* graded A, B, and C. Retail poultry is generally Grade A, with Grades B and C usually reserved for processed foods.

- *Eggs:* graded AA, A, and B. Grades AA and A are almost equal in quality, but Grade A is more commonly sold in retail stores. Because the criteria for grading depends on the appearance of the yolk when broken, Grade B eggs are best used only for cooking and baking.

Fat and Lean Claims

USDA regulations now apply to labeling claims for the fat content of meat and poultry. When these claims are made, the label must specify actual percentages of fat. If frozen dinners or entrées use the term *light* or *lean* fancifully, such as with Lean Cuisine products, they are exempt from these requirements.

- *Lean or low-fat:* The product may contain no more than 10 percent fat.

- *Extra-lean:* This is restricted to products containing no more than 5 percent fat.

- *Light, leaner, or less fat:* These are used for meat products with 25 percent less fat than USDA standards or comparable products specify. *Light* may also refer to a 25-percent reduction in breading, sodium, or calories, and the label must indicate what was reduced.

higher than with fresh or frozen produce, but sodium and sugar is often added during the processing.

Small young vegetables and fruits are often the tastiest and contain more nutrients per pound than do large ones because nutrients are usually concentrated near the surface. The darkest vegetables—deep orange carrots and dark green leafy lettuce, for example—generally have the highest nutrients. Similarly, pink grapefruit has more vitamin A than white grapefruit. While the biggest, prettiest fruits and vegetables are not necessarily the best buys, they often are. The recent controversy over Alar, the ripening agent that was once sprayed on apples to prevent their falling prematurely was an example of a largely baseless consumer scare, as the American Council on Science and Health reported in 1990 (see Chapter 11).

Produce should be purchased individually and not prepackaged and should be limited to amounts that can be used while still fresh. By buying fruits and vegetables in season, prices will be lower and quality higher. Fresh produce that sits unused in the refrigerator for too long will lose taste and nutrition. Therefore, it is best to shop for vegetables twice weekly or use canned and frozen vegetables.

Juice. Because some nutrients and fiber are lost in processing, juice is not as nutritious as fresh fruit, but certainly more so than soft drinks. The consumer should beware, however, that only a product bearing the name *fruit juice* is 100 percent juice. Sugar and water, in varying degrees, are the prime ingredients of many other products, such as fruit drinks, that are packaged like juice.

Dried fruit. Dried fruit offers a convenient alternative for those who do not want to carry the weight of fresh fruit—for example, hikers—or those who prefer its concentrated flavor. Depending on the kind of fruit, it contains the same amounts of vitamins A and C,

copper, fiber, iron, potassium, and other nutrients as its fresh counterpart. Several cautions are in order, however. Not only is dried fruit higher in calories than fresh, more of it is usually consumed in a sitting because it does not contain the water of fresh fruit, which imparts a feeling of fullness. Dried fruit is often treated with sulfite preservatives, harmful to people with sulfite-sensitive asthma. It is also a powerful laxative. Eating sticky dried fruit demands the same dental care as sweets.

Choosing Foods in the Bread and Cereal Group

Breads. The most nutritious breads are the least refined. Whole grains provide the best sources of minerals, vitamins, and fiber, while in bread that has been enriched, the niacin, iron, riboflavin, and thiamine that was destroyed in processing is restored. Bread labeled *whole wheat* must be baked from 100 percent whole-wheat flour (and thus contain all of the natural constituents of wheat in unaltered proportions), whereas that labeled *wheat* is made from a blend of enriched white and whole-wheat flours. Darker breads are not always more nutritious; caramel color is

USDA Standards for Fruits and Vegetables

- *Fresh produce:* graded Fancy, no. 1 and no. 2. Most retail produce is graded no. 1, although consumers rarely see the grading.

- *Canned, frozen, and dried produce:* graded A or Fancy, B, and C. While equally nutritious, Grade A products are most uniform in size and color; only aesthetic appeal declines with grade. Consumers rarely see these grades, although they affect pricing.

often added to give rye, pumpernickel, and wheat breads their characteristically richer coloring.

Cereals. Consumers are faced with a dizzying array of hot and cold breakfast cereals, many heavily advertised and loaded with sugar, salt, and fat, or a penny's worth of vitamins and a doubled price. Whole-grain cereals, like whole-grain breads, are the most nutritious. They also are higher in fiber than refined products. (Bran products also are high in fiber.) The label will reveal whether whole grains—wheat, oat, rye, corn—are the first item on a cereal's ingredient list. Fat and sugar is often added to granola, making it seldom the health bargain its promoters claim. Cereals that require cooking, such as rolled oats, toasted wheat, and Cream of Rice, are better buys and usually retain the vitamins and fiber of the natural grain. Checking a cereal's price per serving can result in savings. The additional packaging usually makes individual-sized boxes the most expensive per serving.

Grains and pasta. Carbohydrate-rich rice and pasta are consumed in abundance in the United States, while other grains, such as bulgur, cracked wheat, couscous, wheat berries, or oats, that are found in health-food stores and supermarkets are popular elsewhere in the world but have been relatively neglected here. Brown rice is slightly more nutritious than polished white rice; converted white rice has fewer nutrients than the polished variety; and instant white rice has the fewest of all.

Choosing Foods in the Milk Group

Milk has long been touted as nature's most perfect food. However, whole milk is too high in fat for many adults, although it is ideal for most young children. By definition, 3.5 percent of whole milk must be fat, and since milk is mostly water, this means that almost half (72 of 150) of the calories in whole milk come from fat. A better choice for many adults is low-fat milk, which usually has a fat content of either 1 percent or 2 percent, or skim milk, which contains less than 1 percent fat. Many manufacturers return some of the vitamin A that is lost in the skimming process along with the addition of vitamin D.

Nonfat dry milk. Less costly than skim milk but with equal amounts of nutrients and a much longer shelf life, nonfat dry milk is a good choice for the thrifty consumer. It is excellent for cooking and can be combined with skim milk to provide the flavor some people prefer.

Evaporated milk. Evaporated or condensed milk has been heated, vacuum-concentrated to remove 60 percent of the water, homogenized, and canned. It contains at least 7.5 percent milk fat. The nutrient value of reconstituted evaporated milk is similar to that of fresh milk. Evaporated skim milk is now more commonly available than it was. Sweetened evaporated milk is much higher in calories than regular condensed milk because it must contain at least 8 percent milk fat and enough sweetener to prevent spoilage.

Chocolate-flavored milk. Chocolate syrup or cocoa and sweetener is added to whole, low-fat, or skim milk to give it a chocolate taste.

Chocolate-flavored milk drink. Chocolate syrup or cocoa and sweeteners are added to low-fat or skim milk to give it a chocolate taste.

Raw milk. Raw milk is milk that has not been pasteurized (heated) to kill microorganisms that transmit disease. Milk leaves the cow in a relatively pure state but is a ready breeding ground for bacteria. The Food and Drug Administration has concluded that consuming unpasteurized milk poses health risks. Certification does not guarantee purity. There have been incidences of the bacterial infections campylobacteriosis and fatal salmonellosis from the bacteria in raw milk and cheese made from it, with the danger particularly great to the elderly, the young, and the infirm. Assays reveal vitamin loss in pasteurized milk does not exceed 10 percent, refuting those who say the pasteurization process excessively destroys nutrients in milk. Heat cannot destroy minerals. About 25 states ban the sale of raw milk within their borders, and the FDA opposes its interstate movement.

Pasteurized milk. Pasteurized milk, except for skim milk, is processed by a homogenizer, a stainless-steel pump that forces whole milk through nozzles under high pressure to break up fat globules into small particles that will not rise to the top but, instead, remain evenly suspended throughout. Before homogenization became the norm, bottled milk naturally separated, with the cream on top and the skim milk on the bottom. Homogenization guarantees that milk is consistently creamy white, has a smooth taste, and contains no clumps of butterfat. There is no evidence that homogenization effects either nutrients or the healthfulness of milk.

Sweet acidophilus milk. The *Lactobacillus acidophilus* bacteria, which thrive in milk, are normally present in the human intestine. The process of deliberately growing them in milk is called culturing. Yogurt, cultured buttermilk, and the sour kind of acidophilus milk are true bacterial cultures. The sweet version of acidophilus milk is a low-fat cold milk to which precultured bacteria have been added, without further fermentation. It tastes like regular low-fat milk, whereas naturally cultured acidophilus milk has a sour taste re-

sembling cultured buttermilk and yogurt. It is often recommended for those who are lactose-intolerant. No specific health claims are made by the producers of sweet acidophilus milk, although promoters suggest it has health-maintaining properties.

Buttermilk. Buttermilk is milk to which lactic acid has been added to either skim or low-fat pasteurized milk. It has a thicker consistency than regular milk and a tart taste. Cultured buttermilk is low in calories (99 for an 8-ounce cup), but has 257 milligrams of sodium (compared to about 125 milligrams in skim or low-fat milk), which may preclude it from a low-salt diet.

Ultrahigh-temperature (UHT) milk. UHT milk has been subjected to temperatures of 285 degrees F. (140 degrees C.) for one to three seconds and sealed in germ-free containers. These packages can be held unopened at room temperatures for three to six months with insignificant vitamin losses. UHT milk is convenient for campers, people living in remote areas, and those with limited refrigerator space. Popular in Europe, this milk is also available in the United States.

Filled milk, imitation milk, and nondairy creamers. Filled-milk manufacturers replace the butterfat of whole milk with a vegetable oil, usually coconut. Imitation milk is a blend, usually consisting of soy protein, corn syrup, coconut oil, vitamins, and minerals, which is useful mostly for people who can't drink regular milk. Nondairy creamers, either powdered or liquid, may also contain coconut oil. While imitation milk products sometimes boast that they contain no cholesterol, they often contain coconut oil or hydrogenated oils that are saturated. Dietary saturated fats tend to raise blood cholesterol more than does dietary cholesterol. When buying any imitation milk product, read the label carefully. In terms of quality protein, fat, and vitamin and mineral content, imitation milk products also are usually nutritionally inferior to real milk.

Yogurt. Yogurt is a mixture of milk, skim milk, and/or cream that has been cultured with friendly bacteria (*Lactobacillus bulgaricus* and *Streptococcus thermophilus*). It is more nutritious and economical to buy plain yogurt and add fresh fruit or other flavorings at home than to purchase the fruited variety, which is laden with sugars and calories.

Cheese. Cheese purchased at supermarkets can be divided into three broad categories: unripened—such as cottage, mozzarella, cream, and ricotta—which are the lowest in fats and cholesterol and come in low-fat versions; ripened, which includes cheddar, Swiss, Muenster, and Parmesan; and hard cheese, which is high in fats. Processed cheese, cheese food, and cheese spread all include additives such as thickeners, stabilizers, gums, and extra fat. FDA standards of identity specify ingredients, fat and moisture content, pasteurization requirements, and manufacturing procedures for many different types of cheeses. (See Chapter 33 for further information for those who are lactose-intolerant.)

Imitation cheese. Like other dairy products, imitation cheese is not nutritionally equivalent to real cheese and is likely to be made with hydrogenated vegetable oils. These products are most often adjacent to real cheese in the dairy case.

Choosing Fats and Sweets

Budget-conscious shoppers should look seriously for ways to cut their consumption of fats and sweets, which contribute calories and appetite appeal to the diet but do not deliver many nutrients.

Fats. Vegetable oils are divided among saturated, monounsaturated, and polyunsaturated fats. The best general-purpose oils are polyunsaturated and monounsaturated. Safflower, soybean, peanut, sesame, sunflower, and olive oils have distinctive tastes and are good alternatives to corn oil when choosing an all-purpose polyunsaturated oil. Hydrogenation converts polyunsaturated fatty acids to saturated fats, making hardened margarines and vegetable shortening. Hydrogenation is the process of making an unsaturated oil more saturated (saturated means saturated with hydrogen). Palm, palm-kernel, and coconut oil are highly saturated vegetable oils. A product with a flexible label that reads. ''Contains one of the following oils: corn, sunflower, or coconut'' is likely to contain coconut oil, especially as it is

---

USDA Standards for the Milk Group

- *Milk:* Milk is classified Grade A if it is produced on a farm and in a dairy processing plant meeting Grade A standards (which are agreed upon by government and industry officials).

- *Butter:* It is graded AA, A, and B depending on the number of flavor and body defects it contains. Grade AA is allowed the least number of defects, and Grade A has fewer than Grade B. Cheddar cheese is graded U.S. AA, A, B, or C, depending on the number of its attributes.

- *Instant nonfat dry milk:* U.S. Extra Grade indicates that the milk dissolves readily and tastes sweet and pleasant.

- *Cottage cheese and processed cheese:* There are no grade standards, only standards of identity. If cottage cheese is labeled Grade A, it means it was made from Grade A milk and produced on a farm that met Grade A standards.

the least expensive. Of the fatty acids in hydrogenated coconut oil, 90 to 95 percent are saturated.

Margarine, usually a blend of vegetable oils, is a better source of polyunsaturates than butter, which is 80 percent milk fat. Many consumers, however, prefer the flavor of butter, although butter-flavored margarines are available. It is important to note, however, that margarine and butter are equal in calories despite their different fat composition. In selecting margarine, read nutrition labels carefully to compare polyunsaturated fatty acids to saturated fatty acids in a margarine. (See also Chapter 6 and the end of Chapter 26.)

Sweets. Sweets are not an essential component of any diet, but they do add to the pleasure of eating. Few people tend to forego them, and often there is no need to do so.

On Guard Against Excess Fats and Sugars

Saturated fats and sugars have an insidious way of sneaking into processed foods. Read labels and watch for the following ingredients.

More Saturated Fats
Beef fat
Butter
Cocoa butter
Coconut oil
Hydrogenated oil
Hydrogenated vegetable oil
Lard
Palm oil
Shortening
Sour cream
Suet
Sweet cream
Whole milk
Whole-milk cheese

Higher in Monounsaturated Fats
Olive oil
Peanut oil
Canola oil

Mostly Polyunsaturated Fats
Corn oil
Cottonseed oil
Safflower oil
Sesame oil
Soybean oil
Sunflower oil

Sugars
Beet sugar
Brown sugar
Cane sugar
Corn sugar
Corn sweetener
Corn syrup
Dextrin
Dextrose
Fructose
Galactose
Glucose
High-fructose corn syrup (HFCS)
Honey
Invert sugar
Lactose
Levulose
Maltose
Mannitol
Maple syrup
Molasses
Sorbitol
Sucrose
Turbinado sugar

Note: Whether or not partially hydrogenated corn, cottonseed, safflower, sesame, soybean, and sunflower oils are high or low in unsaturated fatty acids depends on the degree of hydrogenation. See the end of Chapter 26.

Again, moderation is the key—an occasional small ice cream cone or other "indulgence" does no harm as long as it is included as part of your day's calorie allowance.

Fortunately, there are many healthful desserts that will satisfy a "sweet tooth" without adding excessive calories or fats to the diet. Often it's a matter of artful substitution—sherbet or sorbet instead of ice cream, a fruit crisp instead of pie, or an oatmeal cookie instead of a candy bar or brownie.

Even people with dietary restrictions who must limit their intake of sugar, fat, or cholesterol can still enjoy a variety of sweet-tasting foods. Some of these may be made with sugar substitutes, but there also are many fruit-based desserts and low-fat or skim milk products that are low in calories and high in nutrition. Examples are frozen fruit bars, low-fat frozen desserts, fresh-fruit compotes, and home-made banana, date, or other such breads baked with negligible amounts of fat. Both the American Heart Association and the American Diabetes Association offer cookbooks with recipes for a variety of tasty and nutritious desserts. (For a more complete discussion and specific suggestions, see Chapter 8.)

CONCLUSION

It is in wise food shopping that you have an opportunity to put into practice the myriad lessons of this book. In this chapter, we have attempted to give a broad overview of how to go about making smart decisions when food shopping. With practice, you will soon find that you can sort through misleading advertising claims and select those foods that give you the most for your nutrition dollar.

41

Food Storage and Preparation

Rosalinda Lawson, R.D., Elyse Sosin, R.D., M.A., and
Fran C. Grossman, R.D., M.S.

■

INTRODUCTION

An understanding of proper storage, preparation, and cooking techniques will help a consumer serve nutritious and appetizing meals. In this chapter, guidelines are provided for refrigerating and freezing perishables, storing canned and dried goods, and preparing foods prior to cooking. A description of the cooking methods that best conserve nutrients is also included here, along with tips on using leftovers, preventing food poisoning, and packing lunch boxes and picnics. Light, heat, moisture, and air—all can rob food of many nutrients. By following certain guidelines and taking appropriate precautions, however, the loss can be minimized and foods kept fresh and safe from the time they are purchased until they are eaten.

STORAGE GUIDELINES

The storage guidelines that follow are designed to maximize safety and minimize nutrient loss. Consumers should know which foods should be refrigerated and which should be kept at room temperature, how to wrap food to extend its useful life, and the length of time food can be kept safely. Proper storage is important, since light can destroy vitamins A, K, and B_2 (riboflavin); heat dissipates vitamin C, vitamin B_1 (thiamine), and folic acid; and air destroys vitamins C, E, and K.

The Refrigerator

The danger zone for food spoilage is between 45 and 140 degrees F. In this temperature range, bacteria, molds, and yeast grow freely. Food should not be left at these temperatures for more than two hours. The refrigerator should be set between 35 and 40 degrees F. (a setting at Normal usually suffices); the meat keeper should be just above freezing. Self-defrosting refrigerators usually have a uniform temperature throughout. In other models, the shelves on the back of the door and the bottom of the refrigerator are usually the warmest places and should not be used to store highly perishable foods. The area closest to the freezing unit usually stays the coldest. An appliance thermometer helps verify temperatures.

Air will not circulate freely when a refrigerator is packed too tightly: as a result, food will not be cooled evenly. Allow adequate space between storage containers and try to distribute items fairly evenly among shelves. Food should usually be stored in the smallest possible container, because contact with air speeds deterioration. Airtight containers, aluminum foil, or plastic wrap prevent foods from being dried out. To minimize handling and exposure, food should be left in its store wrappings until used. An exception is whole poultry, which should be unwrapped and the bag of giblets removed. It can then be rewrapped in plastic. Meat can be left in its store wrapper if it is going to be used in a day or so; otherwise, rewrap in plastic or foil to prevent drying. The refrigerator should be inspected regularly for food that has deteriorated and should be thrown out; it should be cleaned periodically with a mixture of water and baking soda.

Dry Storage

Dry goods and cans should be stored in a cool, dark, dry, and insect-free pantry or cupboard. An ideal temperature is 50 degrees F., although 60 to 70 degrees F. is more common and quite acceptable. The risk of spoilage increases greatly at higher temperatures; in fact, special manufacturing procedures are used for canned goods sold in tropical climates. Dry goods should be stored in containers with tight-fitting lids to reduce exposure to moisture, air, and insects. Foods should not be stored near the stove or the refrigerator exhaust or under the kitchen sink. Cleaning products should always be kept away from edibles and cans should be dust-free.

Most experts recommend one-year storage for canned foods even though most usually retain their quality and nutrients for longer periods. Some canned foods lose their color or undergo a change in taste with long storage. For example, canned products with a high acid content, such as tomato, citrus, or other acidic fruits or vinegars, tend to react with the can when stored for a long time, giving food a metallic taste. Eventually cans rust or corrode, allowing bacterial agents to enter, with the consequent danger of food poisoning (see Food Poisoning on page 695). Consumers should check labels to be sure that canned products do not require refrigeration; canned hams, for example, need cold storage.

Newly purchased cans of food should be placed behind older cans so that they are used in proper sequence. Once a can is opened, its contents should be transferred to a glass or plastic container (to prevent metal toxicity, which can result from eating food in a metal can that is exposed to air) and refrigerated.

Root cellars can be used to store produce in regions where winter temperatures average 30 degrees F. or lower. Vegetables and fruits—carrots, potatoes, beets, and turnips, apples, pears, and grapes, for example—can all be wintered over in a cool basement or an outdoor root cellar. Since fruits can absorb vegetable odors, they should be stored away from onions, garlic, and other vegetables.

Home canning, preserving, and drying are other good ways to store food for long periods of time. However, improperly canned foods have been implicated in cases of botulism (see the discussion on page 700). Detailed instructions for proper canning can be found in many cookbooks.

The Meat Group

Meat, poultry, and fish stay freshest in the coldest part of the refrigerator, especially where air circulates freely. They should be loosely wrapped in butcher's paper or plastic; usually the original packaging is adequate unless there is a great deal of blood. Meat that is frozen shouldn't be wrapped in plastic, as it is more prone to freezer burn (resulting from loss of moisture due to prolonged contact with air). Bruised fish spoils quickly and should be handled with particular care. Shellfish will not keep in the refrigerator for more than a few hours; it should be stored on ice or at temperatures below freezing. In these conditions, it keeps for two or three days.

When hot dogs and luncheon meats are refrigerated in their original vacuum-sealed packages, they stay fresh for two weeks; once opened, they should be rewrapped tightly and used within a few days. Cured and smoked meats also store best in their original wrappings. With the exception of hard salami, meat that shows any sign of mold should be discarded. Salami can be saved if the moldy area and the surrounding inch of meat are cut away.

The following are tips for storing other foods in the meat group.

- Unshelled nuts keep well at room temperature for up to six months; other nuts should be refrigerated or frozen so that they do not become rancid. Moldy nuts must be discarded.

- Dried beans stored in glass jars lose light-sensitive riboflavin.

- Eggs should be refrigerated in their original carton, with the larger end pointing up to keep the yolk centered. Although most refrigerators have an egg rack on the door, it is best to store eggs away from the door where the temperature is more constant.

The Fruit and Vegetable Group

The vitamin content of raw fruit and vegetables is diminished if produce is kept at normal room temperature. The vegetable crisper of a refrigerator hydrates produce, keeping it fresh for several days, although some vitamins are gradually lost. Crispers are most effective when they are at least two-thirds full. Fruit and vegetables stored in a refrigerator without a hydrator should be kept in unsealed plastic bags. Fruit should always be treated with particular care to avoid crushing or bruising. Small spots of mold can be cut off firm produce, such as cabbage, peppers, and carrots. Soft vegetables, such as leafy greens, tomatoes, and cucumbers, should be discarded if mold appears.

To prevent rot related to dampness, most produce should not be washed until it is ready to be used. Lettuce and other green leafy vegetables are exceptions. These can be washed and dried ahead of time and stored in plastic bags with a paper towel to absorb moisture.

Fresh peas and lima beans should be left in their pods during refrigeration; berries should keep their stems. However, the tops of carrots, beets, parsnips, radishes, rutabagas, and turnips should be removed before storage.

Sweet potatoes, hard-rind squash, eggplant, rutabagas, and onions (but not scallions) are best stored in the refrigerator or another cool, dry, and dark place. Light lowers the nutritional value of potatoes, and high temperatures cause them to sprout or shrivel: they should be kept cool, moist, and in the dark. Onions also sprout and decay when the temperature or humidity is high.

Fruit and tomatoes ripen best at room temperature; when they are fully ripe, they should be refrigerated. When bananas are refrigerated, their skin will darken but the flavor is not affected. Citrus fruits can be stored either at room temperature or in the refrigerator. Cut melons and pineapple should be wrapped and kept refrigerated. Dried fruit stored in a tightly closed container keeps well at room temperature except in humid weather. Juice should be refrigerated in the smallest container possible so that vitamins are not destroyed by exposure to oxygen.

The Bread and Cereal Group

Whole-grain flours and crackers can ordinarily be stored at room temperature except when the weather is hot. Cereals, rice, bulgur, and most other grains do not need to be refrigerated, but because they are susceptible to insects, they should be stored in airtight containers. Like beans, however, they will lose riboflavin if they are stored in glass jars that are exposed to light.

Yeast bread stays freshest when it is wrapped in foil or plastic and stored in a cool, dark place, such as a bread box. In hot and humid weather, however, bread is better protected against mold in the refrigerator, although it will dry out more quickly. Moldy bread, cereal, and grain products should be discarded.

The Milk Group

Fresh milk and cream should be closed tightly so that they do not absorb the odors or flavors of other foods in the refrigerator. Milk and cream sold in opaque containers retain nutrients longer than those in plastic jugs because the fluorescent lights in food stores destroy some of the vitamin A and riboflavin. Keeping nonfat dry milk in a tightly closed container at room temperature prevents it from becoming lumpy or stale.

Soft cheese should be tightly covered and refrigerated; hard cheese lasts well in a cool, dark place. Hard cheese remains edible even when mold develops if an inch around the mold is cut off. Moldy cottage cheese, sour or sweet cream, yogurt, or soft cheeses should not be saved.

Fats and Sweets

Warm temperatures turn oil rancid and destroy some vitamins A, D, and E, so most fats should be refrigerated or used quickly. It may be wise to avoid buying gallon-size containers, since the oil may turn rancid before you have chance to use it all. (Rancid oil will have a characterisic bitter smell.) Some oils become cloudy or solid when kept cold but quickly return to clear liquid at room temperature. To prevent deterioration on exposure to air, oils should fill the containers in which they are stored. Mayonnaise and oil-based salad dressing should always be stored in the refrigerator.

Margarine and butter should be wrapped tightly; quantities for immediate use can be stored conveniently in the refrigerator and the rest should be frozen. Margarine and butter both turn rancid when left too long at room temperature.

Syrup should be stored at room temperature until opened, then refrigerated to prevent mold. If it crystallizes, it can be restored to liquid form by placing the jars in hot water.

(For a more complete list of how, where, and for how long to store specific food items, see Table 41.1.)

PREPARING SAFE, NUTRITIOUS FOODS

In general, more nutrients are lost from fresh foods in the final preparation for the table than in commercial processing. Frozen and commercially canned foods usually are prepared quickly at the height of their nutritional value. In contrast, foods you buy fresh may have been picked before fully ripe (when most foods are at peak nutrition) and then traveled for long distances or been stored for long periods, causing further nutritional decline.

The stability of nutrients varies widely. Carbohydrate, fat, and fat-soluble vitamins are not greatly affected by ordinary preparation methods, but the water-soluble vitamins are much more vulnerable. Vitamin C is more easily destroyed than any other nutrient, so the conservation of that vitamin is often used as a measure of the conservation of other nutrients. If vitamin C is protected, other nutrients will be also. Overcooking and the use of too much liquid or too high a heat will have an adverse effect on many nutrients and on the flavor, texture, and appearance of most foods.

Meat

In general, poultry, veal, fish, and lean meat are healthier than fat-laced cuts of beef, lamb, and pork. Visible fat should always be trimmed off red meats before cooking. Poultry skin is unquestionably flavorful but it is also a source of fat. When the skin is removed before cooking, the loss of flavor can be minimized by the use of herbs and spices. Meat and poultry can be washed under cold running water before cooking; fish should be wiped with a damp cloth.

Poultry should be stuffed just before it is ready to be cooked—never ahead of time—to avoid bacterial contamination of the stuffing. Stuffing should be loosely packed in order to cook all the way through.

Meats should be cooked at relatively low heat (about 300 degrees F.) to reduce shrinkage, preserve juiciness, and safeguard the B vitamins. Dry-heat cooking methods—roasting, baking, broiling, and grilling—are most commonly used for tender cuts of meat. Moist-heat methods—boiling, poaching, stewing, steaming, and braising—use a liquid

(water, soup stock, or wine) and slow cooking to soften the connective tissue in tougher, leaner cuts of meat. Some vitamins and minerals will be lost to the cooking liquid, but the loss can be minimized by using the liquid as a gravy or sauce.

A meat thermometer, which measures the internal temperature of a piece of meat, helps determine when meat is properly cooked. Medium and rare beef is pink in the center; well-done meat is light brown. The center of a roast cooked to the rare stage will barely reach 140 degrees F., the temperature at which most food-borne bacteria are killed. Hamburger, which is particularly susceptible to bacteria because it is handled so frequently, should not be eaten rare; the meat should be brown or brownish pink in the center. Pork should have no pink color. Poultry is thoroughly cooked when its juices are clear, its leg joints move easily, and the thigh meat is soft to the touch. Fish should flake easily with a fork when it is ready to eat. Fresh hams should be thoroughly cooked; precooked or fully cooked hams can be eaten cold or reheated. The label will provide directions. (For a timetable for broiling meats, see Table 41.2.)

Fat from cooking bacon or sausage should never be reused as it has been associated with an increased cancer risk.

Vegetables

Valuable nutrients are lost if vegetables are not prepared properly. All vegetables should be washed under running water (never soaked) to remove dirt, insects, water-soluble pesticides, and other contaminants. If necessary, a very dilute solution of dish detergent and water may be used to help clean the vegetables, after which wash thoroughly.

A concentration of a vegetable's nutrients is in the skin or just below it. The skin of tomato, for example, contains three times more vitamin C than the flesh. While the wax coating and pesticide residues on some of to-day's produce often make washing, and sometimes even peeling, necessary, there is no need to peel root vegetables (potatoes, beets, carrots, turnips, etc.), tomatoes, or unwaxed cucumbers. It is better to cook vegetables with the peel intact; it can be removed before serving, if necessary.

The coarse outer leaves of lettuce and cabbage have more calcium, iron, and vitamin A than the inside leaves. Broccoli leaves have more vitamin A than the stalks or florets; the leafy parts of collard greens, turnip greens, and kale are richer in vitamin A than the stems or mid-ribs; and the oft-discarded cabbage core is loaded with vitamin C. Parsley is much more than just a garnish; it is flavorful, rich in vitamins A and C, and freezes well.

Roughly two-thirds of the water-soluble nutrients in canned vegetables are contained

Table 41.1. Pantry and Refrigerator Storage

Food	Recommended Storage Time	Handling Hints
STAPLES		
Baking powder	1 year	Keep dry and very tightly covered.
Baking soda	2 years +	Keep dry and covered.
Bouillon cubes	1 year	Keep dry and tightly covered.
Bread	5 days	Refrigerate in hot weather.
Bread crumbs, dried	6 months	Keep dry and covered.
CANNED FOODS		
Unopened canned goods	1 year	Keep cool and dry.
DRIED FOODS		
Fruits	1 year	
Cereals		
ready-to-eat, unopened	6–12 months or expiration date	
ready-to-eat, opened	2–3 months	Refold package liner tightly after opening.
cereal to be cooked	6 months	Keep dry and tightly closed.
Cornmeal	12 months	Keep tightly closed.
Cornstarch	18 months	Keep tightly closed.
Flour		
white	2 years +	Keep in airtight container
whole-wheat	6–8 months	Keep refrigerated. Store in moisture-proof airtight container.
Gelatin, all types	18 months	Keep in original container.
Grits	12 months	Keep in covered, airtight container.
Honey	12 months	If crystals form, warm jar in pan of hot water.
Jams, jellies	12 months	Refrigerate after opening.
Milk, dry		
nonfat, unopened	12 months	
nonfat, opened	6 months	Keep in airtight container.
Pasta	2 years +	
Rice		
white	2 years +	Keep tightly closed.
brown or rice mixes	4–6 months	Keep tightly closed.
Salad dressings		
bottled, unopened	10–12 months	
bottled, opened	3 months	Refrigerate after opening.
made from mix	2 weeks	Refrigerate prepared dressing.

in the vegetables themselves; the remaining nutrients have dissolved into the vegetable liquid, which should always be used. Commercially canned vegetables should be thoroughly warmed, not recooked. Home-canned vegetables with low-acid content, however, should be boiled for ten minutes, in order to destroy any microorganisms that may be present.

Vegetables should not be chopped, peeled, shelled, or, as with lettuce, torn up until they are ready to be cooked. Bruised vegetables rapidly lose vitamins A and C; the more surfaces that are exposed to the air, the more nutritional value is lost. If possible, fruit and vegetables should be cooked whole, or at least in large pieces.

Vegetables are usually prepared with moist heat or a variety of frying techniques. Steaming and stir-frying are the cooking techniques of choice for the nutrition-conscious consumer, because they are least damaging to

Table 41.1. Pantry and Refrigerator Storage *(cont.)*

Food	Recommended Storage Time	Handling Hints
DRIED FOODS		
Salad oils		
unopened	6 months	
opened	3 months	Refrigerate large quantities for longer storage.
Shortenings, solid	8 months	Do not refrigerate.
Sugar		
white	2 years +	Cover tightly.
brown	6 months	Refrigerate in airtight container.
Syrups	12 months	Refrigerate after opening.
Vinegar	2 years +	
SPICES, HERBS, CONDIMENTS		
Catsup, chili sauce		
unopened	12 months	
opened	6 months	Refrigerate after opening.
Mustard, prepared		
unopened	2 years	
opened	6–8 months	Refrigerate after opening.
Spices and herbs	6–12 months	Keep in airtight containers away from light and heat.
OTHERS		
Nuts in shell	6 months	Refrigerate after opening. Freeze for longer storage. Unsalted and blanched nuts keep longer than salted.
Peanut butter	6–9 months	
Peas and beans, dried	12 months	Keep in airtight container in cool, dry place.
Vegetables, fresh		Store in ventilated containers
onions	6–7 months	—in cool, dry, dark place.
potatoes, white	4–9 months	—in cool, moist, dark place.
MEAT, POULTRY, FISH, EGGS		
Meats		
beef, lamb, pork, and veal roasts, chops, steaks	3–5 days	All meat, poultry, and fish, when bought in plastic wrapping (from self-service counters) should be stored in original packages.
ground meat, stew meat	1–2 days	
variety meats (liver, heart, etc.)	1–2 days	At home, poke a small hole in the wrapper of prepackaged, uncured meats to allow air circulation.

vitamin content. Boiling, poaching, and stewing vegetables cause water-soluble vitamins and minerals—particularly vitamins B and C, potassium, and iron—to leach into the cooking liquid. If vegetables must be boiled, the water should be brought to a boil before adding the vegetables; a tight lid reduces the amount of water that is needed. As little water and as short a cooking time as possible is best. Nutritional loss can be further minimized by using the vegetable cooking liquid in another dish. Waterless cooking, in which vegetables are cooked slowly in their own juices and the small amount of water that remains on them

Table 41.1.   Pantry and Refrigerator Storage *(cont.)*

Food	Recommended Storage Time	Handling Hints
MEAT, POULTRY, FISH, EGGS		
Poultry		
chicken, duck, turkey	1–2 days	
Fish	1 day	
Cured and smoked meats		
hard sausage	2 weeks	
frankfurters, hot dogs	1 week	
hams, whole	1 week	
hams, canned, unopened	6–12 months	Check label: most require refrigeration.
luncheon meats	3 days	Keep tightly wrapped.
Eggs		
in shell	1–2 weeks	Time limit for best quality; safe longer. Store covered. Keep small ends down to center yolks.
DAIRY PRODUCTS		
Butter, margarine	2 weeks	Freeze for longer storage.
Cheese		
cottage	7–10 days	Keep all cheese tightly wrapped. If mold forms, discard entire package.
cream	10–14 days	
natural, hard	1–3 weeks	
processed	5 weeks	
Cream		
fresh	1 week	Check pull date for keeping time unopened.
sour	1 week	
Milk	1 week	Check for signs of spoilage: cream and milk will start to smell; yogurt begins to separate.
Yogurt	3 weeks	
OTHER		
Opened canned foods	3 days	After a few days, transfer to glass, ceramic, or plastic container to avoid metallic taste. Keep covered.
tomato-based	5 days	
Fresh or reconstituted juices	1 week	Keep covered.
Leftover gravy and broth	1–2 days	Keep covered.
Mayonnaise	3 months	Refrigerate after opening; keep covered.
Nuts, unshelled	6 months	Freeze for longer storage.

Reprinted with permission from the Division of Agriculture and Natural Resources, State of California, Sacramento, California.

from being washed, does not conserve nutrients any better than quick cooking in the small amount of water needed to prevent scorching.

Generally, the most nutritious vegetables are those that are cooked the least. Vegetables should be tender but retain an edge of crispness; soggy or mushy vegetables may have had most of the vitamins and minerals cooked out. Although baking soda (sodium bicarbonate) gives green vegetables a bright, fresh color, it destroys a significant amount of their vitamin C and thiamine.

When cooked, vegetables should be served as quickly as possible. Nutrients are lost when vegetables are left too long at room temperature. If a meal is delayed, vegetable dishes should be covered and refrigerated.

Other Foods

Soaking or rinsing certain foods can cause nutrient loss. For example, when dried peas and beans are soaked overnight, vitamins leach out into the water. It is better to boil them in water for two minutes, then allow them to stand for an hour before continuing with the recipe. Similarly, rinsing rice or pasta before cooking washes away many of the valuable B vitamins and minerals that cling to their surfaces. The amount of water required

---

Table 41.2. Timetable for Broiling Meats, Poultry, and Fish

Item and Cut	Thickness	Distance from Heat*	Approximate Broiling Time
	INCHES	INCHES	MINUTES
Beef:			
Patties, ground	1	2 to 3	15 to 25
Steaks: rib, club, T-bone,	1 to 1½	3 to 5	15 to 35
porterhouse, sirloin	1½ to 2	3 to 5	35 to 55
Lamb:			
Chops: loin, rib, shoulder	1 to 1½	3 to 5	12
	1½ to 2	3 to 5	22
Patties, ground	1	2 to 3	18
Pork:			
Chops: rib or loin	¾ to 1	2 to 3	30 to 35
Bacon, regular		2 to 3	4 to 5
Canadian bacon	¼ to ½	2 to 3	6 to 10
Cured ham slice	½ to 1	2 to 3	10 to 20
Poultry:			
Chicken, young: halves, quarters, and meaty pieces	Laid flat	About 5	35 to 50
Turkey, fryer-roaster pieces	Laid flat	About 5	60 to 75
Fish:			
Fillets and steaks		3	10 to 15
Pan-dressed		3	10 to 16
King crab legs		4	8 to 10
Spiny lobster tails		4	10 to 15

*Thicker cuts should be placed farther from the heat source than thin cuts. Frozen meat or fish should also be placed farther from the heat source to ensure doneness throughout each piece.

From the U.S. Department of Agriculture *Home Economics Research Report*, number 46.

to cook rice and other grains should always be measured. When excess cooking water is poured off, nutrients drain away, too.

Contrary to popular belief, it is more nutritious to eat the whole fresh fruit than to drink freshly squeezed fruit juices, because the nutrients and fiber in fruit pulp are lost when they are squeezed.

COOKING TECHNIQUES

Roasting. Roasting thick cuts of meat and whole poultry at a constant moderate temperature (about 300 degrees F.) helps retain moisture and many of the nutrients. About one-third of the thiamine, biotin, and vitamin B_{12} is lost, but less than ten percent of the riboflavin and niacin. Roasted meat cooks most evenly when it is placed on a rack in a shallow pan so that heat penetrates all sides but the meat does not cook in its own drippings. Overcooking destroys thiamine, and salting during cooking dries the meat out. The pan drippings from roast meat are rich in the B vitamins; the fat should be skimmed off and the juices poured over the meat when it is served.

Baking. Baking is a dry-heat method, identical to roasting. However, by convention, the word *baking* is used for ham and fish dishes, soufflés, and bread and cakes, among others. Baking cereal products allows much of the thiamine to be retained. The surface in contact with heat should be limited as much as possible and bread baked only until the top is light brown. Bread baked in pans has a higher thiamine content than cookies baked on a sheet.

Broiling and grilling. Broiling, in a conventional gas or electric stove, and grilling, over an outdoor or indoor grill, is suitable for the thinner cuts of meat, poultry, and fish, for vegetables such as tomatoes and peppers, and even for some fruit. Cooking temperatures can be regulated by altering the distance between the food and the heat source. When meat is broiled, most of the riboflavin and between 60 and 80 percent of the thiamine is preserved.

Charcoal broiling burns up much of the fat on meat, but the smoke that is generated when the fat drips into the fire contains potent carcinogens. Although there is little concern about occasional charcoal broiling, any danger can be minimized by using only lean meats, placing meat on foil above the coals, and keeping the grill lid open to disperse the smoke. Charcoal smoke will also be reduced if meat is first partially baked or parboiled.

Braising. Braising is a moist-heat method particularly useful for cooking tougher cuts of meat and poultry, but it is also popular for vegetables. Food is either wrapped in foil or placed in a covered container, then cooked with a small amount of water, stock, or other appropriate liquid. A richer flavor can be obtained by browning meats before they are braised. Nonfat browning techniques include broiling meat briefly and pan-frying in nonstick pans. For crispness, braised poultry can be uncovered for a few minutes at the end of the cooking time.

Steaming. When food is steamed, it never touches the cooking water, making this process among the most nutritious cooking methods. Fish and vegetables are placed in a steamer basket, then over simmering water. Steaming is fast, fat-free, and causes minimal nutrient loss. For example, broccoli when boiled loses more than 60 percent of its vitamin C; when steamed, only 20 percent.

Stir-frying. Equally good for producing food low in fat and high in nutritional content is stir-frying, the traditional method of cooking Chinese food. Uniformly cut pieces of meat and vegetables are tossed quickly at high temperatures with very little oil.

Deep-fat frying. Food does not absorb a great amount of fat if the fat is first heated to a very high temperature and food is cooked rapidly. As heated fat decomposes, however, it forms acrolein, an irritating gas, believed by some to be carcinogenic. Deep-fat frying can also be expensive, particularly if the oil is discarded after one use, as is sometimes recommended.

Pressure cooking. Pressure cookers use steam under pressure to cut cooking times by half or more. Because food is cooked quickly and without much water, nutrients are preserved. Meats and one-pot dinners are well suited to this method of cooking, although it is important to time dishes accurately to avoid overcooking. Pressure cookers can be dangerous when used improperly, so consumers should always follow the manufacturer's instructions carefully.

Crock pots. This long, slow cooking method makes last-minute food preparation unnecessary but destroys many B vitamins. The nutrient-rich cooking liquid should be used.

Microwave ovens. Nearly 70 percent of American households now have microwave ovens. Not only do these appliances save cooking time, they reduce the need for fats and preserve the nutritional value of vegetables. They do have drawbacks, however. Nutrients are lost in the drippings from meat, and food is not always cooked evenly. To ensure that food is thoroughly cooked, some recipes require that it stands at room temperature, or is covered with foil to retain heat, for 10 to 15 minutes after it is removed from the oven. Meat should be pierced with a thermometer in several places to check for consistent temperature. Lower temperatures and periodic turning of the food also help to ensure that meat is thoroughly cooked. Bones should be removed before cooking, since they may shield part of the meat from the high-frequency electromagnetic waves.

Burns of the hands, lips, and mouth from microwave ovens are a growing problem. Although containers are not directly heated by microwaves, heat from the food inside them can make them very hot. Consumers can prevent their hands from being burned by using pot holders. Scald burns on the mouth and lips occur because microwaves do not heat food uniformly, especially liquids, with the result that hot and cold spots typically develop. Hot spots may be undetected, even if the food is tested first. (For this reason, baby bottles should never be heated in a microwave, nor should the oven be used for home canning.) Stirring food during and after cooking will help evenly distribute the heat. Heating pasteurized, homogenized milk for about two minutes at full power in a microwave oven extends its shelf life to three weeks (from the usual seven to ten days) and preserves protein, calcium, riboflavin, and vitamin A. Anyone who microwaves milk at home needs a temperature probe to be sure that the milk in all parts of the container has been heated to 160 degrees F. Microwaving food placed on paper towels or napkins should be avoided because recycled paper products contain chemicals that may promote cancer. Also, plastic wrap should not come in contact with the food because it may melt at high temperatures. (See Modifying a Recipe and Using Leftovers on pages 691 and 692.)

COOKWARE

There are many different kinds of cookware, each with different advantages and drawbacks. In general, the heavier the cookware, the more evenly heat is distributed and the less likelihood there is of burning. The following are advantages and disadvantages of different types of cookware.

Nonstick pots. Using nonstick pots and pans is an easy way to cut down on fat consumption. The heavier grades are the most durable. Only plastic, rubber, and wooden utensils should be used with nonstick pans because they will not scratch the surface.

Iron pots. The iron that leaches out from iron pots can add significantly to daily iron intakes, although the pots can also destroy some vitamins. Acidic foods, such as tomatoes, will be discolored if they are cooked in iron pots.

Copper. This metal conducts heat better than all others commonly used in the manufacture of cookware. Copper pots are lined—usually with tin—to prevent corrosion and food from absorbing copper. They should be retinned when the lining wears. But cooking in copper, even when lined, can destroy some important vitamins.

Glass. Riboflavin can break down when food is cooked in glass baking dishes. Cooking times may be reduced when using glass or pyrex in the oven.

Stainless steel. People with allergies to certain metals may be unable to use stainless steel, which is a blend of iron, chromium, and, sometimes, nickel.

Aluminum. The speculated link between Alzheimer's disease and the use of aluminum pots remains pure speculation, but aluminum should be avoided when cooking salty, acidic, and alkaline foods, because the metal may dissolve, discoloring food or giving it a strong odor.

FROZEN FOODS

Foods that have been frozen properly, wrapped correctly, and stored at the appropriate temperature are second only to fresh foods in nutritional value. In fact, since vitamins are lost rapidly at temperatures above freezing, frozen vegetables may well contain more nutrients than their fresh counterparts, if the latter have been held for several days in the supermarket and the home refrigerator. The freezing process itself does not significantly affect the vitamin content of vegetables. Some nutrients, however, may be lost in the preparatory steps—chopping and blanching, for example.

Freezers and refrigerator freezer units expand a consumer's range of food options by providing a way to preserve food at its seasonal peak, save leftovers, take advantage of food sales, and prepare meals well before they will be eaten. To minimize nutritional loss and curb the growth of bacteria, frozen foods should be stored at temperatures at or below 0 degrees F., which is easy to do in a freezer or in a refrigerator-freezer with a separate outside door. Freezer compartments inside refrigerators cannot usually be kept much below 15 degrees F., without freezing the food inside the refrigerator, as well. Foods stored at that temperature quickly lose vitamins and should not be kept longer than a few days.

Freezing preserves food quality and halts the growth of microorganisms, but it does not improve food or kill bacteria, although it does prevent them from multiplying. Materials used for packaging frozen food should be moisture- and vapor-proof, greaseless, and odorless. Heavy aluminum foil, plastic containers with tight-fitting lids, muffin tins, milk cartons, freezer bags or freezer paper are all fine; however, aluminum foil should not come in direct contact with acidic foods, such as tomatoes and fruit juices. Microwave trays

Modifying a Recipe

Many recipes call for large amounts of fat, sugar, and salt. Modifying a recipe to retain flavor while improving nutritional value requires an understanding of three basic principles: elimination, reduction, and substitution. Lighter, healthier dishes can be created by learning which ingredients can be dropped altogether, how to cut back on the use of certain foods, and when to substitute one product for a more nutritious one. The following are tips on modifying recipes.

- To reduce fats, reduce the amount by at least one-third. If there is no discernible loss in flavor, the dish can be made with even less fat. If a casserole isn't moist enough, broth, wine, or vegetable juice can be added.

- Instead of butter or margarine, a vegetable spray can be used to coat pans.

- Low-fat dairy products can almost always substitute for richer ones. Low-fat yogurt, or low-fat cottage cheese blended with yogurt or skim milk, works well in lieu of sour cream. A little flour or cornstarch can be stirred into the yogurt to avoid a watery texture when heated. Skim or low-fat milk can replace whole milk, and evaporated skim milk is a good substitute for cream.

- Onions and mushrooms can be cooked in a little broth rather than sautéed in butter.

- When making sauces, blend cold milk or juice instead of fat with flour to make a smooth paste.

- Skim fat from soup stock, stews, and casseroles by chilling a dish to allow the fat to harden and then removing it with a spoon.

- Whip potatoes with skim milk or the water in which the potatoes are cooked instead of butter.

- There are numerous low-fat, water-whipped margarine, mayonnaise, and salad-dressing products on the market today that can be substituted for the traditional product in casserole, grain, and vegetable dishes. Note that because these products have a substantial water content, they may not react to heat in the same way as the originals. They may not be flavorful enough to be appropriate substitutes for baked goods.

- Marinate food in lemon or lime juice, wine, broth, tomato juice, or low-fat yogurt instead of oil.

- Use pureed vegetables and low-fat dry milk to thicken soups instead of cream. Use pureed vegetables instead of cream-based sauces on fish, pasta, and poultry.

- Two or more egg whites can often be substituted for one whole egg.

- Salt can be eliminated from any recipe except baked goods made with yeast, in which it is necessary to control the rising of the dough.

- Substitute herbs and spices, lemon juice, garlic, and onions for salt. Salt is an acquired taste from which most people need to be weaned gradually; zesty flavor substitutes make it easier.

- Salty foods, such as sauerkraut, capers, and corned beef, can be soaked in cold water for at least 15 minutes before cooking or eating; if the food is extremely salty, the water can be changed several times. This desalting method results in some loss of flavor, but is important for those concerned about salt intake.

- Sugar can be reduced by one-third in most recipes without loss of flavor.

- Flavor extracts (such as vanilla or almond), spices (including cinnamon and nutmeg), or sweet fruits (such as pears and bananas), can be substituted for some of the sugar in a recipe.

- Fresh fruit or preserves should be added to yogurt instead of using the presweetened product.

and aluminum containers from store-bought frozen foods may also be reusable (check the label). The smaller a container, the more quickly—and more safely—food will freeze and thaw. Since ordinary glass can become dangerously brittle in the freezer, specially tempered glass freezer jars should be used instead.

Air should be excluded as far as possible to reduce oxidation and loss of nutrients, flavor, and color. Containers of solid food should be filled to the top; containers of liquids should be filled to within half an inch of the top, to allow for expansion when frozen; flexible wrappings should be shaped and squeezed to drive out air. Food that is not tightly wrapped may suffer freezer burn— white dried-out patches on the surface and an off flavor, the result of moisture loss. All packages should be sealed with freezer tape, with date and contents clearly labeled with a felt pen or wax pencil.

Since foods should be frozen as rapidly as possible, it is important not to add too much to the freezer at any one time, because it can strain the motor. The addition of three or four pounds of food per cubic foot of freezer space allows for quick freezing, which should be completed in 2 to a maximum of 24 hours, depending on the size of the package and the density of the food. Once frozen solidly, the packages should be arranged compactly, while allowing for circulation of air.

What to Freeze

Uncooked meats, poultry, fish, soup stocks, and prepared and precooked dishes are common freezer items. Hard cheese, milk,

Using Leftovers

- Do not cool leftover dishes at room temperature, because bacteria grow rapidly in warm food. Instead, transfer food into shallow containers, cover them tightly, label, date, and refrigerate immediately.

- Use refrigerated leftovers within two to four days and thoroughly reheat before use. Any food that is questionable in smell or appearance should be discarded.

- Reheat leftovers in a microwave oven to retain most of their vitamins, color, texture, and flavor. Vitamin loss can also be minimized by reheating food in a double boiler. Wrap large pieces of meat in foil and reheat in the oven at 350 degrees F.

- Simmer leftover meat, poultry, or fish bones for a stock rich in calcium and B vitamins; enrich with celery leaves, parsley stems, and other vegetable scraps. Stock adds flavor and nutrients to rice, soup, stew, or sauce and can be frozen in ice-cube trays for later use.

- Always remove leftover stuffing from poultry and refrigerate separately.

- Cracked eggs should be used only when they are cooked thoroughly to kill bacteria. In fact, it is a good idea always to cook eggs thoroughly. Cool cooked eggs quickly, then use immediately or refrigerate.

- Egg-based or creamed dishes should be refrigerated immediately after cooking and consumed within a few days. Any food containing raw eggs should be eaten on the same day or discarded.

- Overripe bananas and other fruits can be added to pancake batter, breads, cakes, plain yogurt, milk shakes, blender drinks, or to a sauce for ice cream.

- The liquid from canned or cooked fruits and vegetables is rich in leached nutrients and can be used in desserts, soups, stews, chowders, and casseroles.

whipped-cream rosettes, butter, margarine, egg whites and yolks, chopped herbs and onions, many fruits and vegetables, nuts, dried fruit, bread crumbs, cooked grains, pastry shells, cookies, and wine also freeze well. Breads can be frozen sliced or unsliced.

The packaged meats and poultry purchased at the supermarket are seldom wrapped adequately for safe freezer storage. Meats need to be repacked in a moisture- or vapor-resistant material and then wrapped tightly to keep out air. They can be frozen in meal-size portions—a quarter-pound of boned meat or a half-pound of meat with bones per person is average—or cut into suitable sizes for cooking dishes such as stews. When bones are frozen, they should be wrapped carefully so that holes are not poked through the wrappings.

Fresh produce should be frozen as soon as possible after being harvested, to prevent loss of vitamins and the growth of bacteria. Vegetables should be blanched (cooked briefly in boiling water, then plunged into cold water) to destroy enzymes that alter color, texture, and flavor. Fresh berries and some firm-textured fruits can be frozen on a cookie sheet, then transferred to a closed container. Fruits that tend to oxidize and discolor, such as apples and pears, should be sprinkled with lemon juice and ascorbic-acid powder, or frozen in a syrup to which ascorbic acid has been added.

Eggshells crack in the freezer, but raw egg whites and yolks can be beaten together and frozen. Egg yolks freeze poorly unless they are mixed with corn syrup, sugar, or salt; egg whites can be frozen alone.

Foods that don't do well in the freezer include the following.

- Foods with a high water content, such as salad greens, cucumbers, watermelon, celery, cantaloupe, and to-matoes, radishes, and potatoes; they become mushy when frozen.

- Certain dairy products, including cream-based sauces, heavy cream, and soft cheese, which lose texture.

- Sour cream and yogurt, which tend to separate when they are defrosted.

- Mayonnaise, salad dressing, and any product in which these are used; baked goods made with egg whites, custard, meringue, and cake batter; jellies and jams; products with gelatin; luncheon meats.

- Hard-boiled eggs, which become tough when frozen.

- Fried foods, which become soggy when reheated.

Home-Cooked Foods

A nutritious, economical, and timesaving use of the freezer is to stock it with home-cooked dishes. Some small changes to the recipe may be necessary. Dishes to be frozen should be slightly undercooked so that they will remain crisp when reheated. Some spices intensify in flavor or become bitter after they have been frozen, so it is best to season lightly and correct after reheating. Flour-based sauces tend to separate when frozen, so it may be best to use arrowroot or cornstarch.

Dinners that will be reheated in a microwave oven should be stored in containers that can be popped directly into the oven. Metal containers or aluminum foil cannot be used.

The Freezer Timetable

Food will not keep indefinitely, even at the coldest temperatures. Commercially packaged foods are generally flash frozen or packaged with preservatives so they last longer in the freezer than home-prepared foods do. The accompanying guide shows how long food can be frozen without appreciable loss of quality and nutrients. (See Table 41.3 for a guide to storing food at 0 degrees F., or below.)

Thawing

Many experts believe that nutrients are lost in the juices that drip from frozen meats, fish, and poultry as they thaw, so they are best cooked without thawing if sufficient time is available. Other studies, however, have found that the quality of the meat is not substantially affected if it is thawed before cooking.

Frozen roasts, steaks, and chops take about 150 percent longer to cook than unfrozen cuts of the same weight and shape; whole frozen poultry needs about 125 percent of normal cooking time. Individual servings of frozen fish need twice the cooking time of fresh or thawed pieces.

A microwave oven can be used to quickly defrost meats that must be thawed in advance. If meat is thawed in the refrigerator, it should be timed to be ready just before cooking. The following is a list of thawing times needed for different meats and fish.

Table 41.3. Cold Storage of Meat and Poultry

Product	Refrigerator (Days at 40°F)	Freezer (Months at 0°F)	Product	Refrigerator (Days at 40°F)	Freezer (Months at 0°F)
FRESH MEATS			**PROCESSED MEATS** *(cont.)*		
Roasts (beef)	3 to 5	6 to 12	Ham (slices)	3 to 4	1 to 2
Roasts (lamb)	3 to 5	6 to 9	Luncheon meats	3 to 5*	1 to 2
Roasts, (pork, veal)	3 to 5	4 to 8	Sausage (smoked)	7	1 to 2
Steaks (beef)	3 to 5	6 to 12	Sausage (dry, semi-dry)	14 to 21	1 to 2
Chops (lamb)	3 to 5	6 to 9	**FRESH POULTRY**		
Chops (pork)	3 to 5	3 to 4	Chicken and turkey (whole)	1 to 2	12
Hamburger, ground and stew meats	1 to 2	3 to 4	Chicken pieces	1 to 2	9
Variety meats (tongue, brain, kidneys, liver, and heart)	1 to 2	3 to 4	Turkey pieces	1 to 2	6
			Duck and goose (whole)	1 to 2	6
Sausage (pork)	1 to 2	1 to 2	Giblets	1 to 2	3 to 4
COOKED MEATS			**COOKED POULTRY**		
Cooked meat and meat dishes	3 to 4	2 to 3	Covered with broth, gravy	1 to 2	6
Gravy and meat broth	1 to 2	2 to 3	Pieces not in broth or gravy	3 to 4	1
PROCESSED MEATS (Frozen, cured meat loses quality rapidly and should be used as soon as possible.)			Cooked poultry dishes	3 to 4	4 to 6
			Fried chicken	3 to 4	4
Bacon	7	1	**GAME**		
Frankfurters	7*	1 to 2	Deer	3 to 5	6 to 12
Ham (whole)	7	1 to 2	Rabbit	1 to 2	12
Ham (half)	3 to 5	1 to 2	Duck and goose (whole, wild)	1 to 2	6

*Once a vacuum-sealed package is opened. Unopened vacuum-sealed packages can be stored in the refrigerator for 2 weeks.

Reprinted from *The Safe Food Book: Your Kitchen Guide*, U.S. Department of Agriculture, Food Safety and Inspection Service, October 1988.

- Small roasts (five pounds or less) take three to five hours per pound to thaw; larger roasts, four to seven hours.

- A one-pound fish takes one day to thaw.

- Poultry under four pounds will thaw in one-half to two-thirds of a day.

- Birds 4 to 12 pounds need one to two days to thaw.

- Birds 12 to 20 pounds need two to three days.

- Birds weighing more than 20 pounds should defrost for three or four days.

Allowing frozen dinners to thaw at room temperature invites bacterial growth. Cooked food can usually be reheated from the frozen state, or allowed to defrost overnight in the refrigerator. Commercially prepared foods are usually cooked without thawing, but the package instructions should be followed. Frozen fruits and vegetables should be cooked without thawing to minimize loss of nutrients.

When Is Refreezing Safe?

Food in a full freezer will remain thoroughly frozen for two days, if the power fails; a half-full freezer is safe for one day only. Dry ice (25 pounds for a ten-cubic-foot freezer) will hold a full freezer for an additional three or four days; a half-full one, for two or three. Some foods that have thawed can be refrozen without danger; others are more susceptible to bacterial growth and should be discarded unless they can be eaten immediately. (See Table 41.4.)

If wrapped food feels hard to the touch or its ice crystals are still intact, it can usually be safely refrozen. Many foods that have reached refrigerator temperature (40 degrees F.) can be put back in the freezer, but there are exceptions: fish and seafood; precooked meals that contain fish, meat, or poultry; organ meats; ice cream and any dishes that contain cream; and garden vegetables. These should be cooked and served immediately, or discarded. Most foods that have warmed to room temperature should be discarded or consumed immediately, although grains, beans, herbs, and spices often can be refrozen. If there is a hint of odor or discoloration, the food should be discarded.

FOOD POISONING

Well over 2 million cases of bacterial food poisoning are reported every year. Although foods may be contaminated while being processed, transported, and displayed for sale in food markets, most cases of bacterial food poisoning can be traced to careless handling and preparation at home (20 percent) and in restaurants, cafeterias, and other food-service establishments (77 percent). (See Foods to Go on page 699.) Among the bacteria most commonly implicated are *Salmonella, Staphylococcus aureus, Clostridium botulinum,* and *Clostridium perfringens,* but there are many others that may cause both isolated cases and near-epidemics of poisoning. Food poisoning is rarely fatal but can be extremely debilitating, especially for those who are also the most vulnerable: young children, the elderly, and the chronically ill. Foods should never be tasted if food poisoning is suspected.

The foods most often found to be contaminated are those of animal origin: meat, poultry, fish, shellfish, and raw (unpasteurized) milk. Special precautions should be taken when handling these foods. Although the bacteria present in raw meat and

Table 41.4. Frozen Food—When to Save and When to Throw It Out

	Still contains ice crystals and feels as cold as if refrigerated	Thawed. Held above 40°F for over 2 hours
MEAT, POULTRY, SEAFOOD		
Beef, veal, lamb, pork and ground meats	Refreeze	Discard
Poultry and ground poultry	Refreeze	Discard
Variety meats (liver, kidney, heart, chitterlings)	Refreeze	Discard
Casseroles, stews, soups, convenience foods, pizza	Refreeze	Discard
Fish, shellfish, breaded seafood products	Refreeze. However there will be some texture and flavor loss.	Discard
DAIRY		
Milk	Refreeze. May lose some texture.	Discard
Eggs (out of shell) and egg products	Refreeze	Discard
Ice cream, frozen yogurt	Discard	Discard
Cheese (soft and semisoft), cream cheese, ricotta	Refreeze. May lose some texture.	Discard
Hard cheeses (cheddar, Swiss, Parmesan)	Refreeze	Refreeze
Casseroles containing milk, cream, eggs, soft cheeses	Refreeze	Discard
Cheesecake	Refreeze	Discard
FRUITS		
Juices	Refreeze	Refreeze. Discard if mold, yeasty smell or sliminess develops.
Home or commercially packaged	Refreeze. Will change in texture and flavor.	Refreeze. Discard if mold, yeasty smell or sliminess develops.
VEGETABLES		
Juices	Refreeze	Discard after held above 40°F for 6 hours.
Home or commercially packaged or blanched	Refreeze. May suffer texture and flavor loss.	Discard after held above 40°F for 6 hours.
BREADS, PASTRIES		
Breads, rolls, muffins, cakes (without custard fillings)	Refreeze	Refreeze
Cakes, pies, pastries with custard or cheese filling	Refreeze	Discard
Pie crusts	Refreeze	Refreeze
Commercial and homemade bread dough	Refreeze. Some quality loss may occur.	Refreeze. Considerable quality loss.
OTHER		
Casseroles—pasta, rice based	Refreeze	Discard
Flour, cornmeal, nuts	Refreeze	Refreeze
	Food still cold, held at 40°F or above under 2 hours	**Held above 40°F for over 2 hours**
DAIRY		
Milk, cream, sour cream, buttermilk, evaporated milk, yogurt	Safe	Discard
Butter, margarine	Safe	Safe
Baby formula, opened	Safe	Discard
EGGS		
Eggs, fresh	Safe	Discard
Hard-cooked in shell	Safe	Discard
Egg dishes	Safe	Discard
Custards and puddings	Safe	Discard

Table 41.4. Frozen Food—When to Save and When to Throw It Out *(cont.)*

	Food still cold held at 40°F or above under 2 hours	Held above 40°F for over 2 hours
CHEESE		
Hard cheeses, processed cheeses	Safe	Safe
Soft cheeses, cottage cheese	Safe	Discard
FRUITS		
Fruit juices, opened	Safe	Safe
Canned fruits, opened	Safe	Safe
Fresh fruits, coconut, raisins, dried fruits, candied fruits, dates	Safe	Safe
VEGETABLES		
Vegetables, cooked	Safe	Discard after 6 hours
Vegetable juice, opened	Safe	Discard after 6 hours
Baked potatoes	Safe	Discard
Fresh mushrooms, herbs and spices	Safe	Safe
Garlic, chopped in oil or butter	Safe	Discard
Casseroles, soups, stews	Safe	Discard
MEAT, POULTRY, SEAFOOD		
Fresh or leftover meat, poultry, fish or seafood	Safe	Discard
Thawing meat or poultry	Safe	Discard if warmer than refrigerator temperatures
Meat, tuna, shrimp, chicken, egg salad	Safe	Discard
Gravy, stuffing	Safe	Discard
Lunch meats, hot dogs, bacon, sausage, dried beef	Safe	Discard
Pizza—meat topped	Safe	Discard
Canned meats (*not* labeled "Keep Refrigerated") but refrigerated after opening	Safe	Discard
Canned hams labeled "Keep Refrigerated"	Safe	Discard
PIES, PASTRY		
Pastries, cream filled	Safe	Discard
Pies—custard, cheese filled or chiffons	Safe	Discard
Pies, fruit	Safe	Safe
BREAD, CAKES, COOKIES, PASTA		
Bread, rolls, cakes, muffins, quick breads	Safe	Safe
Refrigerator biscuits, rolls, cookie dough	Safe	Discard
Cooked pasta, spaghetti	Safe	Discard
Pasta salads with mayonnaise or vinegar base	Safe	Discard
SAUCES, SPREADS, JAMS		
Mayonnaise, tartar sauce, horseradish	Safe	Discard if above 50°F for over 8 hours
Peanut butter	Safe	Safe
Opened salad dressing, jelly, relish, taco and barbeque sauce, mustard, catsup, olives	Safe	Safe

Reprinted from *Food News for Consumers,* Summer 1989, U.S. Department of Agriculture, Food Safety and Inspection Service.

poultry will be killed at the high temperatures reached by most cooking methods, they can easily spread to other foods via utensils and chopping blocks. Hands, countertops, and utensils should be washed in hot soapy water between each step in food preparation. Dishcloths, which can harbor bacteria, should be washed regularly; sponges should be rinsed thoroughly with hot water.

As emphasized above, foods should never be left for more than two hours at temperatures between 45 and 140 degrees F., because bacteria multiply rapidly in such conditions. If food is not to be eaten right after it is cooked, it should be refrigerated or frozen. Food that is discolored or malodorous and containers that are damaged or disfigured should be discarded immediately. Suspicious foods should never be tasted and, when possible, not even sniffed.

Salmonella

The numerous strains of the toxic Salmonella microorganism are responsible for more incidents of food poisoning than any other bacteria. Raw or undercooked meats, poultry, poultry stuffing, unrefrigerated or cracked eggs, dairy products left at room temperature, unpasteurized milk, and fish and shellfish taken from contaminated waters may contain the Salmonella bacteria. The bacteria are also present in human and animal feces and can spread easily from food handlers who are healthy carriers.

The flavor, odor, and taste of food give no hint of contamination, but usually within 24 hours after being ingested, Salmonella bacteria multiply rapidly in the intestines, causing headaches, abdominal discomfort, diarrhea, chills, and sometimes vomiting. Severe cases of salmonella poisoning may cause dehydration. The illness usually lasts two to four days, although young children, the elderly, and the infirm can be much more seriously ill.

Improper cooking and food storage and poor hygienic standards among those who handle foodstuffs are the most common causes for the spread of microorganisms. Salmonella bacteria thrive in temperatures between 44 and 115 degrees F.; they cannot live in temperatures above 140 degrees F. longer than ten minutes. Therefore, cooking foods thoroughly, not letting them sit at room temperature, and storing them properly in the refrigerator are three important ways to prevent salmonella poisoning. Thorough washing of hands and dishes also helps reduce the risk.

To avoid the possibility of cross-contamination, raw foods should always be kept away from other foods. Starchy foods and dairy products are especially vulnerable to cross-contamination. Special care should be taken when handling poultry and stuffing, pork, roast beef, and hamburger.

To help prevent the spread of salmonella, the following should be observed.

- Hands, countertops, cutting boards, and all cooking utensils should be washed with hot soapy water between each step of the preparation of chicken and other foods, and after completing preparation.

- Chicken should always be cooked until its internal temperature reaches 180 degrees F., or until the juices run clear when the thickest part of the inner thigh is probed with a fork. If blood is still dripping from a chicken, it has not been heated enough to kill the bacteria.

- To avoid recontamination, cooked meat should never be returned to the unwashed plate or chopping board where it was prepared in its raw state.

- Poultry, meat, and stuffing should be served quickly after being cooked, and refrigerated soon afterward.

- Ready-to-eat food should be stored apart from raw foods in the refrigerator.

Staphylococcus aureus

Staphylococcus bacteria occur naturally on the skin and in the nasal passages of humans and animals, particularly in wounds and skin eruptions. The organism may also be expelled into the air while breathing, talking, coughing, and sneezing, and it is frequently passed along by food handlers. *Staphylococcus* bacteria are killed when subjected to temperatures above 140 degrees F. for ten minutes. However, if they are permitted to multiply in food left at room temperature, they produce enterotoxins that are highly resistant to heat, freezing, and chemicals.

Staphylococcus bacteria toxins can be found in meats, poultry, cheese and egg prod-

Foods to Go

To keep a day's picnic as safe as it is enjoyable, these safety precautions should be followed.

- A lunch box should be washed after every use to prevent bacterial growth. Only clean paper bags that have not been used to carry other foods should be used as lunch bags.

- A prepared lunch should be refrigerated until it is time to leave for work or school in the morning, and, if possible, refrigerated again at the job or classroom site.

- Sandwiches can be frozen overnight; they will be ready to eat by noon. Sandwiches should be made with coarse bread; fillings that freeze poorly, such as egg salad, should be avoided. Those that freeze well, such as chicken and tuna-fish salads, are good choices.

- A clean thermos bottle will preserve hot liquids and semiliquid foods for several hours if the seal is tight. Pouring boiling water into the thermos just before use lengthens the time hot foods can be safely stored. Conversely, a thermos should be rinsed with cold water if it is to be used for milk or juice.

- Contrary to myth, commercial mayonnaise is not a common cause of food poisoning. Mayonnaise usually contains lemon juice, or another acidic flavoring, and salt, which actually impede bacterial growth. Homemade mayonnaise, if prepared without lemon juice or vinegar, can be risky.

- On a picnic, perishable food—especially meats, prepared salads, eggs, and milk products—should be kept in a well-insulated, ice-packed cooler. Cold canned drinks can also be used to help cool food. The cooler should be kept in the shade and opened as rarely as possible.

- Although keeping clean is harder outside, it is important to wash up before preparing food—especially between handling raw meat or poultry and handling other foods. Disposable Handi-Wipes may be useful.

- Insulating a heated casserole dish will help to keep food safe and warm. The dish should be wrapped first in aluminum foil, then newspapers, and then a towel.

- It is seldom wise to drink stream or river water, which may be heavily contaminated. Water can be boiled for 20 minutes, then allowed to stand for one-half hour to allow foreign matter to settle; water can also be treated with commercial purification tablets. For short trips, it is easier to carry bottled water—about one gallon per day per person.

ucts, sandwich spreads, coleslaw, dairy products, starchy salads, custards, and cream-filled desserts that have been improperly refrigerated. No change in the odor, taste, or appearance of food is discernible. The symptoms of food poisoning—sudden and violent nausea, vomiting, diarrhea, abdominal cramps, and prostration—occur within two to four hours of ingestion and last a day or two.

Adhering to the basic principles of cooking and storing foods will help prevent a staph infection.

Clostridium perfringens

These bacteria grow in anaerobic (reduced oxygen) conditions. They commonly inhabit the intestinal tracts of humans and other warm-blooded animals, and are therefore also found in soil and sewage. *Perfringens* bacteria are themselves toxic; they also produce heat-resistant spores that contaminate food left in the temperature danger zone. Meat, poultry, and other high-protein foods that are improperly cooked or stored, and foods kept for long periods on steam tables (which has given the bacteria the nickname "cafeteria germ"), are susceptible to the *perfringens* spores.

Symptoms—gas pain and diarrhea are common; vomiting and nausea occur only rarely—appear from 8 to 24 hours after eating contaminated foods and usually subside within 24 hours. The risk of *perfringens* contamination can be reduced with standard precautions, with particular attention given to poultry, gravy, stews, and casseroles. Dividing large quantities of cooked foods into smaller portions exposes more food to the air, discouraging the growth of the bacteria.

Clostridium botulinum

A very dangerous and sometimes fatal form of food poisoning, botulism is associated with contaminated canned foods. Botulism spores are widespread in the environment. However, they are inactive in the presence of oxygen, germinating mainly in anaerobic, low-acid conditions—as within sealed cans and containers of low-acid food. Commercially canned foods and vacuum-packed meats are seldom contaminated, nor are home-canned foods that are prepared properly.

Active botulism spores release a toxin that affects the nervous system, producing general weakness, headache, double vision, impaired speech, and difficulty in chewing, swallowing, and breathing. The symptoms usually occur in 18 to 36 hours but may take as long as eight days to develop. Unless a victim seeks immediate treatment, botulism can be fatal within three to seven days.

To prevent the virulent organism, meats and poultry, and low-acid vegetables such as string beans, corn, beets, and peas, which may have been contaminated by botulism in the soil, should be processed in a pressure cooker or canner for up to 75 minutes at 10 pounds of pressure in order to kill botulism spores. Containers of high-acid foods, such as tomatoes and acidic fruits, should be processed in a boiling-water bath according to canning instructions in a reliable cookbook. As a precaution, all home-canned foods should be boiled before serving—10 minutes for high-acid foods and 20 minutes for low-acid ones. Consumers should avoid eating from cans that leak, bulge, or spurt liquid upon opening. Health authorities should be notified if there is a reason to suspect botulism, especially if the source appears to be a commercial product or a meal eaten in a restaurant.

Trichinosis

Although it has become quite rare in this country, trichinosis is a very common and dangerous disease worldwide. The infection results from eating raw or undercooked pork or such pork products as liver, sausage (or, very rarely, bear meat) that contain the larvae of the *Trichinella* worms.

Fever and diarrhea may occur within a day or two of eating infected meat. More severe symptoms appear within 7 to 15 days, as the larvae mature into worms, mate, and discharge thousands of new larvae into the bloodstream. These larvae invade the skeletal muscles, causing pain and fever and occasionally grave respiratory problems.

Although relief is available for many of the symptoms of trichinosis, there is no known cure. However, *Trichinella* larvae cannot survive heat, and thus pork is safe to eat when its internal temperature reaches 160 degrees F. Pork and pork products should never be eaten when they are even slightly pink.

Paralytic Shellfish Poisoning

Periodically, marine microorganisms appear along the coast in such numbers as to color the water in a phenomenon known as red tide. Mussels, clams, scallops, and oysters may ingest this microorganism, which produces a toxin that survives cooking. The symptoms of poisoning, discernible within 30 minutes, are facial numbness, difficulty in breathing, muscle weakness, and sometimes partial paralysis. Shellfish taken from red-tide areas should never be consumed.

GLOSSARY

Acne. A condition in which the sebaceous (oil) glands become inflamed or blocked, or both. The predisposition is hereditary but the increase in androgens, male hormones present in both sexes that increase during adolescence, may promote it.

Acquired Immune Deficiency Syndrome (AIDS). A variably progressive viral disease transmitted by direct sexual contact and exposure to infected blood. The HIV virus attacks the immune system, leaving the patient vulnerable to certain cancers and "opportunistic" infections and disorders, including starvation due to an inability to absorb and utilize dietary nutrients.

Acrodermatitis enteropathica. A hereditary disorder. A defect in the absorption of zinc results in zinc deficiency.

Adipocytes. Fat cells.

Adrenocorticotrophic hormone (ACTH). A hormone that the pituitary gland releases to initiate the release of corticoids from the adrenal glands.

Affective disorders. Mood disorders with secondary disturbances in thinking and behavior; manic and depressive disorders.

Aflatoxin. A naturally occurring toxin produced by molds. Found mainly on peanuts, cottonseed, and corn.

Albumin. Any protein that is soluble in water and concentrated salt solutions, and that coagulates because of heat, found in almost all animal and in many vegetable tissues.

Aldosterone. A hormone that the adrenal cortex secretes. It regulates the kidneys' retention of sodium and secretion of potassium.

Allele. An alternative form of a gene that occupies corresponding sites on chromosomes.

Allergen. A foreign substance (i.e., not from your own body) that causes an allergic reaction.

Alopecia. Baldness.

Alzheimer's disease. A progressive form of presenile dementia, with deterioration of brain cells.

Amenorrhea. Failure to menstruate.

Amino acids. Organic (carbon-containing) acids containing one or more amino (NH_2) groups. The body links these acids together to make proteins. The diet must provide nine necessary amino acids, which are therefore called *essential* (meaning that it is essential that we eat them); the body manufactures the remaining eleven amino acids as needed.

Amniotic fluid. The fluid that surrounds the fetus in the uterus.

Amphetamines. Drugs that stimulate the central nervous system, often used as anticongestant inhalants, as well as for their ability to combat fatigue and suppress appetite, and (illegally) for their euphoric effects.

Anabolic steroids. Synthetic derivatives of testosterone, the male sex hormone that helps the body build muscle and synthesize proteins. Some athletes take them to enhance strength and improve performance, and anabolic steroids may do so, but while producing long-term damage to health and longevity.

Anaphylaxis. A severe and immediate hypersensitivity reaction that can result in death. The reaction is an extreme response to a repeat exposure to an antigen to which one is sensitive.

Anemia. A deficiency in the number or volume of red blood cells, or of hemoglobin.

Angina. Severe pain. Angina pectoris is the severe chest pain that occurs when the oxygen flow to the heart muscle is insufficient, usually the result of narrowing of the coronary arteries.

Anorexia nervosa. An eating disorder most common in adolescent and young women characterized by preoccupation with body image, self-induced starvation, and excessive exercising.

Antibodies. Proteins contained in blood and body fluids that are part of the body's immune response. Antibodies attach to invading organisms or foreign substances to help defend the body.

Antigens. A foreign substance that stimulates the body to produce an immune response.

Arrhythmia. An irregularity in the heartbeat.

Arteriosclerosis. A condition in which the walls of the arteries harden.

Arthritis. Inflammation of joints, a characteristic of over 100 disorders.

Aspartame. An artificial sweetener created by linking two amino acids, aspartic acid and phenylalanine, that is 200 times sweeter than sugar. It is widely found in soft drinks, cereal, gelatin, desserts, instant coffee, and tea and cocoa mixes.

Atherosclerosis. A form of arteriosclerosis in which, in addition to a hardening of the walls of the arteries, fatty deposits build up on the inner arterial walls and interfere with blood flow.

Attention-deficient hyperactivity disorder. A term applied to certain children with learning problems and impaired visual and spatial coordination. Its characteristics include excessive motor activity, inattentiveness, impulsiveness, impatience, poor tolerance for frustration, and distractibility. National Institute of Mental Health studies indicate that it rarely relates to dietary additives and never to sugar.

Azotemia. A buildup of urea and other nitrogen-containing waste products in the blood.

Barbiturates. Sedative-hypnotic drugs that are often prescribed as sleeping pills or tranquilizers because of their ability to reduce anxiety and induce sleep.

Basal metabolic rate (BMR). The energy required to carry on vital continuous processes such as circulation, respiration, thermogenesis, and other functions.

Beriberi. A disease caused by thiamine (vitamin B_1) deficiency.

Bilirubin. Bile pigment that can cause jaundice when normal bile excretion from liver to gut is blocked.

Biotin. A vitamin of the B complex group that is essential for many of the body's chemical processes, and for the metabolism of glucose and the formation of some fatty acids. All the biotin that we need is usually manufactured by our intestinal bacteria; it is also found in meats, poultry, fish, eggs, nuts, seeds, legumes, and some vegetables.

Blood plasma. Fluid part of the blood that contains specific proteins for clotting.

Blood platelets. Structures in the blood that are involved in blood clotting.

Blood pressure. The force or tension that the blood exerts against artery walls as it circulates. Systolic pressure reflects the maximum force (with the heart muscle contracted) and diastolic pressure reflects the minimum force (with the heart muscle relaxed).

Blood serum. Blood plasma from which the clotting agents have been removed.

Botulism. A dangerous and sometimes fatal form of food poisoning caused by the growth of *Clostridium botulinum* bacteria in anaerobic (without oxygen) conditions of low acidity such as in improperly canned vegetables and fruits. The toxin damages the nervous system, producing headache, weakness, double vision, impaired speech, and difficulty in chewing, swallowing, and breathing.

Bradycardia. A slowing of the heartbeat.

Bulimia. An eating disorder characterized by alternating episodes of gorging and then purging, usually by vomiting or abusing laxatives.

Cachexia. A wasting of the body. It occurs in people with tumors of the liver, pancreas, and digestive tract and widespread malignancies. It appears to be related to the body's release of tumor necrosis factor (TNF), also called cachectin.

Caffeine. A central nervous system stimulant that belongs to a group of drugs called methylxanthines, found in more than 60 species of plants, including coffee, tea, and cocoa plants.

Calcitonin. A hormone that the thyroid gland secretes. It blocks the action of the hormone parathormone, preventing the release of calcium from bone. It is used in the treatment of osteoporosis to prevent bone resorption.

Calcium. The most plentiful mineral in the human body, making up much of the bones and teeth, with some in the soft tissues and body fluids. It is necessary for proper nerve and muscle function, for blood clotting, and to activate enzymes necessary for the conversion of food to energy. Good sources include milk and milk products, sardines (particularly when eaten with the bones), oysters, green leafy vegetables, citrus fruits, tofu, and dried peas and beans.

Carbohydrates. Organic molecules, composed primarily of carbon, hydrogen, and oxygen atoms, that provide energy for the brain, central nervous system, and muscle cells. They are divided into three groups: monosaccharides, disaccharides, and polysaccharides. See separate headings.

Caries. Decay of the teeth and bone.

Carotene. A group of pigments, one of which, beta carotene, is a precursor of vitamin A and is found mostly in sweet potatoes, carrots, leafy vegetables, egg yolk, milk, and body fat. The body can convert beta carotene into vitamin A. All carotenoids trap singlet oxygen; beta carotene represents only 10 percent of all plant carotenoids.

Catecholamine. A class of neurotransmitters (transmitters of nerve signals) that includes norepinephrine, epinephrine, and dopamine.

Celiac sprue. Diarrhea and poor food absorption due to an intolerance to gluten, a protein found in wheat, rye, oats, and barley. Also called "gluten-induced enteropathy."

Chlorine. A nonmetallic element (halogen) that is a necessary part of body cells and fluids, and also a component of hydrochloric acid, an acid found in gastric juice and important in digestion. Good dietary sources include salt, processed foods, milk, and salt water.

Cholesterol. A fatty substance that is a major component of all cell membranes and myelin. From it our cells make adrenal and sex hormones, bile acids, and vitamin D in the skin (with the aid of sunlight). The body produces and stores it mainly in the liver. It is also found in foods from animal sources (egg yolks, meat, milk, etc.). It is essential for life in moderate amounts; harmful in excess.

Chromium. A trace mineral that becomes a part of the body's "glucose tolerance factor," which works with insulin for proper glucose metabolism. Good sources include whole-grain breads and cereals, brewer's yeast, beer, and peanuts.

Cirrhosis. A disease of the liver characterized by extensive scarring and inflammation. It can result in progressive destruction of the tissues of the organ. The term also has a largely obsolete use to describe scarring in any organ.

Cleft palate. A groove in the mouth that results from a congenital defect in the development of the mouth in the womb, as a result of which the bones of the palate do not fuse.

Closed date. A production code which manufacturers stamp on a food product to assure quality and monitor distribution.

Cobalamin (vitamin B_{12}). One of the B complex vitamins necessary for normal DNA and fatty acid synthesis, the formation of blood cells, and proper nerve function. Good sources include almost any animal product (dairy products, eggs, meats, fish), but no plant products.

Cocaine. A highly addictive, toxic alkaloid derived from the leaves of the coca plant that has narcotic and euphoric effects.

Collagen. Connective tissue that helps hold cells together.

Colostomy. A surgical procedure in which a pathway for wastes is made leading from the colon through the wall of the abdomen.

Complementary proteins. Those protein-containing plant foods which alone are deficient in one or more of the essential amino acids, but when paired with a plant food deficient in a different essential amino acid, "complement" each other to provide a complete protein. (Example: beans and rice). See incomplete proteins.

Complete protein. A protein that contains all the essential amino acids in the appropriate proportions for human use. Found in single animal foods such as milk, cheese, meat, and fish, and can be constructed by appropriate combination of two or more complementary plant foods (such as beans and rice).

Copper. A trace mineral. It is necessary for the production of red blood cells, connective tissues, and nerve fibers, and is a component of several enzymes. Good dietary sources include chocolate, nuts, seafood, organ meats, dried peas and beans, prunes, raisins, and avocados.

Coronary thrombosis. A blood clot (thrombosis) blocking a coronary artery. A common cause of heart attack.

Cortisol. A hormone that the adrenal glands release. It helps increase the level and availability of glucose to provide energy for the muscles, brain, and heart.

Cretinism. A severe type of mental retardation caused by the lack of thyroid tissue or a severe deficiency in thyroid hormone in early infancy, usually resulting from dietary lack of iodine, which is a necessary part of thyroid hormone.

Crohn's disease. A condition in which areas of the intestine become inflamed and swollen. Regional enteritis. First described by Dr. B. B. Crohn and two other Mount Sinai physicians.

Cushing's syndrome. A disease characterized by overproduction of adrenal hormones.

Cystic fibrosis. A hereditary disorder of the mucus-producing glands in the pancreas, bronchi, intestines, and liver.

Cystitis. Inflammation of the bladder, which occurs more often in women than men.

Dandruff. A condition in which dead cells excessively flake off the skin of the scalp and sometimes from the nose, behind the ears, in the genital region, and under the arms. A form of seborrheic dermatitis.

Delirium tremens (DTs). A neuropsychiatric disorder due to acute withdrawal from prolonged abuse of alcohol. Symptoms include low-grade fever, hallucinations, confusion, nausea, and trembling of the hands.

Deoxyribonucleic acid (DNA). The basic genetic material ("genetic blueprint") of all human cells.

Dermis. The layer of skin beneath the epidermis.

Dermatitis. Inflammation of the skin.

Desirable weight. The weight range for height and body build associated with the lowest frequency of disease and death.

Dextrin. A soluble carbohydrate made by the hydrolysis of starch en route to becoming glucose.

Dextrose. Glucose produced from cornstarch that has been treated with heat and acids or enzymes.

Diabetes mellitus. Sugar in the urine, with excessive urination, due to too much sugar in the blood, caused either by an insufficiency of insulin or by a defect in the body's ability to utilize insulin.

Dietetic. A term on a food label indicating the product is appropriate for restricted diets, such as a low-sodium regimen, or that it is of low or reduced caloric content.

"Direct" food additives. Substances intentionally added to food to improve flavor, texture, or color, or to prevent spoilage.

Disaccharides. Simple carbohydrates (sugars) that are composed of two monosaccharide (sugar) units; this group includes maltose, sucrose, and lactose.

Diuretic. A substance that causes the body to excrete urine.

Diverticulosis. A condition in which diverticula (sacs which bulge outward from the walls of the intestine) form, sometimes causing inflammation which can result in bleeding, pain, inflammation (diverticulitis), and perforation of the diverticula.

Down's syndrome. A congenital defect caused by a chromosomal abnormality, marked by varying degrees of mental retardation and characteristic physical features, such as slanting eyes ("mongolism").

Duodenal ulcer. An open sore in the duodenum.

Eczema. A condition in which the skin becomes inflamed, scaly, and itchy.

Edema. Retention of fluid causes this swelling of any part of the body, especially the arms, legs, ankles, and feet.

Eicosanoids. Prostaglandins (PGEs, PGFs, prostacyclin), thromboxanes, and leucotrienes. The body makes them from polyunsaturated fatty acids in the diet.

Electrolytes. Substances that, when dissolved, separate into ions capable of conducting electricity. In the body, the elements sodium, potassium, magnesium, and chloride are electrolytes that are instrumental in transmitting nerve impulses, contracting muscles, and maintaining a proper fluid level and acid-base balance of fluids.

"Empty" calories. Calories from sources largely devoid of essential nutrients such as vitamins and minerals. A pejorative term applied to fats, sweets, and alcohol.

Endorphins. A group of substances which the brain makes that help in the tolerance of pain.

Enkephalin. A naturally occurring opiate involved in the perception of pain and the integration of emotional experiences.

Enriched. A legal labeling definition for foods indicating the addition of nutrients either to replace those lost in processing or to add nutrients the food does not naturally contain. The same definition applies to the term *fortified*. Basically meant adding more of the same.

Enteral feeding. Food that is supplied directly to the intestine through a tube rather than by being eaten.

Enzymes. Protein molecules that are specific catalysts for many of the chemical reactions that take place in the body.

Epidermis. The outermost layer of skin.

Erythrocytes. Red blood cells. Their main function is to transport oxygen from the lungs to the rest of the body.

Escherichia coli. A bacteria species found in the intestine of humans and other animals. One of the most common causes of urinary tract infections and epidemics of diarrhea, especially in children.

Esophagitis. Inflammation of the esophagus.

Essential amino acids. Nine necessary amino acids found together in meats, eggs, and milk (i.e., in all animal protein) that the body cannot manufacture and must obtain from the diet.

Essential nutrient. A nutrient necessary for health that one must obtain in food because the body either does not make it at all or does not make enough of it.

Estrogen. A feminizing sex hormone made in both sexes, but in much greater quantities in women. It is produced by the ovaries, adrenal glands, the placenta, and by the enzyme aromatase in fatty tissue.

Ethyl acetate. A chemical that occurs naturally in some fruits and vegetables. Some manufacturers use it in decaffeinated coffees instead of methylene chloride because the latter may cause cancer in laboratory animals.

Evaporated milk. Milk that has been heated, vacuum concentrated, homogenized, and canned.

Expiration date. A date stamped on a product to indicate the last date on which one should use it.

Fat-soluble vitamins. Vitamins A, D, E, and K. The body absorbs them with the aid of fat and stores them in fat. Each is a chemical, as well as a vitamin, and megadoses can be harmful.

Fatty liver disease. A condition in which fat collects in the cells of the liver, distorting it. It can result from excessive alcohol intake, kwashiorkor (protein malnutrition), diabetes, Reye's syndrome, and the toxicity of some drugs.

Fetal Alcohol Syndrome (FAS). A number of physical and mental defects produced in the fetus because of alcohol consumption by the mother.

Fluoridation of water. A process in which the essential trace mineral fluoride is added to the water supply to reduce the frequency of dental cavities. Fluoride is harmful in megadoses, as are all essential nutrients.

Fluorine. A halogen (nonmetallic element) that helps maintain and harden bones and teeth and improves the body's uptake of calcium. Many municipalities add it to water supplies; in some places it is naturally present in the water in safe and adequate quantities (4 parts per million).

Fluorosis. A discoloring of the tooth enamel due to a high concentration of fluoride prior to tooth eruption.

Folic acid. One of the B-complex vitamins. The body needs it to help make the genetic materials DNA and RNA and manufacture blood cells. Good sources include liver and other meats, green leafy vegetables and legumes, fruits, nuts, seeds, whole-grain cereals and breads, dairy products, and eggs.

Food. Any usually animal or plant product that provides nourishment when ingested.

Food and Drug Administration. The U.S. federal agency in charge of enforcing the provisions of the U.S. Food, Drug, & Cosmetic Act. Known by its acronym, "FDA."

Food grades. A system by which the U.S. Department of Agriculture (USDA) measures the quality of appearance, uniformity, texture, and sometimes taste of some meat, poultry, eggs, dairy products, and fresh and canned produce.

Food supplement. A concentrate of one or more nutrient substances, used to supplement a nutritionally inadequate diet. Some "food supplements" are in fact "unsafe food additives," by the definition of U.S. law. Most "food supplements" are a waste of money.

Fortified. A legal labeling definition indicating that nutrients have been added to a food either to replace those lost in the processing or to enrich or increase the nutritive value of the product. The same definition applies to the label *enriched*. Basically meant adding a new ingredient.

Free radicals. By-products of oxygen metabolism that can attack cell components and irreversibly damage them. Necessary for health in small quantities; harmful in large quantities.

Fructose. A naturally occurring fruit sugar. It is a monosaccharide.

Fructosemia. A hereditary intolerance to fructose.

Galactosemia. A disorder in which any or all of three enzymes that help the body to utilize the sugar called galactose are defective. Early nutritional therapy can prevent serious, potentially fatal, complications.

Gallbladder. The pear-shaped sac connected to the liver that stores and concentrates bile, the mixture of acids and salts the liver produces to help digest fat in the small intestine.

Gallstones. Stones composed chiefly of cholesterol or bilirubin and calcium that form in the gallbladder or in the gallbladder's ducts.

Gastric ulcer. An ulcer that forms in the stomach.

Gastroesophageal reflux. A disorder in which the lower esophageal sphincter does not stay closed when the stomach is full or under pressure, with the result that food and acidic digestive juices back up (or reflux) into the esophagus, causing heartburn.

Gastrostomy. Surgical procedure in which a tube is placed through the abdominal wall directly into the stomach for feeding.

Genetics. The study of heredity. Genes are hereditary units constituting blueprints for all our proteins, which, in turn, direct all our cell activity.

Gestational diabetes. Diabetes mellitus that appears during some pregnancies, triggered by the increase in hormones during pregnancy, which partially blocks the action of insulin.

Gingivitis. Inflammation of the gums.

Glomerulonephritis. Inflammation of the glomerulus, the tuft of blood capillaries in the kidneys.

Glucose. A monosaccharide (simple sugar) that the body uses directly for energy.

Glycogen. Large chains of glucose molecules that are stored in the liver and muscles for future energy use, when they will be converted back to glucose for the body's direct energy needs.

Glycosuria. Sugar in the urine; a major sign of diabetes mellitus.

Gonadotropins. Hormones that stimulate the gonads to produce the male and female sex hormones.

Gout. A disorder producing excessive uric acid, some of which forms as crystals around joints, causing pain and inflammation.

Granulocytes. White blood cells containing granules.

Graves' disease. A condition in which the thyroid is hyperactive; characterized by increased metabolism.

Guar. A water-soluble dietary fiber that can modestly lower blood cholesterol.

Halogen. A nonmetallic element that forms a saltlike compound with sodium. The halogens are bromine, chlorine, fluorine, and iodine.

"Hard" water. Water with relatively high levels of calcium and magnesium, which leave a residue on tubs and appliances.

Hashimoto's disease. A chronic noninfectious inflammation and infiltration with lymphoid tissue of the thyroid gland; believed to be an autoimmune disorder.

Heart attack. See **myocardial infarction.**

Heme iron. The nonprotein oxygen-binding, iron-containing part of hemoglobin found in animal products, especially red meat, liver, and organ meats. The body absorbs heme iron five times better than plant iron.

Hemochromatosis. An inborn metabolic error, due to the inheritance of two iron-loading genes (one from each parent), in which the intestine absorbs more iron from food than the body can safely store, causing iron destruction of the pancreas, liver, and other organs.

Hemodialysis. A procedure in which an artificial kidney machine cleans waste products from the blood.

Hemoglobin. The oxygen-carrying molecule in red blood cells that delivers oxygen to all the cells that need it.

Hemolytic anemia. An anemia in which red blood cells are hemolyzed (broken down) faster than they are replaced. Any of a variety of hereditary disorders or drugs can produce this condition. Fava beans produce it in genetically predisposed people.

Hemorrhoids. An abnormal enlargement of veins in the anal area, often provoked by increased pressure from straining during defecation. The condition produces pain, bleeding, and itching.

Hepatitis. Inflammation of the liver, usually due to a viral infection, but also the result of alcohol and drug abuse, or certain bacterial infections. Hepatitis A virus is found in fecal matter and is spread by improper food handling or by contaminated seafood. Hepatitis B is spread by direct blood contact, such as with blood transfusions or use of contaminated needles. Hepatitis C, or non-A, non-B hepatitis, is also transmitted through blood contact.

Heredity. The means by which parents transmit family characteristics to their offspring.

Heroin. A highly addictive, powerful chemical derivative of morphine made from the opium poppy. People inject, snort, or take it orally for its euphoric effects.

Hiatal hernia. A condition in which a portion of the stomach protrudes through the diaphragm into the chest.

High-density lipoproteins (HDL). The smallest and densest of the lipoproteins. The cholesterol on them is nicknamed "good" cholesterol. They retrieve cholesterol from the body's tissues and transport it to the liver, which excretes much of it in the bile.

Homogenization. A process by which the particles in a fluid are broken up and evenly distributed. It usually refers to milk in which the fat globules are broken up and dispersed to prevent the cream from separating from the milk. Raw milk zealots incorrectly represent this process as harmful. It does *not* cause absorption of xanthine oxidase.

Hormones. Substances that various glands in the endocrine system secrete; the bloodstream carries them to different organs that they affect.

Human chorionic gonadotropin (HCG). A hormone secreted by the placenta that aids the implantation of the fertilized egg in the uterine wall. Tests to detect pregnancy determine its presence as a positive indication.

Hydrogenation. The process of transforming a soft or liquid polyunsaturated fatty acid into a harder, more saturated fat by adding hydrogen, usually accomplished by bubbling hydrogen gas through the liquid oil. "Saturated fat" means "hydrogenated fat."

Hypercalciuria. Excess calcium in the urine.

Hypercholesterolemia. A metabolic disorder, usually inherited, characterized by excessive amounts of cholesterol in the blood. If you have the "right" genes, your body can process large amounts of cholesterol without buildup, and you can eat all the cholesterol you want; if you have the "wrong" genes, you must restrict cholesterol intake.

Hyperglycemia. A buildup of glucose in the blood; the result of a condition (usually diabetes) in which the body is unable to utilize glucose properly.

Hyperinsulinemia. Excessive amounts of insulin in the blood.

Hyperlipidemia. High levels of lipids in the blood.

Hypernatremia. Increased blood sodium caused by excessive water loss from the body or excessive sodium retention.

Hyperthyroidism. Also known as Graves' disease or toxic goiter, a condition in which the thyroid is overactive, excessively increasing metabolism.

Hypertriglyceridemia. Elevation of blood triglycerides.

Hyperuricemia. Excess uric acid in the blood.

Hypoglycemia. Low blood sugar. In most cases of "low blood sugar," levels prove to be normal when measured during an "attack," and the condition is an example of psychogenic symptomology. The American Diabetes Association calls this "nonhypoglycemia."

Hypokalemia. A deficiency of potassium that affects muscle function.

Hyponatremia. Low levels of sodium in the blood that can produce headache, nausea, muscle weakness, twitching or cramping, mental confusion, seizure, or coma.

Hypothalamus. A portion of the brain that regulates sleep, sexual desire, appetite, and body temperature and controls endocrine gland secretion, body temperature, water balance, and sugar and fat metabolism.

Hypothyroidism. A disorder in which the activity of the thyroid is decreased. Also known as myxedema or an underactive thyroid gland.

Ileitis. Inflammation of the ileum, the lower part of the small intestine. Regional ileitis is a chronic condition known as Crohn's disease, named for one of the Mount Sinai physicians who first described it. Reduces nutrient absorption.

Ileocolitis. Inflammation of the small and large intestines. Often present in Crohn's disease. Reduces nutrient absorption.

Ileostomy. A surgical procedure in which an opening is made through the abdominal wall into the ileum. May be part of a treatment for ulcerative colitis, Crohn's disease, or other intestinal tract conditions that do not respond to medication.

Ileum. Lower part of the small intestine.

Imitation foods. A federal labeling definition for those foods that contain a lower percentage of the specific food than specified by the federal government for the standard product.

Immunoglobin. Forms of proteins that function as antibodies.

Incomplete proteins. Proteins, such as those from most single vegetable sources, that are deficient in one or more essential amino acids. Also called **lower quality proteins.** See **complementary proteins.**

"Indirect" food additives. More than 10,000 substances that unintentionally enter foods during growing, processing, packaging, or preparing. For example: chemicals in some plastic packaging that may leach into food during microwaving.

Insoluble fibers. Those substances that pass through the digestive tract without being digested. Some are broken down by fermentation in the intestine and absorbed across the colon as free fatty acids.

Inspection stamp. A stamp from the U.S. Department of Agriculture that must be placed on meat, poultry, and packaged, processed meat products before sale to consumers to indicate that the food is wholesome and was prepared (slaughtered, packaged, processed) under sanitary conditions.

Insulin. A hormone that the beta cells of the pancreas produces. Insulin regulates the metabolism of carbohydrates and is necessary for the utilization of glucose in body cells with insulin receptors.

Iodine. A halogen. An essential part of thyroid hormones. Good dietary sources include iodized salt, seafood, and vegetables grown in iodine-rich soil.

Iron. A trace mineral essential as part of hemoglobin and myoglobin. Good sources include red meat, liver, fish, green leafy vegetables, enriched bread, dried prunes, apricots and raisins. Humans absorb the iron from animal sources on average five times better than that from plant sources.

Iron-deficiency anemia. Anemia caused by a deficiency of iron; most often a result of a loss of blood from menstruation, ulcers, malignancies, or of increased iron needs during pregnancy or infancy.

Irritable bowel syndrome. A group of symptoms, including abdominal pain and cramping, constipation, diarrhea, bloating, and stomach distress, which emotional stress or anxiety may trigger.

Jaundice. A condition in which excessive bilirubin (bile pigment) causes the skin, the whites of the eyes, and other parts of the body to take on a yellowish hue. Distinguished from carotenemia (too much carotene in the blood), in which condition the whites of the eyes stay white.

Keratin. An insoluble protein that is the main constituent of hair, nails, the epidermis of the skin, and the enamel of the teeth.

Ketoacidosis. An excess of ketones in the blood. It can lead to a life-threatening coma if allowed to persist. May be a complication of untreated diabetes.

Ketogenic diets. A diet high in protein and low in carbohydrates. It causes the body to produce ketones and can lead to ketosis and potentially serious side effects.

Ketones. These potentially toxic by-products are the partially burned fatty acids that the body uses as an alternative fuel source when carbohydrates are not available.

Ketosis. A condition in which ketones accumulate in the blood, making it more acidic and upsetting the body's chemical balance. It can cause headaches, dizziness, fatigue, nausea, and an increase in the risk of heart disease in susceptible people. Especially dangerous for people who are diabetic and women who are pregnant.

Kidneys. Two organs that filter the blood; maintain fluid, electrolyte, and acid-alkaline balance; and excrete as urine the waste products of metabolism. They also help regulate blood pressure, help produce red blood cells, and help reabsorb and metabolize several nutrients.

Kidney stones. Stones composed of calcium (oxalate or phosphate), uric acid, cystine, magnesium or ammonium phosphate that form in the kidney or the ureter (tract leading to the bladder). They can cause a great deal of pain in the small of the back or the groin.

Kwashiorkor. A condition resulting from a severe deficiency in protein. Characteristics include growth retardation, edema (fluid retention and swelling of the extremities), changes in the skin and hair (often to a rust color), and liver problems. Most often occurs in the tropics and subtropics, but can be seen in impoverished areas around the world.

Lactase. An enzyme on the surface of cells lining the small intestine necessary to digest lactose.

Lactose. The principal sugar found in milk; also used as a "filler" in pharmaceutical products.

Lactose intolerance. The inability to digest milk sugar, caused by a lack of lactase.

Lactovegetarians. Those vegetarians who do not eat meat or eggs but do eat dairy products.

Laetrile. A trade name for a chemical called amygdalin, isolated from the almond-shaped pits of stone-bearing fruits (apricots, etc.). It is 6 percent cyanide by weight and a lucrative fake cancer remedy, heavily promoted by organized quackery. It is illegal to sell in the U.S.

Lecithin. A naturally occurring emulsifier in cell protoplasm that helps stabilize cholesterol in the bile and prevents gallstones from forming. It is found in some foods (eggs, soybeans) and manufactured by the body. Commercial lecithin is about 6 percent pure.

Leukemia. A form of cancer in which the leukocytes (white blood cells) proliferate and spread throughout the body.

Leukocytes. White blood cells.

Light. See *lite*.

Linoleic acid. An essential polyunsaturated fatty acid.

Lipid. A fatty substance composed of different proportions of hydrogen, carbon, and oxygen. Examples include triglycerides, cortisol, and cholesterol.

Lipofuscin. A brown pigment that causes "liver spots" on the skin and in the brain. It is produced when free radicals (by-products of oxygen metabolism) attach to cell membranes, and is related to aging.

Lipoprotein. A combination of a lipid (fat) and a protein. Some lipoproteins transport cholesterol in the blood. The three main types are high-density (HDL); low-density (LDL); and very low-density (VLDL).

Liposuction. A procedure of cosmetic surgery in which special tubing sucks fat out of unsightly stores.

Lite. A food label with various meanings: that a food contains fewer calories, less fat, or less sodium, or is a lighter color than the standard product. Also spelled "light."

Lithium. A soft silvery metallic element, necessary in trace amounts for blood formation. In large amounts, a drug that reduces mania and depression. Highly toxic in excess.

Low calorie. A label applied to foods that contain no more than 40 calories per serving and no more than 0.4 calories per gram. A "serving size" can be whatever the seller chooses. This label cannot be applied to certain foods naturally low in calories, such as celery.

Low-density lipoprotein (LDL). The most abundant of the lipoproteins, these usually carry about 65 percent of the circulating cholesterol to cells. High levels are often associated with atherosclerosis.

Lower esophageal sphincter (LES). A ringlike muscle circling the base of the esophagus that opens to admit food to the stomach and closes to prevent the stomach's contents from backing up.

Lymphocytes. White blood cells that are produced chiefly in the lymph nodes.

Lymphoma. A term that denotes a "solid tumor" cancer of the lymphoid system.

Lysergic acid (LSD). A synthetic hallucinogenic drug, also known as "acid," that was a popular "recreational drug" during the 1960s.

Magnesium. A mineral that the body needs to build bones, transmit nerve impulses, ensure proper muscle function, manufacture protein and DNA, and activate enzymes needed to release energy from glycogen stored in muscles. Good sources include green leafy vegetables, whole grains, meat, poultry, dried beans and peas, and nuts.

Maltose. A disaccharide that is made up of two molecules of glucose; present in plants during seed germination. Also called malt sugar.

Manganese. A trace mineral needed for normal tendon and bone structure, and the component of certain enzymes important for metabolism. Good dietary sources include tea, coffee, bran, dried peas and beans, and nuts.

Mannitol. A sugar alcohol, obtained from fruits or dextrose. It is often found in products for diabetics.

Marijuana. The cannabis or hemp plant, whose leaves and flowering tops are smoked or ingested for their euphoric effect.

Megaloblastic anemia. A giant germ cell anemia, usually caused by a deficiency of vitamin B_{12} or of folic acid (a B vitamin).

Melanocytes. Cells of the epidermis that produce melanin, the main pigment in the skin.

Menarche. The pubertal onset of menstruation.

Menkes' disease. A hereditary abnormality of copper absorption that causes a degeneration of the brain and retardation of growth in infants and leads to death.

Menopause. The time of a woman's life during which ovulation and menstruation stop, after which time she is unable to conceive.

Metabolism. Physical and chemical processes in the body, including the use of energy, that are necessary to maintain life.

Methylene chloride. A chemical that removes caffeine from coffee beans. Although it may cause cancer in laboratory animals when significant amounts are inhaled, the FDA has allowed it to remain as an agent in the decaffeination process because the beans retain so little of it. See **Ethyl acetate.**

Micronutrients. Nutrients that the body requires in trace or very small quantities.

Migraine headache. Migraine literally means "one side of the head." A severe headache that results from the abnormal dilation of the blood vessels on the scalp, the neck or around the eye, causing visual disturbances, pain, nausea, vomiting, and sensitivity to light.

Minimum standards of quality. Mandatory standards that the Food and Drug Administration has set pertaining to the color, tenderness, and allowable freedom from defects permissible for many canned fruits and vegetables.

Molybdenum. A trace mineral that helps regulate iron storage and is a component of some enzymes needed in metabolism. Good sources include dried peas and beans, organ meats, whole-grain breads and cereals, and dark leafy vegetables.

Monosaccharides. The simplest of sugars, containing one sugar molecule (usually on a six-carbon-atom backbone). They include glucose, fructose, and galactose.

Monosodium glutamate (MSG). A flavor enhancer for food, used especially in Chinese food, ingestion of which may be associated with headache, facial flushing, chest pressure and pain ("Chinese restaurant syndrome") in some individuals and with asthma in some asthmatics.

Monounsaturated fats. Fats, such as those found in olive and peanut oils, that are liquid at room temperature and semisolid or solid when refrigerated. Most do not raise serum cholesterol and are, therefore, preferable to saturated fats for people with high serum cholesterol.

Morning sickness. Nausea and vomiting during pregnancy that actually can occur at any time of the day. Although it is most typical during the first three months of pregnancy, some women experience it for the entire nine months and some women don't experience it at all.

Multiple sclerosis. A disease in which the fatty myelin sheaths that surround and protect the nerves deteriorate, interfering with the ability of the nerve to function and causing a wide range of symptoms, which include involuntary oscillation of the eyeballs, weakness, tremor, loss of coordination, and instability in walking. May result from an interplay of genetic, viral, and immunologic factors. Often waxes and wanes, rather than steadily progressing.

Myocardial infarction. A heart attack; an interruption of blood flow in one or more coronary arteries that results in lack of oxygen and damages the heart muscle.

Myoglobin. The substance that stores oxygen in muscles.

Natural. A term that, when applied to meat or poultry products, usually indicates that they contain no preservatives, artificial flavors, or colors and are minimally processed. There is no federal definition for the term, and different states have different (or no) definitions.

Natural vitamins. Vitamins that contain extracts from foods rather than synthetic sources. There are no completely natural vitamins on the market. For example, "rose hips vitamin C" is 2 percent natural and 98 percent synthetic. If it were 100 percent rose hips, each pill would be the size of a golf ball.

Nephritis. Inflammation of the kidney.

Nephron. The functional unit of the kidney that filters waste products from the blood and excretes some waste products concentrated in urine.

Nephrotic syndrome. Loss of protein into the urine due to a malfunction of the capillaries in the glomeruli of the kidneys.

Neurotransmitters. The chemical substances that help transmit messages from one cell to another.

Niacin (vitamin B_3). One of the vitamins in the B complex. Certain enzymes need it to convert food to energy, and it promotes normal appetite, digestion, and proper nerve function. In large doses, lowers blood cholesterol, but has some toxicity. Good sources include meat, poultry, legumes, milk, eggs, and peanuts.

Nicotine. A highly addictive, poisonous substance in tobacco leaves. Nicotine addiction is the force that drives smokers to smoke, to maintain a high level of nicotine in their blood.

Nocturia. Excessive urination during the night; sometimes an indication of the kidneys' inability to form a concentrated urine, and sometimes an indication of an enlarged prostate gland.

Nonessential amino acids. Those amino acids that the body can manufacture as it needs them.

Nonheme iron. Dietary iron from plant sources. Relatively poorly absorbed. Vitamin C (ascorbic acid) and some other acids enhance absorption. Also called inorganic iron.

Norwalk virus. A viral agent that most commonly causes epidemics of diarrhea in camps, schools, and families.

Nutrient. Any of a wide variety of food substances that nourish the body.

Obesity. Defined as more than 20 percent above desirable weight for height, age, sex, and body build (bone structure and muscularity).

Oligomenorrhea. Reduced frequency of menstrual cycles.

Open date. A date stamped on a product so that the consumer can determine its freshness.

Osteoarthritis. The most common form of degenerative joint disease, in which a breakdown of joint cartilage occurs, causing joint pain and stiffness. It has no relation to nutrition, except in the fact that obesity worsens it because of excess weight on the joints.

Osteomalacia. The adult form of rickets, a disease in which low levels of calcium and phosphate in the blood prevent bone calcification. Caused by a deficiency of vitamin D in the diet (or lack of skin exposure to sunlight) or by conditions inhibiting vitamin D absorption or use.

Osteoporosis. A condition in which bones lose mass and become porous and fragile, markedly increasing susceptibility to fractures. Results over a period of years from a complex interplay of genetic, hormonal, nutritional (intake of calcium, phosphorus, magnesium, fluoride, amino acids, etc.), and other factors. Adequate dietary calcium while bone is being laid down (birth to age 35) delays its onset.

Ovolactovegetarians. Those vegetarians who abstain from meat, poultry, and fish, but eat dairy products and eggs.

Oxalic acid. A chemical substance found in spinach, chard, beet greens, rhubarb and other foods, which in excess can form kidney stones. The body makes it from excess vitamin C, which also can produce oxalate kidney stones.

Pack date. A date stamped on frozen or canned items to indicate when the food was processed, manufactured, or packaged.

Pantothenic acid (vitamin B_5).One of the B complex vitamins. It is involved in the metabolism of lipids, carbohydrates, and some amino acids, and is necessary for the manufacture of the adrenal hormones and chemicals that regulate nerve function. Bacteria in the intestine manufacture it. Therefore, the body needs little, if any, from food sources, where it is abundant in animal products, legumes, and whole-grain breads and cereals.

Paralytic shellfish poisoning. A food poisoning that occurs after one eats shellfish contaminated with the Gonyaulax protozoan, which are found in waters where the phenomenon of "red tide" appears. Symptoms develop within 30 minutes of ingestion, and include facial numbness, difficulty in breathing, muscle weakness, and, sometimes, partial paralysis.

Parathormone. A hormone that the four parathyroid glands secrete. Parathormone regulates the levels of calcium and phosphorus in the body.

Parenteral nutrition. The intravenous (directly into the bloodstream) administration (via tubing) of nutrient fluids, amino acids, carbohydrates, fats, vitamins, and/or minerals.

Parkinson's disease. A disorder of the central nervous system that occurs most frequently in people aged 50 to 65. It causes tremors, slowed movement, muscular rigidity, and other symptoms.

Passive smoking. Nonsmokers' inhalation of cigarette, pipe, or cigar smoke. Exposes the nonsmoker to the same components (and hazards) of tobacco smoke as smokers. Also called secondary or involuntary smoking.

Pasteurization. Heating of milk and other fluids to destroy disease-transmitting microorganisms.

Pectin. A gummy, water-soluble dietary fiber that can modestly lower blood cholesterol.

Peptic ulcer. An open sore in the lining of the stomach or duodenum related to acidic gastric secretions penetrating the protective mucosal lining of the gastrointestinal wall, thereby reaching the underlying muscular layers. Some recent work suggests the possible involvement of a microorganism.

Periodontitis. Inflammation and destruction of the periodontal membrane, the tissue that surrounds the roots of the teeth and holds them to the jaw.

Peripheral vascular disease. The narrowing of vessels that carry blood to the arms and legs.

Peristalsis. The wavelike contractions of the intestine that propel nutrients forward.

Pernicious anemia. Vitamin B_{12} deficiency anemia that results from a lack of adequate stomach secretion of "intrinsic factor," a substance that enables the body to absorb vitamin B_{12}.

Phenylketonuria. A genetic defect blocking the metabolism of the amino acid phenylalanine. The buildup of phenylalanine in the body can result in mental retardation, seizures, and hyperactivity.

Phospholipids. Waxy or greasy compounds containing phosphoric acid. Constituents of cell membranes.

Phosphorus. An abundant mineral in the body. It helps build and maintain bones and teeth, promotes proper nerve and muscle function, helps to maintain the body's chemical balance, and is needed by certain enzymes to convert food into energy. Good sources include dairy products, egg yolks, meat, poultry, fish, and legumes.

Pica. The craving and ingestion of unusual substances such as earth, clay, cornstarch, ice, baking soda, ashes, paint, paraffin, coffee grounds, etc. Often a symptom of iron deficiency.

Placebo. An inert substance, either by nature or because an adequate body pool of it already exists (such as sugar or vitamin B_{12}), which has no known effect on a particular condition being studied, given as part of a research study, or to satisfy a patient, if the positive psychological effect it confers gives the same relief as an allegedly helpful nutrient or drug, then the helpful nutrient or drug is also a placebo. See **suggestion.**

Placenta. The organ that develops within the pregnant uterus about the third month of pregnancy, through which the fetus receives nourishment and oxygen and the mother's body removes fetal waste products.

Polypeptides. Chains of linked amino acids.

Polysaccharides. Chains of linked saccharides (starches, glycogen, etc.).

Polyunsaturated fats. Fatty acids, such as those found in fish and corn or soybean oils, with two or more unsaturated (double; no hydrogen) bonds. They are liquid at room temperature and when refrigerated. They tend to modestly lower blood cholesterol. They are subdivided into omega-3 and omega-6 depending on whether their first double bond occurs 3 or 6 carbons from the methyl carbon.

Polyuria. Excessive urination.

Potassium. A trace mineral. With sodium, it helps regulate the body's fluid balance, promotes transmission of nerve impulses and proper muscle contraction, and is needed for proper metabolism. Rich dietary sources include bananas, oranges, apricots, avocados, potatoes, bran, peanuts, and dried peas and beans.

Pre-eclampsia. A condition during pregnancy characterized by hypertension, headache, edema, and excess protein in the blood. Also called toxemia.

Premenstrual syndrome (PMS). A set of physical and emotional symptoms that occur before each menstrual period in some women. They are related to hormonal changes and water retention. Vitamin B_6 has been used to relieve the symptoms; it gives the same relief as a sugar pill (80 percent). Unlike a sugar pill, 50 or more mg daily of vitamin B_6 may produce sensory nerve damage.

"Proof." A term that refers to the concentration of alcohol in an alcoholic beverage. In the United States, "proof" is two times the alcohol content (e.g., 10 percent alcohol is 20 proof alcohol).

Prostaglandin. A family of hormonelike compounds derived from long-chain unsaturated fatty acids that have a wide range of actions in the body, which may be good or bad depending on the situation, including stimulating uterine contractions during childbirth, helping lower blood pressure and open airways, and regulating body temperature and acid secretion in the stomach. Aspirin and other NSAIDs (*non*steroid *anti*inflammatory *d*rugs) inhibit their production.

Protein. An organic substance composed of amino acids. Necessary for life. Second to water as the most abundant substance in the body. A primary component of all cells. Proteins play a role in all cell activity as nutrient carriers, enzymes, etc.

Psoriasis. A common chronic skin condition in which the epidermal cells grow rapidly, causing the skin to become thickened, red, and scaly.

Purified water. Water that has had its minerals removed.

Pyridoxine (vitamin B_6). One of the B complex vitamins; essential for protein, lipid, and carbohydrate metabolism, and important for the formation of red blood cells and the promotion of proper nerve function. Megadoses (50 mg or more daily) may damage nerves. Good sources include liver, nuts, brown rice, wheat germ, black strap molasses, fish, and butter.

Raw milk. Milk that is not pasteurized.

Recommended Dietary Allowances (RDAs). Standards created by nutrition experts and adopted by the Food and Nutrition Board of the National Research Council of the National Academy of Sciences for levels of average daily intake of essential nutrients, which levels not only encompass the nutritional needs of essentially all healthy persons, but also include a slight excess to allow the buildup of a reserve against future need. Issued about every five years since World War II. U.S. RDAs are derived by the Food and Drug Administration from the high 1968 RDAs, and appear on food and vitamin and mineral pill labels.

Recommended Dietary Intakes (RDIs). Standards set by the World Health Organization for the level of average daily nutrient intake to encompass the nutritional needs of essentially all healthy persons, plus some extra for storage. RDIs are international RDAs.

"Reduced calorie." A term indicating that a food contains at least one-third fewer calories than the standard product.

Renin. An enzyme that the kidneys synthesize, store, and secrete. It is instrumental in controlling blood pressure.

Retinoic acid. A derivative of vitamin A sometimes prescribed to topically treat difficult cases of acne. Excesses of vitamin A or its derivative can produce deformities in babies if women who are pregnant take it.

Rheumatoid arthritis. A form of arthritis that can also affect parts of the body other than joints. In addition to joint pain, symptoms can include low-grade fever, loss of appetite, fatigue, and anemia. An autoimmune disease in which the body attacks its own joints.

Rhinitis. Inflammation of and watery discharge from the mucous membrane of the nose. Usually from an allergic response or cold.

Riboflavin (vitamin B_2). One of the eight water-soluble vitamins in the vitamin B complex. It is instrumental in the metabolism of food and the release of energy to cells, and is important for the maintenance of skin, mucous membranes, the cornea of the eye, and nerve sheaths. Good sources include whole-grain or enriched grain products, liver, milk, meat, eggs, and green leafy vegetables.

Rickets. A deficiency of vitamin D, due either to inadequate exposure to sunlight or to dietary or metabolic problems, causes this childhood disease. Bone does not adequately calcify, causing pain, bowed legs, and rounding or misalignment of the spine.

Rosacea. A chronic skin condition usually afflicting those over the age of 30 in which the facial capillaries dilate, acne develops, and the skin on the nose sometimes thickens.

Rotavirus. A virus responsible for most of the acute diarrhea in babies and young children.

Saccharides. The scientific term for sugars, which are a group of carbohydrates composed of carbon, hydrogen, and oxygen, with a 2:1 ratio of hydrogen to oxygen. Most sugars have a sweet taste.

Salmonella. A toxic bacterium that occurs in raw or undercooked meat, poultry, stuffing, eggs, unpasteurized milk, fish, and shellfish from fecally contaminated waters, and other foods handled, cooked, and stored in unsanitary conditions. Symptoms of salmonella poisoning include headaches, watery diarrhea, vomiting, nausea, and chills. Can be fatal if untreated, especially in hot weather.

Saturated fats. Hydrogenated fats. Fatty acids in which hydrogen atoms replace double bonds between carbon atoms. These are solid or hard at room temperature and are found in animal and milk fats (with the exception of liquid palm and coconut, tropical plant oils). Dietary saturated fats raise blood cholesterol levels more than does dietary cholesterol, since the liver converts them to cholesterol.

Scurvy. A severe deficiency of vitamin C causes this disease, characterized by bleeding gums, hemorrhages, and extreme weakness.

Selenium. An essential trace mineral with antioxidant properties that help prevent the breakdown of fats and body chemicals. Food sources include chicken, egg yolks, seafood, whole-grain breads and cereals, mushrooms, onions, and garlic. Highly toxic in megadoses.

Sell-by date. A date stamped on a food product to indicate the last day a product should be sold.

Serotonin. A neurotransmitter that helps promote sleep and regulate secretion of pituitary hormones and pain perception.

Shelf date. A date stamped on some food products, usually baked goods, to indicate the date of placement on the shelf.

Sickle cell anemia. A hereditary disorder in which the red blood cells become sickle-shaped when deprived of oxygen, causing anemia and pain (a "sickle cell crisis"). It mostly affects blacks. Being strongly antioxidant, megadoses of vitamin C have produced such crises.

Sodium. A trace mineral that helps maintain body fluid balance. Good sources include salt, processed foods, milk, and, in some areas, water.

Sodium propionate. A substance naturally present in Swiss cheese and commonly added to bread and other baked goods to retard the growth of molds.

"Soft" water. Water with high levels of sodium.

Soluble fibers. Those fibers that are "sticky" when wet and seem to dissolve (but actually just suspend) in water.

Sorbitol. The most common sugar alcohol. See **mannitol** and **xylitol**.

Standards of composition. The minimum percentages of meat and poultry that the United States Department of Agriculture allows in foods labeled as meat and poultry products.

Standards of fill of containers. Food and Drug Administration requirements specifying the minimum amounts of food that a package of a given size can contain.

Standards of identity. Governmental regulations stating mandatory ingredients in certain combinations for a seller to call a product "cheese," "catsup," etc., which allow manufacturers of some 300 foods to omit a list of ingredients.

Staphylococci. A bacteria that causes food poisoning, "staph" infections, and some skin infections.

Substitute food. A legal labeling definition for those foods nutritionally equivalent to another, more common product.

Sucrose. A disaccharide composed of chemically bonded molecules of glucose and fructose. Its most common sources are beets and sugarcane, but honey, many fruits, and some vegetables also contain some.

"Sugar-free." A food label indicating that the product contains no saccharide sweetener, such as sucrose. The product may contain any of the sugar alcohols, sorbitol, xylitol, or mannitol, even though they contain similar calories as sugar.

"Sugarless." See **"sugar-free."**

Suggestion. A potent psychological force that can relieve physical as well as psychological pain and other discomforts. It accounts for pain relief by placebos, by hypnosis, and some of the relief from acupuncture. See also **placebo.**

Sulfites. A group of sulfur-containing agents used as food preservatives, especially on salad bars in restaurants, processed potatoes, and some convenience foods. They can cause mild to severe allergy symptoms in individuals sensitive to them, particularly sulfite-sensitive asthmatics.

Sulfur. A trace mineral that is a component of several amino acids needed to make hair and nails. Good dietary sources include wheat germ, dried peas and beans, beef, peanuts, and clams.

Tannin. A component of tea that can irritate the digestive tract, cause constipation, and reduce iron absorption.

Tay-Sachs disease. Cerebral spongolipidosis. A hereditary, fatal brain disease striking mostly Ashkenazic Jewish infants of Eastern European descent.

Telogen effluvium. A condition in which more hair than usual enters the telogen (resting or final) phase, resulting in hair loss. Can follow severe shock, such as that which occurs during major surgery, starvation, high fever, or extreme stress, or can result from hormonal fluctuations following childbirth.

Temporomandibular joint disorder (TMD). A group of disorders related to the jaw joint and the muscles that control the jaw. These disorders are associated with psychological stress or trauma to the jaw. Symptoms can include muscle or joint pain, headaches, restriction of the jaw's opening, and clicking. Sometimes a spurious diagnosis followed by expensive, unnecessary therapy.

Testosterone. A hormone produced primarily by the testes that is responsible for the male secondary sex characteristics.

Theobromine. The major xanthine in cocoa and chocolate that, with properties similar to those of caffeine, acts as a diuretic, relaxes smooth muscles, and dilates blood vessels.

Theophylline. A xanthine central nervous system stimulant, similar to caffeine, found in tea.

Thermogenesis. The production of body heat.

Thiamine (vitamin B₁). One of the eight water-soluble compounds in the vitamin B complex. It is needed for conversion of carbohydrates into energy and fat, for proper nerve function, and for digestion. Found in greatest quantity in whole-grain and enriched cereals and breads, pork, liver, and soybeans.

Toxemia. A condition affecting some pregnant women characterized by edema, hypertension, and excess protein in the urine. Also called pre-eclampsia.

Trace minerals. Nutrients that the body needs in very small amounts.

Trichinosis. A parasitic infection that results from eating raw or undercooked pork or such products as pork sausage (or, rarely, bear meat) containing the larvae of the trichinella worms. Fever and diarrhea are the initial symptoms; pain, fever, and respiratory problems may occur as the parasites pass through the lungs and lodge in muscle, including the diaphragm.

Triglyceride. The most common lipid (fat) in the diet and in body fat.

Tryptophan. An essential amino acid found in meat, milk, and eggs. A precursor of the neurotransmitter serotonin. Deficiency produces pellagra. Use as a "food supplement" has been associated with over 2000 cases of eosinophilia-myalgia syndrome (EMS) in 1989–1990, with over 20 deaths by early 1990.

Tryosinemia. A hereditary enzyme defect resulting in kidney and liver damage.

Ulcerative colitis. A condition of inflammation of the intestine and ulceration of the colon and rectum. It causes diarrhea, which often contains blood, and abdominal pain.

Unit price. The price per unit (an ounce, pint, quart, gallon, etc.) of a product.

Urea. A by-product of protein breakdown excreted in the urine.

Uremia. A condition in which toxic by-products of protein metabolism remain in the blood when the kidneys are unable to filter and excrete them. Symptoms may include nausea, vomiting, coma, or convulsions.

Urticaria (hives). Itchy welts on the skin triggered by insect stings or allergy-causing tissue histamine releases.

Vasopressin. A hormone that the pituitary gland secretes, vasopressin is instrumental in raising blood pressure, increasing peristalsis, and in causing the kidneys to concentrate urine when water is in short supply in the body.

Vegans. Strict vegetarians who use no animal products. They eat no animal protein at all, not even eggs or dairy products, and wear no leather.

Ventricular fibrillation. Uncontrolled quivering of the heart muscle that prevents it from pumping blood through the body. If not controlled, it can result in death.

Very low-density lipoproteins (VLDL). These lipoproteins normally carry about 15 percent of the circulating cholesterol to cells. High levels are associated with atherosclerosis.

Vitamin A. One of the four fat-soluble vitamins. Necessary for vision, reproduction, and the formation and maintenance of skin, mucous membranes, bones, and teeth. Megadoses produce birth defects. Good sources include liver, eggs, and butter. A precursor, beta carotene, is found in a number of yellow, orange, and dark green vegetables and fruit.

Vitamin C. A water-soluble vitamin, also called ascorbic acid, that is important in the production of collagen and the maintenance of capillaries, cartilage, bones, and teeth. Promotes healing and helps the body fight infection. Good sources include citrus fruits and juices, green or leafy vegetables, potatoes, cabbage and cauliflower. As a chemical, it is a potent antioxidant and large amounts can deprive tissues of oxygen and cause oxalate deposits that can harm the kidneys, heart, and joints.

Vitamin D. One of the four fat-soluble vitamins. Necessary for the body's absorption and metabolism of calcium and phosphorus, and important for the maintenance of teeth and bones. Good sources include egg yolks, fish, cod liver oil, fortified milk, and butter. The body can also derive it from exposure to sunlight. Megadoses are toxic.

Vitamin K. One of the four fat-soluble vitamins. It enables the liver to manufacture prothrombin and other proteins that bind calcium and are necessary for normal blood clotting and bone crystal formation. Intestinal bacteria manufacture it to provide part of the body's requirement; dietary sources, such as spinach and other green leafy vegetables, milk products, meats, eggs, cereals, fruits, and vegetables, provide the rest.

Water-soluble vitamins. Vitamin C and the eight B vitamins. Organic compounds, they are vital for life in small amounts. Body stores last months (e.g., folic acid) to years (e.g., vitamin B_{12}). Each is a chemical as well as a vitamin; therefore, megadoses can be harmful.

Wernicke-Korsakoff syndrome. Central nervous system disorder characterized by weakness, eye muscle paralysis, inability to walk unaided, confusion, and confabulation. Excessive alcohol intake and severe deficiency of B vitamins, particularly thiamine, cause it.

Wilson's disease. A hereditary disease that produces toxic accumulations of copper, damaging the liver and brain.

Xanthines. A group of alkaloid drugs called methylxanthines that occurs in over 60 species of plants, including coffee (caffeine), cocoa (caffeine and theobromine), tea leaves (caffeine, some theobromine, and theophylline), and cola acuminata (guru) nuts (caffeine).

Xanthinuria. An inherited enzyme deficiency that results in reduced conversion of xanthines to uric acid in the body and can cause recurrent kidney stones.

Xylitol. One of the sugar alcohols, derived from fruits or made from dextrose. See also **mannitol** and **sorbitol.**

Zinc. A trace mineral that is an essential component of more than 100 enzymes needed for proper digestion and metabolism. Well absorbed dietary sources include meats, fish, milk, egg yolks, soy products, and peanut butter. Poorly absorbed sources include bran and whole-grain breads and cereals.

REFERENCES

Herbert, V. "Vitamins." In *The World Book Encyclopedia.* Chicago: World Book-Childcraft International, Inc., 1988.

M. E. Shils and V. R. Young, editors. *Modern Nutrition in Health and Disease,* seventh edition. Philadelphia: Lea and Febiger, 1988.

Recommended Dietary Allowances, tenth edition. Washington, D.C.: National Academy Press, 1989.

Nutrient Values

Food (Portion)	Calories	Carbohydrates (gm.)	Sodium (mg.)	Alcohol (gm.)
ALCOHOL				
Beer, regular (12 oz.)	145	13	19	13
Beer, light (12 oz.)	100	5	10	11
Bloody Mary (1 cocktail, 5 oz.)	115	5	332	14
Daiquiri (1 cocktail, 2 oz.)	110	4	3	14
Gin, rum, vodka, whiskey, 80 proof (1.5 oz.)	95	Tr	Tr	14
Gin, rum, vodka, whiskey, 86 proof (1.5 oz.)	105	Tr	Tr	15
Gin, rum, vodka, whiskey, 90 proof (1.5 oz.)	110	Tr	Tr	16
Gin and tonic (1 cocktail, 7.5 oz.)	170	16	10	16
Martini (1 cocktail, 2.5 oz.)	155	Tr	2	22
Piña colada (1 cocktail, 4.5 oz.)	260	40	9	14
Screwdriver (1 cocktail, 7 oz.)	175	18	2	14
Tom Collins (1 cocktail, 7.5 oz.)	120	3	39	16
Whiskey sour (1 cocktail, 3 oz.)	125	5	10	15
Wine, dessert (3.5 oz.)	155	12	9	16
Wine, red (3.5 oz.)	75	2	6	10
Wine, white (3.5 oz.)	70	1	5	10

Food (Portion)	Calories	Fats (gm.)	Saturated (gm.)	Monounsaturated (gm.)	Polyunsaturated (gm.)	Cholesterol (mg.)	Vitamin A (IU)
COOKING OILS AND BUTTERS							
Bacon fat (1 T)	125	14	NA	NA	NA	NA	NA
Butter (1 T)	100	11	7.1	3.3	0.4	31	430
Canola oil (1 T)	124	14	1.0	8.2	4.1	0	0
Chicken fat (1 T)	115	13	3.8	5.7	2.7	11	NA
Coconut oil (1 T)	120	14	1.8	0.8	0.2	0	0
Corn oil (1 T)	125	14	1.8	3.4	8.2	0	0
Cottonseed oil (1 T)	120	14	3.5	2.4	7.1	0	0
Lard (1 T)	115	13	5.1	5.9	1.5	12	NA
Margarine, imitation, soft, diet (1 T)	50	5	1.1	2.2	1.9	0	460
Margarine, regular, hard (1 T)	100	11	2.2	5.0	3.6	0	460
Margarine, regular, soft (1 T)	100	11	1.9	4.0	4.8	0	460
Margarinelike spread, soft (1 T)	75	9	1.8	4.4	1.9	0	460
Olive oil (1 T)	125	14	1.9	10.3	1.2	0	0
Safflower oil (1 T)	125	14	1.3	1.7	10.4	0	0
Soybean oil (1 T)	120	14	2.0	3.2	7.9	0	0
Sunflower oil (1 T)	125	14	1.4	2.7	9.2	0	0
Vegetable shortening (1 T)	115	13	3.3	5.8	3.4	0	0

Food (Portion)	Calories	Carbohydrates (gm.)	Protein (gm.)	Fats (gm.)	Calcium (mg.)	Iron (mg.)
BEEF						
Brisket, fat and lean (3 oz.)	330	0	20	28	7	1.9
Brisket, lean only (3 oz.)	205	0	25	11	5	2.4
Chuck, roast braised, fat and lean (3 oz.)	310	0	22	24	10	2.6
Chuck, roast, lean only (3 oz.)	215	0	27	11	9	3.2
Corned beef (brisket) (3 oz.)	215	Tr	15	16	7	1.6
Flanksteak, broiled, fat or lean (3 oz.)	215	0	21	14	5	2.1
Flanksteak, broiled, lean only (3 oz.)	205	0	22	13	5	2.2
Ground beef, extra-lean, broiled or pan-fried (3 oz.)	225	0	24	14	7	2.4
Ground beef, lean (3 oz.)	235	0	24	15	10	2.1
Ground beef, regular, broiled or pan-fried (3 oz.)	245	0	23	16	10	2.3
Porterhouse steak, broiled, fat and lean 3 oz.)	255	0	21	18	7	2.3
Porterhouse steak, broiled, lean only (3 oz.)	185	0	24	9	6	2.6
Rib, roasted, fat and lean (3 oz.)	325	0	19	27	10	1.8
Rib, roasted, lean only (3 oz.)	205	0	23	12	9	2.2
Round, broiled, fat and lean (3 oz.)	235	0	22	16	6	2.0
Round, broiled, lean only (3 oz.)	165	0	24	7	5	2.3
Shortribs, braised, fat and lean (3 oz.)	400	0	18	36	10	2.0
Shortribs, braised, lean only (3 oz.)	250	0	26	15	9	3.0
Sirloin, broiled, fat and lean (3 oz.)	240	0	23	15	9	2.6
Sirloin, broiled, lean only (3 oz.)	175	0	26	7	9	2.9
T-bone, broiled, fat and lean (3 oz.)	275	0	20	21	8	2.2
T-bone, broiled, lean only (3 oz.)	180	0	24	9	6	2.6
Tenderloin, broiled, fat and lean (3 oz.)	225	0	22	15	7	2.8
Tenderloin, broiled, lean only (3 oz.)	175	0	24	8	6	3.0
BEVERAGES						
Club soda (12-oz. can)	0	0	0	0	17	NA
Coffee, brewed (6 oz.)	5	1	Tr	Tr	3	0.1
Coffee, instant (6 oz.)	5	1	Tr	Tr	6	0.1
Cola, diet (12-oz. can)	Tr	Tr	0	0	14	0.2
Cola, regular (12-oz. can)	150	38	0	0	9	0.1
Dr. Pepper-type (12-oz. can)	150	38	0	0	12	0.1
Fruit juices: *See* Fruits and Fruit Juices						
Fruit-punch drink, canned (8 oz.)	110	30	Tr	0	16	0.5
Gatorade (8 oz.)	39	10.5	0	0	23	NA
Ginger ale (12-oz. can)	125	32	Tr	0	12	0.7

NA: Not available in references used.

*Crude fiber.

**Cooked and drained unless otherwise stated.

***Based on typical recipe; ingredients and nutrients may vary among recipes.

$: Varies depending on amount of salt added.

$$: Varies depending on type of oil used for frying.

TR: Trace.

	Sodium (mg.)	Potassium (mg.)	Thiamine (mg.)	Riboflavin (mg.)	Niacin (mg.)	Vitamin C (mg.)	Vitamin A (IU)	Cholesterol (mg.)	Fiber (gm.)
BEEF									
	52	195	.05	.15	2.6	0	NA	79	0
	61	244	.06	.18	3.2	0	NA	79	0
	52	198	.06	0.2	2.3	0	NA	86	0
	58	234	.07	.24	2.7	0	NA	88	0
	964	123	.02	.14	2.6	0	NA	83	0
	70	338	.09	.16	4.1	0	NA	60	0
	70	344	.09	.16	4.2	0	NA	60	0
	70	310	.06	.26	4.8	0	NA	82	0
	75	292	.05	0.2	4.8	0	NA	84	
	79	280	.34	.18	0	0	NA	84	0
	52	303	.08	.18	3.5	0	NA	70	0
	56	346	.09	.21	3.9	0	NA	68	0
	54	250	.06	.15	2.8	0	NA	72	0
	63	320	.07	.18	3.5	0	NA	68	0
	51	311	.08	.18	3.2	0	NA	71	0
	54	352	.09	.20	3.5	0	NA	70	0
	43	191	.04	.13	2.1	0	NA	80	0
	50	266	.06	.17	2.7	0	NA	79	0
	53	306	0.1	.22	3.3	0	NA	77	0
	56	342	.11	.25	3.6	0	NA	76	0
	51	288	.08	.18	3.3	0	NA	71	0
	56	346	.09	.21	3.9	0	NA	68	0
	52	323	0.1	.23	3.1	0	NA	73	0
	54	356	.11	.25	3.3	0	NA	72	0
BEVERAGES									
	75	6	0	0	0	0	0	0	0
	4	96	0	0	0.4	0	0	0	0
	6	64	0	Tr	0.5	0	0	0	0
	32	7	0	0	0	0	0	0	0
	14	4	0	0	0	0	0	0	0
	38	2	0	0	0	0	0	0	0
	56	64	.06	.06	Tr	74	32	0	0
	123	23	NA	NA	NA	NA	NA	NA	NA
	25	5	0	0	0	0	0	0	0

NA: Not available in references used.
*Crude fiber.
**Cooked and drained unless otherwise stated.
***Based on typical recipe; ingredients and nutrients may vary among recipes.
$: Varies depending on amount of salt added.
$$: Varies depending on type of oil used for frying.
TR: Trace.

Food (Portion)	Calories	Carbohydrates (gm.)	Protein (gm.)	Fats (gm.)	Calcium (mg.)	Iron (mg.)
BEVERAGES *(cont.)*						
Grape-juice drink, canned (8 oz.)	130	32	Tr	0	8	0.2
Grape soda (12-oz. can)	160	42	0	0	12	0.3
Kool-Aid, all flavors, with sugar added, prepared (8 oz.)	100	25	0	0	0	0
Lemonade (prepared from concentrate) (8 oz.)	100	26	Tr	Tr	8	0.4
Lemon-lime soda (12-oz. can)	150	38	0	0	9	0.2
Limeade (prepared from concentrate) (8 oz.)	100	27	Tr	Tr	7	0.1
Milk beverages (milk, cocoa, eggnog, milk shake): *See* Milk						
Orange drink, canned (8 oz.)	125	32	0	0	16	0.7
Orange-flavor drink, breakfast-type from powder (6 oz.)	85	22	0	0	46	0.2
Orange soda (12-oz. can)	175	46	0	0	19	0.2
Pineapple and orange-juice drink, canned (8 oz.)	125	29	3	0	13	0.7
Root beer (,12-oz. can)	150	39	Tr	0	19	0.2
Tea, brewed (6 oz.)	2	Tr	0	0	0	Tr
Tea, low-calorie from instant (8 oz.)	5	1	Tr	0	5	0.2
Tea, sweetened from instant (8 oz.)	85	22	Tr	Tr	6	Tr
Tonic water (12-oz. can)	125	32	0	0	5	NA
Vegetable juices: *See* Vegetables						
BREADS/ROLLS						
Bagel (1 med.)	200	38	7	2	29	1.8
Biscuit (from mix, 1, 2-in. diam.)	95	14	2	3	58	0.7
Biscuit (from refrigerated dough, 1, 2-in. diam.)	65	10	1	2	4	0.5
Biscuit (homemade, 1, 2 in.)	100	13	2	5	47	0.7
Bread crumbs, dry (1 cup)	390	73	13	5	122	4.1
Bread crumbs, soft (1 cup)	120	22	4	2	57	1.3
Corn bread (homemade, 1 piece)	200	29	4	7	90	1.2
Corn bread (from mix, 1 piece, 2 × 2 in.)	130	20	3	3	60	1.1
Cracked wheat (1 slice)	65	12	2	1	16	0.7
Dinner roll (1 med.)	85	14	2	2	33	0.8
Frank/burger roll (1)	115	20	3	2	54	1.2
French (1 slice)	100	18	3	1	39	1.1
French toast	155	17	6	7	72	1.3
Hard roll (1 med.)	155	30	5	2	24	1.4
Hoagie, or enriched submarine (1 roll, 3 3/4 in. round, 2 in. high)	400	72	11	8	100	3.8

NA: Not available in references used.

*Crude fiber.

**Cooked and drained unless otherwise stated.

***Based on typical recipe; ingredients and nutrients may vary among recipes.

$: Varies depending on amount of salt added.

$$: Varies depending on type of oil used for frying.

TR: Trace.

Sodium (mg.)	Potassium (mg.)	Thiamine (mg.)	Riboflavin (mg.)	Niacin (mg.)	Vitamin C (mg.)	Vitamin A (IU)	Cholesterol (mg.)	Fiber (gm.)
BEVERAGES *(cont.)*								
2	88	.02	.02	0.2	40	5	0	0
57	3	0	0	0	0	0	0	0
0	0	0	0	0	NA	0	0	0
8	38	.02	.05	Tr	10	53	0	NA
41	4	0	0	Tr	0	0	0	0
6	33	Tr	Tr	0.1	7	NA	0	NA
41	44	.01	Tr	Tr	85	44	0	0
9	37	Tr	.03	0	91	1,376	0	0
46	9	0	0	0	0	0	0	0
9	116	.08	.05	.52	56	1,328	0	0
49	3	0	0	0	0	0	0	0
5	66	0	.02	0	0	0	0	0
24	41	0	.01	0.1	0	0	0	0
13	50	0	.05	0.1	0	0	0	0
15	1	0	0	0	0	0	0	0
BREADS/ROLLS								
245	50	.26	.20	2.4	0	0	0	NA
262	56	.12	.11	0.8	Tr	20	Tr	Tr
249	18	.08	.05	0.7	0	0	1	Tr
195	32	.08	.08	0.8	Tr	10	Tr	Tr
736	152	.35	.35	4.8	0	0	5	0.3
231	50	.21	.14	1.7	Tr	Tr	0	0.3
232	78	.15	.15	1.2	Tr	110	0	1.7
480	65	NA	NA	NA	NA	NA	0	NA
106	34	0.1	.09	0.8	Tr	Tr	0	2.1
155	36	.14	.09	1.1	Tr	Tr	Tr	NA
241	56	0.2	.13	1.6	Tr	Tr	Tr	NA
203	32	.16	.12	1.4	Tr	Tr	0	1.3
257	86	.12	.16	1	Tr	110	112	0.1
313	49	0.2	.12	1.7	0	0	Tr	NA
683	128	.54	.33	4.5	0	0	Tr	NA

NA: Not available in references used.

*Crude fiber.

**Cooked and drained unless otherwise stated.

***Based on typical recipe; ingredients and nutrients may vary among recipes.

$: Varies depending on amount of salt added.

$$: Varies depending on type of oil used for frying.

TR: Trace.

Food (Portion)	Calories	Carbohydrates (gm.)	Protein (gm.)	Fats (gm.)	Calcium (mg.)	Iron (mg.)
BREADS/ROLLS *(cont.)*						
Italian (1 slice)	85	17	3	Tr	5	0.8
Mixed-grain (1 slice)	65	12	2	1	27	0.8
Pita (1)	165	33	6	1	49	1.4
Pumpernickel (1 slice)	80	16	3	1	23	0.9
Raisin (1 slice)	65	13	2	1	25	0.8
Rye (1 slice)	65	12	2	1	20	0.7
Rye roll (1 small)	55	9	1	2	6	0.5
Taco/tostada shell (1)	50	7	1	2	16	0.3
Tortilla, corn (1)	65	13	2	1	42	1.4
Tortilla, flour (1)	95	17	2	2	46	1.1
Wheat (1 slice)	65	12	2	1	32	0.9
White (1 slice)	65	12	2	1	32	0.7
Whole-wheat (1 slice)	70	13	3	1	20	1.0
Whole-wheat roll (1 med.)	90	18	4	1	34	0.8
CAKES						
Angel food (1/12 cake)	125	29	3	Tr	44	0.2
Banana cake (1/12 cake)	260	36	3	11	NA	NA
Boston cream pie (3 1/8-in. arc)	310	50	5	10	70	0.5
Caramel with caramel icing (1/16 cake)	265	42	3	10	59	1.0
Carrot cake with cream cheese frosting (1/16 cake)	385	48	4	21	44	1.3
Cheese cake, plain (1/12 cake)	280	26	5	18	52	0.4
Chocolate with chocolate icing (1/16 cake)	235	40	3	8	41	1.4
Coconut (1/16 cake)	260	42	3	9	31	0.2
Fruit cake, dark (2/3-in. arc of tube cake)	165	25	2	7	41	1.2
German chocolate (1/16 cake)	195	27	2	8	NA	NA
Gingerbread (2 3/4 × 2 3/4 × 1 3/8 in.)	175	32	2	4	57	1.2
Marble with white icing (1/16 cake)	215	40	3	6	51	0.5
Pineapple upside-down (1 piece)	235	37	2	9	54	1.2
Plain (1 piece, 3 × 3 × 2 in.)	315	48	4	12	55	1.3
Pound (1 slice, 1/17 of loaf)	120	15	2	5	20	0.5
Shortcake, plain (1 piece)	85	12	1	2	10	0.1
Spice with icing (1/16 cake)	270	47	3	8	55	0.6
Sponge (1/16 cake)	120	22	3	2	12	0.5
White with frosting (1/16 cake)	260	42	3	9	33	1.0
Yellow with chocolate frosting (1/16 cake)	245	39	2	11	23	1.2

NA: Not available in references used.
*Crude fiber.
**Cooked and drained unless otherwise stated.
***Based on typical recipe; ingredients and nutrients may vary among recipes.
$: Varies depending on amount of salt added.
$$: Varies depending on type of oil used for frying.
TR: Trace.

Sodium (mg.)	Potassium (mg.)	Thiamine (mg.)	Riboflavin (mg.)	Niacin (mg.)	Vitamin C (mg.)	Vitamin A (IU)	Cholesterol (mg.)	Fiber (gm.)
BREADS/ROLLS *(cont.)*								
176	22	.12	.07	1.0	0	0	0	Tr
106	56	0.1	0.1	1.1	Tr	Tr	0	0.2
339	71	.27	.12	2.2	0	0	0	NA
177	141	.11	.17	1.1	0	0	0	4.3
92	59	.08	.15	1.0	Tr	Tr	0	0.4
175	51	0.1	.08	0.8	0	0	0	0.9
120	16	.21	.06	0.8	NA	7	NA	0.1*
72	25	.03	.02	0.2	NA	NA	NA	0.2*
53	52	0.2	.14	1.5	NA	NA	NA	0.3*
NA	NA	.01	.08	1.0	Tr	0	NA	NA
138	35	.12	.08	1.2	Tr	Tr	0	0.2
129	28	.12	.08	0.9	Tr	Tr	0	0.5
180	50	.10	.06	1.1	Tr	Tr	0	1.4
197	102	.12	.05	1.1	Tr	Tr	NA	0.6*
CAKES								
269	71	.03	.11	0.1	0	0	0	NA
305	NA	NA	NA	NA	NA	NA	NA	NA
192	92	.03	.11	0.2	Tr	220	NA	NA
178	46	.02	.05	0.1	Tr	140	NA	NA
279	108	.11	.12	0.9	1	140	74	NA
204	90	.03	.12	0.4	5	230	170	NA
181	90	.07	0.1	0.6	Tr	100	37	NA
178	74	.01	.04	0.2	Tr	15	NA	NA
67	194	.08	.08	0.5	16	50	20	NA
315	NA	NA	NA	NA	NA	NA	NA	NA
192	173	.09	.11	0.8	Tr	0	1	NA
168	79	.01	.05	0.1	Tr	60	NA	NA
179	128	.12	.08	0.8	4	290	0	NA
258	68	.14	.15	1.1	Tr	150	61	NA
96	28	.05	.06	0.5	Tr	200	32	NA
NA	NA	.03	.03	0.1	Tr	85	NA	NA
189	63	.02	.07	0.2	Tr	120	NA	NA
68	36	.02	.06	0.1	Tr	185	NA	NA
176	52	.20	.13	1.7	0	40	3	NA
192	123	.05	.14	0.6	0	120	38	NA

NA: Not available in references used.
*Crude fiber.
**Cooked and drained unless otherwise stated.
***Based on typical recipe; ingredients and nutrients may vary among recipes.
$: Varies depending on amount of salt added.
$$: Varies depending on type of oil used for frying.
TR: Trace.

Food (Portion)	Calories	Carbohydrates (gm.)	Protein (gm.)	Fats (gm.)	Calcium (mg.)	Iron (mg.)
CANDY						
Butterscotch (1 oz., 6 pieces)	115	27	Tr	1	5	0.4
Caramels, plain or chocolate (1 oz., 3 pieces)	115	22	1	3	42	0.4
CHOCOLATE						
Chocolate, milk, plain (1 oz.)	145	16	2	9	50	0.4
Chocolate, milk, with almonds, peanuts (1 oz.)	155	14	4	10	57	0.4
Chocolate, semi-sweet chips (1/4 cup, 15 chips)	215	24	2	15	13	1.4
Chocolate disks, sugar-coated (M & M's) (1 oz., 31 pieces)	130	21	2	6	38	0.4
Fondant, chocolate-covered (1 oz.)	115	23	0.5	3	16	0.3
Fondant, mint and candy corn, etc. (1 oz.)	105	27	Tr	0	2	0.1
Fudge, chocolate w/nuts (1 oz.)	120	20	1	5	22	0.3
Fudge, plain chocolate (1 oz.)	115	21	1		22	0.3
Gum drops (1 oz.)	100	25	Tr	Tr	2	0.1
Hard candy (1 oz., 6 pieces)	110	28	0	0	Tr	0.1
Jelly beans (1 oz., 10 pieces)	105	26	Tr	Tr	1	0.3
Marshmallows (1 oz.)	90	23	1	0	1	0.5
Peanut bars (1 oz.)	145	13	5	9	12	0.5
Peanut brittle (1 oz.)	120	23	2	3	10	0.7
Peanuts, red, chocolate-covered (1 oz.)	155	13	5	9	23	0.7
Raisins, chocolate-covered (1 oz.)	115	20	1	4	27	0.5
CEREALS, COLD						
All-Bran (13/ cup)	70	21	4	1	23	4.5
Apple Jacks (1 cup)	110	26	2	Tr	3	4.5
Bran (1/2 cup)	80	26	4	1	26	2.9
Bran Buds (1/3 cup)	70	22	4	1	19	4.5
Bran Chex (2/3 cup)	90	23	3	1	17	4.5
Bran flakes (40% bran) (1 cup)	105	28	4	1	19	12.4
Cap'n Crunch (3/4 cup)	120	23	1	3	5	7.5
Cheerios (1 1/4 cup)	110	20	4	2	48	4.5
Cookie Crisp (1 cup)	115	25	1	1	5	4.5
Corn Bran (2/3 cup)	100	24	2	1	33	9.6
Corn Chex (1 cup)	110	25	2	Tr	3	1.8
Corn flakes, plain (1 cup)	100	21	2	Tr	NA	0.6
Corn flakes, coated (1 cup)	155	36	2	Tr	1	1.0
Corn Flakes, Kellogg's (1 cup)	110	24	2	Tr	1	1.8
Corn, puffed, cocoa-flavored (1 cup)	115	26	2	1	6	3.5

NA: Not available in references used.

*Crude fiber.

**Cooked and drained unless otherwise stated.

***Based on typical recipe; ingredients and nutrients may vary among recipes.

$: Varies depending on amount of salt added.

$$: Varies depending on type of oil used for frying.

TR: Trace.

Sodium (mg.)	Potassium (mg.)	Thiamine (mg.)	Riboflavin (mg.)	Niacin (mg.)	Vitamin C (mg.)	Vitamin A (IU)	Cholesterol (mg.)	Fiber (gm.)
CANDY								
19	1	0	Tr	Tr	0	40	NA	NA
64	54	.01	.05	0.1	Tr	Tr	1	NA
CHOCOLATE								
23	96	.02	0.1	0.1	Tr	30	6	NA
21	132	.04	0.1	0.8	Tr	30	5	NA
6	148	.02	.07	0.2	Tr	10	0	NA
20	71	.02	.06	0.1	Tr	30	0	NA
52	26	.01	.02	Tr	Tr	Tr	0	NA
57	1	Tr	Tr	Tr	0	0	0	NA
48	50	.01	.03	0.1	Tr	Tr	1	NA
54	42	.01	.03	0.1	Tr	Tr	1	NA
10	1	0	Tr	Tr	0	0	0	NA
7	1	0.1	0	0	0	0	0	NA
7	11	0	0	Tr	Tr	0	0	NA
25	2	0	Tr	Tr	0	0	0	NA
3	127	.12	.02	2.7	0	0	0	NA
9	43	.05	.01	1.0	0	0	0	NA
NA	NA	.02	.06	2.1	NA	50	NA	NA
NA	NA	.02	.12	0.2	NA	50	0	NA
CEREALS, COLD								
320	350	.37	.43	5.0	15	1,250	0	8.6
125	23	0.4	0.4	5.0	15	1,250	0	0.3
246	233	.44	.53	4.4	13	1,410	0	2.0
174	474	0.4	0.4	5.0	15	1,250	0	7.7
263	228	0.4	.15	5.0	15	62	0	5.7
207	137	.41	.49	4.1	12	1,650	0	1.0
213	37	0.5	.55	6.6	0	40	0	0.3
307	101	.37	.43	5.0	15	1,250	0	1.6
195	28	0.4	0.4	5.0	15	1,250	0	0.1
244	55	0.3	.55	8.6	NA	NA	0	5.9
271	23	0.4	0.1	5.0	15	143	0	0.3
251	30	.29	.35	2.9	9	1,180	0	.08
267	27	.46	.56	4.6	14	1,880	0	0.1
351	26	.37	.43	5.0	15	1,250	0	0.4
255	NA	.35	.42	3.5	11	0	0	0.1

NA: Not available in references used.

*Crude fiber.

**Cooked and drained unless otherwise stated.

***Based on typical recipe; ingredients and nutrients may vary among recipes.

$: Varies depending on amount of salt added.

$$: Varies depending on type of oil used for frying.

TR: Trace.

Food (Portion)	Calories	Carbohydrates (gm.)	Protein (gm.)	Fats (gm.)	Calcium (mg.)	Iron (mg.)
CEREALS, COLD *(cont.)*						
Corn, puffed, shredded (1 cup)	95	22		Tr	1	0.6
Cracklin' Oat Bran (1/2 cup)	110	20	3	4	15	1.8
40% Bran Flakes (3/4 cup)	95	22	4	1	14	8.1
Froot Loops (1 cup)	110	25	2	1	3	4.5
Fruit & Fibre (1/2 cup)	85	22	3	Tr	14	4.4
Fruit & Fibre, with dates, raisins, walnuts (1/2 cup)	85	21	3	1	15	4.4
Granola (1 oz.)	140	16	4	8	18	1.1
Grape-nuts (1/4 cup)	100	23	3	Tr	11	1.2
Quaker 100% Natural Cereal (1/ cup)	135	18	3	6	38	0.8
Nature Valley Granola (1/3 cup)	125	19	3	5	18	0.9
Lucky Charms (1 cup)	110	23	3	1	32	4.5
Nutri-Grain, corn (2/3 cup)	110	24	2	1	1	0.6
Nutri-Grain, wheat (3/4 cup)	105	24	2	Tr	8	0.8
Product 19 (3/4 cup)	110	24	3	Tr	3	18.0
Puffed Rice (1 cup)	55	13	1	Tr	1	0.2
Puffed Wheat (1 cup)	50	11	2	Tr	4	0.7
Raisin Bran (3/4 cup)	90	21	3	1	10	3.5
Rice, crisped (1 cup)	115	26	2	Tr	6	0.8
Rice, puffed (1 cup)	60	13	1	Tr	3	0.3
Rice Krispies (1 cup)	110	25	2	Tr	4	1.8
Special K (1 1/3 cup)	110	21	6	Tr	8	4.5
Sugar Frosted Flakes (3/4 cup)	110	26	1	Tr	1	1.8
Shredded Wheat (2/3 cup)	100	23	3	1	11	1.2
Sugar Smacks (3/4 cup)	105	25	2	1	3	1.8
Total (1 cup)	100	22	3	1	48	18.0
Wheat, puffed (1 cup)	55	12	2	Tr	4	0.6
Wheat, shredded, without sugar, salt (1 cup)	90	20	2	Tr	11	0.9
Wheat, shredded, without sugar, salt, spoonsize biscuits (1 cup)	175	40	5	1	22	1.8
Wheat germ (1 oz., 1/4 cup)	110	14	8	3	13	2.6
Wheaties (1 cup)	100	23	3	1	43	4.5
CEREALS, HOT, COOKED						
Corn grits (3/4 cup)	110	24	3	Tr	1	1.2
Corn grits, instant, plain (1 packet)	80	18	2	Tr	7	1.0
Cream of Rice (3/4 cup)	95	21	2	Tr	6	0.3
Cream of Wheat (3/4 cup)	105	22	3	Tr	40	8.2
Farina, cooked (3/4 cup)	85	18	2	Tr	3	0.9

NA: Not available in references used.

*Crude fiber.

**Cooked and drained unless otherwise stated.

***Based on typical recipe; ingredients and nutrients may vary among recipes.

$: Varies depending on amount of salt added.

$$: Varies depending on type of oil used for frying.

TR: Trace.

Sodium (mg.)	Potassium (mg.)	Thiamine (mg.)	Riboflavin (mg.)	Niacin (mg.)	Vitamin C (mg.)	Vitamin A (IU)	Cholesterol (mg.)	Fiber (gm.)
CEREALS, COLD *(cont.)*								
269	NA	.11	.05	0.5	0	0	0	0.1
150	160	NA	NA	NA	NA	NA	0	4.0
264	180	0.4	0.4	5.0	NA	1,250	0	6.0
145	26	.37	.43	5.0	15	1,250	0	0.3
193	151	.37	.42	4.9	0	1,235	0	3.0
68	149	.37	.42	4.9	0	1,235	0	3.0
3	142	.17	.07	0.5	0	10	0	0.4*
197	95	.37	.43	5.0	0	1,250	0	2.2
11	150	.08	.15	0.6	NA	NA	0	1.0
58	98	0.1	.05	0.2	0	20	0	1.0*
201	59	.37	.43	5.0	15	1,250	0	0.6
187	66	0.4	0.4	5.0	15	1,250	0	2.0
193	77	0.4	0.4	5.0	15	1,250	0	2.1
325	44	1.5	1.7	20.0	60	5,000	0	1.2
0	16	Tr	Tr	0.4	NA	NA	0	0.2
1	49	.03	.03	1.5	NA	NA	0	0.9
207	147	.28	.34	3.9	0	960	0	3.6
283	29	.35	.42	3.5	11	1,410	0	0.4
Tr	15	.07	.01	0.7	0	0	0	0.1
340	29	.37	.43	5.0	15	1,250	0	Tr
265	49	0.4	0.4	5.0	15	1,250	0	0.4
230	18	.37	.43	5.0	15	1,250	0	0.2
3	102	.07	.08	1.5	0	0	0	3.3
75	42	.37	.43	5.0	15	1,250	0	0.3
352	106	1.5	1.7	20.0	60	5,000	0	2.5
1	51	.08	.03	1.2	0	0	0	0.5
1	87	.06	.03	1.1	0	0	0	2.2
2	174	.11	.06	2.2	0	0	0	2.6
1	268	.47	.23	1.6	2	NA	0	0.7
354	106	0.4	0.4	5.0	15	1,250	0	2.6
CEREALS, HOT, COOKED								
0	40	.18	.11	1.5	NA	0	0	0.1*
343	29	.18	.08	1.3	0	0	0	0.1*
1	37	0.1	0	0.8	NA	NA	0	0.1*
4	34	.18	.05	1.1	NA	0	0	0.6
1	22	.14	.09	1.0	NA	NA	0	0.1*

NA: Not available in references used.

*Crude fiber.

**Cooked and drained unless otherwise stated.

***Based on typical recipe; ingredients and nutrients may vary among recipes.

$: Varies depending on amount of salt added.

$$: Varies depending on type of oil used for frying.

TR: Trace.

Food (Portion)	Calories	Carbohydrates (gm.)	Protein (gm.)	Fats (gm.)	Calcium (mg.)	Iron (mg.)
CEREALS, HOT, COOKED *(cont.)*						
Oatmeal (3/4 cup)	108	19	4	2	15	1.2
Oatmeal, instant, fortified, flavored (1 packet)	160	31	5	2	168	6.7
CHEESE, NATURAL						
American (1 oz.)	105	Tr	6	9	174	0.1
American, spread (1 T)	47	1	3	3	91	Tr
Blue (1 oz.)	100	1	6	8	150	0.1
Brick (1 oz.)	105	1	7	8	191	0.1
Brie (1 oz.)	95	Tr	6	8	52	0.1
Camembert (1 oz.)	85	Tr	6	7	110	0.1
Cheddar (1 oz.)	115	Tr	7	9	204	0.2
Cheddar (1 cup shredded)	455	1	28	37	815	0.8
Cheshire (1 oz.)	110	1	7	9	182	0.1
Colby (1 oz.)	110	1	7	9	94	0.2
Cottage, creamed (1/2 cup)	110	3	13	5	53	0.1
Cottage, low-fat, 2% (1/2 cup)	100	4	16	2	78	0.2
Cream cheese (1 oz.)	100	1	2	10	23	0.3
Edam (1 oz.)	100	Tr	7	8	207	0.1
Feta (1 oz.)	75	1	4	6	140	0.2
Gouda (1 oz.)	100	1	7	8	198	0.1
Gruyère (1 oz.)	115	Tr	8	9	287	NA
Monterey (1 oz.)	105	Tr	7	9	212	0.2
Mozzarella, part skim (1 oz.)	80	1	8	5	207	0.1
Mozzarella, whole milk (1 oz.)	80	1	6	6	147	0.1
Muenster (1 oz.)	105	Tr	7	9	203	0.1
Parmesan (1 cup, grated)	455	4	42	30	1,376	1.0
Parmesan (1 oz.)	130	1	12	9	390	0.3
Parmesan (1 T, grated)	25	Tr	2	2	69	Tr
Provolone (1 oz.)	100	1	7	8	214	0.1
Ricotta, part skim (1/2 cup)	170	6	14	10	337	0.6
Ricotta, whole milk (1/2 cup)	215	4	14	16	254	0.4
Romano (1 oz.)	110	1	9	8	302	NA
Roquefort (1 oz.)	105	1	6	9	188	0.2
Swiss (1 oz.)	105	1	8	8	272	Tr
CHEESE, PROCESSED						
American, cold pack (1 oz.)	94	2	6	7	141	0.2
Cheddar, cold pack (1 oz.)	93	2	6	7	139	0.2
Port wine, cold pack (1 oz.)	100	Tr	5	9	50	NA
Swiss (1 oz.)	95	1	7	7	219	0.2

NA: Not available in references used.

*Crude fiber.

**Cooked and drained unless otherwise stated.

***Based on typical recipe; ingredients and nutrients may vary among recipes.

$: Varies depending on amount of salt added.

$$: Varies depending on type of oil used for frying.

TR: Trace.

Sodium (mg.)	Potassium (mg.)	Thiamine (mg.)	Riboflavin (mg.)	Niacin (mg.)	Vitamin C (mg.)	Vitamin A (IU)	Cholesterol (mg.)	Fiber (gm.)
CEREALS, HOT, COOKED *(cont.)*								
1	99	.04	.23	0.4	NA	30	0	2.8
254	137	.53	.38	5.9	Tr	1,530	0	2.3
CHEESE, NATURAL								
406	46	.01	0.1	Tr	0	340	27	0
218	39	Tr	Tr	Tr	0	127	9	0
396	73	.01	.11	0.3	0	200	21	0
159	38	Tr	.10	Tr	0	307	27	0
178	43	.02	.15	Tr	0	189	28	0
239	53	Tr	.14	0.2	0	262	20	0
176	28	.01	.11	Tr	0	300	30	0
701	111	.03	.42	0.1	0	1,200	119	0
198	27	.01	.08	NA	0	279	29	0
171	36	Tr	.11	Tr	0	293	27	0
425	88	.02	.17	0.1	Tr	171	16	0
459	108	.02	.21	0.2	Tr	80	10	0
84	34	Tr	.06	Tr	0	405	31	0
274	53	.01	.11	Tr	0	260	25	0
316	18	.04	.24	0.3	0	130	25	0
232	34	0.1	0.1	Tr	0	183	32	0
95	23	.02	0.1	Tr	0	346	31	0
152	23	NA	.11	NA	0	269	NA	0
150	27	.01	0.1	Tr	0	180	15	0
106	19	Tr	.07	Tr	0	220	22	0
178	38	Tr	.09	Tr	0	320	27	0
1,861	107	.05	.39	0.3	0	700	79	0
528	30	.01	.11	0.1	0	200	22	0
93	5	Tr	.02	Tr	0	40	3	0
248	39	.01	.09	Tr	0	230	20	0
155	155	.03	.23	0.1	0	536	38	0
104	128	.02	.24	0.2	0	605	62	0
340	NA	NA	0.1	Tr	0	162	29	0
513	26	.01	.17	0.2	0	297	26	0
74	31	Tr	0.1	Tr	0	240	26	0
CHEESE, PROCESSED								
274	103	.01	.12	Tr	0	200	18	0
270	102	.01	.12	Tr	0	197	18	0
250	75	NA	NA	NA	0	NA	20	0
388	61	Tr	.08	Tr	0	230	24	0

NA: Not available in references used.
*Crude fiber.
**Cooked and drained unless otherwise stated.
***Based on typical recipe; ingredients and nutrients may vary among recipes.
$: Varies depending on amount of salt added.
$$: Varies depending on type of oil used for frying.
TR: Trace.

Food (Portion)	Calories	Carbohydrates (gm.)	Protein (gm.)	Fats (gm.)	Calcium (mg.)	Iron (mg.)
COMBINATION FOODS***						
Beans, baked, homemade (1/2 cup)	190	27	7	6	77	2.5
Beans, baked, with franks (1/2 cup)	182	20	9	8	61	2.2
Beef potpie, home recipe (1/3 of 9-in. pie)	515	39	21	30	29	3.8
Beef vegetable stew (1 cup)	20	15	16	11	29	2.9
Chicken and noodles, homemade (1 cup)	365	26	22	18	26	2.2
Chicken parmigiana, homemade (7 oz.)	308	22	22	15	174	6.3
Chicken potpie, homemade (1/3 of 9-in. pie)	545	42	23	31	70	3.0
Chili with beans, canned (1 cup)	340	31	19	16	82	4.3
Corned beef hash (1 cup)	290	29	22	10	28	2.9
Macaroni and cheese (1 cup)	430	40	17	22	362	1.8
Quiche lorraine (1/8 pie)	600	29	13	48	211	1.0
Spaghetti with tomato sauce and cheese, canned (1 cup)	190	39	6	2	40	2.8
Spaghetti with tomato sauce and cheese, homemade (1 cup)	260	37	9	9	80	2.3
Spaghetti with meatballs and tomato sauce, canned (1 cup)	260	29	12	10	· 53	3.3
Spaghetti with meatballs and tomato sauce, homemade (1 cup)	330	39	19	12	124	3.7
Spinach soufflé (1/2 cup)	110	1	5	9	115	0.7
Tuna noodle casserole, homemade (1 cup)	200	25	18	12	NA	NA
CONDIMENTS						
Catsup (1 T)	15	4	Tr	Tr	3	0.1
Mayonnaise (imitation) (1 T)	35	2	Tr	3	Tr	0
Mayonnaise (regular) (1 T)	100	Tr	Tr	11	3	0.1
Mustard, prepared, yellow (1 T)	5	Tr	Tr	Tr	4	0.1
Soy sauce (1 T)	10	2	2	0	3	0.5
Steak sauce (1 T)	20	3	Tr	Tr	6	0.4
Tartar sauce (1 T)	75 ·	1	Tr ·	8	3	0.1
Worcestershire sauce (1 T)	10	3	Tr	0	15	0.9
COOKIES						
Animal crackers (15)	120	22	2	3	3	0.9
Brownie, commercial with nuts and frosting (1 small)	100	16	1	4	13	0.6
Brownie, homemade with nuts (1, 1 3/4 × 1 3/4 × 7/8 in.)	95	11	1	6	9	0.4
Butter (1 small)	25	4	Tr	1	6	Tr

NA: Not available in references used.

*Crude fiber.

**Cooked and drained unless otherwise stated.

***Based on typical recipe; ingredients and nutrients may vary among recipes.

$: Varies depending on amount of salt added.

$$: Varies depending on type of oil used for frying.

TR: Trace.

Sodium (mg.)	Potassium (mg.)	Thiamine (mg.)	Riboflavin (mg.)	Niacin (mg.)	Vitamin C (mg.)	Vitamin A (IU)	Cholesterol (mg.)	Fiber (gm.)
COMBINATION FOODS ***								
532	452	.17	.06	.51	2	0	6	0.9*
551	301	.07	.07	1.15	3	200	8	1.2*
596	334	.29	.29	4.8	6	4,220	42	NA
292	613	.15	.17	4.7	17	5,690	71	NA
600	149	.05	.17	4.3	Tr	430	103	NA
358	342	.16	.18	4.8	16	1,388	NA	NA
594	343	.32	.32	4.9	5	7,220	56	NA
1,354	594	.08	.18	3.3	8	150	28	NA
40	NA	.15	.21	4.6	21	30	NA	0.6*
1,086	240	0.2	0.4	1.8	1	860	44	NA
653	283	.11	.32	Tr	Tr	1,640	285	NA
955	303	.35	.28	4.5	10	930	3	NA
955	408	.25	.18	2.3	13	1,080	8	NA
1,220	245	.15	.18	2.3	5	100	23	NA
1,009	665	.25	0.3	4.0	22	159	89	NA
381	101	.04	.15	0.2	1	1,730	92	0.8*
NA	NA	NA	NA	NA	NA	NA	NA	NA
CONDIMENTS								
56	54	.01	.01	.01	2	210	0	NA
75	2	0	0	0	0	0	4	NA
80	5	0	0	Tr	0	40	8	NA
63	7	Tr	0.1	Tr	Tr	0	NA	NA
1,029	64	.01	.02	0.6	0	0	0	NA
149	64	.01	.07	Tr	11	50	NA	NA
182	11	Tr	Tr	0	Tr	30	4	NA
147	120	Tr	.03	Tr	27	50	NA	NA
COOKIES								
113	26	.08	.13	1.1	0	0	0	0.1*
59	50	.08	.07	0.3	Tr	70	14	NA
51	35	.05	.05	0.3	Tr	20	18	NA
21	3	Tr	Tr	Tr	0	30	NA	NA

NA: Not available in references used.

*Crude fiber.

**Cooked and drained unless otherwise stated.

***Based on typical recipe; ingredients and nutrients may vary among recipes.

$: Varies depending on amount of salt added.

$$: Varies depending on type of oil used for frying.

TR: Trace.

Food (Portion)	Calories	Carbohydrates (gm.)	Protein (gm.)	Fats (gm.)	Calcium (mg.)	Iron (mg.)
COOKIES *(cont.)*						
Butterscotch (1 small)	115	16	1	5	31	0.5
Chocolate (1)	93	15	2	3	11	0.2
Chocolate chip, commercial (1 med.)	45	7	0.5	2	3	0.2
Chocolate chip, homemade (1 med.)	45	6	0.5	3	3	0.2
Coconut bar (1)	110	14	1	5	16	0.3
Fig bar (1)	55	11	0.5	1	10	0.3
Gingersnaps (3 small)	50	10	1	1	9	0.3
Graham cracker (chocolate covered) (1, 2 × 2 in.)	60	9	1	3	15	0.3
Marshmallow with chocolate coating (1)	55	9	0.5	2	3	0.1
Macaroons (1)	65	9	1	3	4	0.1
Molasses (1)	70	10	1	3	15	0.5
Oatmeal raisin (1 med., 2 5/8-in. diam.)	60	9	1	2	4	0.5
Peanut butter cookie, homemade (1 med., 2 5/8-in. diam.)	60	7	1	4	5	0.3
Peanut butter, sandwich type (1)	60	8	1	2	5	0.1
Sandwich-type (1 med., 3/4-in. diam.)	50	7	0.5	2	3	0.4
Shortbread, homemade (1 large)	70	8	1	4	3	0.3
Sugar, (1 med.)	60	8	0.5	3	12	0.2
Sugar wafer (2)	55	8	0.5	2	4	Tr
Vanilla wafers (3 small)	50	8	1	2	4	Tr
Vienna finger sandwich (1)	70	11	1	3	6	0.3
CRACKERS						
Goldfish (12)	30	4	Tr	2	4	0.2
Graham (2)	60	11	1	1	6	0.4
Melba toast (1 piece)	20	4	1	Tr	6	0.1
Oyster (15)	60	10	1	2	2	0.6
Saltines (4)	50	9	1	1	3	0.5
Whole-wheat wafers (2)	35	5	1	2	3	0.2
Zwieback (1 piece)	30	5	1	1	1	Tr
CREAM AND IMITATION CREAMERS						
Half and half (1 T)	20	1	Tr	2	16	Tr
Half and half (1 cup)	315	10	7	28	254	0.2
Heavy (1 T)	50	Tr	Tr	6	10	Tr
Heavy (1 cup)	820	7	5	88	154	0.1
Imitation coffee creamer (liquid) (1 T)	20	2	Tr	1	1	Tr
Imitation coffee creamer (dry) (1 T)	10	1	Tr	1	Tr	Tr
Light (1 T)	30	1	Tr	3	14	Tr

NA: Not available in references used.

*Crude fiber.

**Cooked and drained unless otherwise stated.

***Based on typical recipe; ingredients and nutrients may vary among recipes.

$: Varies depending on amount of salt added.

$$: Varies depending on type of oil used for frying.

TR: Trace.

Sodium (mg.)	Potassium (mg.)	Thiamine (mg.)	Riboflavin (mg.)	Niacin (mg.)	Vitamin C (mg.)	Vitamin A (IU)	Cholesterol (mg.)	Fiber (gm.)
COOKIES (cont.)								
98	88	.01	.02	Tr	0	NA	NA	NA
29	27	.01	.02	0.1	NA	30	NA	0.1*
35	17	.02	.05	0.2	Tr	10	1	NA
20	20	.02	.02	0.2	0	5	4	NA
33	50	.01	.01	0.1	0	35	NA	0.1*
45	41	.02	.02	0.2	Tr	20	7	0.2*
69	55	Tr	Tr	Tr	NA	10	NA	NA
53	42	.01	.04	0.2	0	10	0	0.1*
27	12	Tr	.01	Tr	Tr	35	NA	NA
5	65	.01	.02	0.1	Tr	0	NA	0.3*
58	21	.03	.02	0.2	0	10	NA	Tr*
74	22	.02	.02	0.2	0	10	Tr	NA
36	28	.02	.02	0.5	0	5	6	NA
21	21	.01	.01	0.4	0	25	NA	NA
47	16	.02	.02	0.2	0	0	0	NA
62	9	.04	.03	0.4	Tr	150	0	NA
65	8	.02	.02	0.3	0	10	7	NA
21	7	Tr	Tr	0.1	0	15	NA	Tr*
28	8	Tr	.01	Tr	0	10	8	Tr*
NA	NA	NA	NA	NA	NA	NA	NA	NA
CRACKERS								
50	12	0	.02	0.2	0	1	NA	NA
86	36	.02	.03	0.6	0	0	0	2.8
4	11	.01	.01	0.1	0	0	0	NA
153	17	.05	.07	0.8	0	0	NA	0.1
165	17	.06	.05	0.6	0	0	4	0.5
59	31	.02	.03	0.4	0	0	NA	0
18	11	Tr	Tr	NA	0	NA	0	0
CREAM AND IMITATION CREAMERS								
6	19	.01	.02	Tr	Tr	70	6	0
98	314	.08	.36	0.2	2	1,050	89	0
6	11	Tr	.02	Tr	Tr	220	21	0
89	179	.05	.26	0.1	1	3,500	326	0
12	29	0	0	0	0	10	0	0
4	16	0	Tr	0	0	Tr	0	0
6	18	Tr	.02	Tr	Tr	110	10	0

NA: Not available in references used.

*Crude fiber.

**Cooked and drained unless otherwise stated.

***Based on typical recipe; ingredients and nutrients may vary among recipes.

$: Varies depending on amount of salt added.

$$: Varies depending on type of oil used for frying.

TR: Trace.

Food (Portion)	Calories	Carbohydrates (gm.)	Protein (gm.)	Fats (gm.)	Calcium (mg.)	Iron (mg.)
CREAM AND IMITATION CREAMERS *(cont.)*						
Light (1 cup)	470	9	6	46	231	0.1
Light whipping (unwhipped) (1 T)	45	Tr	Tr	5	10	Tr
Light whipping (unwhipped) (1 cup)	700	7	5	74	166	0.1
Sour (1 T)	25	1	Tr	3	14	Tr
Sour (1 cup)	495	10	7	48	268	0.1
Whipped topping (1 T)	10	Tr	Tr	1	3	Tr
Whipped topping (1 cup)	155	7	2	13	61	Tr
EGGS						
Boiled (1 large)	75	0.6	6.25	5.0	25	0.7
Fried, with margarine and salt (1 large)	91	.63	6.23	6.9	25	.72
Scrambled, with whole milk and salt (1 large)	101	1.34	6.77	7.45	44	.73
White (1 large)	17	.34	3.5	0	2	.01
Yolk (1 large)	50	0.3	2.78	5.12	23	.59
FAST FOODS						
Apple pie (1)	280	37	3	13	16	0.9
Biscuit with bacon, eggs, cheese (1)	485	33	16	32	2	2.6
Biscuit with sausage, egg (1)	555	35	18	37	144	3.7
Cheeseburger, regular (1)	300	28	15	15	135	2.3
Cheeseburger, 4 oz. patty (1)	525	40	30	31	236	4.5
Cheeseburger, double (1)	680	44	37	40	218	6.3
Chicken, fried: *See* Poultry						
Chicken, nuggets (6 pieces)	265	12	20	16	14	1.0
Chicken sandwich (1)	615	49	28	34	87	3.0
Cole slaw (1 average serving)	125	10	1	9	NA	NA
Croissant, with egg, cheese, bacon or ham (1)	345	20	16	22	136	2.1
Enchilada (1)	235	24	20	16	322	11.0
English muffin, with egg, cheese, bacon (1)	360	31	18	18	197	3.1
Fish sandwich, regular with cheese (1)	420	39	16	23	132	1.8
Fish sandwich, large without cheese (1)	470	41	18	27	61	2.2
French fries (1 regular serving)	230	28	3	12	NA	0.8
Ham/cheese sandwich (1)	400	38	24	22	201	2.9
Hamburger, regular (1)	245	28	12	11	56	2.2
Hamburger, 4 oz. patty (1)	445	38	25	21	75	4.8
Hamburger, double (1)	685	42	44	39	NA	7.3
Hot dog (1)	280	21	11	16	80	1.4
Hot dog with cheese (1)	330	21	15	21	220	1.4
Hot dog with chili (1)	320	23	13	20	150	1.8

NA: Not available in references used.

*Crude fiber.

**Cooked and drained unless otherwise stated.

***Based on typical recipe; ingredients and nutrients may vary among recipes.

$: Varies depending on amount of salt added.

$$: Varies depending on type of oil used for frying.

TR: Trace.

Sodium (mg.)	Potassium (mg.)	Thiamine (mg.)	Riboflavin (mg.)	Niacin (mg.)	Vitamin C (mg.)	Vitamin A (IU)	Cholesterol (mg.)	Fiber (gm.)
CREAM AND IMITATION CREAMERS *(cont.)*								
95	292	.08	.36	0.1	2	1,730	159	0
5	15	Tr	.02	Tr	Tr	170	17	0
82	231	.06	.3	0.1	1	2,690	265	0
6	17	Tr	.02	Tr	0	90	5	0
123	331	.08	.34	0.2	2	1,820	102	0
4	4	Tr	Tr	Tr	0	30	2	0
78	88	.02	.04	Tr	0	550	46	0
EGGS								
63	60	.03	.25	.04	0	317	213	0
162	61	.026	.24	.035	0	394	223	0
171	84	.032	.27	.048	0.1	416	226	0
55	48	Tr	.15	.031	0	0	0	0
7	16	.028	.06	Tr	0	323	213	0
FAST FOODS								
405	NA	.11	.07	.07	40	NA	7.1	NA
1,269	NA	0.3	.43	2.32	2.0	650	263	NA
1,167	NA	.47	.43	3.4	1.4	590	289	NA
672	219	.26	.24	3.7	1.0	340	44	NA
1,224	407	.33	.48	7.4	3.0	670	104	NA
1,240	NA	.44	.54	9.2	NA	545	NA	NA
574	NA	.12	.12	7.3	NA	100	60	NA
998	NA	.32	0.4	7.6	NA	NA	68	NA
NA	NA	NA	NA	NA	NA	NA	NA	NA
874	219	0.4	.31	2.5	NA	430	255	NA
4,451	2,180	.18	.26	Tr	Tr	2,270	19	NA
832	201	.46	0.5	3.7	1.0	650	213	NA
667	274	.32	.26	3.3	2	160	56	NA
621	375	.35	.23	3.5	1	110	91	NA
NA$	NA	0.1	.03	1.8	10	NA	$$	NA
1,419	NA	.74	.56	4.8	NA	NA	60	NA
463	202	.23	.24	3.8	1	80	32	NA
763	404	.38	.38	7.8	1	160	71	NA
903	NA	.46	.48	9.4	NA	NA	121	NA
830	80	.12	.14	3.0	NA	NA	45	NA
990	150	.12	.17	3.0	NA	100	55	NA
985	150	.15	.26	4.0	NA	NA	55	NA

NA: Not available in references used.

*Crude fiber.

**Cooked and drained unless otherwise stated.

***Based on typical recipe; ingredients and nutrients may vary among recipes.

$: Varies depending on amount of salt added.

$$: Varies depending on type of oil used for frying.

TR: Trace.

Food (Portion)	Calories	Carbohydrates (gm.)	Protein (gm.)	Fats (gm.)	Calcium (mg.)	Iron (mg.)
FAST FOODS *(cont.)*						
Onion rings (1 regular serving)	260	27	4	15	NA	0.7
Pizza, cheese (1 slice)	290	39	15	9	220	1.6
Potato, baked, stuffed with bacon and cheese (1)	570	57	19	30	160	2.7
Potato, baked, stuffed with broccoli and cheese (1)	520	63	13	24	250	2.7
Potato, baked, stuffed with chili and cheese (1)	510	63	22	20	200	3.6
Roast beef sandwiches (1)	345	34	22	13	60	4.0
Taco (1)	195	15	9	11	109	1.2
Tostada (1)	270	28	10	13	186	3.1
Tostada, beef (1)	360	29	18	19	204	5.0
Submarine sandwich, ham, salami, cheese (1, 6 in.)	450	61	14	17	50	2.1
Submarine sandwich, roast beef (1, 6 in.)	370	56	22	7	39	1.5
Submarine sandwich, tuna (1, 6 in.)	580	61	21	28	83	1.2
FISH/SHELLFISH						
Anchovy, canned (3 fillets)	20	Tr	2	1	20	0.3
Black bass, baked (3 oz.)	210	2	17	14	70	0.9
Bass (3 oz.)	117	Tr	20	4	27	0.7
Bluefish, boiled (3 oz.)	135	0	22	4	24	0.6
Bluefish, fried (3 oz.)	170	4	19	8	29	0.8
Clams, raw (3 oz.)	65	2	11	1	59	2.6
Clams, canned, drained (3 oz.)	85	2	13	2	47	3.5
Cod, broiled (3 oz.)	145	0	23	4	26	0.8
Cod, dried, salted (3 oz.)	110	0	24	1	189	3.0
Crabmeat, canned (3 oz.)	85	1	14	2	38	0.7
Crab leg, steamed (1 med.)	40	Tr	7	1	18	0.3
Crabmeat, steamed (3 oz.)	80	Tr	14	2	36	0.5
Crab, softshell (1 med.)	213	12	12	13	41	1.2
Flounder/sole, baked without fat (3 oz.)	80	Tr	17	1	13	0.3
Haddock, broiled (3 oz.)	120	Tr	17	6	11	0.4
Haddock, fried (3 oz.)	175	7	17	9	34	1.0
Halibut, broiled with butter (3 oz.)	140	Tr	20	6	14	0.7
Herring, pickled (3 oz.)	190	0	17	13	29	0.9
Herring, Atlantic, broiled (3 oz.)	215	0	21	14	NA	1.2
Lobster tail, cooked (1 med.)	100	Tr	19	1	68	0.8
Lobster, canned or cooked (3 oz.)	80	Tr	16	1	55	0.7
Mackerel, Atlantic (3 oz.)	200	0	18	13	5	1.0

NA: Not available in references used.

*Crude fiber.

**Cooked and drained unless otherwise stated.

***Based on typical recipe; ingredients and nutrients may vary among recipes.

$: Varies depending on amount of salt added.

$$: Varies depending on type of oil used for frying.

TR: Trace.

Sodium (mg.)	Potassium (mg.)	Thiamine (mg.)	Riboflavin (mg.)	Niacin (mg.)	Vitamin C (mg.)	Vitamin A (IU)	Cholesterol (mg.)	Fiber (gm.)
FAST FOODS (cont.)								
$	NA	NA	NA	NA	NA	NA	$$	NA
699	230	.34	.29	4.2	2	750	56	NA
1,180	1,380	.22	.17	3.0	36	750	22	NA
452	NA	.30	.30	5.0	76.5	NA	23	NA
610	1,590	0.3	.26	4.0	36	750	22	NA
757	338	0.4	.33	6.0	2	240	55	NA
456	263	.09	.07	1.4	1	420	21	NA
534	NA	NA	NA	NA	NA	NA	10	NA
714	NA	NA	NA	NA	NA	NA	49	NA
1,032	145	NA	NA	NA	NA	NA	NA	0.6*
482	294	NA	NA	NA	NA	NA	NA	0.8*
824	160	NA	NA	NA	NA	NA	NA	0.6*
FISH/SHELLFISH								
99	71	NA	NA	NA	NA	NA	7	0
50	187	.05	.12	2.5	0	71	NA	0
375	317	0.1	0.1	3.0	2	97	56	0
87	353	.09	.09	1.6	NA	42	59	0
123	353	.09	.09	0.1	NA	NA	51	0
102	154	.09	.15	1.1	9	90	43	0
102	119	.01	.09	0.9	3	90	54	0
93	341	.07	.09	2.5	NA	150	72	0
6,888	135	.07	.38	NA	NA	NA	69	0
840	93	.07	.07	1.6	0	31	84	0
NA	NA	.07	.03	1.2	1	924	43	0
177	151	.13	.06	2.4	2	1,811	79	0
300	126	0.1	0.1	2.1	1	16	87	0.3
101	286	.05	.08	1.7	1	30	59	0
60	299	.03	.06	1.8	3	232	NA	0
123	270	.06	0.1	2.9	0	70	75	0
103	441	.06	.07	7.7	1	610	62	0
850	85	.04	.18	2.8	0	110	85	0
NA	NA	.01	.15	3.3	0	130	NA	0
218	187	0.1	.07	2.3	0	NA	88	0
176	151	.03	.06	1.9	0	NA	71	0
62	353	.01	.13	2.8	0	109	85	0

NA: Not available in references used.

*Crude fiber.

**Cooked and drained unless otherwise stated.

***Based on typical recipe; ingredients and nutrients may vary among recipes.

$: Varies depending on amount of salt added.

$$: Varies depending on type of oil used for frying.

TR: Trace.

Food (Portion)	Calories	Carbohydrates (gm.)	Protein (gm.)	Fats (gm.)	Calcium (mg.)	Iron (mg.)
FISH/SHELLFISH *(cont.)*						
Mussel, steamed (3 oz.)	138	3	14	7	90	3.0
Oysters, raw (3 oz.)	55	3	7	1	79	5.5
Oysters, breaded, fried (1 med.)	90	5	5	5	49	3.0
Salmon, red (3 oz.)	140	0	21	5	26	0.5
Salmon, canned (3 oz.)	120	0	17	5	167	0.7
Sardines, canned in oil (3 oz.)	175	0	20	9	371	2.6
Scallops, steamed (3 oz.)	95	12	19	1	97	2.5
Scallops, frozen, breaded, fried (6 med.)	195	10	15	10	39	2.0
Shrimp, raw (10 large)	65	Tr	14	Tr	67	1.8
Shrimp, fried (7 med.)	200	11	16	10	61	2.0
Sturgeon, smoked (3 oz.)	125	0	26	2	11	0.6
Sturgeon, steamed (3 oz.)	135	0	21	5	37	1.7
Swordfish (3 oz.)	145	0	24	5	23	1.1
Trout (3 oz.)	175	Tr	21	9	26	1.0
Tuna, canned in oil, drained (3 oz.)	165	0	24	7	7	1.6
Tuna, canned in water, drained (3 oz.)	135	0	30	1	17	0.6
Tuna salad (1/2 cup)	190	10	16	10	16	1.2
FROZEN DESSERTS						
Fruit ice/sorbet (1/2 cup)	123	30	Tr	Tr	NA	NA
Ice cream, chocolate (1/2 cup)	150	16	3	8	93	NA
Ice cream, sandwich (1 med.)	167	26	3	6	73	0.1
Ice cream, strawberry (1/2 cup)	125	16	2	6	73	NA
Ice cream, vanilla, 11% fat (1/2 cup)	135	16	2	7	88	Tr
Ice cream, vanilla, 16% fat (1/2 cup)	175	16	2	12	76	Tr
Ice cream, vanilla, soft (12/ cup)	190	19	4	12	118	0.2
Ice milk, chocolate or strawberry (1/2 cup)	100	16	3	3	112	NA
Ice milk, vanilla (1/2 cup)	90	15	2	3	88	0.1
Popsicle (3 oz.)	70	18	0	0	0	Tr
Pudding pop (1)	95	16	2	3	76	Tr
Sherbet (1 cup)	135	30	1	2	52	0.2
Tofu, frozen dessert (1/2 cup)	220	21	3	13	NA	NA
Yogurt, frozen (1 bar)	65	12	2	1	NA	NA
Yogurt, frozen, chocolate-coated (1)	135	12	2	8	NA	NA
Yogurt, frozen, fruit varieties (1/2 cup)	110	21	4	1	NA	NA
FRUITS AND FRUIT JUICES						
Apple (1 med.)	80	21	Tr	Tr	10	0.2
Apple, without skin (2 3/4-in. diam.)	70	19	Tr	Tr	5	0.1

NA: Not available in references used.

*Crude fiber.

**Cooked and drained unless otherwise stated.

***Based on typical recipe; ingredients and nutrients may vary among recipes.

$: Varies depending on amount of salt added.

$$: Varies depending on type of oil used for frying.

TR: Trace.

Sodium (mg.)	Potassium (mg.)	Thiamine (mg.)	Riboflavin (mg.)	Niacin (mg.)	Vitamin C (mg.)	Vitamin A (IU)	Cholesterol (mg.)	Fiber (gm.)
FISH/SHELLFISH *(cont.)*								
569	281	0.2	0.2	1.2	0	465	42	0
61	102	.12	.15	2.1	8.4	259	42	0
70	64	.07	.10	1.3	4.0	150	35	0
55	305	.18	.14	5.5	NA	290	60	0
443	307	.03	.15	6.8	NA	60	34	0
425	349	.03	.17	4.6	NA	190	85	0
223	400	NA	NA	NA	NA	NA	45	0
298	369	.11	.11	1.6	0	70	70	0
81	71	.01	.02	1.9	NA	NA	87	0
384	189	.06	.09	2.8	0	90	168	0
5,234	132	NA	NA	NA	NA	NA	80	0
91	197	NA	NA	NA	NA	NA	65	0
113	441	.03	.04	9.2	NA	1,722	67	0
122	297	.07	.07	2.3	1	230	71	0
303	298	.04	.09	10.1	0	70	55	0
468	255	.03	0.1	13.4	0	110	48	0
438	266	.03	.07	6.6	3	115	40	NA
FROZEN DESSERTS								
NA	NA	NA	NA	NA	NA	NA	0	0
38	NA	.04	.14	0.1	NA	280	NA	NA
92	102	.02	0.1	0.5	NA	190	NA	NA
30	NA	.02	0.1	Tr	NA	250	NA	NA
58	128	.02	.16	Tr	Tr	270	30	0
54	110	.02	.14	Tr	Tr	450	44	0
76	169	.04	.22	0.1	Tr	395	76	0
47	NA	.04	.16	0.1	NA	NA	NA	NA
52	132	.04	.18	Tr	Tr	105	9	0
11	4	0	0	0	0	0	0	0
63	83	.03	.11	Tr	Tr	100	1	NA
44	99	.02	.09	Tr	2	95	7	0
105	29	NA	NA	NA	NA	0	0	NA
15	NA	NA	NA	NA	NA	NA	5	NA
15	NA	NA	NA	NA	NA	NA	5	NA
25	NA	NA	NA	NA	NA	NA	5	NA
FRUITS AND FRUIT JUICES								
1	159	.02	.02	.11	8	74	0	2.8
0	144	.02	.01	0.1	5	56	0	2.6

NA: Not available in references used.

*Crude fiber.

**Cooked and drained unless otherwise stated.

***Based on typical recipe; ingredients and nutrients may vary among recipes.

$: Varies depending on amount of salt added.

$$: Varies depending on type of oil used for frying.

TR: Trace.

Food (Portion)	Calories	Carbohydrates (gm.)	Protein (gm.)	Fats (gm.)	Calcium (mg.)	Iron (mg.)
FRUITS AND FRUIT JUICES *(cont.)*						
Apple, dried, sulfured (10 rings)	155	42	1	Tr	9	0.9
Apple juice, bottled or canned (4 oz.)	110	15	Tr	Tr	8	0.5
Applesauce, sweetened (1/2 cup)	95	25	Tr	Tr	5	0.4
Apricots (3 raw fruits)	50	12	1	Tr	15	0.6
Apricots, canned, fruit and liquid (1/2 cup)	60	15	1	Tr	15	0.4
Apricots, canned, heavy syrup, fruit and liquid (1/2 cup)	105	28	1	Tr	11	0.8
Apricots, dried, sulfured (10 halves)	85	22	1	Tr	16	1.6
Avocado, California (1)	305	12	4	30	19	2.0
Avocado, Florida (1)	340	27	5	27	33	1.6
Banana, without peel (1)	105	27	1	1	7	0.4
Blackberries, raw (1/2 cup)	35	9	1	Tr	23	0.4
Blueberries (1/2 cup)	40	10	Tr	Tr	4	0.1
Cantaloupe (1/2)	95	22	2	1	28	0.6
Cantaloupe (1 cup cubes)	55	13	1	Tr	17	0.3
Cherries, sweet (10)	50	11	1	1	10	0.3
Cherries, sweet, canned (1/2 cup)	105	27	1	Tr	12	0.5
Cranberries, raw (1 cup whole)	45	12	Tr	Tr	7	0.2
Cranberry juice cocktail (4 oz.)	75	19	Tr	Tr	4	0.2
Cranberry sauce, canned, sweetened (1/4 cup)	105	27	Tr	Tr	2	0.2
Dates, dried (2)	45	12	Tr	Tr	5	0.2
Figs, dried (1)	50	12	1	Tr	27	0.4
Fruit cocktail, canned, juice (1/2 cup)	55	15	1	Tr	10	0.3
Fruit cocktail, heavy syrup (1/2 cup)	95	24	1	Tr	8	0.4
Grapes, sweet, seedless (10)	35	9	Tr	Tr	6	0.1
Grapes, seeded (10)	40	10	Tr	Tr	6	0.1
Grape juice, canned or bottled, unsweetened (1/2 cup)	80	19	1	Tr	11	0.3
Grape juice, sweetened from frozen concentrate (1/2 cup)	65	16	Tr	Tr	4	0.1
Grapefruit, white (1/2)	40	10	1	Tr	14	0.1
Grapefruit, red (1/2)	40	10	1	Tr	14	0.1
Grapefruit, canned, syrup (1/2 cup)	75	20	1	Tr	18	0.5
Grapefruit juice, unsweetened fresh, canned, or frozen (1/2 cup)	50	12	1	Tr	10	0.2
Grapefruit juice, sweetened (1/2 cup)	60	14	1	Tr	10	0.4
Honeydew cubes (1)	60	16	1	Tr	10	0.1

NA: Not available in references used.
*Crude fiber.
**Cooked and drained unless otherwise stated.
***Based on typical recipe; ingredients and nutrients may vary among recipes.
$: Varies depending on amount of salt added.
$$: Varies depending on type of oil used for frying.
TR: Trace.

Sodium (mg.)	Potassium (mg.)	Thiamine (mg.)	Riboflavin (mg.)	Niacin (mg.)	Vitamin C (mg.)	Vitamin A (IU)	Cholesterol (mg.)	Fiber (gm.)
FRUITS AND FRUIT JUICES *(cont.)*								
56	288	0	.01	0.6	2	0	0	1.8*
4	148	.03	.02	0.1	1	0	0	Tr*
4	78	.02	.04	0.2	2	14	0	2.0
1	313	.03	.04	0.6	11	2,769	0	2.2
4	204	.02	.02	0.4	6	2,098	0	3.0
5	180	.03	.03	0.5	4	1,587	0	.5*
3	482	Tr	.05	1.0	1	2,534	0	1.0*
21	1,097	.19	.21	3.3	14	1,060	0	3.6*
15	1,484	.33	.37	5.8	24	1,860	0	6.4*
1	451	.05	.11	0.6	10	92	0	2.1
0	141	.02	.03	0.3	15	119	0	4.5
4	64	.03	.03	0.3	9	72	0	2.5
23	825	0.1	.06	1.5	113	8,608	0	2.7
14	494	.06	.03	0.9	68	5,158	0	1.5
0	152	.03	.04	0.3	5	146	0	1.2
3	187	.03	.05	0.5	5	199	0	0.4*
1	67	.03	.02	0.1	13	44	0	4.0
5	30	.06	.02	Tr	54	NA	0	NA
20	17	.01	.01	Tr	1	14	0	0.2*
Tr	108	.02	.02	0.4	0	8	0	1.6
2	133	.01	.02	0.1	Tr	25	0	3.7
4	118	.02	.02	0.5	3	378	0	0.4*
7	112	.02	.02	0.5	2	262	0	0.6*
1	93	.05	.03	0.2	5	40	0	NA
1	105	.05	.03	0.2	6	40	0	NA
4	167	.03	.05	0.3	Tr	10	0	NA
2	26	.02	.03	0.2	30	10	0	NA
Tr	167	.04	.02	0.3	41	10	0	1.7
Tr	167	.04	.02	0.3	41	310	0	1.7
2	164	.05	.02	0.3	27	0	0	0.4*
1	186	.05	.02	0.2	42	10	0	NA
2	202	.05	.03	0.4	34	10	0	NA
17	461	.13	.03	1.0	42	68	0	1.4

NA: Not available in references used.

*Crude fiber.

**Cooked and drained unless otherwise stated.

***Based on typical recipe; ingredients and nutrients may vary among recipes.

$: Varies depending on amount of salt added.

$$: Varies depending on type of oil used for frying.

TR: Trace.

Food (Portion)	Calories	Carbohydrates (gm.)	Protein (gm.)	Fats (gm.)	Calcium (mg.)	Iron (mg.)
FRUITS AND FRUIT JUICES *(cont.)*						
Kiwi fruit (1 med.)	45	11	1	Tr	20	0.3
Lemon, without peel (1 med.)	15	5	1	Tr	15	0.3
Lemon juice, raw (1/4 cup)	15	5	Tr	Tr	4	Tr
Lemon juice, bottled (1/4 cup)	15	4	Tr	Tr	6	0.1
Lime (1)	20	7	Tr	Tr	22	0.4
Lime juice, raw (1/4 cup, 4 T)	15	6	Tr	Tr	6	0.2
Mango (1 med.)	135	35	1	Tr	21	0.3
Nectarine, raw (1)	65	16	1	1	6	0.2
Orange, raw (1 med.)	60	15	1	Tr	52	0.1
Orange, raw sections without membrane (1/2 cup)	40	11	1	Tr	36	0.1
Orange juice, fresh raw (1/2 cup)	55	13	1	Tr	14	0.2
Orange juice, canned, unsweetened (1/2 cup)	50	12	1	Tr	10	0.6
Orange juice, from frozen (1/2 cup)	55	13	1	Tr	11	0.1
Orange-grapefruit juice, canned (1/2 cup)	55	13	1	Tr	10	0.6
Papaya (1 cup cubed pieces = 1/2 fruit)	55	14	1	Tr	33	0.1
Peaches (1 2-1/2-in. diam., approx. 1/2 cup sliced)	35	10	1	Tr	5	0.1
Peaches, canned juice (1/2 cup)	55	14	1	Tr	8	0.3
Peaches, canned, heavy syrup (1/2 cup)	95	26	1	Tr	4	0.3
Peaches, dried uncooked (5 halves)	155	40	2	Tr	18	2.6
Pears (1 med.)	100	25	1	1	19	0.4
Pears, canned, juice (1/2 cup)	60	16	Tr	Tr	10	0.6
Pears, canned, heavy syrup (1/2 cup)	95	24	Tr	Tr	6	0.3
Pineapple (1/2 cup diced)	40	10	Tr	Tr	6	0.3
Pineapple, canned, juice (1 slice)	35	9	Tr	Tr	8	0.2
Pineapple, canned, juice (1/2 cup chunks/tidbits)	75	20	Tr	Tr	17	0.4
Pineapple, canned, heavy syrup (1 slice)	45	12	Tr	Tr	8	0.2
Pineapple, canned, heavy syrup (1/2 cup chunks/tidbits)	100	26	Tr	Tr	18	0.5
Pineapple juice, canned (1/2 cup)	70	17	Tr	Tr	21	0.3
Pineapple juice from concentrate (1/2 cup)	65	16	Tr	Tr	14	0.4
Plum (1 med.)	35	9	1	Tr	2	0.1
Plum, canned light syrup (3 fruits)	85	22	Tr	Tr	13	1.1
Pomegranate (1)	105	26	1	Tr	5	0.5
Prunes, dried (5 large)	115	31	1	Tr	25	1.2
Prunes, cooked, unsweetened (1/2 cup)	115	30	1	Tr	24	1.2

NA: Not available in references used.

*Crude fiber.

**Cooked and drained unless otherwise stated.

***Based on typical recipe; ingredients and nutrients may vary among recipes.

$: Varies depending on amount of salt added.

$$: Varies depending on type of oil used for frying.

TR: Trace.

Sodium (mg.)	Potassium (mg.)	Thiamine (mg.)	Riboflavin (mg.)	Niacin (mg.)	Vitamin C (mg.)	Vitamin A (IU)	Cholesterol (mg.)	Fiber (gm.)
FRUITS AND FRUIT JUICES *(cont.)*								
4	252	.02	.04	0.4	74	133	0	0.84*
1	80	.02	.01	0.1	31	17	0	0.2*
0	76	.02	Tr	0.1	28	12	0	NA
12	62	.02	.01	0.1	15	9	0	NA
1	68	.02	.01	0.1	20	7	0	NA
Tr	67	.01	.01	0.1	18	6	0	NA
4	322	.12	.12	1.2	57	8,060	0	2.9
0	288	.02	.06	1.3	7	1,001	0	1.9
Tr	237	.11	.05	0.4	70	270	0	1.6
Tr	163	.08	.04	0.3	48	184	0	0.4*
1	248	.11	.03	0.5	62	248	0	0.1*
3	218	.07	.04	0.4	43	218	0	0.1*
1	237	.08	.02	0.2	48	97	0	0.1*
4	195	.07	.04	0.4	36	146	0	NA
4	359	.04	.04	0.5	86	2,819	0	1.7
0	171	.02	.04	0.9	6	465	0	1.4
6	158	.01	.02	0.7	4	472	0	0.3*
8	117	.01	.03	0.8	4	424	0	0.4*
4	648	Tr	.14	2.8	3	1,406	0	1.9*
1	208	.03	.07	.17	7	33	0	5.0
5	119	.01	.01	.25	2	7	0	1.2*
6	82	.01	.02	0.3	1	0	0	1.5*
Tr	88	.07	.03	0.3	12	18	0	1.2
1	70	.06	.01	0.2	6	22	0	0.2*
2	152	.12	.02	0.4	12	48	0	0.2*
1	60	.05	.02	0.2	4	8	0	0.2*
2	132	.11	.03	0.4	9	18	0	0.6*
1	167	.07	.02	0.3	13	6	0	0.1*
2	170	.09	.02	0.2	15	12	0	0.1*
0	113	.03	.06	0.3	6	213	0	1.4
26	123	.02	.05	0.4	1	352	0	0.4*
5	399	.05	.05	0.5	9	NA	0	0.3*
2	365	.04	.08	1.0	2	970	0	7.9
2	354	.02	.11	0.8	3	324	0	8.6

NA: Not available in references used.

*Crude fiber.

**Cooked and drained unless otherwise stated.

***Based on typical recipe; ingredients and nutrients may vary among recipes.

$: Varies depending on amount of salt added.

$$: Varies depending on type of oil used for frying.

TR: Trace.

Food (Portion)	Calories	Carbohydrates (gm.)	Protein (gm.)	Fats (gm.)	Calcium (mg.)	Iron (mg.)
FRUITS AND FRUIT JUICES *(cont.)*						
Prune juice (1/2 cup)	90	22	1	Tr	15	1.5
Raisins (1/2 cup not packed)	220	58	2	Tr	36	1.5
Raisins (seedless, packet 1 1/2 oz. or 1 1/2 T)	40	11	Tr	Tr	7	0.3
Strawberries (1 cup)	45	10.5	0.9	0.6	21	.57
Strawberries, frozen, sweetened (1 cup)	245	66.1	1.4	0.3	28	1.49
Strawberries, frozen, unsweetened (1 cup)	52	13.6	0.6	0.2	23	1.12
Tangerine (1 med.)	37	9.4	.05	0.2	12	.09
Watermelon (1 cup)	50	11.5	1.0	0.7	13	.28
GAME						
Frog legs, flour-coated, fried (4 large)	280	8	17	19	19	1.3
Rabbit, stewed (3 oz.)	185	0	25	9	18	1.3
Venison, roasted (3 oz.)	125	0	25	1.9	17	3.0
GRAVIES						
Beef, canned (2 T)	15	1	1	1	2	0.2
Brown, from dry mix (2 T)	10	2	Tr	Tr	8	Tr
Chicken, canned (2 T)	25	2	1	2	6	0.1
Chicken, from dry mix (2 T)	10	2	Tr	Tr	5	NA
Mushroom, canned (2 T)	15	2	Tr	1	2	0.2
HONEYS, JAMS/PRESERVES, AND JELLIES						
Honey (1 cup)	1,030	279	1	0	17	1.7
Honey (1 T)	65	17	Tr	0	1	0.1
Jams/preserves (1 T)	55	14	Tr	Tr	4	0.2
Jams/preserves (1 packet)	40	10	Tr	Tr	3	0.1
Jellies (1 T)	50	13	Tr	Tr	2	0.1
Jellies (1 packet)	40	10	Tr	Tr	1	Tr
LAMB						
Leg, lean and fat, roasted (3 oz.)	235	0	22	16	9	1.4
Leg, lean only (3 oz.)	160	0	24	6	11	1.9
Loin chop, lean and fat, broiled (1 large chop)	340	0	21	28	9	1.2
Loin chop, lean only (1 large chop)	120	0	18	5	8	1.3
Rib chop, lean and fat, broiled (1 large chop)	360	0	18	32	8	1.0
Rib chop, lean only (1 large chop)	120	0	16	6	6	1.1
LEGUMES						
Black beans, cooked (1/2 cup)	115	20	8	Tr	24	1.8
Blackeyed peas, dry, cooked (1/2 cup)	95	18	7	Tr	22	1.6

NA: Not available in references used.
*Crude fiber.
**Cooked and drained unless otherwise stated.
***Based on typical recipe; ingredients and nutrients may vary among recipes.
$: Varies depending on amount of salt added.
$$: Varies depending on type of oil used for frying.
TR: Trace.

Sodium (mg.)	Potassium (mg.)	Thiamine (mg.)	Riboflavin (mg.)	Niacin (mg.)	Vitamin C (mg.)	Vitamin A (IU)	Cholesterol (mg.)	Fiber (gm.)
FRUITS AND FRUIT JUICES *(cont.)*								
6	353	.02	.09	1.0	5	4	0	Tr*
8	544	.11	.06	0.6	2	6	0	4.9
2	105	.02	.01	0.1	Tr	Tr	0	1.0
2	247	.03	.10	0.3	85	41	0	0.8
8	249	.04	.13	1.02	106	61	0	1.6
3	220	.03	.06	.07	61	66	0	1.2
1	132	.09	.02	0.1	26	77	0	0.3
3	186	.13	.03	0.3	15	58	0	0.5
GAME								
NA	NA	.11	.23	1.2	NA	NA	50	0
35	313	.04	.06	9.5	0	0	55	0
60	286	.31	.24	6.3	0	0	55	0
GRAVIES								
15	24	.01	.01	0.2	0	0	1	NA
143	7	Tr	.01	0.1	NA	NA	Tr	.11*
172	32	Tr	Tr	0.1	0	110	1	NA
142	NA	NA	.02	NA	NA	NA	Tr	.06*
170	32	.01	.02	0.2	0	0	0	NA
HONEYS, JAMS/PRESERVES, AND JELLIES								
17	173	.02	.14	1.0	3	0	0	0
1	11	Tr	.01	0.1	Tr	0	0	0
2	18	Tr	.01	Tr	Tr	Tr	0	NA
2	12	Tr	Tr	Tr	Tr	Tr	0	NA
5	16	Tr	.01	Tr	1	Tr	0	NA
4	13	Tr	Tr	Tr	1	Tr	0	NA
LAMB								
53	241	.13	.23	4.7	NA	Tr	83	0
60	273	.14	.26	5.3	NA	Tr	85	0
51	234	.11	.22	4.8	NA	Tr	93	0
45	205	0.1	.18	4.0	NA	Tr	65	0
44	200	.11	.19	4.1	NA	Tr	83	0
38	174	.09	.15	3.4	NA	Tr	85	0
LEGUMES								
1	306	.21	.05	0.4	0	Tr	0	1.75*
10	286	.20	.05	0.5	0	15	0	12.4

NA: Not available in references used.

*Crude fiber.

**Cooked and drained unless otherwise stated.

***Based on typical recipe; ingredients and nutrients may vary among recipes.

$: Varies depending on amount of salt added.

$$: Varies depending on type of oil used for frying.

TR: Trace.

Food (Portion)	Calories	Carbohydrates (gm.)	Protein (gm.)	Fats (gm.)	Calcium (mg.)	Iron (mg.)
LEGUMES *(cont.)*						
Chickpeas, canned (solids and liquids) (1/2 cup)	143	27	6	1	39	1.6
Chickpeas, cooked (1/2 cup)	135	22	7	2	40	2.4
Kidney beans, red, canned (solids and liquids) (1/2 cup)	110	20	7	Tr	31	1.6
Kidney beans, red, cooked (1/2 cup)	110	20	8	Tr	25	2.6
Lentils, cooked (1/2 cup)	115	20	9	Tr	19	3.3
Pinto beans, canned (solids and liquids) (1/2 cup)	95	17	5	Tr	44	1.9
Pinto beans, cooked (1/2 cup)	115	22	7	Tr	41	2.2
Split peas, cooked (1/2 cup)	115	21	8	Tr	13	1.3
Tofu, raw (1/2 cup)	95	2	10	6	130	6.6
White beans, canned (liquids and solids) (1/2 cup)	155	29	10	Tr	96	4.0
White beans, cooked (1/2 cup)	125	23	9	Tr	81	3.3
MILK/MILK PRODUCTS						
1% (1 cup)	100	10	8	3	300	0.1
2% (1 cup)	120	12	8	5	297	0.1
Buttermilk (1 cup)	100	12	8	2	285	0.1
Skim (1 cup)	85	12	8	Tr	302	0.1
Whole (1 cup)	150	11	8	8	291	0.1
Chocolate milk (1 cup)	210	26	8	8	280	0.6
Cocoa, homemade (1 cup)	220	26	9	9	298	0.8
Cocoa, (mix/water) (1 cup)	100	22	3	1	90	0.3
Condensed, sweet (1 cup)	980	166	24	27	868	0.6
Eggnog (nonalcoholic) (1 cup)	340	34	10	19	330	0.5
Evaporated, skim (1 cup)	200	29	19	1	738	0.7
Milkshake, chocolate (10 oz.)	335	60	9	8	374	0.9
Milkshake, vanilla (10 oz.)	315	50	11	9	413	0.3
Yogurt, lowfat, plain (8 oz.)	145	16	12	4	415	0.2
Yogurt, lowfat, coffee or vanilla (8 oz.)	195	31	11	3	389	0.2
Yogurt, lowfat, with fruit (8 oz.)	230	43	10	2	345	0.2
Yogurt, whole milk, flavored with coffee, vanilla, lemon (8 oz.)	270	43	8	7	284	0.7
Yogurt, whole milk, plain (8 oz.)	140	11	8	7	274	0.1
Yogurt, whole milk, with fruit (8 oz.)	249	45	8	5	227	0.7
MUFFINS						
Blueberry (1 med.)	135	3	20	5	54	0.9

NA: Not available in references used.

*Crude fiber.

**Cooked and drained unless otherwise stated.

***Based on typical recipe; ingredients and nutrients may vary among recipes.

$: Varies depending on amount of salt added.

$$: Varies depending on type of oil used for frying.

TR: Trace.

Sodium (mg.)	Potassium (mg.)	Thiamine (mg.)	Riboflavin (mg.)	Niacin (mg.)	Vitamin C (mg.)	Vitamin A (IU)	Cholesterol (mg.)	Fiber (gm.)
LEGUMES *(cont.)*								
359	206	.04	.04	0.2	5	30	0	1.6*
6	239	.09	.05	0.4	1	20	0	2.0*
437	329	.13	.11	0.6	2	0	0	7.9
2	355	.14	.05	0.5	1	0	0	5.8
2	366	.17	.07	0.6	2	10	0	2.0
499	362	.12	.08	0.4	1	Tr	0	1.51*
1	398	.16	.08	0.3	2	Tr	0	5.3
2	355	.19	.06	0.9	Tr	10	0	5.1
9	150	0.1	.06	.24	0.1	105	0	0.1*
7	595	.13	.05	0.2	0	0	0	0.9*
6	505	.11	.04	0.1	0	0	0	5.0
MILK/MILK PRODUCTS								
123	381	0.1	.41	0.2	2	500	10	0
122	377	0.1	.40	0.2	2	500	18	0
257	371	.08	.38	0.1	2	80	9	0
126	406	.09	.34	0.2	2	500	4	0
120	370	.09	.40	0.2	2	310	33	0
149	417	.09	.40	0.3	2	302	30	0
123	480	0.1	.44	0.4	2	318	33	0
139	223	.03	.17	0.2	Tr	Tr	1	0
389	1,136	.28	1.27	0.6	8	1,000	104	0
138	420	.09	.48	0.3	4	890	149	0
293	845	.11	.79	0.4	3	1,000	9	0
314	634	.13	.63	0.4	0	240	30	0
270	517	.08	.55	0.4	0	320	33	0
159	531	0.1	.49	0.3	2	150	14	0
149	498	0.1	.46	0.2	2	123	11	0
133	442	.08	0.4	0.2	1	100	10	0
136	NA	NA	NA	NA	NA	NA	45	0
105	351	.07	.32	0.2	1	280	29	0
159	NA	NA	NA	NA	NA	NA	45	0
MUFFINS								
198	47	0.1	.11	0.9	0	40	19	0.2

NA: Not available in references used.
*Crude fiber.
**Cooked and drained unless otherwise stated.
***Based on typical recipe; ingredients and nutrients may vary among recipes.
$: Varies depending on amount of salt added.
$$: Varies depending on type of oil used for frying.
TR: Trace.

Food (Portion)	Calories	Carbohydrates (gm.)	Protein (gm.)	Fats (gm.)	Calcium (mg.)	Iron (mg.)
MUFFINS *(cont.)*						
Bran (1 med.)	125	3	19	6	60	1.4
Corn (1 med.)	145	3	21	5	66	0.9
English (1 med.)	140	27	5	1	96	1.7
NUTS AND SEEDS						
Almonds, whole (1 oz., approx. 23)	165	6	6	15	75	1.0
Almonds, slivered (1/4 cup)	200	7	7	18	90	1.2
Brazil nuts, (1 oz., approx. 8 med.)	185	4	4	19	50	1.0
Cashew nuts, dry-roasted, salted (1 oz.)	165	9	4	13	13	1.7
Cashew nuts, oil-roasted, without salt (1 oz., 18 med.)	165	8	5	14	12	1.2
Coconut, dried, sweetened, flaked (1/2 cup)	175	18	1	12	5	0.7
Coconut, raw (1 piece, 2 × 2 × 1/2 in.)	160	7	2	15	6	1.1
Filberts (hazelnuts), unsalted (1 oz.)	180	4	4	18	53	0.9
Macadamia nuts, oil-roasted, salted (1 oz., 10–12 whole)	205	4	2	22	13	0.5
Mixed nuts, oil-roasted, salted (1 oz.)	175	6	5	16	31	0.9
Peanut butter, salted (1 T)	95	3	5	8	5	0.3
Peanuts, oil-roasted, salted (1 oz.)	165	5	8	14	24	0.5
Pecans (1 oz., about 1/4 cup halves)	190	5	2	19	10	0.6
Pistachio nuts, dried, shelled (1 oz., approx. 47 kernels)	165	7	6	14	38	1.9
Sesame seeds, dry, hulled (1 oz.)	45	1	2	4	10	0.6
Sunflower seeds, dried, hulled (1 T)	160	5	6	14	33	1.9
Walnuts, English (approx. 14 halves)	180	5	4	18	27	0.7
ORGAN MEATS						
Brains, beef (3 oz.)	135	0	9	11	8	1.9
Brains, pork (3 oz.)	115	0	10	8	8	1.6
Chicken gizzards (3 oz.)	130	1	23	3.1	8	3.5
Heart, beef or pork, braised or simmered 3 oz.)	135	Tr	22	4	6	5.7
Kidneys, beef, simmered (3 oz.)	120	1	22	3	15	6.2
Kidneys, pork, braised (3 oz.)	130	0	22	4	11	4.5
Liver, beef, braised (3 oz.)	135	3	21	4	6	5.8
Liver, beef, pan-fried (3 oz.)	185	7	23	7	9	5.3
Liver, chicken, simmered (3 oz.)	135	1	21	5	12	7.2
Liver, pork, braised (3 oz.)	140	3	22	4	9	15.2
Sweetbread, beef (thymus), braised (3 oz.)	270	0	19	21	NA	1.3
Tongue, beef, simmered (3 oz.)	240	Tr	19	18	6	2.9

NA: Not available in references used.
*Crude fiber.
**Cooked and drained unless otherwise stated.
***Based on typical recipe; ingredients and nutrients may vary among recipes.
$: Varies depending on amount of salt added.
$$: Varies depending on type of oil used for frying.
TR: Trace.

Sodium (mg.)	Potassium (mg.)	Thiamine (mg.)	Riboflavin (mg.)	Niacin (mg.)	Vitamin C (mg.)	Vitamin A (IU)	Cholesterol (mg.)	Fiber (gm.)
MUFFINS *(cont.)*								
189	99	.11	.13	1.3	0	230	24	0.5
169	57	.11	.11	0.9	0	80	23	0.2
378	331	.23	.19	2.2	NA	0	0	0.3
NUTS AND SEEDS								
3	208	.06	.22	1.0	Tr	0	0	4
4	247	.07	.26	1.1	Tr	0	0	4.8
0	170	.28	.04	0.5	Tr	NA	0	2.4
181	160	.06	.06	0.4	0	0	0	0.2*
5	151	.12	.05	0.5	0	0	0	0.4*
94	117	.01	.01	0.1	0	0	0	0.8*
9	160	.03	.01	0.2	2	0	0	2*
1	126	.14	.03	0.3	Tr	20	0	1.1*
74	94	.06	.03	0.6	0	3	0	0.5*
185	165	.14	.06	1.4	Tr	10	0	0.6*
75	110	.02	.02	2.1	0	0	0	0.5*
122	199	.08	.03	4.2	Tr	0	0	2.6
Tr	111	.24	.04	0.3	1	40	0	2.6
2	310	.23	.05	0.3	Tr	70	0	.53*
3	33	.06	.01	0.4	Tr	10	0	.24*
1	196	.65	.07	1.3	NA	20	0	1.2*
3	142	.11	.04	0.3	1	35	0	1.5
ORGAN MEATS								
102	204	.07	.14	1.9	1	0	1,746	0
77	166	.07	.19	2.8	12	0	2,169	0
57	152	1.4	.02	.21	3.34	160	165	0
42	187	0.3	1.40	4.3	2	9	176	0
114	152	.16	3.45	5.1	1	1,055	329	0
68	121	.34	1.35	4.9	9	221	408	0
60	200	.17	3.48	9.1	19	30,327	331	0
90	309	.18	3.52	12.3	19	30,689	410	0
43	119	.13	1.48	3.8	13	13,919	536	0
42	128	.22	1.87	7.2	20	15,297	302	0
99	368	NA	NA	NA	26	0	250	0
51	153	.03	0.3	1.83	Tr	NA	91	0

NA: Not available in references used.
*Crude fiber.
**Cooked and drained unless otherwise stated.
***Based on typical recipe; ingredients and nutrients may vary among recipes.
$: Varies depending on amount of salt added.
$$: Varies depending on type of oil used for frying.
TR: Trace.

Food (Portion)	Calories	Carbohydrates (gm.)	Protein (gm.)	Fats (gm.)	Calcium (mg.)	Iron (mg.)
ORGAN MEATS *(cont.)*						
Tongue, pork, braised (3 oz.)	230	0	20	16	16	4.2
Tripe, beef, raw (4 oz.)	110	0	16	4	NA	2.2
PANCAKES						
Buckwheat (1, 4-in. diam.)	55	6	2	2	59	0.4
Pancakes, plain (1 med.)	60	8	2	2	31	0.6
PASTA, ENRICHED, COOKED, AND DRAINED						
Macaroni, firm, hot (1 cup)	190	39	7	1	14	2.1
Macaroni, soft, cold (1 cup)	115	24	4	Tr	8	1.3
Noodles, chow mein (1/2 cup)	110	13	3	6	7	0.2
Noodles, egg (1 cup)	200	37	7	2	16	2.6
Spaghetti, firm (1 cup)	190	39	7	1	14	2.0
Spaghetti, soft (1 cup)	155	32	5	1	11	1.7
PASTRIES						
Coffee cake, crumb, homemade (1 piece)	230	38	5	7	44	1.2
Coffee cake (1/8 cake)	145	18	2	7	9	0.7
Cream puff with custard (1)	245	22	7	15	85	0.7
Eclair (1)	315	39	8	15	90	1.3
Danish pastry, plain, round (4 1/4-in. diam. 1-in. high)	220	26	4	12	60	1.1
Danish pastry, fruit, round (1 pastry, 4 1/4-in. diam. ⟋ 1-in. high)	235	28	4	13	17	1.3
Doughnut, cake type, plain (3 1/4-in. diam.)	210	24	3	12	22	1.0
Doughnut, yeast-leavened, glazed (3 1/4-in. diam.)	235	26	4	13	17	1.4
Doughnut, yeast, jelly center (1)	225	30	3	9	28	0.8
Sweet roll (1)	155	21	3	7	11	0.8
Toaster pastry (various flavors) (1)	195	35	2	6	96	2.0
Turnover (various flavors) (commercial) (1 large)	325	32	2	20	3	1.0
Turnover (various flavors) (from mix) (1 small)	175	23	2	8	NA	NA
PICKLES, OLIVES, RELISHES						
Pickles, dill (1 med., 3 3/4 in. long)	5	1	Tr	Tr	17	0.7
Pickles, sweet gherkin (1 small, 2 1/2 in. long)	20	5	Tr	Tr	2	0.2
Olives, green (4 med.)	15	Tr	Tr	2	8	0.2
Olives, ripe (35 med./21 large)	15	Tr	Tr	2	10	0.2
Relish, chopped, sweet (1 T)	20	5	Tr	Tr	3	0.1

NA: Not available in references used.

*Crude fiber.

**Cooked and drained unless otherwise stated.

***Based on typical recipe; ingredients and nutrients may vary among recipes.

$: Varies depending on amount of salt added.

$$: Varies depending on type of oil used for frying.

TR: Trace.

Sodium (mg.)	Potassium (mg.)	Thiamine (mg.)	Riboflavin (mg.)	Niacin (mg.)	Vitamin C (mg.)	Vitamin A (IU)	Cholesterol (mg.)	Fiber (gm.)
ORGAN MEATS *(cont.)*								
93	201	.27	.43	4.54	1	0	124	0
52	305	Tr	.19	.07	4	0	107	0
PANCAKES								
125	66	.04	.05	0.2	Tr	60	20	0.2
138	38	0.8	0.1	0.6	Tr	30	16	Tr
PASTA, ENRICHED, COOKED, AND DRAINED								
1	103	.23	.13	1.8	0	0	0	1.2
1	64	.15	.08	1.2	0	0	0	NA
225	16	.02	.02	0.3	0	0	2	NA
3	70	.22	.13	1.9	0	110	50	1.7
1	103	.23	.13	1.8	0	0	0	1.6
1	85	0.2	.11	1.5	0	0	0	NA
PASTRIES								
310	78	.14	.15	1.3	Tr	120	47	NA
141	28	.09	0.1	0.9	Tr	60	NA	NA
87	127	.04	.12	0.1	0	370	NA	0
NA	NA	.12	.24	1.0	0	730	NA	0
218	53	.16	.17	1.4	Tr	60	49	NA
233	57	.16	.14	1.4	Tr	40	56	NA
192	58	.12	.12	1.1	Tr	20	20	NA
222	64	.28	.12	1.8	0	Tr	21	NA
NA	NA	.12	0.1	0.9	Tr	120	NA	NA
170	47	.16	.13	0.9	Tr	Tr	NA	NA
229	84	.16	.17	2.1	NA	480	NA	NA
250	49	.17	.06	0.8	4	NA	NA	NA
307	NA	NA	NA	NA	NA	NA	NA	NA
PICKLES, OLIVES, RELISHES								
928	130	Tr	.01	Tr	4	70	NA	NA
107	30	Tr	Tr	Tr	1	10	NA	NA
312	7	Tr	Tr	Tr	0	40	NA	NA
68	2	Tr	Tr	Tr	0	10	NA	NA
107	30	Tr	Tr	0	1	20	NA	NA

NA: Not available in references used.

*Crude fiber.

**Cooked and drained unless otherwise stated.

***Based on typical recipe; ingredients and nutrients may vary among recipes.

$: Varies depending on amount of salt added.

$$: Varies depending on type of oil used for frying.

TR: Trace.

Food (Portion)	Calories	Carbohydrates (gm.)	Protein (gm.)	Fats (gm.)	Calcium (mg.)	Iron (mg.)
PIES†						
Apple (1/6 pie)	405	60	3	18	13	1.6
Banana custard (1/6 pie)	335	47	7	14	100	1.3
Blueberry (1/6 pie)	380	55	4	17	17	2.1
Cherry (1/6 pie)	410	61	4	18	22	1.6
Chocolate meringue (1/6 pie)	385	51	8	18	105	1.7
Coconut custard (1/6 pie)	355	38	9	19	143	1.6
Lemon meringue (1/6 pie)	355	53	5	14	20	1.4
Mincemeat (1/6 pie)	430	65	4	18	44	3.0
Peach (1/6 pie)	405	60	4	17	16	1.9
Pecan (1/6 pie)	575	71	7	32	65	4.6
Pumpkin (1/6 pie)	320	37	6	17	78	1.4
Strawberry (1/6 of pie)	245	38	2	10	20	1.3
Sweet potato (1/6 pie)	325	36	7	17	105	1.3
POPCORN						
Air-popped, unsalted (1 cup)	30	6	1	Tr	1	0.2
Popped in veg. oil, salted (1 cup)	55	6	1	3	3	0.3
PORK						
Bacon (3 slices)	110	Tr	6	9	2	0.3
Canadian bacon (2 slices)	85	1	11	4	5	0.4
Fresh ham (leg), lean with fat, roasted (3 oz.)	250	0	21	18	5	0.8
Fresh ham (leg), lean only, roasted (3 oz.)	185	0	24	9	6	1.0
Ham, cured, canned, roasted (3 oz.)	140	Tr	18	7	6	0.9
Ham, lean only (3 oz.)	135	0	21	5	6	0.8
Ham, with fat (3 oz.)	205	0	18	14	6	0.7
Loin chop, lean only, broiled (1 med.)	165	0	23	8	4	0.7
Loin chop, lean and fat, fried (1 med.)	335	0	21	27	4	0.7
Loin chop, lean only, fried (1 med.)	180	0	19	11	3	0.7
Loin chop, with fat (1 med.)	275	0	24	19	3	0.7
Sirloin, braised or broiled, lean and fat (3 oz.)	290	0	22	22	4	0.8
Sirloin, braised or broiled, lean only (3 oz.)	215	0	26	11	6	0.9
Tenderloin, lean only, roasted (3 oz.)	140	0	24	4	7	1.3
Shoulder (picnic or butt), lean and fat, roasted (3 oz.)	277	0	19	22	6	1.1
Shoulder (picnic or butt), lean only, roasted (3 oz.)	206	0	21	12	7	1.3
Spareribs, with fat, braised (3 oz.)	338	0	25	26	40	1.6

†Portion based on 9-in. pie

NA: Not available in references used.
*Crude fiber.
**Cooked and drained unless otherwise stated.
***Based on typical recipe; ingredients and nutrients may vary among recipes.
$: Varies depending on amount of salt added.
$$: Varies depending on type of oil used for frying.
TR: Trace.

Sodium (mg.)	Potassium (mg.)	Thiamine (mg.)	Riboflavin (mg.)	Niacin (mg.)	Vitamin C (mg.)	Vitamin A (IU)	Cholesterol (mg.)	Fiber (gm.)
PIES†								
476	126	.17	.13	1.6	2	50	0	NA
295	309	.11	0.2	1.1	2	380	NA	NA
423	158	.17	.14	1.7	6	140	0	NA
480	166	.19	.14	1.6	0	700	0	NA
389	211	0.1	.23	0.9	Tr	290	NA	NA
375	248	.14	.34	1.0	0	350	NA	NA
395	70	0.1	.14	0.8	4	240	143	NA
708	281	.16	.11	1.1	2	Tr	0	NA
423	235	.17	.16	2.4	5	1,150	0	NA
305	170	0.3	.17	1.1	0	220	95	NA
325	243	.14	0.2	1.2	0	3,750	109	NA
241	149	.06	.09	0.9	31	50	NA	NA
331	248	.13	.23	1	6	3,640	NA	NA
POPCORN								
Tr	20	.03	.01	0.2	0	10	0	NA
86	19	.01	.02	0.1	0	20	0	NA
PORK								
303	92	.13	.05	1.4	6.4	0	16	0
719	181	.38	.09	3.2	10	0	27	0
51	280	.54	.27	3.9	0.3	0	79	0
55	317	.59	0.3	4.2	0.3	0	80	0
908	298	.82	.21	4.3	0	0	35	0
1,128	269	.58	.22	4.3	0	0	47	0
1,009	243	.51	.19	3.8	0	0	52	0
56	302	.83	.22	4.0	Tr	10	71	0
64	323	.91	.24	4.6	Tr	10	92	0
57	305	.84	.22	4.0	Tr	10	72	0
61	312	.87	.24	4.3	Tr	10	84	0
46	313	.66	.27	4.0	0.2	8	86	0
50	373	.76	.32	4.4	0.3	6	88	0
57	457	0.8	.33	4.0	0.3	6	79	0
58	258	.46	.27	3.4	0.2	7	81	0
65	300	0.5	.31	3.7	0.3	6	82	0
79	272	.35	.32	4.7	Tr	9	103	0

†Portion based on 9-in. pie

NA: Not available in references used.
*Crude fiber.
**Cooked and drained unless otherwise stated.
***Based on typical recipe; ingredients and nutrients may vary among recipes.
$: Varies depending on amount of salt added.
$$: Varies depending on type of oil used for frying.
TR: Trace.

Food (Portion)	Calories	Carbohydrates (gm.)	Protein (gm.)	Fats (gm.)	Calcium (mg.)	Iron (mg.)
POULTRY						
Chicken breast without skin, fried (1/2 breast)	160	Tr	29	4	14	1.0
Chicken breast without skin, roasted (1/2 breast)	140	0	27	3	13	0.9
Chicken breast without skin, stewed (1/2 breast)	145	0	28	3	12	0.8
Chicken breast with skin, batter-dipped, fried (1/2 breast)	365	13	35	18	28	1.8
Chicken breast with skin, flour-coated, fried (1/2 breast)	220	2	31	9	16	1.2
Chicken breast with skin, roasted (1/2 breast)	195	0	29	8	14	1.0
Chicken breast with skin, stewed (1/2 breast)	200	0	30	8	14	1.0
Chicken, dark meat without skin, roasted (3 oz.)	175	0	23	8	13	1.1
Chicken dark meat with skin, roasted (3 oz.)	215	0	22	13	13	1.2
Chicken drumstick without skin, fried (1)	80	0	12	3	5	0.6
Chicken drumstick without skin, roasted (1)	75	0	12	2	5	0.6
Chicken drumstick without skin, stewed (1)	80	0	13	3	5	0.6
Chicken drumstick with skin, batter-dipped, fried (1)	195	6	16	11	12	1.0
Chicken drumstick with skin, flour-coated, fried (1)	120	1	13	7	6	0.7
Chicken drumstick with skin, roasted (1)	110	0	14	6	6	0.7
Chicken drumstick with skin, stewed (1)	115	0	14	6	7	0.8
Chicken, light meat without skin, roasted (3 oz.)	145	0	26	4	13	0.9
Chicken, light meat with skin, roasted (3 oz.)	190	0	25	9	13	1.0
Chicken thigh without skin, fried (1)	115	1	15	5	7	0.8
Chicken thigh without skin, roasted (1)	110	0	13	6	6	0.7
Chicken thigh without skin, stewed (1)	105	0	14	5	6	0.8
Chicken thigh with skin, batter-dipped, fried (1)	240	8	19	14	16	1.2
Chicken thigh with skin, flour-coated, fried (1)	160	2	17	9	8	0.9
Chicken thigh with skin, roasted (1)	155	0	16	10	8	0.8
Chicken thigh with skin, stewed (1)	160	0	16	10	8	0.9
Chicken wing without skin, fried (1)	40	0	6	2	3	0.2
Chicken wing without skin, roasted or stewed (1)	45	0	6	2	3	0.3
Chicken wing with skin, batter-dipped, fried (1)	160	5	10	11	10	0.6
Chicken wing with skin, flour-coated, fried (1)	105	1	8	7	5	0.4
Chicken wing with skin, roasted or stewed (1)	100	0	9	7	5	0.4

NA: Not available in references used.

*Crude fiber.

**Cooked and drained unless otherwise stated.

***Based on typical recipe; ingredients and nutrients may vary among recipes.

$: Varies depending on amount of salt added.

$$: Varies depending on type of oil used for frying.

TR: Trace.

Sodium (mg.)	Potassium (mg.)	Thiamine (mg.)	Riboflavin (mg.)	Niacin (mg.)	Vitamin C (mg.)	Vitamin A (IU)	Cholesterol (mg.)	Fiber (gm.)
POULTRY								
68	237	.07	.11	12.7	0	20	78	0
63	220	.06	0.1	11.8	0	18	73	0
59	178	.04	.11	8.0	0	18	73	0
385	282	.16	0.2	14.7	0	94	119	Tr*
75	253	.08	.13	13.5	0	49	88	Tr*
69	240	.06	.12	12.5	0	91	83	0
68	195	.04	.13	8.6	0	90	83	0
79	204	.06	.19	5.6	0	61	79	0
74	187	.06	.18	5.4	0	173	77	0
40	105	.03	0.1	2.6	0	26	40	0
42	108	.03	0.1	2.7	0	26	41	0
37	92	.02	0.1	2.0	0	26	40	0
194	134	.08	.16	3.7	0	62	62	Tr*
44	112	.04	.11	3.0	0	41	44	0
47	119	.04	.11	3.1	0	52	48	0
43	105	.03	.11	2.4	0	52	48	0
65	210	.06	0.1	10.6	0	25	72	0
64	193	.05	0.1	9.5	0	94	72	0
49	134	.05	.13	3.7	0	37	53	0
46	124	.04	.12	3.4	0	34	49	0
41	101	.03	.12	2.9	0	34	49	0
248	165	0.1	0.2	4.9	0	82	80	Tr*
55	147	.58	.15	4.3	0	61	60	Tr*
52	137	.04	.13	3.9	0	102	58	0
49	115	.04	.13	3.3	0	103	57	0
18	42	.01	.03	1.5	0	12	17	0
18	40	.01	.03	1.4	0	13	18	0
157	68	.05	.07	2.6	0	55	39	Tr*
25	57	.02	.04	2.1	0	40	26	0
28	59	.02	.04	2.1	0	54	28	0

NA: Not available in references used.

*Crude fiber.

**Cooked and drained unless otherwise stated.

***Based on typical recipe; ingredients and nutrients may vary among recipes.

$: Varies depending on amount of salt added.

$$: Varies depending on type of oil used for frying.

TR: Trace.

Food (Portion)	Calories	Carbohydrates (gm.)	Protein (gm.)	Fats (gm.)	Calcium (mg.)	Iron (mg.)
POULTRY *(cont.)*						
Duck, flesh only, roasted (3 oz.)	170	0	20	10	10	2.3
Duck, with skin, roasted (3 oz.)	285	0	16	24	9	2.3
Turkey, light meat without skin, roasted (3 oz.)	135	0	25	3	16	1.1
Turkey, light meat with skin, roasted (3 oz.)	165	0	24	7	18	1.2
Turkey, dark meat without skin, roasted (3 oz.)	160	0	24	6	27	2.0
Turkey, dark meat with skin, roasted (3 oz.)	190	0	23	10	28	1.9
PRETZELS						
Stick, 2 1/4 in., long (10)	10	2	Tr	Tr	1	0.1
Twisted (1 med.)	65	13	2	1	4	0.3
PUDDINGS						
Banana (1/2 cup)	170	30	4	4	147	0.1
Butterscotch (1/2 cup)	170	30	4	4	147	0.1
Chocolate from mix (1/2 cup)	150	25	4	4	146	0.2
Custard (1/2 cup)	150	14	7	8	148	0.6
Lemon (1/2 cup)	150	31	4	4	147	0.1
Rice (1/2 cup)	155	27	4	4	133	0.5
Rice and raisins (1/2 cup)	140	26	3	3	95	0.2
Tapioca (1/2 cup)	145	25	4	4	131	0.1
Vanilla, from mix (1/2 cup)	145	27	4	4	129	0.1
Vanilla, instant (1/2 cup)	150	27	4	4	129	0.1
RICE						
Brown (1/2 cup)	115	25	2	1	12	0.5
Instant, enriched, cooked (1/2 cup)	90	20	2	0	2	0.7
White, enriched (1/2 cup)	110	25	2	Tr	10	0.9
SALAD DRESSING						
Blue cheese (low-cal.) (1 T)	11	1	Tr	1	9	Tr
Blue cheese (regular) (1 T)	75	1	1	8	12	Tr
Caesar (regular) (1 T)	70	1	0	7	NA	NA
French (low-cal.) (1 T)	25	2	Tr	2	6	Tr
French (regular) (1 T)	85	1	Tr	9	2	Tr
Green Goddess (1 T)	70	1	Tr	7	2	NA
Italian (low-cal.) (1 T)	5	2	Tr	Tr	1	Tr
Italian (regular) (1 T)	80	1	Tr	9	1	Tr
Mayonnaise-type (low-cal.) (1 T)	20	1	Tr	2	NA	NA
Mayonnaise-type (regular) (1 T)	60	4	Tr	5	2	Tr
Oil and vinegar (home recipe) (1 T)	70	Tr	0	8	NA	NA

NA: Not available in references used.

*Crude fiber.

**Cooked and drained unless otherwise stated.

***Based on typical recipe; ingredients and nutrients may vary among recipes.

$: Varies depending on amount of salt added.

$$: Varies depending on type of oil used for frying.

TR: Trace.

Sodium (mg.)	Potassium (mg.)	Thiamine (mg.)	Riboflavin (mg.)	Niacin (mg.)	Vitamin C (mg.)	Vitamin A (IU)	Cholesterol (mg.)	Fiber (gm.)
POULTRY *(cont.)*								
55	214	.22	0.4	4.3	0	65	76	0
50	173	.15	.23	4.1	0	178	71	0
54	259	.05	.11	5.8	0	0	59	0
54	242	.05	.11	5.3	0	0	65	0
67	246	.05	.21	3.1	0	0	72	0
65	233	.05	0.2	3.0	0	0	76	0
PRETZELS								
48	3	.01	.01	0.1	0	0	0	NA
258	16	.05	.04	0.7	0	0	0	NA
PUDDINGS								
441	187	.05	0.2	0.1	1	150	17	Tr*
478	187	.05	0.2	0.1	1	150	17	Tr*
167	190	.05	0.2	0.1	1	140	15	NA
104	194	.06	.25	0.2	Tr	265	139	NA
387	192	.05	0.2	0.1	1	154	17	0.1*
140	165	0.1	.18	0.6	1	140	15	NA
69	171	.03	.13	0.2	Tr	110	NA	Tr*
152	167	.04	.18	0.1	1	140	15	NA
178	166	.04	.18	0.1	1	140	15	NA
375	164	.04	.17	0.1	1	140	15	NA
RICE								
0	68	.09	.02	1.4	0	0	0	2.4
0	0	.16	.01	0.9	0	0	0	NA
0	28	.12	.01	1.0	0	0	0	0.1
SALAD DRESSING								
155	5	NA	.01	Tr	Tr	20	NA	0
164	6	Tr	.02	Tr	Tr	30	3	0
NA	NA	NA	NA	NA	NA	NA	NA	NA
306	3	Tr	Tr	Tr	Tr	Tr	0	0
188	2	Tr	Tr	Tr	Tr	Tr	0	0
150	9	NA	NA	NA	NA	NA	NA	NA
136	4	Tr	Tr	Tr	Tr	Tr	0	0
162	5	Tr	Tr	Tr	Tr	30	0	0
NA	NA	Tr	Tr	Tr	NA	30	NA	0
107	1	Tr	Tr	Tr	0	30	4	0
Tr	1	NA	NA	NA	NA	NA	NA	NA

NA: Not available in references used.
*Crude fiber.
**Cooked and drained unless otherwise stated.
***Based on typical recipe; ingredients and nutrients may vary among recipes.
$: Varies depending on amount of salt added.
$$: Varies depending on type of oil used for frying.
TR: Trace.

Food (Portion)	Calories	Carbohydrates (gm.)	Protein (gm.)	Fats (gm.)	Calcium (mg.)	Iron (mg.)
SALAD DRESSING *(cont.)*						
Oil and vinegar (regular) (1 T)	70	1	Tr	8	2	NA
Ranch-style (prepared from dry mix and mayonnaise) (1 T)	55	1	Tr	6	NA	NA
Russian (low-cal.) (1 T)	25	4	Tr	1	3	0.1
Russian (regular) (1 T)	75	2	Tr	8	3	0.1
Thousand Island (low-cal.) (1 T)	25	2	Tr	2	2	0.1
Thousand Island (regular) (1 T)	60	2	Tr	6	2	0.1
SAUCES						
Barbeque sauce (1 T)	10	2	Tr	Tr	3	0.1
Cheese, sauce (prepared from dry mix and milk) (2 T)	40	3	2	2	71	Tr
Hollandaise sauce (prepared from dry mix and water) (2 T)	30	2	1	2	16	0.1
White sauce (prepared from dry mix and milk) (2 T)	30	3	1	2	53	Tr
White sauce, homemade, med. (2 T)	50	6	2	4	36	0.1
SAUSAGES AND CURED MEATS						
Bologna (1 oz.)	90	1	4	8	3	0.4
Bologna, turkey (1 oz.)	55	Tr	4	4	24	0.4
Frankfurter (1)	145	1	5	13	5	0.5
Frankfurter, turkey (1 oz.)	100	1	6	8	48	0.8
Cooked ham, extra lean (1 oz.)	35	1	6	2	2	0.2
Cooked ham, regular (1 oz.)	50	1	5	3	2	0.3
Liverwurst (1 oz.)	60	Tr	3	5	5	1.2
Luncheon meat, pork, beef (1 oz.)	100	1	4	9	3	0.2
Pâté, liver (1 T)	40	Tr	2	4	9	0.7
Pepperoni (1 slice)	25	Tr	1	2	1	0.1
Pork sausage (1 small link)	50	Tr	3	4	4	0.2
Salami, cooked (1 slice)	70	1	4	6	4	0.8
Salami, hard, dried (1 slice)	42	Tr	2	3	1	0.2
Smoked link sausage, pork and beef (1 small link)	54	Tr	2	5	2	0.2
Sandwich spread, pork, beef (1 T)	35	2	1	3	2	0.1
Vienna sausage (1)	45	Tr	2	4	2	0.1
SOUPS						
Asparagus, canned and milk (1 cup)	160	16	6	8	175	0.9
Bean and bacon, canned and water (1 cup)	170	23	8	6	81	2.0

NA: Not available in references used.

*Crude fiber.

**Cooked and drained unless otherwise stated.

***Based on typical recipe; ingredients and nutrients may vary among recipes.

$: Varies depending on amount of salt added.

$$: Varies depending on type of oil used for frying.

TR: Trace.

Sodium (mg.)	Potassium (mg.)	Thiamine (mg.)	Riboflavin (mg.)	Niacin (mg.)	Vitamin C (mg.)	Vitamin A (IU)	Cholesterol (mg.)	Fiber (gm.)
SALAD DRESSING *(cont.)*								
244	4	NA	NA	NA	NA	NA	NA	0
97	NA	NA	NA	NA	NA	NA	NA	NA
141	26	NA	NA	NA	NA	NA	1	0.1*
133	24	.01	.01	0.1	1	110	NA	0
150	7	Tr	Tr	Tr	0	50	2	0.2*
112	18	Tr	Tr	Tr	0	50	4	0.3*
SAUCES								
130	28	Tr	Tr	0.1	1	140	0	NA
196	69	.02	.07	Tr	Tr	50	7	NA
196	16	Tr	.02	Tr	Tr	90	7	NA
100	55	.01	.06	Tr	Tr	40	4	NA
111	48	.02	.05	0.1	Tr	150	4	NA
SAUSAGES AND CURED MEATS								
290	52	.05	.04	0.8	6	0	16	0
249	56	.02	.05	1.0	NA	0	28	0
504	75	.09	.05	1.2	12	0	23	0
642	80	.18	.08	1.9	NA	NA	48	0
408	100	.26	.06	1.4	8	0	14	0
376	94	.24	.07	1.5	8	0	16	0
NA	NA	.05	.18	NA	NA	NA	45	0
367	57	.09	.04	0.8	4	NA	15	0
91	18	Tr	.08	0.4	0	429	NA	0
112	19	.02	.01	0.3	NA	NA	NA	0
47	168	.10	.03	0.6	0	0	11	0
302	56	.07	.11	1.0	3	0	18	0
186	38	.06	.03	0.5	3	0	8	0
151	30	.04	.03	0.5	3	0	11	0
152	17	.03	.02	0.3	0	10	6	0
152	16	.01	.02	0.3	0	0	8	0
SOUPS								
1,041	359	0.1	.28	0.9	4	600	22	0.8*
951	402	.09	.03	0.6	2	890	3	6.0

NA: Not available in references used.

*Crude fiber.

**Cooked and drained unless otherwise stated.

***Based on typical recipe; ingredients and nutrients may vary among recipes.

$: Varies depending on amount of salt added.

$$: Varies depending on type of oil used for frying.

TR: Trace.

Food (Portion)	Calories	Carbohydrates (gm.)	Protein (gm.)	Fats (gm.)	Calcium (mg.)	Iron (mg.)
SOUPS *(cont.)*						
Beef consommé, homemade (1 cup)	15	Tr	3	1	14	0.4
Black bean, canned and water (1 cup)	115	20	6	2	45	2.2
Bouillon, unprepared, dehydrated (1 packet)	15	1	1	1	4	0.1
Cheese, canned and milk (1 cup)	230	16	9	15	288	0.8
Chicken and rice, homemade (1 cup)	60	7	4	2	17	0.8
Chicken broth, homemade (1 cup)	40	1	5	1	9	0.5
Chicken noodle, homemade (1 cup)	75	9	4	2	17	0.8
Chicken noodle, prepared dehydrated and water (1 packet, 6 fl. oz.)	46	6	2	1	24	0.4
Clam chowder, Manhattan, homemade (1 cup)	80	12	4	2	34	1.9
Clam chowder, New England, canned and milk (1 cup)	165	17	9	7	187	1.5
Cream of celery, canned and milk (1 cup)	165	15	6	10	186	0.7
Cream of chicken, canned and milk (1 cup)	190	15	7	11	180	0.7
Cream of mushroom, canned and milk (1 cup)	205	15	6	14	178	0.6
Cream of mushroom, homemade (1 cup)	130	9	2	9	46	0.5
Cream of potato, canned and milk (1 cup)	150	17	6	6	166	0.5
Minestrone, homemade (1 cup)	85	11	4	3	34	0.9
Onion, homemade (1 cup)	55	8	4	2	26	0.7
Onion, prepared dehydrated and water (1 packet, 6 fl. oz.)	20	4	1	Tr	9	0.1
Onion, unprepared dehydrated (1 packet)	20	4	1	Tr	10	0.1
Split pea and ham, homemade (1 cup)	190	28	10	4	22	2.3
Tomato, homemade (1 cup)	85	17	2	2	13	1.8
Tomato bisque, canned and milk (1 cup)	200	29	6	7	186	0.9
Tomato vegetable, prepared dehydrated and water (1 packet, 6 fl. oz.)	40	8	1	1	6	0.5
Vegetable and beef, homemade (1 cup)	80	10	6	2	17	1.1
Vegetable, vegetarian, homemade (1 cup)	70	12	2	2	21	1.1
SUGARS						
Brown (1 cup packed)	820	212	0	0	187	4.8
White, granulated (1 cup)	770	199	0	0	3	0.1
White, granulated (1 T, 3 t)	45	12	0	0	Tr	Tr
White, granulated (1 packet)	25	6	0	0	Tr	Tr
White, powdered (sifted, spooned into cup) (1 cup)	385	100	0	0	1	Tr

NA: Not available in references used.

*Crude fiber.

**Cooked and drained unless otherwise stated.

***Based on typical recipe; ingredients and nutrients may vary among recipes.

$: Varies depending on amount of salt added.

$$: Varies depending on type of oil used for frying.

TR: Trace.

Sodium (mg.)	Potassium (mg.)	Thiamine (mg.)	Riboflavin (mg.)	Niacin (mg.)	Vitamin C (mg.)	Vitamin A (IU)	Cholesterol (mg.)	Fiber (gm.)
SOUPS *(cont.)*								
782	130	Tr	.05	1.9	0	0	Tr	NA
1,198	273	.08	.05	0.5	1	510	0	4.0
1,019	27	Tr	.01	0.3	0	Tr	1	NA
1,020	340	.06	.33	0.5	1	1,240	48	NA
814	100	.02	.02	1.1	Tr	660	7	Tr*
776	210	.01	.07	3.3	0	0	1	Tr*
1,107	55	.05	.06	1.4	Tr	710	7	0.2*
957	23	.05	.04	0.7	Tr	50	2	0.3*
1,808	261	.06	.05	1.3	3	920	2	NA
992	300	.07	.24	1.0	4	160	22	NA
1,010	309	.07	.25	0.4	1	460	32	0.4*
1,046	273	.07	.26	0.9	1	710	27	0.1*
1,076	270	.08	.28	0.9	2	150	20	0.2*
1,032	100	.05	.09	0.7	1	0	2	0.5*
1,060	323	.08	.24	0.6	1	440	22	NA
911	312	.05	.04	0.9	1	2,340	2	0.7*
1,053	69	.03	.02	0.6	1	0	0	0.5*
635	48	.02	.04	0.4	Tr	Tr	0	0.2*
627	47	.02	.04	0.4	Tr	Tr	Tr	NA
1,008	400	.15	.08	1.5	1	440	8	4.0
872	263	.09	.05	1.4	66	690	0	0.5*
1,108	604	.11	.27	1.3	7	880	22	NA
856	78	.04	.03	0.6	5	140	0	0.4*
957	173	.04	.05	1.0	2	1,890	5	1.0
823	209	.05	.05	0.9	1	3,000	0	2.0
SUGARS								
97	757	.02	.07	0.2	0	0	0	0
7	5	0	0	0	0	0	0	
Tr	Tr	0	0	0	0	0	0	0
Tr	Tr	0	0	0	0	0	0	0
2	4	0	0	0	0	0	0	0

NA: Not available in references used.

*Crude fiber.

**Cooked and drained unless otherwise stated.

***Based on typical recipe; ingredients and nutrients may vary among recipes.

$: Varies depending on amount of salt added.

$$: Varies depending on type of oil used for frying.

TR: Trace.

Food (Portion)	Calories	Carbohydrates (gm.)	Protein (gm.)	Fats (gm.)	Calcium (mg.)	Iron (mg.)
SYRUPS						
Chocolate-flavored thin type (1 T)	42	11	Tr	Tr	3	0.4
Molasses, blackstrap (1 T)	42	11	0	0	137	5.0
Table syrup (corn and maple) (1 T)	61	16	0	0	Tr	Tr
VEGETABLES**						
Asparagus (6 med. spears)	20	4	2	Tr	22	0.6
Bamboo shoots, canned, drained (1/2 cup)	15	2	1	Tr	5	0.2
Beans, lima, boiled, drained (1/2 cup)	105	20	6	Tr	27	2.1
Beans, snap, green, yellow, or Italian (1/2 cup)	20	5	1	Tr	29	0.8
Bean sprouts, raw (mung) (1/2 cup)	15	3	2	Tr	7	0.5
Beets, boiled, drained (1/2 cup)	25	6	1	Tr	9	0.5
Beets, pickled, canned (1/2 cup sliced)	75	19	1	Tr	13	0.5
Beet greens, broiled, drained (1/2 cup)	20	4	2	Tr	82	1.4
Broccoli, boiled, drained (1/2 cup chopped)	25	4	2	Tr	89	0.9
Broccoli, boiled, drained (1 med.)	55	10	5	Tr	205	2.1
Brussel sprouts, boiled, drained (1/2 cup, 4 sprouts)	30	7	2	Tr	28	0.9
Cabbage, boiled, drained (1/2 cup)	15	4	1	Tr	25	0.3
Cabbage, raw, shredded (1/2 cup)	10	2	Tr	Tr	16	0.2
Cabbage, red, boiled, drained (1/2 cup shredded)	15	3	1	Tr	28	0.3
Cabbage, red, raw (1/2 cup shredded)	10	2	Tr	Tr	18	0.2
Carrot, raw (1 med.)	30	7	1	Tr	19	0.4
Carrot juice (1/2 cup)	50	11	1	Tr	29	0.6
Carrot slices, boiled, drained (1/2 cup)	35	8	1	Tr	24	0.5
Cauliflower, boiled, drained (1/2 cup)	15	3	1	Tr	17	0.3
Cauliflower, raw (3 florets)	15	3	1	Tr	16	0.3
Celery, boiled, drained (1/2 cup diced)	10	3	Tr	Tr	27	0.1
Celery, raw (1 stalk)	5	1	Tr	Tr	14	0.2
Collards (1/2 cup chopped)	15	3	1	Tr	74	0.4
Corn, boiled, drained (1/2 cup)	90	21	3	1	2	0.5
Corn, boiled (1 ear)	85	19	3	1	2	0.5
Cucumber, raw (1/2 cup slices)	5	2	Tr	Tr	7	0.1
Corn, yellow, canned, cream-style (1/2 cup)	95	23	2	1	4	0.5
Eggplant cubes, boiled, drained (1 cup)	25	6	1	Tr	5	0.3
Ginger root, raw (5 slices, 1/8-in. slices)	10	2	Tr	Tr	2	Tr
Kale, boiled, drained (1/2 cup chopped)	20	4	1	Tr	47	0.6
Leeks, boiled, drained (1/2 cup chopped)	15	4	Tr	Tr	16	0.6

NA: Not available in references used.

*Crude fiber.

**Cooked and drained unless otherwise stated.

***Based on typical recipe; ingredients and nutrients may vary among recipes.

$: Varies depending on amount of salt added.

$$: Varies depending on type of oil used for frying.

TR: Trace.

Sodium (mg.)	Potassium (mg.)	Thiamine (mg.)	Riboflavin (mg.)	Niacin (mg.)	Vitamin C (mg.)	Vitamin A (IU)	Cholesterol (mg.)	Fiber (gm.)
SYRUPS								
18	42	Tr	.02	0.1	0	Tr	0	0
19	586	.02	.04	0.4	0	0	0	0
10	4	0	0	0	0	0	0	0
VEGETABLES **								
4	279	.09	.11	0.9	18	746	0	2.2
4	52	.03	.03	0.2	1	10	0	.44*
14	485	.12	.08	0.9	9	315	0	4.4
2	185	.05	.06	0.4	6	413	0	2.1
3	77	.04	0.6	0.4	7	11	0	1.6
42	266	.03	.01	0.2	5	11	0	2.2
301	169	.03	.05	0.3	3	7	0	0.7*
173	654	.08	.21	0.4	18	3,672	0	0.8*
8	127	.06	.16	0.6	49	1,099	0	2.0
19	293	.15	.37	1.4	113	2,537	0	4.5
17	247	.08	.06	0.5	48	561	0	3.9
14	154	.04	.04	0.2	18	64	0	2.0
6	86	.02	.01	0.1	16	4	0	0.7
6	105	.03	.02	0.2	26	20	0	0.6*
4	72	.02	.01	0.1	20	14	0	1.2
25	233	.07	.04	0.7	7	20,253	0	2.4
36	360	.11	.07	0.5	10	31,673	0	1.2*
52	177	.03	.04	0.4	2	19,152	0	2.3
4	200	.04	.03	0.3	34	9	0	1.6
8	199	.04	.03	0.4	40	9	0	1.9
48	266	.02	.02	0.2	4	81	0	1.4
35	114	.01	.01	0.1	2	51	0	0.7
18	88	.02	.04	0.2	9	2,109	0	2.2
14	204	.18	.06	1.3	5	178	0	3.9
13	192	.17	.06	1.2	5	167	0	3.6
1	78	.02	.01	0.2	2	23	0	0.5
365	172	.03	.07	1.2	6	124	0	5.1
3	238	.07	.02	0.6	1	61	0	0.9*
1	46	Tr	Tr	0.1	1	0	0	0.1*
15	148	.03	.05	0.3	27	4,810	0	2.8
46		.01	.01	0.1	2	24	0	1.6

NA: Not available in references used.
*Crude fiber.
**Cooked and drained unless otherwise stated.
***Based on typical recipe; ingredients and nutrients may vary among recipes.
$: Varies depending on amount of salt added.
$$: Varies depending on type of oil used for frying.
TR: Trace.

Food (Portion)	Calories	Carbohydrates (gm.)	Protein (gm.)	Fats (gm.)	Calcium (mg.)	Iron (mg.)
VEGETABLES** *(cont.)*						
Lettuce, butterhead (Boston and Bibb) (1/2 head)	10	2	1	Tr	0	0.2
Lettuce, iceberg, raw (wedge, 1/4 head)	20	3	1	Tr	26	0.7
Lettuce, leaf (1 cup chopped)	10	2	1	Tr	38	0.8
Mushrooms, canned, drained (1/2 cup pieces)	20	4	1	Tr	1	NA
Mushrooms, raw (1/2 cup)	10	2	1	Tr	2	0.4
Mustard greens, boiled, drained (1/2 cup chopped)	10	1	2	Tr	52	0.5
Mixed vegetables, canned, drained (1/2 cup)	40	8	2	Tr	22	0.9
Mixed vegetables, frozen, boiled, drained (1/2 cup)	55	12	3	Tr	22	0.8
Okra, boiled, drained (1/2 cup slices, 7–8 pods)	25	6	1	Tr	50	0.4
Onion, boiled, drained (1/2 cup chopped)	30	7	1	Tr	29	0.2
Onion, dehydrated flakes (1 T)	15	4	Tr	Tr	13	0.1
Onion, raw (1/2 chopped)	25	6	1	Tr	20	0.3
Onion, raw (1/2 cup sliced)	20	4	Tr	Tr	14	0.2
Onions, spring (3)	5	1	Tr	Tr	9	0.3
Parsley, freeze-dried (1 T)	Tr	Tr	Tr	Tr	1	0.2
Parsley, raw (1/2 cup chopped)	10	2	1	Tr	39	1.9
Parsnips, boiled, drained (1/2 cup sliced)	65	15	1	Tr	29	0.4
Peas, Chinese, boiled, drained (1/2 cup)	35	6	3	Tr	33	1.6
Peas, green, boiled, drained (1/2 cup)	65	13	4	Tr	22	1.2
Peas and carrots, frozen, cooked, drained (1/2 cup)	40	8	2	Tr	18	0.8
Peas and onions, frozen, cooked, drained (1/2 cup)	40	8	2	Tr	13	0.8
Pepper, green, raw (1 med.)	20	4	1	Tr	4	0.9
Pepper, sweet, green, boiled, drained (1/2 cup chopped)	12	3	Tr	Tr	3	0.6
Pepper, sweet, red, boiled, drained (1/2 cup chopped)	12	3	Tr	Tr	3	0.6
Pepper, sweet, red, raw (1 med.)	20	4	1	Tr	4	0.9
Potato, baked, without skin (1 med.)	145	34	3	Tr	8	0.5
Potato, baked, with skin (1 med.)	220	51	5	Tr	20	2.7
Potato, boiled, peeled (1 med.)	115	27	2	Tr	9	0.4
Potatoes, French-fried, frozen (oven-heated) (10)	110	17	2	4	5	0.7

NA: Not available in references used.
*Crude fiber.
**Cooked and drained unless otherwise stated.
***Based on typical recipe; ingredients and nutrients may vary among recipes.
$: Varies depending on amount of salt added.
$$: Varies depending on type of oil used for frying.
TR: Trace.

Sodium (mg.)	Potassium (mg.)	Thiamine (mg.)	Riboflavin (mg.)	Niacin (mg.)	Vitamin C (mg.)	Vitamin A (IU)	Cholesterol (mg.)	Fiber (gm.)
VEGETABLES** *(cont.)*								
4	208	.05	.05	0.2	6	790	0	1.2
12	213	.06	.04	0.3	5	450	0	1.4
5	148	.03	.04	0.1	10	1,060	0	1.2
NA	NA	NA	NA	NA	NA	0	0	NA
1	130	.04	.16	1.4	1	0	0	0.9
11	141	.03	.04	0.3	18	2,122	0	1.6
122	239	.04	.04	0.5	4	9,551	0	1.1*
32	154	.06	.11	0.8	3	3,892	0	1.1*
4	257	.11	.04	0.7	13	460	0	2.6
8	159	.04	Tr	0.1	6	0	0	2.2
1	81	.02	Tr	Tr	4	4	0	0.2*
2	124	.05	.01	0.1	7	0	0	2.6
1	89	.03	Tr	Tr	5	0	0	1.8
Tr	38	.01	.02	Tr	7	750	0	0.5
2	25	Tr	.01	Tr	1	250	0	Tr*
12	161	.02	.03	0.2	27	1,560	0	1.2
8	287	.06	.04	0.6	10	0	0	3.1
3	192	0.1	.06	0.4	38	10	0	1.3
2	217	.21	.12	1.6	11	478	0	4.1
55	127	.18	.05	0.9	6	6,209	0	1.1*
NA	NA	.14	.06	0.9	6	313	0	NA
2	144	.06	.04	0.4	95	392	0	0.8
1	88	.04	.02	0.2	76	264	0	1.2
1	88	.04	.02	0.2	76	2,557	0	NA
2	144	.06	.04	0.4	141	4,218	0	0.8
8	610	.16	.03	2.2	20	0	0	3.7
16	844	.22	.07	3.3	26	0	0	1.3*
6	479	.14	.03	1.9	14	0	0	2.7
16	229	.06	.02	1.2	5	0	0	34*

NA: Not available in references used.

*Crude fiber.

**Cooked and drained unless otherwise stated.

***Based on typical recipe; ingredients and nutrients may vary among recipes.

$: Varies depending on amount of salt added.

$$: Varies depending on type of oil used for frying.

TR: Trace.

Food (Portion)	Calories	Carbohydrates (gm.)	Protein (gm.)	Fats (gm.)	Calcium (mg.)	Iron (mg.)
VEGETABLES** *(cont.)*						
Potatoes, French-fried, frozen (in vegetable oil) (10)	160	20	2	8	10	0.4
Potatoes, hash browns, from frozen (1/2 cup)	170	22	3	9	12	1.2
Potatoes, mashed, with milk (1/2 cup)	80	18	2	1	28	0.3
Potatoes, mashed, from flakes, with milk, butter, and salt added (1/2 cup)	105	16	2	6	52	0.2
Potato chips (10)	105	10	1	7	5	0.2
Potato salad with mayonnaise (1/2 cup)	180	14	4	10	24	0.8
Pumpkin, canned (1/2 cup)	40	10	1	Tr	32	1.7
Pumpkin, cooked, mashed, drained (1/2 cup)	25	6	1	Tr	18	0.7
Radish, raw (4 med.)	5	1	Tr	Tr	4	0.1
Rutabagas, boiled, drained (1/2 cup cubes)	30	7	1	Tr	36	0.4
Sauerkraut, canned (1/2 cup)	20	5	1	Tr	36	1.7
Spinach, frozen, boiled (1/2 cup)	30	5	3	Tr	139	1.4
Spinach, frozen, uncooked (1 cup chopped)	10	2	2	Tr	54	1.5
Spinach soufflé (1/2 cup)	110	1	6	9	165	0.7
Squash, summer, boiled, drained (1/2 cup)	20	4	1	Tr	24	0.3
Squash, winter, baked (1/2 cup)	40	9	1	1	14	0.3
Succotash, frozen, boiled, drained (1/2 cup)	80	17	4	1	13	0.8
Sweet potato, baked, flesh only (1, 5 in. long, 2 in. diameter)	120	28	2	Tr	32	0.5
Sweet potatoes, boiled, without skin (1/2 cup mashed)	170	40	3	Tr	35	1.0
Sweet potatoes, candied (1, 2 1/2 × 2 in.)	145	29	1	3	27	1.2
Tomato, canned, solid and liquid (1/2 cup)	25	5	1	Tr	31	0.8
Tomato juice (1/2 cup)	20	5	1	Tr	10	0.7
Tomato paste, canned (1 T)	15	3	1	Tr	6	0.5
Tomato puree, canned (1/2 cup)	50	12	2	Tr	18	1.2
Tomato, raw (1 med.)	25	5	1	Tr	9	0.6
Tomato sauce, canned (1/2 cup)	85	9	2	Tr	17	0.9
Turnips, boiled, drained (1/2 cup cubes)	15	4	1	Tr	18	0.2
Turnip greens, boiled, drained (1/2 cup chopped)	15	3	1	Tr	99	0.6
Vegetable juice, cocktail (1/2 cup)	20	6	1	Tr	13	0.5
Watercress, raw (1/2 cup chopped)	Tr	Tr	Tr	Tr	20	Tr
Yam, boiled, drained, or baked (1/2 cup cubes)	80	19	1	Tr	9	0.4
WAFFLES						
Homemade (1, 7 in.)	245	26	7	13	154	1.5
From mix (1, 7 in.)	205	27	7	8	179	1.2

NA: Not available in references used.

*Crude fiber.

**Cooked and drained unless otherwise stated.

***Based on typical recipe; ingredients and nutrients may vary among recipes.

$: Varies depending on amount of salt added.

$$: Varies depending on type of oil used for frying.

TR: Trace.

Sodium (mg.)	Potassium (mg.)	Thiamine (mg.)	Riboflavin (mg.)	Niacin (mg.)	Vitamin C (mg.)	Vitamin A (IU)	Cholesterol (mg.)	Fiber (gm.)
VEGETABLES** *(cont.)*								
108	366	.09	.01	1.6	5	0	0	.34*
26	340	.17	.03	3.8	10	0	0	NA
318	314	.09	.04	1.2	7	20	0	1.7
348	244	12	05	0.7	10	190	14	NA
94	260	.03	Tr	0.4	8	0	0	0.3*
661	317	0.1	Tr	1.1	13	261	86	0.5*
6	251	.03	.07	0.4	5	26,908	0	2.2
2	280	.04	0.1	0.5	6	1,320	0	1.0*
4	42	Tr	.01	0.1	4	Tr	0	0.5
15	244	.06	.03	0.5	19	0	0	1.7
780	201	.02	.03	0.2	17	21	0	2.4
82	283	.06	.16	0.4	12	7,395	C	2.1
43	307	.04	0.1	0.4	15	3,690	0	1.4
381	101	.04	.15	0.2	1	1,730	0	0.4*
1	173	.04	.04	0.5	5	259	0	.7
1	445	.08	.02	0.7	10	3,628	0	3.6
38	225	.06	.06	1.1	5	196	0	0.9*
12	397	.08	.14	0.7	28	24,877	0	2.7
21	301	.09	.23	1.0	28	27,968	0	3.8
74	198	.02	.04	0.4	7	4,400	8	0.4*
196	265	.06	.04	0.9	18	725	0	NA
441	268	.06	.04	0.8	22	678	0	0.5*
11	153	.02	.03	0.5	7	404	0	0.2*
25	526	.09	.07	2.2	44	1,701	0	1.0*
10	255	.07	.06	0.7	22	1,390	0	1.0
738	452	.08	.07	1.4	16	1,195	0	0.9*
39	106	.02	.02	0.2	9	0	0	1.7
21	146	.03	.05	0.3	20	3,959	0	2.8
442	234	.05	.03	0.9	34	1,416	0	0.3*
7	56	.02	.02	Tr	7	799	0	0.6
6	455	.06	.02	0.4	8	0	0	2.6
445	129	.18	.24	1.5	Tr	140	102	NA
512	146	.14	.23	0.9	Tr	170	59	NA

NA: Not available in references used.
*Crude fiber.
**Cooked and drained unless otherwise stated.
***Based on typical recipe; ingredients and nutrients may vary among recipes.
$: Varies depending on amount of salt added.
$$: Varies depending on type of oil used for frying.
TR: Trace.

Sources

Nutrient values in these tables are derived from a number of sources, which are listed below:

Anderson, James, W. M.D. *Plant Fiber in Foods*. Lexington, Kentucky: HCF Diabetes Foundation, P.O. Box 22124, Lexington, Kentucky, 1986.

Hill, Lynne. *People's Nutritive Encyclopedia*. New York: Putnam Publishing Group, 1987.

International Life Science Institute/Nutrition Foundation. *Present Knowledge in Nutrition*. 6th Edition. Washington, D.C., 1990.

Leveille, Gilbert, et al. *Nutrients in Foods*. Cambridge, Massachusetts: Nutrition Guild, 1983.

National Livestock & Meat Board. "Nutrient Value of Meat." *Food & Nutrition News*. Vol. 59, no. 2. March/April 1987.

Pennington, Jean, and Church, Helen. *Food Values of Portions Commonly Used*. 14th ed. New York: Harper and Row, 1985.

Roth Laboratories. "Fast Foods 1986. Nutrient Analysis." *Dietetic Currents*. Vol. 13, no. 6. 1986.

USDA. "Nutritive Value of American Foods in Common Units." *Agriculture Handbook*. No. 456. 1975.

USDA. "Composition of Foods." *Agriculture Handbook*. No. 8/1–8/16. 1976–1981.

USDA. "Nutritional Value of Foods." *Home Garden Bulletin*. No. 72. 1985.

Index